A Practical Guide for
MEDICAL TEACHERS
Fifth Edition

Edited by

John A Dent MMEd MD FAMEE FHEA FRCS(Ed)
International Relations Officer, Association for Medical Education in Europe; Honorary
Reader in Medical Education and Orthopaedic Surgery, University of Dundee, Dundee, UK

Ronald M Harden OBE MD FRCP(Glas) FRCPC FRCSEd
General Secretary of AMEE, Editor of Medical Teacher and Professor (Emeritus), Medical
Education, University of Dundee; Formerly Director of the Centre for Medical Education,
Teaching Dean and Consultant Physician, Dundee, UK

Dan Hunt MD MBA
Assistant Secretary, Liaison Committee on Medical Education; Senior Director of Accreditation
Services, Association of American Medical Colleges, Washington DC, USA

Foreword by

Brian D Hodges PhD MD FRCPC
Executive Vice-President Education, University Health Network; Professor,
Department of Psychiatry, University of Toronto; Scientist, Wilson Centre for Research in
Education; Richard and Elizabeth Currie Chair in Health Professions Education Research;
Senior Fellow, Massey College; Senior Strategy Advisor, The AMS Phoenix Project, Toronto,
Canada

ELSEVIER
Edinburgh   London   New York   Oxford   Philadelphia   St Louis   Sydney   Toronto   2017

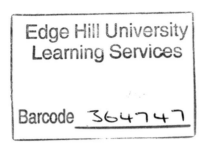
ELSEVIER

First edition 2001
Second edition 2005
Third edition 2009
Fourth edition 2013
Fifth edition 2017

ISBN   9780702068911

Notices

Knowledge and best practice in this field are constantly changing. As new research and experience broaden our understanding, changes in research methods, professional practices, or medical treatment may become necessary.

Practitioners and researchers must always rely on their own experience and knowledge in evaluating and using any information, methods, compounds, or experiments described herein. In using such information or methods they should be mindful of their own safety and the safety of others, including parties for whom they have a professional responsibility.

With respect to any drug or pharmaceutical products identified, readers are advised to check the most current information provided (i) on procedures featured or (ii) by the manufacturer of each product to be administered, to verify the recommended dose or formula, the method and duration of administration, and contraindications. It is the responsibility of practitioners, relying on their own experience and knowledge of their patients, to make diagnoses, to determine dosages and the best treatment for each individual patient, and to take all appropriate safety precautions.

To the fullest extent of the law, neither the publisher nor the authors, contributors, or editors, assume any liability for any injury and/or damage to persons or property as a matter of products liability, negligence or otherwise, or from any use or operation of any methods, products, instructions, or ideas contained in the material herein.

Printed in Great Britain

Last digit is the print number: 9 8 7 6 5 4

Contents

SECTION 5 ASSESSMENT

SECTION 6 STAFF

SECTION 7 STUDENTS

SECTION 8 MEDICAL SCHOOL

Foreword

It is an honour to provide the foreword to this fine book, the fifth edition of what has become a trusted companion for medical educators. This revised edition brings new chapters and introduces new authors who will inspire a wide international audience. Recent years have seen a greater focus in medical schools on social sciences and medical humanities, increased attention to social accountability and globalization, widespread uptake of longitudinal integrated clerkships and recognition of the importance of student engagement. All of these topics have been included in this new edition, creating an indispensable resource at a time of considerable change.

The medical education literature is enormous and can be daunting. This book serves as a place to start and a source to dip into for support and wisdom. It has a decidedly international flavor, given its team of over one hundred authors from fifteen countries. In our globalizing world, students, educators as well as practices traverse borders quickly. Yet resources are unevenly available to those who carry the responsibility of education, making a trusted single source valuable.

I had the pleasure recently to witness the birth of the first masters of health sciences education in the country of Ethiopia. As the members of the class grappled with the challenging issues facing education, *A Practical Guide for Medical Teachers* served as an entry point to the larger literature, a map of the terrain on their journey to becoming health professional educators, a source of inspiration for research topics and a companion in the classroom and clinic. It will serve you in all of these ways as well.

This fifth edition is organized in eight sections, each designed with a focused, practical theme. The first section sketches out the horizon of medical education, underscoring the importance of thinking of learning as a lifelong commitment from the first day of medical school to the last day of practice. Here, the 'hidden curriculum' that perplexes and undoes so many good intentions is highlighted. The second section of the book addresses the many contexts in which medical education takes place. The chapters in this section remind us that one size does not fit all. Today medical education increasingly involves simulation centres, video conferencing, distance learning and a wide variety of settings from the largest of urban centres to rural or remote settings.

An expanded third section builds on the second, by exploring the amazing range of strategies and technologies available to educators. Alongside well-established approaches such as problem-based and outcomes-based education the reader has a valuable guide to the emerging areas of integrated education, team-based learning and a growing, and at times overwhelming, array of digital technologies. The fourth section is where educators can turn for help with what can feel at times like an endless demand for curriculum time. Here, cogent arguments can be found to help with the why, how and how much in areas such as basic and social science, ethics, professionalism, evidence-based medicine and patient safety and the humanities. This section also gives consideration to the forces of integration, globalization and the ubiquity of information that is transforming healthcare in every country.

The fifth section provides a terrific, much sought-after reference for assessing students.

This selection of experts has created a helpful resource that serves to reduce what is often an overwhelming sense that there are too many tools, approaches and controversies in the literature on assessment. These authors underscore the shift away from a focus on individual tests and tools towards a more comprehensive understanding of systems of assessment that should be built to foster learning. Section six, though a short section, is in some ways the anchor of the book. Taking up the essential task of staff development and the scholarship of education, these two chapters address a foundation on which all good education rests. High quality education requires on the one hand an engaged, creative and constantly learning community of educators, and on the other a supportive institutional environment that fosters professional and educational development.

The seventh section turns to the important issue of making the student experience the best it can be. Chapters on student selection, support, engagement and peer-assisted learning lay out a blue print for education that is welcoming, supportive and learner-centred. The final section looks at the biggest picture, asking, what is a medical school for? The chapters in this section explore teachers as change agents, concepts of leadership, social accountability and one of today's hottest topics - the learning environment. The section concludes with a well-placed last chapter calling for research to examine the assumptions, practices, effects and outcomes of education. It will whet the appetite of budding education researchers.

The fifth edition of *A Practical Guide for Medical Teachers* is many things: a rich resource, a trusted companion, a source of wisdom, and a map of our vast and expanding field. Perhaps what it represents most is an invitation. To the newest in our field, it is an invitation to join the global community of medical educators. For those who have been around for a while, it is an invitation to become a little better, as a teacher, scholar or leader. Simply put, no matter where one is on the journey of medical education, we are all teaching and we are all learning.

Brian D. Hodges MD PhD FRCPC
Toronto 2017

Preface

As was said in the preface to previous editions the aim of *A Practical Guide for Medical Teachers* is to help colleagues in the healthcare professions to teach and to help students to learn. Our intention in this new edition remains the same.

An important hallmark of this fifth edition is that the book has retained its original size and shape during the last 16 years and so remains a manageable and practical handbook. Thanks to the expertise of individual authors, it has been possible to keep the majority of chapters to the eight-to-nine page limit with the exception of instances where chapters from the previous edition have been combined. As a result, we hope that we have enabled the reader to learn a great deal about a specific topic in a relatively short reading span.

The last three editions of the book have contained around 50 chapters. We again sought to remain within this limit while seeking to accommodate emerging or expanded topics. Some chapters have therefore been either omitted or combined this time. For example, while it is still true that study guides are an important teaching tool, that chapter has been discontinued to allow fresh approaches to learning to be included. It goes without saying that the many authors and co-authors deserve high praise for their willingness to tolerate the well-meant nagging of the editors. As we all know it takes a lot longer to write a short document than it does to write a long one. We are pleased that, as a result, it has been possible to add nine new chapters and make substantial revisions of a further fourteen chapters without unduly expanding the length of the book.

From the first edition of *A Practical Guide for Medical Teachers* onwards a section has been devoted to curriculum themes. It is here that one sees a dramatic change in the number of chapters. In the first edition, this section had six chapters – and it is gratifying to see that the principles of evidence-based medicine were there from the start. However, for this fifth edition, this section has blossomed from six to eleven chapters. These new chapters highlight more important developments in medical education.

The continuing growth of interest in professionalism and scholarship in medical education, as well as in staff development and academic standards has been pointed out in previous editions. This interest now includes teachers from a range of healthcare professions and also students.

We hope that the book can serve as a useful resource for a larger group of multi-professional colleagues at all stages of their personal professional development.

There has been increasing internationalization of medical education over the last 16 years. While the first edition had fewer chapters, it averaged around one author per chapter. This time the average is two authors per chapter and we now welcome 21 new authors. This expansion of authorship reflects the growing contribution of experts from all over the world. The first edition had authors from just six countries. This fifth edition draws authors from 15 different countries including Australia, Brazil, Canada, Estonia, France, Great Britain, Hong Kong, India, the Netherlands, Portugal, Singapore, the Republic of South Africa, Sweden, the United Arab Emirates and the United States of America. While to some extent, this expanded list of contributors reflects the development of the global relevance of the book, it also reflects the growing number of medical education scholars from around the world. This international appeal has been highlighted by translations of recent editions into Classical Chinese, Japanese, Korean, Vietnamese and Arabic.

As part of this international development we welcome a co-editor from the United States of America. As Senior Director of Accreditation Services at the Association of American Medical Colleges and Assistant Secretary of the Liaison Committee on Medical Education, Dan Hunt brings a wealth of experience in medical education and highlights the increasing transatlantic interest in *A Practical Guide for Medical Teachers*. For the second time we would like to thank Professor Brian Hodges from the Wilson Centre for Research in Education at the University of Toronto for writing a Foreword for a new edition. Prof. Hodges has innovative theories on many topics in medical education and is a frequent speaker at international conferences.

Finally, having worked with the staff of Elsevier now for several years, we are increasingly grateful to Laurence Hunter and his team for their support, patience and steady guidance during the preparation of this new edition.

JA Dent
RM Harden
D Hunt
Dundee, 2017

Contributors

Shelley R Adler PhD
Interim Director & Director of Education, Osher Center for Integrative Medicine, University of California, San Francisco, San Francisco, CA, USA

Susan Ambrose DA
Senior Vice Provost for Undergraduate Education & Experiential Learning, Northeastern University, Boston, MA, USA

Raja C Bandaranayake MBBS PhD MSEd FRACS
Visiting Professor & Consultant, Medical Education, Gulf Medical University, Ajman, UAE

Amanda Barnard BA(HONS) BMED(HONS) FRACGP SFHEA
Associate Dean, Rural and Indigenous Health, and Head, Rural Clinical School, Australian National University Medical School, Canberra, ACT, Australia

Barbara Barzansky PhD MHPE
LCME Co-Secretary, American Medical Association, Chicago, IL, USA

Fernando Bello
Director, Centre for Engagement and Simulation Science, Surgery & Cancer, Imperial College London, London, UK

Charles Boelen MD DPH MSc
International Consultant in Health System and Personnel, Sciez-sur-Léman, France

Katharine Boursicot BSc MBBS MRCOG MAHPE NTF SFHEA
Director, Health Professional Assessment Consultancy, Singapore

Clarence H Braddock III MD MPH MACP
Professor of Medicine, Maxine and Eugene Rosenfeld Chair in Medical Education, Vice Dean for Education, David Geffen School of Medicine at UCLA, Los Angeles, CA, USA

John E Carr PhD ABPP
Professor Emeritus, Psychiatry and Behavioral Sciences, University of Washington School of Medicine, Seattle, WA, USA

Julie Y Chen MD FCFPC
Department of Family Medicine & Primary Care and Bau Institute of Medical and Health Sciences Education, The University of Hong Kong, Hong Kong SAR, China

Jacqueline Chin BPhil DPhil (Oxon)
Associate Professor, Centre for Biomedical Ethics, Yong Loo Lin School of Medicine, National University of Singapore, Singapore

Jennifer Cleland BSc(Hons) MSc PhD DClinPsychol
John Simpson Chair of Medical Education Research, Institute of Education for Medical and Dental Sciences, University of Aberdeen, Aberdeen, UK

Richard M Conran MD PhD JD FCAP
Professor of Pathology and Anatomy, Eastern Virginia Medical School, Norfolk, VA, USA

Ian D Couper MBBCh MFamMed FCFP(SA)
Director, Ukwanda Centre for Rural Health, and Professor of Rural Health, Centre for Health Professions Education, Faculty of Medicine and Health Sciences, Stellenbosch University, RSA

John A Dent MMEd MD FAMEE FHEA FRCS(Ed)
International Relations Officer, Association for Medical Education in Europe; Honorary Reader in Medical Education and Orthopaedic Surgery, University of Dundee, Dundee, UK

Paul K Drain MD MPH
Assistant Professor, Departments of Global
Health, Medicine (Infectious Diseases),
Epidemiology, University of Washington,
Seattle, WA, USA

Erik W Driessen PhD
Professor, Department of Educational
Development & Research, Maastricht
University, Maastricht, Netherlands

Steven J Durning MD PhD FACP
Professor of Medicine and Pathology,
Uniformed Services University, Bethesda, MD,
USA

Rachel H Ellaway BSc PhD
Professor, Community Health Sciences,
Research, and Director, Office of Health and
Medical Education Scholarship, Cumming
School of Medicine, University of Calgary,
Calgary, AB, Canada

Luci Etheridge MBChB MRCPCH EdD
Consultant Paediatrician and Honorary Senior
Lecturer, Paediatrics, St George's Hospital and
St George's University of London, London,
UK

Jason R Frank MD MA(Ed) FRCPC
Director, Specialty Education, Strategy, and
Standards, Royal College of Physicians and
Surgeons of Canada, Ottawa, ON, Canada

Charles P Friedman PhD
Chair, Learning Health Sciences, University of
Michigan Medical School, Ann Arbor, MI,
USA

Elizabeth H Gaufberg MD MPH
Associate Professor of Medicine and Psychiatry,
Harvard Medical School/Cambridge Health
Alliance, Cambridge, MA, USA

Jeff Gold MD
Chancellor, Office of the Chancellor,
University of Nebraska Medical Center,
Omaha, NE, USA

Janet Grant MSc PhD
Academic Director, Centre for Medical
Education in Context (CenMEDIC), London,
UK

Larry D Gruppen PhD
Professor, Learning Health Sciences, University
of Michigan, Ann Arbor, MI, USA

Frederic W Hafferty PhD
Professor of Medical Education, Division of
Internal Medicine, College of Medicine,
Program on Professionalism and Values, Mayo
Clinic, Rochester, MN, USA

Hossam Hamdy MBChB FRCS PhD
Professor of Surgery and Medical Education,
Chancellor Gulf Medical University, Ajman,
UAE

Aviad Haramati PhD
Professor and Director, Department of
Biochemistry and the Center for Innovation
and Leadership in Education (CENTILE),
Georgetown University School of Medicine,
Washington, DC, USA

Ronald M Harden OBE MD FRCP(Glas) FRCPC
FRCSEd
General Secretary, Association for Medical
Education in Europe; Former Professor of
Medical Education, Director of the Centre for
Medical Education and Teaching Dean,
University of Dundee, UK; Professor of
Medical Education, Al-Imam University,
Riyadh, Saudi Arabia

Jeni Harden MA MPhil PhD
Director of Education, Usher Institute of
Population Health Sciences and Informatics,
University of Edinburgh, Edinburgh, UK

Linda A Headrick MD MS
Senior Associate Dean for Education, Helen
Mae Spiese Professor in Medicine, School of
Medicine, University of Missouri, Columbia,
MO, USA

Sylvia Heeneman PhD
Professor, Department of Pathology School of
Health Professions Education, Maastricht
University, Maastricht, Netherlands

David Hirsh MD
Director, Harvard Medical School Academy
Fellowship in Medical Education, Medicine,
Harvard Medical School / Cambridge Health
Alliance, Cambridge, MA, USA

Anita Ho PhD
Associate Professor and Director of
Undergraduate Ethics Curriculum, Centre for
Biomedical Ethics, Yong Loo Lin School of
Medicine, National University of Singapore,
Singapore

Eric S Holmboe MD
Senior Vice President, Milestones, ACGME,
Chicago, IL, USA

Kathryn N Huggett MA PhD
Assistant Dean and Director, The Teaching
Academy; Professor, Medicine, University of
Vermont Larner College of Medicine,
Burlington, VT, USA

Dan Hunt MD MBA
Assistant Secretary, Liaison Committee on
Medical Education; Senior Director of
Accreditation Services, Association of
American Medical Colleges, Washington, DC,
USA

Abbas Hyderi MD MPH
Associate Professor of Clinical Family Medicine
and Associate Dean for Curriculum, Family
Medicine, University of Illinois at Chicago
College of Medicine, Chicago, IL, USA

William B Jeffries III MS PhD
Senior Associate Dean for Medical Education,
and Professor, Pharmacology, University of
Vermont, Larner College of Medicine,
Burlington, VT, USA

Benjamin Kligler MD MPH
Vice Chair and Research Director, Department
of Integrative Medicine, Mount Sinai Beth
Israel; Associate Professor of Family and
Community Medicine, Icahn School of
Medicine at Mount Sinai, New York, NY, USA

Roger Kneebone PhD FRCS FRCSEd FRCGP
Professor of Surgical Education and
Engagement Science, Surgery & Cancer,
Imperial College London, London, UK

Sharon K Krackov MS EdD
Professor, Medical Education, Albany Medical
College, Albany, NY, USA

Nirusha Lachman PhD
Professor of Anatomy, Mayo Clinic College of
Medicine and Science, Mayo Clinic, Rochester,
MN, USA

Joel Lanphear PhD
Professor Interim Senior associate Dean/
Academic Affairs, Central Michigan University,
College of Medicine, Mount Pleasant, MI,
USA

Susan J Lieff MD MEd MMan
Vice-Chair Education, Dept of Psychiatry,
Faculty of Medicine, University of Toronto,
Toronto, ON, Canada

Lauren A Maggio PhD MS(LIS)
Associate Professor, Department of Medicine,
and Associate Director of Distributed Learning
and Technology, Grad Programs in Health
Professions Education, Uniformed Services
University of the Health Sciences, Bethesda,
MD, USA

Kyriaki C Marti DMD MD PhD
Clinical Assistant Professor, Oral and
Maxillofacial Surgery, University of Michigan,
Ann Arbor, MI, USA

Marie Matte PhD
Associate Dean, Compliance, Assessment, and
Evaluation, Office of Medical Education,
Central Michigan University College of
Medicine, Mount Pleasant, MI, USA

Judy McKimm MBA MA(Ed) BA(Hons) SFHEA
Professor of Medical Education, School of
Medicine, Swansea University, Swansea, West
Glamorgan, UK

Danette W McKinley BA MA PhD
Director, Research and Data Resources,
Foundation for Advancement of International
Medical Education and Research, Philadelphia,
PA, USA

I Chris McManus MA MD PhD FRCP(Lon) FRCP(Ed)
FMedSci
Professor of Psychology and Medical
Education, Research Dept of Medical
Education, The Medical School, University
College London, London, UK

Stewart P Mennin BS MS PhD
Mennin Consulting and Associates, Sao Paulo,
Brazil

Larry K Michaelsen PhD
Professor Emeritus, Management, University of
Central Missouri, Warrensburg, MO, USA

Donald Moore PhD
Professor, Medical Education and
Administration, Vanderbilt University School
of Medicine, Nashville, TN, USA

Debra Nestel PhD FAcadMEd CHSE-A
Professor of Surgical Education, Department of
Surgery, Melbourne Medical School, Faculty of
Medicine, Dentistry & Health Sciences,
University of Melbourne, Melbourne, VIC,
Australia; Professor of Simulation Education in
Healthcare, Monash Institute for Health and
Clinical Education, Faculty of Medicine,
Nursing & Health Sciences, Monash University,
Clayton, VIC, Australia

Andre Jacques Neusy MD DTM&H
Senior Director, Training for Health Equity
Network, New York City, NY, USA

John Norcini PhD
President and CEO, Foundation for
Advancement of International Medical
Education and Research, Philadelphia, PA,
USA

Helen M O'Sullivan BSc PhD MBA
Professor, Associate Pro-Vice-Chancellor
(Online Learning), University of Liverpool,
Liverpool, UK

Björg Pálsdóttir MPA
Chief Executive Officer, Training for Health
Equity Network, New York, NY, USA

Dean Parmelee MD
Associate Dean for Academic Affairs, Wright
State University Boonshoft School of
Medicine, Dayton, OH, USA

Johmarx Patton MD MHI
Director, Education Informatics and
Technology, Health Information Technology
and Services, University of Michigan Medical
School, Ann Arbor, MI, USA

Douglas E Paull MD MS
Director of Patient Safety Curriculum and
Medical Simulation, National Center for
Patient Safety, Veterans Health Administration,
Ann Arbor, MI, USA

Wojciech Pawlina MD
Professor of Anatomy and Medical Education,
and Director of Procedural Skills Laboratory,
Mayo Clinic, College of Medicine and Science,
Mayo Clinic, Rochester, MN, USA

Antoinette S Peters PhD
Corresponding member of the faculty,
Department of Population Medicine, Harvard
Medical School, Boston, MA, USA

Rille Pihlak MD
European Junior Doctors, University of Tartu,
Estonia

Henry S Pohl BS MD
Vice Dean for Academic Administration,
Albany Medical College, Albany, NY, USA

Mark Edward Quirk EdD
Professor, Family Medicine and Community
Health, University of Massachusetts Medical
School, Worcester, MA, USA

Subha Ramani MBBS MMEd MPH
Assistant Professor of Medicine, Medicine, Harvard Medical School, Boston, MA, USA

Michael T Ross BSc MBChB EdD MRCGP FRCP(Edin)
Senior Clinical Lecturer, Centre for Medical Education, The University of Edinburgh, Edinburgh, UK

James Rourke MD CCFFP(EM) MClinSci FCFP FRRMS FCAHS LLD
Professor of Family Medicine, Dean of Medicine (2004–16), Memorial University of Newfoundland, St. John's, NL, Canada

Leslie Rourke MD CCFP MClSc FCFP FRRMS
Professor Emerita of Family Medicine, Memorial University of Newfoundland, St. John's, NL, Canada

Michael E Rytting MD
Professor, Pediatrics and Leukemia, The University of Texas M.D. Anderson Cancer Center, Houston, TX, USA

Juliana Sa MD
Invited Assitant, Faculty of Health Sciences, University of Beira Interior, Covilha, Portugal

Joan M Sargeant PhD
Professor and Head, Division of Medical Education, Dalhousie University, Halifax, NS, Canada

Lambert W T Schuwirth MD PhD
Professor of Medical Education, Flinders University Prideaux Centre for Research in Health Professions Education, School of Medicine, Flinders University, Adelaide, SA, Australia

John R Skelton BA MA RSA MRCGP
Professor, College of Medical and Dental Sciences, University of Birmingham, Birmingham, UK

Linda Snell MD MHPE FRCPC MACP
Professor of Medicine, Centre for Medical Education, McGill University, Montreal, QC, Canada

Henry M Sondheimer MD
Former Senior Director, Medical Education, Association of American Medical Colleges, Washington, DC, USA

Malathi Srinivasan MD
Professor of Medicine, Department of Internal Medicine, University of California, Davis School of Medicine, Sacramento, CA, USA

Yvonne Steinert PhD
Director, Centre for Medical Education, Faculty of Medicine, McGill University, Montreal, QC, Canada

Terese Stenfors-Hayes PhD
Senior Researcher, Department of Learning, Informatics, Management and Ethics, Karolinska Institutet, Stockholm, Sweden

Roger Strasser MBBS BMedSc MClSc FRACGP FACRRM FRCG(hon)
Dean and CEO, Northern Ontario School of Medicine, Lakehead and Laurentian Universities, Thunder Bay and Sudbury, ON, Canada

John L Szarek PhD CHSE
Professor and Director Clinical Pharmacology; Education Director for Simulation, Basic Sciences, Geisinger Commonwealth School of Medicine, Scranton, PA, USA

Jill E Thistlethwaite BSc MBBS PhD MMEd FRCGP FRACGP
Health Professions Education Consultant, Adjunct Professor, University of Technology, Sydney, NSW, Australia; Honorary Professor, School of Education, University of Queensland, QLD, Australia

Dario Torre MD PHD MPH
Associate Professor of Medicine, Uniformed Health Services University of Health Sciences, Bethesda, MD, USA

Jeroen J G van Merriënboer PhD
School of Health Professions Education, Maastricht University, Maastricht, Netherlands

Cees P M van der Vleuten PhD
Professor of Education, Department of
Educational Development and Research,
Maastricht University, Maastricht, Netherlands

Peter H Vlasses BSc Pharmacy PharmD
Executive Director, Accreditation Council for
Pharmacy Education, Chicago, IL, USA

Teck Chuan Voo BA MA PhD
Assistant Professor, Director of Graduate
Education, Centre for Biomedical Ethics,
National University of Singapore, Yong Loo Lin
School of Medicine, Singapore

Donna M Waechter PhD
Senior Director and LCME Assistant Secretary,
Association of American Medical Colleges,
Washington, DC, USA

Lucie Kaye Walters MBBS FACRRM PhD
Professor Rural Medical Education, Rural
Clinical School, Flinders University, Mount
Gambier, SA, Australia

Val J Wass OBE BSc FRCGP FRCP PhD MHPE PFHEA FAoME
Emeritus Professor in Medical Education,
Faculty of Health, Keele University, Newcastle
under Lyme, Staffordshire, UK

Kevin B Weiss MD
Senior Vice President for Accreditation,
Institutional Accreditation and CLER,
ACGME, Chicago, IL, USA

Michael S Wilkes MD PhD
Professor of Medicine and Global Health,
Deans Office, University of California, Davis,
CA, USA

Paul S Worley MBBS PhD MBA FACRRM FRACGP
DObstRANZCOG GAICD
Dean of Medicine, School of Medicine,
Flinders University, Adelaide, SA, Australia

Harry Yi-Jui Wu
Medical Ethics and Humanities Unit, Li Ka
Shing Faculty of Medicine, Pokfulam, Hong
Kong, SAR, China

Ann Mary Wylie Ann M Wylie PhD MA FRSPH FAcadMEd
FHEA
Senior Teaching Fellow; Deputy Director of
Community Education; Module Lead for
Global Health and Electives SSC Lead; QI and
Health Promotion Community Lead; King's
Undergraduate Medical Education in the
Community Team (KUMEC), Department of
Primary Care and Public Health Sciences,
King's College London School of Medicine,
London, UK

Geoffrey H Young PhD
Senior Director, Student Affairs and Programs,
Association of American Medical Colleges,
Washington, DC, USA

Anand Zachariah MD DNB
Professor, Medicine Unit 1 and Infectious
Disease, Christian Medical College, Vellore,
Tamil Nadu, India

Section 1

Curriculum development

1

New horizons in medical education

J. A. Dent, R. M. Harden, D. Hunt

Trends

A review of changes in medical education over the last 16 years has revealed several major trends, which are discussed in this fifth edition:

- Integration of information
- Learning situations
- An authentic curriculum
- Authentic assessment
- Our awareness of students

Some things change and others remain the same. With the fifth edition of this book, it is useful to look back to the first edition published in 2001 and track the trends in medical education over the past 16 years by looking at which sections and chapters have come and gone and what are the new ones in this edition. What has not changed, as noted in the first and subsequent editions, is that medical education continues to respond to a variety of challenges. Namely, the increase in medically related information, the role of mobile technologies that allow access to this information, changes in the healthcare delivery models, and the evolving role of the patient who has more information about their illnesses than ever before. These issues shape today's medical education programmes, but, interestingly, they are the same ones that were noted in the first edition as well. So, while these pressures and opportunities may have increased since then, they have been around for a while, and one can look at the chapters of the various editions of this book to see how educational programmes are evolving to adapt to these external forces.

There appear to be four major trends over this 16-year period of time. There is more emphasis on:

1. Integration of information
2. Changing learning situations
3. An authentic curriculum
4. Students and student engagement

INTEGRATION OF INFORMATION

The first edition had a chapter on integration. However, as medical educators have come to incorporate more adult learning principles into their work on curricular design and into their day-to-day teaching, the importance of connecting information to the context that it will be used has become more and more important. The days of large discipline-based courses that served as 'building blocks' are over. It is important to realize that this is not just connecting clinical situations to basic science principles. The concept of integration in medical education has moved beyond earlier clinical exposure to reinforce the relevance of basic science principles to integration in the broadest sense of the word. Schools are now using curriculum mapping and software driven content management systems to ensure that the information is not isolated in a given course but connects to other relevant concepts. For example, the physiology of fluid flowing over a surface needs to be integrated with the anatomically rough surface of a mitral valve, which explains the characteristic heart sound of mitral regurgitation. In the past, those individual principles might have been taught in different courses with the student expected to be the integrating factor. Now, faculty are working to create their educational offerings to maximize the opportunity for students to learn these principles and prepare them to apply them in their ultimate clinical settings.

The concept of a vertically integrated curriculum has been with us for some time, but now the integration of basic sciences with clinical experiences in the later years, and of clinical experience with basic sciences in the early years, is more fully understood. You will still find a chapter in this edition devoted to integration, but notice how it also emerges as a theme in the new chapter on longitudinal integrated clerkships and is echoed in chapters devoted to curriculum design and the undergraduate programme. References to integration between health-care professions and multi-professional education are also present.

 Longitudinal integrated clerkships address four imperatives: connecting educational structures to the sciences of learning, stemming ethical erosion, improving health systems, and meeting societal needs.

CHANGING LEARNING SITUATIONS

Continuing the trend that began in the second edition, there are chapters discussing the value and approach to learning in communities and in rural and remote settings. There is an awareness that more training in the under-served communities is more likely to lead to students choosing to practice in these settings in the future. This increased emphasis is capitalized in the fifth edition with a new chapter on social accountability.

 Social accountability forms the essential foundation for medical practice and medical education.

The experience of the student in the classroom and in the clinical setting has evolved to take advantage of new learning approaches. Traditional methods such as lectures are evolving with the development of the 'flipped' classroom, while new approaches such as simulation and e-learning continue to develop.

 Faculty can be assured that the flipped classroom will likely enhance student engagement and performance.

The first edition had a chapter on problem-based learning and the fifth edition highlights how this concept has evolved over time. Adding to this 'toolbox' of teaching strategies in the classroom is an update on the chapter on team-based learning. This is further augmented by a chapter related to small-group teaching.

AN AUTHENTIC CURRICULUM

The book recognizes the move to a more authentic curriculum, with an emphasis on the learning outcomes as they relate to the competencies of a doctor to practise medicine in the communities that they serve. Chapters on behavioural science, medical humanities, integrative medicine and global awareness account for some of the additional chapters and reflect important topics that need to be covered in an already full curriculum.

 Social and behavioural sciences facilitate students' awareness of their wider roles and address the potential impact of their own values and beliefs on practice.

The responsibility of the curriculum to help students to ask the right question, i.e. to find sources of information to provide an answer and then to evaluate the answer, is also addressed, as is the continuing development of the concept of outcome- and competency-based education and entrustable professional activities (EPAs).

The last of these new additions in this section is consistent with the challenge of trying to cover so much material in such a short period of time; that chapter is titled *Education at a time of ubiquitous information* and seems like a fitting way to close this section.

 Because new evidence is being generated in real time, clinicians need to be able to deal with uncertainty of evidence when making decisions.

The changes taking place in assessment as outlined includes the programmatic approach to assessment and also contributes to an authentic curriculum.

 A holistic view on assessment is emerging in which formative and summative assessment strategies are combined.

STUDENTS AND STUDENT ENGAGEMENT

The importance of selecting students with the appropriate attributes for medicine is discussed as a component of the application of an outcome-based approach to medical education.

Subsequent student engagement with the curriculum is endorsed by professional bodies such as the General Medical Council (GMC) in the UK (GMC, 2011) and is now a popular theme at conferences. It is recognized by the Association for Medical Education in Europe (AMEE) as contributing to its AMEE: Aspire for Excellence Award (Aspire, 2015). There is now a new chapter on this in the book.

Finally, a robust mechanism for student support addressing all aspects of student welfare continues to be required.

 Designing educational programmes that engage the student in the management and improvement enhances the overall learning process.

Summary

This chapter reviews developments in medical education, comparing the current edition to previous versions of this book. Important new learning technologies, situations and themes have been included.

There is increasing realization that student learning must be integrated. There is also a need for an authentic curriculum and themes relating to this have now been masterfully described in new chapters.

Finally, there is a developing awareness of a focus on students as this affects student selection, curriculum participation and student welfare in our medical schools.

References

ASPIRE, 2015. Online. http://www.aspire-to-excellence .org. (Accesssed 27 December 2016).

General Medical Council, 2011. Tomorrow's Doctors. GMC, London.

Curriculum planning and development

M. E. Quirk, R. M. Harden

Trends

- Careful and continuous monitoring of the taught curriculum in relation to the declared curriculum and learner outcomes is necessary.
- Recent curriculum reform targets the process and skills of thinking and the ability to adapt to situations as much as the knowledge base of learners.
- Curriculum planning should require the use of new tools such as predictive analytics and dynamic curriculum mapping.

Introduction

The torrid pace of medical advances mandates a new paradigm for curriculum development. The concept of transformation should be viewed as a continuous process woven into the fabric of grassroots medical teaching and learning, rather than an 'every five-year institutional-level' event. The new paradigm reinforces the age-old features of curriculum development such as defining objectives methods and evaluation. It also introduces novel features such as predicting and tracking outcomes related to the delivered curriculum. The days are now past when the teacher produced a curriculum like a magician produced a rabbit out of a hat, when the lecturer taught whatever attracted his or her interest and when the students' clinical training was limited to the patients who happened to present during a clinical attachment. It is now accepted that careful and continuous planning and monitoring outcomes is necessary if the programme of teaching and learning is to be successful.

 "No one would cheer more loudly for a change than Abraham Flexner ... The flexibility and freedom to change – indeed, the mandate to do so – were part of Flexner's essential message."

Cooke et al., 2006

What is a curriculum?

A curriculum is more than just a syllabus or a statement of content. A curriculum is about what should happen in a teaching programme – about the intention of the teachers, about the way they make this happen and judge the results. This extended vision of a curriculum is illustrated in Fig. 2.1. Curriculum planning can be considered in 10 steps (Harden, 1986b). This chapter looks at these steps and the changes in emphasis since the publication of the fourth edition of the text.

 The 10 steps described provide a useful checklist for planning and evaluating a curriculum.

IDENTIFYING THE NEED

The relevance or appropriateness of educational programmes has been questioned by Frenk et al. (2010), Cooke et al. (2010) and others. The need has been recognized to emphasize not only sickness salvaging, organic pathology and crisis care, but also health promotion and preventative medicine. Increasing attention is being paid to the social responsibility of a medical school and the extent to which it meets and equips its graduates to meet the needs of the population it serves. The medical system in which the learner will practise, and the way they will continuously learn from their practices, are increasingly recognized as important needs.

 "Professional education has not kept pace with these challenges, largely because of the fragmented, outdated, and static curricula that produce ill-equipped graduates."

Frenk et al., 2010

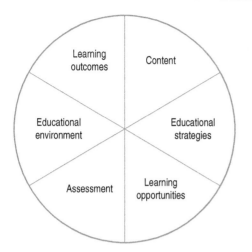

Fig. 2.1 An extended vision of a curriculum.

 "A move from the 'How' and 'When' to the 'What' and 'Whether'. "

Spady, 1994

The idea of learning outcomes is not new. Since the work of Bloom, Mager and others in the 1960s and 1970s, the value of setting out the aims and objectives of a training programme has been recognized. In practice, however, long lists of aims and objectives have proved unworkable and have been ignored in planning and implementing a curriculum. In recent years, the move to an outcome- or competency-based approach to the curriculum with outcome frameworks has gained momentum and is increasingly dominating education thinking.

A range of approaches can be used to identify curriculum needs (Dunn et al., 1985):

- *The 'wise men' approach.* Senior teachers and senior practitioners from different specialty backgrounds reach a consensus.
- *Consultation with stakeholders.* The views of members of the public, patients, government and other professions are sought.
- *A study of errors in practice.* Areas where the curriculum is deficient are identified.
- *Critical-incident studies.* Individuals are asked to describe key medical incidents in their experience that represent good or bad practice.
- *Task analysis.* The work undertaken by a doctor is studied.
- *Study of star performers.* Doctors recognized as 'star performers' are studied to identify their special qualities or competencies.

ESTABLISHING THE LEARNING OUTCOMES

 If you leave this book with only one idea, it should be the concept of outcome-based education.

One of the big ideas in medical education over the past decade has been the move to the use of learning outcomes as the driver for curriculum planning (Harden, 2007). In an outcome-based approach to education, as discussed in Chapter 15, the learning outcomes are defined and the specified, measured outcomes inform decisions about the curriculum and the curriculum development process. This represents a move away from a process model of curriculum planning, where the teaching and learning experiences and methods are the only concerns, to a product-oriented model, where what matters most are the learning outcomes and the product.

AGREEING ON THE CONTENT

The content of a textbook is outlined in the content pages and in the index. The content of a curriculum is found in the syllabus and in the topics covered in lectures and other learning opportunities. Traditionally, there has been an emphasis on knowledge, and this has been reflected in student assessment. Content relating to skills (including thinking) and attitudes is now recognized also as important. Increasing emphasis has been placed on an authentic curriculum – a curriculum where the content is more closely related to the work of the practising doctor. Basic science content, for example, is considered in the context of clinical medicine.

The content of the curriculum can be presented from a number of perspectives:

- subjects or disciplines (a traditional curriculum)
- body systems, e.g. the cardiovascular system (an integrated curriculum)
- the life cycle, e.g. childhood, adulthood, old age
- problems (a problem-based curriculum)
- clinical presentations or tasks (a scenario-based, case-based or task-based curriculum).

These are not mutually exclusive; grids can be prepared, which look at the content of a curriculum from two or more of these perspectives.

No account of curriculum content would be complete without reference to 'the hidden curriculum'. The 'declared' curriculum is the curriculum as set out in the institution's documents. The 'taught' curriculum is what happens in practice. The 'learned' curriculum is what is learned by the student. The 'hidden' curriculum is the students' informal learning that is different from what is taught (Fig. 2.2 and see Chapter 6). Both the taught and learned curricula are embedded in 'the learning environment' that reflects the values, attitudes and educational philosophy of the academic leaders and faculty.

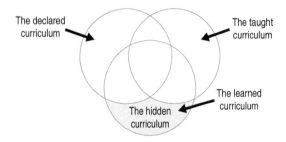

Fig. 2.2 The hidden curriculum.

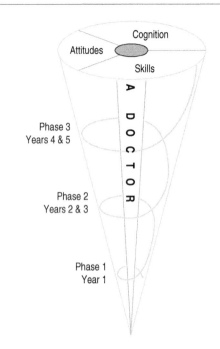

Fig. 2.3 A spiral curriculum.

EXPERIENCE AS CORE CONTENT

 "The student no longer merely watches, listens, memorizes: he does. His own activities in the laboratory and in the clinic are the main factors in his instruction and discipline. An education in medicine nowadays involves both learning and learning how; the student cannot effectively know, unless he knows how."

Flexner, 1910

Knowledge and action provide the foundation upon which metacognitive mental operations define experience and guide learning in both the basic and clinical science curricula. Metacognition is thinking about one's own or another's thinking and feeling. This thinking process underlies several 'higher-order' thinking skills such as clinical decision making, reflection, communication and perspective-taking, self-assessment and planning (Quirk, 2006). Recent curriculum reform targets the process and skills of thinking as much as the medical knowledge base of learners. Referring to the 'new curriculum', Charles Hundert, Dean of Harvard Medical School states: "Medical education is not about the transmission of information but about the transformation of the learner." (Shaw, 2015).

The aim is to prepare a learner to demonstrate mastery of core skills and the ability to adapt to new situations. (Ericsson, 2015; Carbonell et al., 2014)

ORGANIZING THE CONTENT

An assumption in a traditional medical curriculum was that students should first master the basic and then the applied medical sciences before moving on to study clinical medicine. Too often students failed to see the relevance of what was taught to their future career as doctors, and after they had passed examinations in the basic sciences, they tended to forget or ignore what they had learned.

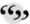 *"Early experience helps medical students socialise to their chosen profession. It helps them acquire a range of subject matter and makes their learning more real and relevant. It can influence career choices."*

Dornan et al., 2006

It has been advocated that the curriculum should be turned on its head, with students starting to think like a health professional from the day they enter medical school. Students at Hofstra Medical School, New York spend their first 8 weeks working as paramedics. On their first day at the University of California, San Francisco Medical School students are assigned to a healthcare team where they will play a significant role and learn about healthcare systems. In a vertically integrated curriculum, students are introduced to clinical medicine and to systems-based practice alongside the basic sciences in the early years of the programme. The need for students to continue their studies of the basic sciences as applied to clinical and population medicine within a systems framework in the later years is now recognized. In a final portfolio assessment, students at Dundee Medical School, for example, are expected to interpret the clinical cases they document in the context of an understanding of the basic sciences.

A spiral curriculum (Fig. 2.3) offers a useful approach to the organization of content (Harden & Stamper 1999). In a spiral curriculum:

• there is iterative revisiting of topics throughout the course

* topics are revisited at different levels of difficulty
* new learning is related to previous learning
* the competence of students increases with each visit to a topic.

DECIDING THE EDUCATIONAL STRATEGY

 In planning a curriculum, ask teachers to identify where they think they are at present on each continuum in the SPICES model and where they would like to go.

Much discussion and controversy in medical education has related to education strategies. The SPICES model (Fig. 2.4) offers a useful tool for planning a new curriculum or evaluating an existing one (Harden et al., 1984). It represents each strategy as a continuum, avoiding the polarizing of opinion and acknowledging that schools may vary in their approach.

Student-centred learning

In student-centred learning, students are given more responsibility for their own education. What the student learns matters, rather than what is taught. This is discussed further in Chapter 18 on independent learning. It is now appreciated that the teacher has an important role as facilitator of learning and that the student should not be abandoned and needs some sort of guidance and support.

With a greater understanding of how students learn and with advances in learning techniques we will see a move to an adaptive curriculum, where the content and the teaching and learning methods and strategies are tailored to the personal needs of the individual learner. This will include the use of new tools for traveling the educational pathway, such as predictive analytics and dynamic curriculum mapping. Students will spend different amounts of time studying a unit depending on their learning needs and milestones achieved. Each student's mastery of the learning outcomes should be continuously assessed during the course, and at times when further study can be arranged depending on the student's needs.

Student-centred ———— Teacher-centred
Problem-based ———— Information-oriented
Integrated or ———— Subject or
interprofessional ———— discipline-based
Community-based ———— Hospital-based
Elective-driven ———— Uniform
Systematic ———— Opportunistic

Fig. 2.4 SPICES model of educational strategies.

Problem-based learning (PBL)

PBL is a seductive approach to medical education, which, as described in Chapter 18 continues to attract attention. Digital technologies can be used to present the problem or as a source of information to guide the student's learning. PBL is used not only with students working in small groups but also in the context of large groups, in individualized learning or with students working at a distance. Eleven steps can be recognized in the PBL continuum between information-orientated and problem-based/task-based learning (Harden & Davis, 1998).

In task-based learning (TBL) the learning is focused on a series of tasks that the doctor may be expected to undertake, such as the management of a patient with abdominal pain. TBL is a useful approach to integration and PBL in clinical clerkships (Harden et al., 2000).

 "TBL offers an attractive combination of pragmatism and idealism: pragmatism in the sense that learning with an explicit sense of purpose is seen as an important source of student motivation and satisfaction; idealism in that it is consonant with current theories of education."

Harden et al., 1996

Integration and interprofessional learning

During the last two decades there has been a move away from structuring the curriculum around basic sciences and medical disciplines. Integrated teaching is now a standard feature of many curricula. It is discussed further in Chapter 16. Eleven steps on a continuum between discipline-based and integrated teaching have been described (Harden, 2000).

There is a move to interprofessional teaching, where integrated teaching and learning involving the different healthcare professions occur and where students look at a subject from the perspective of other professions as well as their own (Hammick et al., 2007). This is discussed further in Chapter 17.

Community-based learning

 "Clinical learning sites may include mental health services, long-term care facilities and family practice clinics, as well as hospitals and health services in remote, rural and urban communities."

Kelly, 2011

There are strong educational and logistical arguments for placing less emphasis on a hospital-based programme and more emphasis on the community as a context for student learning. Many curricula are now community orientated, with students spending 10% or more of their time in the community. This is discussed further in Chapters 10 and 11.

Consider when planning the curriculum which learning outcomes can be achieved more readily in a community-based attachment. Examples may be coping with uncertainty and health promotion.

Community-based clerkships are now more closely integrated into the curriculum as a planned learning experience.

Electives

 "The elective is a traditional and much enjoyed part of most medical courses."

Bullimore, 1998

Electives and student selected components (SSCs) are now firmly established as a valued component of the curriculum in many medical schools. They have moved from being a fringe event to an important educational activity that contributes to the expected exit learning outcomes.

It is no longer possible for students to study in depth all topics in a curriculum. Electives or SSCs provide students with the opportunity to study areas of interest to them, while at the same time developing skills in critical appraisal, self-assessment and time management.

Systematic approach

An opportunistic approach, where in the classroom teachers teach what is of interest to them and in the clinical setting students focus their learning on the patients that happen to be available, is no longer appropriate.

A more systematic approach to curriculum planning is necessary to ensure that students have learning experiences that match the expected learning outcomes and that the core curriculum includes the competences essential for medical practice.

 Think of the curriculum as a planned educational experience.

A range of paper and electronic methods can be used to record encounters students have with patients, and the records can then be analysed to see if there are gaps or deficiencies in the students' experiences.

The future will see greater use made of curriculum maps, where the students' progress through the curriculum is charted across the learning experiences, the assessments and the learning outcomes.

CHOOSING THE TEACHING METHODS

There is no panacea, no magic answer to teaching. A good teacher facilitates the students' learning by making use of a range of methods and applying each method for the use to which it is most appropriate. Chapters in this book describe the tools available in the teacher's toolkit:

- The lecture and whole-class teaching remain powerful tools if used properly. They need not be passive, and their role is more than one of information transfer. New strategies such as team-based learning and 'flipped' classrooms provide guidance for greatly enhancing the learning experience associated with this long-standing method of teaching in large groups.
- Small-group work facilitates interaction between students and makes possible cooperative learning, with students learning from each other. Small-group work is usually an important element in problem-based learning.
- Independent learning can make an important contribution. Students master the area being studied, while at the same time they develop the ability to work on their own and to take responsibility for their own learning.

 There is no holy grail of instructional wizardry that will provide a solution to all teaching problems. The teacher's toolkit should contain a variety of approaches, each with its strengths and weaknesses.

A significant development in recent years has been the application of new learning technologies including simulation and e-learning (Ellaway & Masters, 2008). Computers may be used as a source of information, to present interactive patient simulations, to facilitate and manage learning and to support collaborative or peer-to-peer learning. Synchronous activities such as video conferencing and Massive Open Online Courses (MOOCs), as well as asynchronous interactive methods involving online case-based modules and simulation enable educators to overcome traditional curricular constraints of time and space.

 "The move from desktop PCs to laptops, smart phones and tablets has increased the possibilities of learning closer to clinical patient experience, so called 'near patient learning', where students can access learning resources just prior to or just after seeing and interacting with patients."

Roberts, 2012

Teaching and learning experiences can be rated in terms of:
- authenticity, with theoretical approaches at one end of the spectrum and real-life ones at the other
- formality, with different levels of formality and informality.

Teaching situations can be located in each quadrant of the formality/authenticity grid (Fig. 2.5).

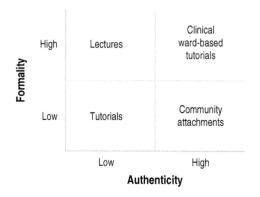

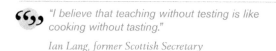

Fig. 2.5 Teaching situations.

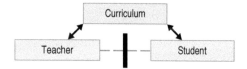

Fig. 2.6 Failure in communication.

PREPARING THE ASSESSMENT

Student assessment is a key component of the curriculum and is addressed in Section 5 of this book. The significant effect that examinations have on student learning is well documented.

> "I believe that teaching without testing is like cooking without tasting."
>
> *Ian Lang, former Scottish Secretary*

Issues that should be addressed in assessment include:
- What should be assessed?
  - A grid or blueprint should be prepared relating the assessment to the specific learning outcomes. This should include knowledge, skills and attitudes.
- How should it be assessed?
  Methods should include:
  - a written approach such as multiple-choice questions (MCQs) or constructed response questions
  - a performance assessment such as an Objective Structured Clinical Examination (OSCE)
  - a collection of evidence such as in a portfolio.
- What are the aims of the assessment process?
  Aims may include:
  - to pass or fail the student
  - to grade the student
  - to provide the student and teacher with feedback
  - to motivate the student
  - to support the learning. There is a move from 'assessment of learning' to 'assessment for learning' and 'assessment as learning'.

- When should students be assessed?
  Students can be assessed:
  - at the beginning of the course to assess what they already know or can do
  - during the course as formative assessment
  - at the end of the course to assess their achievement of the expected learning outcomes.
- Who should assess the student?
  - Depending on the context, the responsibility may rest with a national or international body, the medical school, the teachers or student peers
  - Increasing attention should be paid to self-assessment, with students encouraged to assess their own competence, a skill required for lifelong practice-based learning. The evidence suggests that physicians are not equipped to do so (Davis et al., 2006).

COMMUNICATION ABOUT THE CURRICULUM

Failure of communication between teacher and student is a common problem in medical education (Fig. 2.6).

Teachers have the responsibility to ensure that students have a clear understanding of:
- what they should be learning – the learning outcomes
- their access to the range of learning experiences and opportunities available
- how they can match the available learning experiences to their own personal needs
- whether they have mastered the topic or not, and if not, what further studies and experiences are required.

 Failure to keep staff and students informed about the curriculum is a common recipe for failure.

Communication can be improved by providing students with:
- a clear statement of the learning outcomes expected at each stage of the curriculum
- a curriculum map that matches the learning outcomes to the learning experiences and the assessment

- an electronic or print-based study guide, which helps the students to manage their learning and make the best use of their time.

PROMOTING AN APPROPRIATE EDUCATIONAL OR LEARNING ENVIRONMENT

The educational environment or 'climate' is a key aspect of the curriculum (Genn, 2001). It is less tangible than the content studied, the teaching methods used or the examinations. It is nonetheless of equal importance.

 Measurement of the education environment should be part of a curriculum evaluation.

There is little point in developing a curriculum where an aim is to orientate the student to medicine in the community and to health promotion if the students perceive that what is valued by the senior teachers is hospital practice, curative medicine and research. In the same way, it is difficult to develop in students a spirit of teamwork and collaboration if the environment in the medical school is a competitive rather than a collaborative one.

Tools to assess the educational environment such as the Dundee Ready Education Environment Measure (DREEM) are available. A major study of the learning environment implemented by the American Medical Association involves 28 medical schools and tracks perceptions of faculty and peer support, competition for grades, integration of basic and clinical sciences over 4 years of the medical curriculum (Skochelak et al., 2016).

 "The educational climate is the soul and spirit of the medical curriculum."

Genn, 2001

MANAGING THE CURRICULUM

Attention to curriculum management has become more important with

- increasing complexity of the curriculum including integrated and interdisciplinary teaching
- increasing pressures on staff with regard to their clinical duties, teaching responsibilities and research commitments
- distributed learning on different sites
- increased demands and increased student numbers at a time of financial constraints
- changes in the healthcare system and medical practice
- increasing demands for accountability.

In the context of undergraduate medical schools, it is likely that:

- responsibilities and resources for teaching will be at a faculty rather than departmental level

- an undergraduate medical education committee will be responsible for planning and implementing the curriculum
- a teaching dean or director of undergraduate medical education will be appointed who has a commitment to curriculum development and implementation
- staff will be appointed with particular expertise in curriculum planning, teaching methods and assessment to support work on the curriculum
- time and contributions made by staff to teaching will be recognized
- a staff development programme will be a requirement for all staff
- an independent group will have responsibility for academic standards and quality assurance.

There are similar requirements with respect to postgraduate education.

Curriculum management is data management. Theoretical and technological advances greatly enhance our ability to not only manage the curriculum but transform it into a dynamic, personal learning experience.

 "Analytics marries large data sets, statistical techniques, and predictive modelling ... to produce actionable intelligence."

Campbell et al., 2007

Teachers and learners together transform the educational process by grounding their actions and decisions about direction, meaning and performance in heretofore largely untapped descriptive and predictive data. These data can be used to improve accuracy of self assessments as well as predict future performance in the organic curriculum (Pusic et al., 2015).

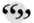 *"Online learning systems – learning management systems, learning platforms, and learning software – have the ability to capture streams of fine-grained learner behaviors, and the tools and techniques described above can operate on the data to provide a variety of stakeholders with feedback to improve teaching, learning, and educational decision-making."*

US Department of Education, 2012

Mining the data of the multifaceted curriculum for analytic purposes is captured in a dynamic interpretation of the curriculum map. The capacity for the curriculum to constitute a whole greater than the sum of its parts and the map to be used to navigate the territory is foreshadowed by Harden (2001). New technologies and approaches to data enable us to 'take a satellite view' of the multidimensional map akin to a Global Positioning System (GPS). This new CPS (Curriculum

Positioning System) offers a dynamic interactive educational tool that enables stakeholders to establish performance destinations and methods of transportation, waypoints and estimated time of arrival, plot courses for learning, create personalized alternative routes, reflect on their journeys and renew future teaching and learning plans.

A final word: in any major curriculum revision, don't expect to get it right first time. The curriculum will continue to evolve and will need to change in response to local circumstances and to changes in medicine.

 "A little known fact is that the Apollo moon missions were on course less than 1% of the time. The mission was composed of almost constant mid-course corrections."

Belasco, 1996

Summary

The concept of curriculum reform should be viewed on a continuum rather than a recurring event. This chapter provides 10 steps that serve as a useful checklist for monitoring the process. The following is a summary of each step.

1. The training programme is intended to fulfil the goals and objectives. These have been expanded to include population medicine and the healthcare system.

2. The expected and explicit student learning outcomes should inform all decisions about curriculum development.

3. The content included should include basic and clinical knowledge plus the values, attitudes and educational philosophy of the academic leaders and faculty. The process and skills of thinking should also be included.

4. The organization of the content, including the sequence in which it is covered, is a critical factor to consider. There is growing sentiment among educational leaders that medical students learn about the healthcare system from the day they enter medical school.

5. The educational strategies should strive to help the learner integrate knowledge for use.

6. The teaching methods used should include an appropriate blend of large-group teaching, small-group teaching and the use of new learning technologies matched to the level of learning objectives. Emphasis on personalized learning has opened the door to asynchronous digital teaching underlying new mobile platforms and group techniques like the flipped classroom.

7. Assessment of the students' progress should tie explicitly to specific learning outcomes related to knowledge, skills and attitudes.

8. The declared curriculum including objectives and assessments should be exposed and readily available to all the stakeholders including the students.

9. The hidden curriculum should be included in the measurement of the educational environment.

10. In this dynamic model, the curriculum map serves as an opportunity to manage and develop the curriculum. It presents an opportunity to compare the declared and the delivered curricula in relation to learning outcomes.

Although there is a loose chronological sequence to these steps, we recognize that process of curriculum development is much more a spiral than a linear process. In addition, any step could mark the 'entry point' to the process depending upon needs and context.

References

Cooke, M., Irby, D.M., O'Brien, B.C., 2010. Educating physicians: a call for reform of medical schools and residency. Jossey-Bass, San Francisco.

Cooke, M., Irby, D.M., Sullivan, W., Ludmerer, K.M., 2006. American Medical Education 100 Years after the Flexner Report. N. Engl. J. Med. 355, 1339–1344.

Campbell, J.P., Oblinger, D.G. Academic analytics. Educause, October, 2007.

Carbonell, K.B., Stalmeijer, R.E., Konings, K.D., et al., 2014. How experts deal with novel situations: a review of adaptive expertise. Educ. Res. Rev. 12, 14–29.

Davis, D.A., Mazmanian, P.E., Fordis, M., et al., 2006. Accuracy of physician self-assessment compared with observed measures of competence. JAMA 296 (9), 1094–1102.

Dornan, T., Littlewood, S., Margolis, S.A., et al., 2006. How can experience in clinical and community settings contribute to early medical education? A BEME systematic review. BEME Guide No 6. Med. Teach. 28, 3–18.

Dunn, W.R., Hamilton, D.D., Harden, R.M., 1985. Techniques of identifying competencies needed by doctors. Med. Teach. 7 (1), 15–25.

Ellaway, R., Masters, K., 2008. AMEE guide 32: e-Learning in medical education Part 1: learning, teaching and assessment. Med. Teach. 30, 455–473.

Ericsson, K.A., 2015. Acquisition and maintenance of medical expertise: a perspective from the expert-performance approach with deliberate practice. Acad. Med. 90, 1471–1486.

Flexner, A., 1910. Medical education in the United States and Canada. Bulletin number 4. The Carnegie Foundation, New York, p. 53.

Frenk, J., Chen, L., Bhutta, Z.A., et al., 2010. Health professionals for a new century: transforming education to strengthen health systems in an interdependent world. Lancet 376, 1923–1958.

Genn, J.M., 2001. AMEE medical education guide no. 23. Curriculum, environment, climate, quality and change in medical education – a unifying perspective. AMEE, Dundee.

Hammick, M., Freeth, D., Koppel, I., et al., 2007. A best evidence systematic review of inter-professional education: BEME Guide no. 9. Med. Teach. 29, 735–751.

Harden, R.M., 1986b. Ten questions to ask when planning a course or curriculum. Med. Educ. 20, 356–365.

Harden, R.M., 2000. The integration ladder: a tool for curriculum planning and evaluation. Med. Educ. 34, 551–557.

Harden, R.M., 2001. AMEE guide number 21: curriculum mapping: a tool for transparent and authentic teaching and learning. Med. Teach. 23 (2), 123–137.

Harden, R.M., 2007. Outcome-based education: the future is today. Med. Teach. 29, 625–629.

Harden, R.M., Crosby, J.R., Davis, M.H., et al., 2000. Task-based learning: the answer to integration and problem-based learning in the clinical years. Med. Educ. 34, 391–397.

Harden, R.M., Davis, M.H., 1998. The continuum of problem-based learning. Med. Teach. 20 (4), 301–306.

Harden, R.M., Sowden, S., Dunn, W.R., 1984. Some educational strategies in curriculum development: the SPICES model. Med. Educ. 18, 284–297.

Harden, R.M., Stamper, N., 1999. What is a spiral curriculum? Med. Teach. 21 (2), 141–143.

Pusic, M., Boutis, K., Hatala, R., Cook, D., 2015. Learning curves in health professions education. Acad. Med. 90 (8), 1034–1042.

Quirk, M., 2006. Intuition and Metacognition in Medical Education; Keys to Expertise. Springer.

Shaw, J. Rethinking the Medical Curriculum. Harvard Magazine. September/October, 2015.

Skochelak, S., Stansfield, R.B., Dunham, L., et al., 2016. Medical student perceptions of the learning environment at the end of the first year: a 28 medical school collaborative. Acad. Med. 91 (9), 1257–1262.

US Department of Education Office of Education Enhancing Teaching and Learning Report. Technology 2012.

The undergraduate curriculum

J. Lanphear, M. Matte

Trends

- Curriculum design has evolved from simply having quality courses as 'stepping stones', to designs that integrate all content across the educational program.

- Making meaningful links between the stages of training from pre-med to undergraduate to postgraduate and into practice is one of the most enduring challenges today.

- Alignment of content along the continuum of medical education through systematic cascade of learning objectives is one tool used to ensure integration of content and transition to the next level of learning.

- Curriculum design models are evolving to insure medical educators are aware of the unique place undergraduate medical education holds along the continuum of medical education.

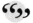
"The undergraduate medical curriculum is often viewed simultaneously as the cause and solution to issues facing medicine today."

Joel Lanphear

Introduction

In Chapter 2 Quirk and Harden defined a new curriculum paradigm as "a process involving definition of objectives, methods and evaluation and includes predicting and tracking curriculum outcomes". When one examines the depth and breadth of a physician's education and training, the objectives, methods, evaluation and the outcome measures should be organized along a continuum that begins with the educational experiences of students prior to matriculation to medical school and leads in many countries to postgraduate or specialty training. In keeping with this definition, the undergraduate medical curriculum occupies a unique space along what is often called a continuum of medical education. A continuum is defined as "a coherent whole characterized as a collection, sequence or progression of values or elements varying by minute degrees"

(Merriam-Webster, 2003). This continuum of medical education includes not only the pre-medical experiences, but the undergraduate medical education, graduate medical education and continuing professional education experiences. The stages in the development of a physician must be sequenced and implemented in such a way as to prepare the learner for a career based in the process of lifelong learning (Kruse, 2013).

Although the continuum appears to represent a rather smooth succession along a linear course, in practice, the stages have been implemented more as separate entities placed upon one another over specified periods of time, more as one would picture building blocks (Petersdorf, 1994). In considering the undergraduate medical curriculum, an awareness and consideration for where students have been in their educational journey must help to inform the tasks that lie ahead in their first foray into medicine, i.e. the creation of as smooth a transition as possible along a complicated and varied continuum.

Medical educators have the responsibility therefore to improve the transition between each stage of learning along the continuum by examining outcome measures for each stage and designing a curriculum that aligns with these measures. Educators recommend working with the 'final product in mind' as each level of competency is developed along the continuum. In many countries, there are different licensing organizations for each stage of the learning continuum rather than one single coordinating agency. Until a more coherent licensing model is created, it is incumbent upon medical educators to facilitate transitions between stages.

In addition to its unique place between pre-professional and postgraduate training, the undergraduate curriculum presents students as learners with challenges and opportunities, many of which are entirely new and unique to them. The rate at which learning occurs, and the amount of information learners are expected to master has been described as the difference between 'drinking from a water fountain and a fire hose'. Many learners enter medical school having performed at high levels of academic achievement in prior pre- and post-secondary courses and have performed well on admissions tests and in interview processes. In fact, they are now among a group of students who for a large part have similar abilities and goals. It may be a unique experience for some to realize that they are among true academic equals. As the medical school experience is demanding and distinctive, medical schools need to provide for student support for these experiences. However, in many instances, learners will realize that their peers all have talents and unique sets of skills that can be drawn upon as support in a positive way.

As part of the medical curriculum, students will encounter illness, disease and death at a very personal level as they engage in some form of simulated or actual patient care encounter. And although each has met their goal of medical school admission each will also respond differently to experiences they have in the laboratory, classroom and clinical contexts (Corrigan et al., 2010). Medical schools and faculty have developed a sensitivity to these issues and have developed active and ongoing systems to assist. It is useful to keep in mind that by explaining to students the intent of the curriculum design, this will draw upon the power of metacognition, which describes the process of a deeper learning experience when we think about what and how we are learning.

A medical school that employs team-based, problem-based and case-based small-group learning as primary curriculum activities often provide some form of orientation to this type of learning, including the opportunity to practice in this learning environment to ensure the greatest productivity for each student can be achieved (McCrorie, 2010).

Finally, it is important for those developing curricular models and content to acknowledge that medical students arrive at medical school with a variety of background experiences, knowledge, skills and attitudes from prior learning. They do not arrive as in Aristotle's words with a *tabula rosa* or blank slate (Aristotle) in their repertoires. It is appropriate to assume that a student's background will have an impact on how they approach their learning, just as the planned learning experiences will impact their achievement of the goals and objectives of the programme in terms of learning, behaviours, clinical decision making and clinical and communication skill development. It is important therefore, during the process of selection of medical students, that a student's previous experiences be considered.

 In designing the undergraduate curriculum, it is important to consider the experiences students bring with them to medical school, and those that lie ahead along the continuum of medical education.

Forces shaping the curriculum

Conceptually, the undergraduate medical curriculum should provide the necessary clinical skills and knowledge to succeed at the next stages of the continuum. At a minimum, this includes a clear understanding of the basic medical, clinical and social sciences as explanatory to the process of wellness and disease in the context of the human body and perhaps more importantly in the context of patient care.

The forces that have and continue to shape the development and direction of this unique undergraduate medical educational experience have come from a variety of sources. Many are internal to the medical school, and many have been supported by external bodies concerned that the medical curriculum deliver its promise of improved healthcare. Change has come as a result of social, cultural, political and economic forces universal to all countries, organizations and governments. Arguably, the undergraduate curriculum is influenced by all, but often unable to control many.

Perhaps the most consequential individual force shaping medical education in general and the undergraduate curriculum specifically was the 1910 report entitled *Medical Education in the United States and Canada: A Report to the Carnegie Foundation for the Advancement of Teaching*. This report, written by Abraham Flexner commonly referred to as the Flexner Report, summarized his findings in visits to 155 medical schools in Canada and the United States in 1909 (Pritchett & Flexner, 1910). Suffice to say, the recommendations of the original report published in 1910 had an enormous impact on bringing medical education into the university scientific setting, establishing standards for medical curricula, and medical education in general. Perhaps the single greatest impact on undergraduate medical education has come from the following quote from the Flexner Report:

 "For purposes of convenience, the medical curriculum may be divided into two parts, according as the work is carried on mainly in laboratories of mainly in the hospital. But the distinction is only superficial, for in the hospital is itself, in the fullest sense Laboratory. In general, the four year curriculum falls into two fairly equal sections: The first two years are devoted to laboratory sciences and the last to clinical work."

Pritchett & Flexner, 1910

Although Flexner clearly believed that the sciences of the first two years were critical to advances in clinical care, the long-term impact on undergraduate medical education worldwide has led in large part to the most prevalent model of medical education. That is, two years of basic science followed by two years of clinical training and education in hospital. While this divide has been eased over the past two decades with clinical skills training and work with patients starting at the beginning of medical school, there is still more of an artificial divide than most desire. Even in countries with 5- and 6-year programmes, the divide between the basic science and clinical experience, even with early clinical skill training, can be profound. The fact that the new Carnegie Foundation Report of 2010 calls for greater integration of the basic science and clinical experiences stands as evidence to this fact as do other recommendations similar to those of the 1910 report (Irby et al., 2010). A similar call for greater integration can be found in the General Medical Council's *Tomorrow's Doctors. Recommendations on Undergraduate Medical Education* (1993).

Another factor shaping undergraduate medical education has been the emergence of research in medical education based upon a rapid expansion of medical and scientific knowledge, changes in the standards of accrediting bodies worldwide, and an increase in demands for accountability from the public. Summarizing three decades of medical education research Norman notes, "Perhaps the most important evidence of progress in the discipline is that we are now more likely than before to demand evidence to guide educational decision making—as a change in educational culture." (Norman, 2002) In specific terms the major impacts from medical education research and thus the development and delivery of the undergraduate curriculum have been:

- a better understanding of how medical expertise is acquired
- development and research in problem-based learning
- improved assessment methods (Norman, 2002)

Concomitant with this, and as part of emerging medical education research, has been the development of cognitive science research. Modern computer and imaging technology have led to the ability to better understand the mind and how it functions to process information. It is generally understood that cognitive science is an interdisciplinary approach involving the fields of psychology, philosophy, linguistics, anthropology, artificial intelligence and neuroscience (Miller, 2003). For medical education this has meant new understanding of the human learning process. The impact of the research in cognitive science upon the undergraduate curriculum will be discussed in greater detail later.

Another force that has influenced the undergraduate curriculum is the nature of the healthcare system in a given country or region, and the nature of medical practice in that system. Imagine a system in which primary healthcare was widely distributed, provided universally to all citizens, and one in which physicians and healthcare providers received the same remuneration regardless of a patient's gender, age, ethnicity or economic status. Imagine that the volume of patients seen in a given day or week was not the determinant of remuneration. Such systems would welcome medical students as learners and physicians would have an adequate amount of time to spend with them and their patients. Such a system may exist today, but a more common system is one in which the distribution of primary care physicians and primary healthcare providers does not match the needs of the population.

More commonly, healthcare is disease oriented rather than prevention and wellness centred, isolationism between and among healthcare providers is common, and large disparities exist between segments of the population. In this model physicians and healthcare providers find themselves pressured to see more and more patients and find students placed in their practices a detriment to their productivity and incomes (Frenk et al., 2010). These are not environments into which medical students should be placed as these curricular experiences become the 'model' for care and perpetuate the current system. In summary, the context in which medical education occurs, nature of the healthcare system, cultural values, the rapid change of the nature of health-care and physician role models all impact the undergraduate curriculum and the students touched by them. As noted earlier, advances in medical education research and the cognitive sciences have also had a large impact on the undergraduate medical curriculum.

In a landmark publication, Papa and Harasym (1999) describe stages of medical schools in North America from a cognitive sciences perspective. They describe five curricular models by year and era of initiation, portions of which exist in medical schools to this day, worldwide. They are:

- Apprenticeship Model (1765)
- Discipline-based Model (1871)
- Organ-System-based Model (1951)
- Problem-based Model (1971)
- Clinical Presentation-based Model (1991)

It can be argued that the discipline-based model was heavily reinforced by interpretation of the Flexner Report of 1910 and that the relative speed of curricular reform between the 1960s and the 1990s was the result of change in our knowledge from the emerging research in medical education heavily influenced by cognitive science research. Each of these models exhibit strengths and weaknesses, and today it is common for undergraduate medical curricula to reflect some of each in a mixed model attempting to draw upon the strengths of each and to compensate for their shortcomings.

Perhaps the most impactful research finding from cognitive research studies related specifically to medical knowledge expertise and diagnostic reasoning. It had been argued that what students learned in a specific problem in a problem-based case would then generalize to different medical problems. The work of Elstein, Schulman and Sprafka (1978) demonstrated that problem solving and diagnostic skills were problem specific and not generalizable. These findings and others led to the development of the clinical presentation model and the realization that medical students would need experience with a large range of specific medical problems to eventually become competent physicians. The development of early clinical experiences for medical students in the curriculum, the use of simulated patients and simulation devices can all be viewed as mechanisms to begin the process of student exposure to a broad range of medical problems. These experiences provide students with foundational experiences that will assist in the transition to postgraduate education and training.

In many countries, the number and distribution of healthcare providers is a significant problem. In the same way that our understanding of the nature of cognitive learning has changed, the context in which undergraduate medical education occurs has been critically examined. It has been shown that the distribution of primary care physicians into rural area for instance, is associated with a rural upbringing, positive educational experiences in rural areas as undergraduate students and postgraduate training in rural areas (Strasser et al., 2016).

 The directions of the undergraduate medical curriculum have been shaped by external influences, internal influences, and advances in understanding the learning process through research in the cognitive sciences.

Critical components of the undergraduate medical education programme as they relate to the continuum of medical education

In order for the undergraduate curriculum to be both effective and meaningful as a component of the continuum of medical education, there are a number of concepts that should be considered in planning the curriculum (Liaison Committee on Medical Education, 2015; General Medical Council, 2015). Among these are:

1. a statement of the mission, vision and goals of the medical school
2. scientific content that is current and appropriate to the mission and includes the major concepts of basic and clinical sciences
3. a curricular model that supports the learning required of each student
4. a system of curriculum management that provides centralized overview of curriculum delivery
5. programmes in place that provide for the assessment of student performance and evaluation of the programme

6. a system that assures faculty are of sufficient quality and preparation for their roles
7. adequate financial and physical resource to deliver the curriculum
8. an educational environment that is safe for students and conducive to learning.

1. Mission, vision and goals

A statement of the medical school's mission serves as a guide to the direction an institution plans to follow in implementing its curriculum. The goals outlined in the mission should also include the concepts of preparing students for whatever medical practice or postgraduate education and training they may select. A mission should reflect the need for a sound basis in science, and the application of these sciences to clinical practice. As such, the mission ultimately should guide the development of over-arching programme objectives that serve as a framework for the design and development of all teaching and learning activities. The over-arching programme objectives in turn guide the development of course goals and objectives and eventually specific learning activities and their outcome measures/assessment. This 'cascade' effect is illustrated in Fig. 3.1.

2. Scientific curriculum content

It is important that the curriculum of the medical school include the basic biomedical, clinical and social sciences content and concepts contributing to the modern and appropriate practice of medicine today. It also should include opportunities to develop the competencies graduates will need in order to be successful in the next stage of training along the continuum of medical education. This includes not only the acquisition of traditional basic and medical sciences knowledge, such as biochemistry, physiology, microbiology, pharmacology, immunology and pathology to name a few, but newer concepts as well. Among these newer

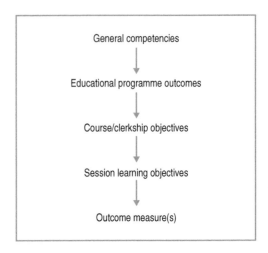

Fig. 3.1 Programme objectives cascade here.

concepts are wellness, translational research and the behavioural and social sciences. The involvement of qualified faculty in developing the curriculum content is essential. It is advisable to use references from national and international organizations, such as the Association for the Study of Medical Education (ASME), the Association of American Medical Colleges (AAMC), and the Association of Faculties of Medicine in Canada (AFMC), in determining content for the undergraduate curriculum. Modern curricula should include concepts in medical ethics, population health, and interpersonal communication skills, all of which are required of a learner engaged in postgraduate learning activities. These concepts are best described and understood in the context of the culture and legal system in which the course is taught and in which medicine will be practiced. The inclusion of this specific curricular content requires faculty leadership and collaboration as, in the end, it is the role of the institutional faculty to determine curricular content and to agree on its sequencing and delivery.

3. A curricular model that supports the learning required of each student

Any curricular model a school chooses must support the mission of the school. For example, if the mission articulates the need for access to high quality healthcare for all populations the school serves, the curriculum must support the provision of learning activities in which students can learn medicine in a context that serves the mission.

In developing an undergraduate medical education curriculum, medical educators must take into account the unusually large volume of medical knowledge, clinical and communication skills required of a medical student, and the need for each student to retain the knowledge and skills as they transition to the next stage along the continuum of medical education. While far beyond the scope of this chapter, suffice it to say, medical educators must consider basic learning theories as they design and develop learning activities in order to meet the learning needs/preferences of the medical students. Typically, these activities would include small- and large-group learning, simulation – to include the use of standardized patients, journal clubs, laboratory experiences and self-directed learning opportunities.

4. Managing the curriculum

Central management and control of the undergraduate curriculum is essential for insuring that the goals of the curriculum and its contents are aligned to the mission. The ultimate responsibility for delivery of a quality curriculum lies with the chief academic officer, usually the dean. Many medical colleges have a vice dean to whom oversight of the curriculum is delegated and a curriculum committee made up of faculty representatives who report to the vice dean. Historically, medical curriculum committees have been composed

of departmentally based representatives whose primary task was to make sure that their department's courses were included. This is the model that existed in the era of the discipline-based curriculum.

More recently, in the era of the problem-based, organ-systems curriculum and the clinical presentation-based model, new structures have arisen to facilitate the integration of multiple and inter-related concepts and content. This has included providing physician input into planning courses in the first years of the curriculum and serving as co-course directors along with their counterparts from the basic sciences. As co-course directors, initial clinically relevant case problems are developed and often presented as a team. The presentation of the clinical case and its related diagnostic reasoning provides a 'scaffold' for better understanding the concepts presented in the organ-systems course (Ambrose, 2010). This model is based on course development teams organized around common themes or organ systems. These groups of faculty from different disciplines represent the clinical and basic science content areas that are focused on the integration of content. These groups are ultimately responsible to the curriculum committee. Themes or threads of curriculum may also be used to provide integration of content around common presenting problems or concepts.

Ensuring the horizontal and vertical integration of content and learning activities is an important concept in the curriculum management process. In this case, 'integrate' is defined as "to form, coordinate or blend into a functioning or unified whole" (Merriam-Webster's Collegiate Dictionary, 2003). In a curricular sense, there are two types of integration. Vertical integration occurs between the content, skills, behaviours and attitudes for those experiences or courses occurring at the same time or between years of the curriculum. Horizontal integration is the integration of content, skills, behaviours and attitudes between course and experiences that proceed or follow.

Perhaps the most powerful tool for insuring that horizontal and vertical integration occurs is through the use of a curriculum map. A curriculum map is built upon the concept of the cascade effect described in Fig. 3.1. It need not require an elaborate electronic system as there are workable models that can be built using a searchable spread sheet. The key is in connecting the components of the cascade in hierarchical fashion from the mission to goals to objective to content and to assessment methods.

Central management of the curriculum is fundamental to ensuring horizontal and vertical integration of course content and sequencing of learning experiences. Mapping curricular objectives to programme goals and outcomes is a critical tool to achieve these tasks.

5. Assessment of student performance and programme evaluation

A number of factors in addition to those mentioned above contribute to the creation of a quality curriculum. Among these are systems in place to assess student progress, to evaluate the faculty performance and to evaluate the program in general. This system is often referred to as continuous quality improvement (CQI). Data of student performance should be comprehensive and measure not only acquisition of content knowledge but skills, attitudes and behaviours reflected in the programme objectives. The methods used to measure performance must be appropriate to the learning context. Information on student progress should be collected systematically and reported within a reasonable time frame to allow learners to correct errors. It is highly desirable that students receive formative feedback, that is, feedback on their performance that is provided during the learning experience and well before a final mark or score is recorded. This gives the student a sense of how they are progressing and also allows them to improve before a summative grade or mark is recorded (Wood, 2010).

Student feedback on the specific learning experience, course or faculty instructor is another source of information on the curriculum. When systematically and anonymously collected, feedback from students is valid and useful in understanding their perspective on the curriculum experience. When student numbers are small, such as in some clinical rotations or seminars, data should be collected over time and bunched to assure anonymity.

Annual reviews of the curriculum by the curriculum committee and any other committees engaged in curriculum oversight are important sources of information. At these review sessions all data relevant to the curriculum should be available for review. Discussion should include student assessments with passing and failing rates, student feedback on their experiences, course director and faculty comments. Data comparing courses across the criterion should be available as well.

6. Preparation of faculty for their roles as teachers

To support the quality of teaching and learning in the curriculum there must be a system in place that insures all faculty teaching and assessing students have proper credentials and training for the task. These will vary from school to school but the qualifications should be published and made available through the normal means that applicants use to make applications. Usually this includes type of degree, areas of specialty, training and levels of experience and a copy of their resume or curriculum vitae. Letters of reference are usually sought for final candidates. It is common to ask final applicants to interview on sight and to provide a presentation of their educational and research area of interest. Review of faculty candidates is most often accomplished by a faculty committee of peers capable of judging the academic merit and eligibility for rank upon appointment. Engagement of faculty in this process is another method to insure quality of the educational programme and decreases the potential of bias in the selection process.

7. Financial and physical resources

The availability of resources both financial and physical vary widely between medical schools around the world. Each institution must ultimately decide what the appropriate levels of financing are and the types of facilities that best fit their mission and learning opportunities designed for the curriculum.

8. Safe learning environment

Assuring students and faculty with a safe environment in which to teach and learn is not only essential to their wellbeing but also for their ability to be successful. For students this means the ability to comment on their experiences and their concerns without fear of reprisal. And since it is called a medical school, it should be expected that students will make mistakes and errors in judgement. The process towards becoming a healthcare professional is a difficult one at best, and students need to be assured that there are processes in place to protect them and their patients. Anonymity in evaluating learning experience is one mechanism, as is the ability to review their records and to appeal actions such as grades and reprimands that they feel unfair. A student handbook or similar document should be available to students, faculty and staff, which states these protections.

Summary

The undergraduate medical education curriculum is unique not only as a medical student's first full-time exposure to medicine but also as a bridge between those experiences prior to medical school and the specialty training that may follow. This continuum of medical education culminating in medical practice and lifelong learning is a journey that is not always as smooth as it could be. Given the enormous amount to be learned by students and the forces constantly affecting the curriculum, it is the responsibility of medical educators to ease the transitions along this continuum. This can best be done by continued vigilance in understanding where students have come from before medical school, where they are headed beyond undergraduate education and training, and always in keeping with the mission, vision and educational goals of the institution. Always start with the end in mind.

References

Ambrose, S., 2010. How learning works. In: Mayer, R. (Ed.), What Kinds of Feedback Enhance Learning? Jossey Boss, Hoboken, p. 146, 121-152.

Aristotle, De anima 429b29-430a1.

Corrigan, O., Ellis, K., Bleakley, A., et al., 2010. Quality in medical education. In: Swanick, T. (Ed.), Understanding Medical Education. Wiley-Blackwell, London, pp. 379–391.

Elstein, A.S., Shulman, L.S., Sprafka, S.A., 1978. Medical Problem Solving: An Analysis of Clinical Reasoning. Harvard University Press, Cambridge, Massachusetts.

Frenk, J., Chen, L., Bhutta, Z.A., et al., 2010. Health professions for a new century: transforming education to strengthen health systems in an interdependent world. Lancet doi:10.1016/S0140-6736(10)61854-5.

General Medical Council, 1993. Tomorrow's Doctors. Recommendations on Undergraduate Medical Education. GMC, London.

General Medical Council, 2015. Promoting Excellence: Standards for Medical Education and Training. GMC, London.

Irby, D.M., Ivens, M., O'Brien, B., 2010. Call for reform of medical education by the Carnegie Foundation for the advancement of teaching: 1910 and 2010. Acad. Med. 85 (2), 220–227.

Kruse, J., 2013. Social accountability across the continuum of medical education. Fam. Med. 45 (5), 208–211.

Liaison Committee on Medical Education, 2015. Functions and Structure of a Medical School. Liaison Committee on Medical Education, Washington, D.C.

McCrorie, P., 2010. Teaching and leading small groups. In: Swanick, T. (Ed.), Understanding Medical Education. Wiley-Blackwell, London, pp. 124–138.

Merriam-Webster's Collegiate Dictionary, eleventh ed. 2003. Springfield, Massachusetts, p. 650.

Miller, G.A., 2003. The cognitive revolution. Trends Cogn. Sci. 7 (3), 141–144.

Norman, G.R., 2002 Research in medical education: three decades of programs. BMJ online 324 (7353), 1560–1562.

Papa, F.J., Harasym, P.H., 1999. Medical curriculum reform in North America, 1765 to the present: a cognitive science perspective. Acad. Med. 74 (2), 154–164.

Petersdorf, R.G., 1994. Medical curriculum training, and the continuum of medical education. Soc. Med. 87 (Suppl. 1 22), 41–49.

Pritchett, H., Flexner, A., 1910. Medical Education in the United States and Canada: A Report for the Carnegie Foundation for the Advancement of Teaching. The Carnegie Foundation, New York, pp. 57–70.

Strasser, R., Couper, I., Wynn-Jones, J., et al., 2016. Education for rural practice in rural practice. Educ. Prim. Care 27 (1).

Wood, T., 2010. Formative assessment. In: Swanich, T. (Ed.), Understanding Medical Education. Blackwell, London, pp. 259–269.

4

Postgraduate medical education: a 'pipeline' to competence

L. Snell, J. R. Frank, R. Pihlak, J. Sa

Trends

- In addition to being learners, postgraduate trainees play critical roles in healthcare systems.

- During residency learning occurs primarily in the workplace: this requires new approaches for teaching and assessment in this setting.

- Outcome-based paradigms of residency education are evolving as models where competency frameworks form the basis of curriculum, learning and assessment.

- Training outside large academic health centers is becoming more common and provides different opportunities and perspectives.

Introduction

 "Residency is when 'doctors come of professional age – acquiring the knowledge and skills of their specialties or subspecialties, forming professional identities, and developing habits, behaviors, attitudes, and values that last a professional lifetime.'"

Ludmerer, 2015

Postgraduate medical education (PGME) is that period of medical training following graduation from medical school and before a physician is thought competent for independent practice. This period, which can last from 1 to 7 or more years, is the time when young doctors improve knowledge, hone skills, develop professional attitudes and cultivate behaviours that prepare them for a career of autonomous practice. The first residency programmes, in the specialties of internal medicine and surgery, were established in the USA in the early 1900s by Osler and Halsted. These were hospital-based programmes where medical school graduates became trainee physicians responsible, under supervision, for patient care; the name 'resident' comes from the fact that these young doctors would often 'reside' in the hospital.

In this chapter we will use the term 'resident' to refer to postgraduate medical trainees. Around the world these individuals have also been called junior doctors, house officers, registrars, (post)graduate trainees or clinical fellows (RCPSC, 2014). To confuse matters further, this phase of training is referred to as graduate medical education in the USA and postgraduate medical education in much of the rest of the world.

This chapter provides a brief overview of the major issues in PGME today, and addresses the following questions:

- What roles do residents play a healthcare system?
- What is the importance of transitions into, through, and out of residency and how are these managed?
- What are the various models of PGME?
- What strategies for teaching, learning and assessment are commonly used?
- How is the quality of residency programmes assured?
- What are some of the current controversies in PGME?

Functions of PGME and postgraduate trainees in a healthcare system

Postgraduate medical trainees are unique entities in healthcare systems in that they are simultaneously both workers and learners, which may be the cause of some confusion (Imrie et al., 2014). Residents perform a major part of the patient care in teaching hospitals and other healthcare institutions, under a variable amount of supervision depending on their level and the context. In most cases, they are paid as practising doctors and have stipulated patient-care tasks. Without postgraduate trainees in this role, most academic health institutions around the world would not be able to provide their current level of care.

Box 4.1 Roles of residents

- Learner
- Clinical practitioner
- Teacher
- Assessor
- Mentor
- Role model
- Researcher
- Contributor to quality improvement
- Administrator
- Leader
- Team member
- Health advocate
- Innovator
- Activist

Residents have other functions besides patient care (Box 4.1). Perhaps the most prominent is teaching medical students and junior trainees. Medical students learn about a third of their knowledge and skills from residents, and residents spend up to one-fourth of their work time teaching (Snell, 2011).

 "Teaching by residents is different from and likely complementary to faculty teaching... Residents tend to teach different things in a different way at different times."

Snell, 2011

Many residents, particularly in their senior years, are also significantly involved in medical research of many types: basic, applied, clinical, translational, and in areas such as medical education, epidemiology and population studies, health services and the field of quality and safety, to name a few. Residents also have major roles as leaders and managers, running teams of more junior trainees, contributing to the organizations in which they work through serving on committees, and effecting change in education and clinical care through their efforts.

Transitions in PGME

ADMISSIONS AND MATCHING

Medical school graduates enter the PGME system through a variety of pathways (see Chapter 42). Most programmes select trainees based on their performance as a medical student, academic records, personal statements, reference letters, interviews, tests of personality or emotional intelligence, or tests of knowledge, situational judgement or skills (Patterson et al., 2015). A

newer form of interview is the MMI (multiple mini-interview), where candidates undertake an OSCE-like series of short interviews, like a multiple stations exam, addressing specific tasks, attributes or competencies (Hofmeister et al., 2008). One commonly used route is a standardized 'match', where trainees rank their choice of programmes, and potential programmes rate and rank all applicants. An electronic match is likely to result in a fair, objective and transparent process of assigning trainees to programmes. In some countries, an individual medical graduate must search for and apply to many posts. The acceptance decision may be made by the department chief, clinical unit director or the residency programme director.

The transition from medical student to junior doctor is often stressful, with different expectations and roles. This transition can be eased with orientation sessions, 'boot camps' (Ambardekar et al., 2016), residency guides and mentoring and peer mentoring programmes.

TRANSITION FROM JUNIOR RESIDENT TO SENIOR RESIDENT

The movement from a novice trainee to a more senior should in theory be a continuous one but is often more of an abrupt event, where the completion of foundational training and a move to the next stage brings greater responsibility and autonomy (Pantaleoni et al., 2014). In particular, adding teaching, supervisory and leadership roles to clinical duties may stress residents. Attention to resident wellbeing, focused education on the new roles aforementioned and mentoring programmes can assist in this transition.

TRANSITION FROM PGME TO PRACTICE

The move to fully autonomous practice brings further new responsibilities, which may go beyond medical expertise. Managing a practice, controlling finances, administrative duties, the skills needed for independent research, leading quality initiatives, continuing lifelong learning and being a consultant to government institutions and organizations are examples of skills and duties that may be newly added to the young physician's roles. To ease the transition, many of these skills can be taught in the later parts of postgraduate education as the resident becomes increasingly autonomous.

Models of PGME

There is great variability of the organization of postgraduate medical training, responsibility and curricula from country to country. Some countries have developed structured programmes, the components of which are planned clinical/practical placements, expert supervision, regular theoretical teaching, research experience, systematic assessments and evaluation

- 1 to 2 internship/foundational years after medical school, followed by specialist training of 3 to 10+ years (UK, Japan, Australia)
- Direct entry from medical school into 2 to 10 years specialist training (USA, Canada)
- Accumulating varied clinical experiences (Nordic countries)
- Fixed-term specialist training (Eastern European countries)
- Mixed programmes – a fixed-term, during which the resident accrues experience
- Competency-based models such as those being implemented in Canada and the USA

of the training programmes. In other countries, the process of postgraduate medical education remains more traditional, based on practical clinical training (WFME, 2015) and time spent learning in the workplace. There are, however, some basic archetypes, as shown in Box 4.2.

As these curricular models are quite diverse, the required length of training is often variable. To attain the equivalent qualifications for practice, training may range from 2 years to 10 years following medical school in various countries.

THE ROLE OF INTERNSHIPS OR FOUNDATIONAL TRAINING

A major variable in these curricula is the existence and length of an internship for training in broad foundational competencies. There are countries where no internship exists, others where an internship is a standalone entity and a physician may not even need further specialization, others where the internship is incorporated into the specialty training and still others where it stands alone, acting as basic medical training before specialty training.

SETTING FOR TRAINING

Where the training takes place varies across countries, with sites of training ranging from isolated, rural place-ments, community clinics, practitioners' outpatient offices to multi-specialty high-acuity tertiary care hospitals. There are educational trade-offs between a one-to-one relationship with a single supervisor and a large academic health centre with a critical mass of trainees and supervisors and a wide range of clinical exposure, but less personal attention and possibly less opportunity for hands-on practice. Exposure to settings outside of major academic centres influences some residents to choose to work in these often under-served areas in their future practice (see Chapter 11).

The setting for training goes beyond education implications and may affect clinical service needs, a resident's choice of eventual practice location, health human resource planning and funding and policy issues.

RESPONSIBILITY FOR CURRICULAR DEVELOPMENT AND MANAGEMENT

Universities, hospitals (academic or community, urban or rural), communities or private organizations may play a role in residency programme development and management. Jurisdictions vary with regards to who sets PGME curricula, and how they are structured. At one end of a spectrum, the 'curriculum' is essentially the scope of practice of the individual supervisor or group of supervising clinicians. In this scenario, trainees' workplace learning allows them to acquire this same scope, akin to a vocational apprenticeship. Individual institutions often design a local curriculum that is semi-structured, with pre-planned and sequenced learning combined with ad hoc learning as part of patient care. Further along this curriculum planning spectrum are the national or international standards set by various institutions such as the Royal Colleges, World Federation of Medical Education (WFME, 2015) or specialty boards around the world. Finally, some specialty societies build their own core curricula for multiple countries or institutions to implement (ESMO – European Society for Medical Oncology; ACOG – the American Congress of Obstetricians and Gynecologists; European Society for Emergency Medicine; some specialties in Brazil). These are often mixed programmes with a minimum length requirement; experience is gained in different areas from different clinical settings. Regardless of the model, clinical experiences with increasing responsibility for patient care (also known as rotations, placements or terms) is the *sine qua non* of PGME.

POST-CERTIFICATION TRAINING

Another characteristic of PGME is the existence of different pathways or special non-clinical areas of concentration within training. These vary greatly around the world and include areas such as research, global health, medical education and healthcare leadership. Many countries also offer clinical fellowships after the postgraduate certification to allow further sub-specialization; in other places, these are considered part of continuing professional development programmes and not postgraduate training.

Teaching, learning and assessment in PGME

For most of the twentieth century, postgraduate educa-tion was based on residents rotating through various clinical settings for a defined period of time. Clinical experience was accepted as the only requirement to attain clinical competence. Recently, there has been an increasing interest in outcome-based or competency-based learning, and several countries started to use competency frameworks to design their postgraduate medical training (see Chapter 15). A number of medical organizations across the globe have defined competencies and outcomes for health professionals. Examples of these frameworks are CanMEDS 2015 in Canada (Frank et al., 2015), Accreditation Council for Graduate Medical Education (Swing, 2007) in United States, The Scottish Doctor, and the Royal Australasian College of Physicians in Australia and New Zealand competencies. These well-defined competencies inform the organization of curricular structure, the choice of learning methods and the use of assessment tools that are consistent with the desired results. They also underlie decisions on when competence is attained and advancement to the next training stage (Frank et al., 2010). Furthermore, competency-based programmes allow trainees to take more responsibility for their own learning process.

"Postgraduate medical education is a unique educational environment, with its emphasis on work-based learning, clinical supervision as a predominant method of training, performance-based assessment, and the challenge of simultaneously delivering education, training and service."

Steinert, 2011

In postgraduate education, much of the learning occurs in a workplace setting while the resident is concurrently caring for a patient or performing other clinical tasks. Postgraduate medical education is an immersive experience in which applied learning is expected to happen in the authentic setting by exposing the trainee to the work they will actually do in the future. The resident's clinical supervisors may coach, direct and teach informally or may use tools to frame their observations and feedback (Table 4.1). In this context, experiences that are not included in the formal curriculum play an important role in learning. 'Informal learning' is described in the literature as unintended, opportunistic and unconstructed since it occurs in surroundings of an unstructured curriculum (Eraut, 2004). Role-modelling is an important educational strategy that occurs at every level of education (Stern-szus et al., 2015) but is particularly important in PGME. In work-based learning it acts as an important method to acquire professional identity as well as to develop knowledge and skills.

As the trainee progresses along the educational path, learning and care activities evolve to approximate the tasks of a practising doctor, with an increasing level of autonomy provided to trainees. In this process, the trainee is included in a community of practice and moves from the periphery of their medical community

Table 4.1 Teaching and learning methods in postgraduate education*

Work-based learning methods	Strategies outside the workplace
Reflection, guided reflection	Lectures and seminars, including flipped classroom formats (see Chapter 7)
Role-modelling	Journal club and critical appraisal sessions
Mentoring	Small group discussions
Bedside teaching and learning: Strategies include 'The one-minute teacher' (Neher & Stevens, 2003), SNAPPS (Wolpaw et al., 2003), observation with feedback; ward rounds	Use of case scenarios, vignettes
Formal frameworks for observation that can provide a basis for feedback, e.g. Mini-CEX (Norcini et al., 2003), P-MEX (Cruess et al., 2006)	Online learning
Interprofessional interactions	Simulation
Portfolios and logbooks	Workshops, academic half-days
Case presentations	University courses
Morbidity and mortality rounds	Conferences, congresses

*For more details see the chapters in Section 2 Learning Situations, Section 3 Education Strategies and Technologies, and Glover-Takahashi et al., 2015.

towards the centre by developing competence and professional identity (Lave & Wenger, 1991).

As well as work-based learning, resident education may occur in non-clinical settings through problem-based learning activities, workshops, lectures, journal clubs, case-based discussions and in simulation contexts (Table 4.1). In many programmes, there is an attempt to balance clinically based education and patient care with protected study time and formal education activities. There are great differences around the world – some programmes have fixed times for formal learning during the week or month, others collect credit points during a residency programme, and still others have no mandatory formal teaching or study time. According to the WFME (World Federation of Medical Education) Postgraduate Medical Education Global Standards as well as clinical work, the programme provider(s) must include relevant theory of basic biomedical, clinical, behavioural and social sciences; clinical decision making; communication skills; medical ethics; public health; medical jurisprudence; managerial disciplines and as

> **Box 4.3 Examples of strategies for assessment in the workplace (see Chapter 35)**
>
> - Direct observation of resident performance
> - Tools to structure observation and feedback of clinical performance (OScore, MiniCEX, etc.)
> - Review of work products (clinical documents that form part of the medical record)
> - Multi-source feedback (360-degree assessments)
> - Learning portfolios (e.g. records of performance achievements)
> - Logbooks (e.g. records of activities or procedures)
> - Encounter cards (e.g. daily shift assessment card)

> **Box 4.4 Markers of PGME quality found in various systems**
>
> - Programme mission and goals
> - Complete sets of competencies to be achieved
> - Programme blueprint mapping learning goals, instructional methods and assessment by activity
> - Positive learning environment
> - Effectiveness of teaching
> - Learner scores on standardized testing
> - Numbers of resident and faculty research publications
> - Adequacy of resources for the programme (e.g. financing, personnel, infrastructure, dedicated time, patients)
> - Resident wellbeing
> - Graduate competence or performance
> - Quality of patient care

well must organize the educational programme with appropriate attention to patient safety (WFME, 2015).

As part of work-based learning, residents undergo ongoing assessment, both formative and summative. The common assessment strategies are listed in Box 4.3. Formative assessment or feedback is critical to the development of knowledge, skills and expertise in all competencies (see Chapter 37). Residents are assessed through direct observation of their interactions with patients, but also on the quality of their case presentations, written work and clinical outcomes (see Chapter 35). They may be assessed by their clinical supervisors, more senior residents, other health professionals, their students and patients.

External assessment in PGME: summative, certification

In most PGME systems around the world, there are a number of formal, summative, external assessments that serve as gateways to further career stages. As opposed to the formative feedback or summative decisions within the programme, these often involve a third-party institution or process to assess competence at a key stage of training. The most common of these processes are licensing and certification examinations at the end of training. These tend to focus heavily on knowledge and are usually designed as written tests, with or without a component of a structured oral exam. Their purpose is to provide an independent summative decision on competence to proceed to the next career stage (e.g. certification in a discipline before independent practice) or to obtain a licence in a jurisdiction. Occasionally, they are also used for programme evaluation purposes, comparing learner performance between training institutions or sites. Nevertheless, when

well-designed, these exams are predictive of future performance. (Wenghofer et al., 2009)

PGME quality, accreditation and CQI

What does it mean to have 'quality' PGME? This varies with perspective, and most likely has changed over the history of medical education. Quality PGME has at times involved such markers as the number of trainees in a programme, the academic performance of incoming or outgoing residents, the research published by participants in a programme, the awards won by residents or teachers, the type of and stature of jobs that graduates obtain or the examination scores of trainees. These perspectives have evolved to provide a greater focus on 'good educational practices' and programme outcomes in the form of graduate performance. Some of these markers of PGME quality are in Box 4.4.

Good education practice would also involve the continuous quality improvement (CQI) of PGME itself. The enterprise related to external programme evaluation of PGME institutions is called accreditation in most jurisdictions. Accreditation typically involves some kind of third-party oversight or evaluation of the local resident education process, environment or outcomes. Often, but not always, this involves designated reviewers (aka surveyors) visiting the programme and interviewing participants to create a report on local training as compared to pre-established standards. Accreditation can have both a formative and summative role in PGME systems, enhancing CQI and making decisions on the future viability of training programmes.

Controversies in PGME

There are a number of controversial issues in PGME – we highlight a selected few in detail here and others are listed in Table 4.2.

THE DEBATE ABOUT GENERALISM VERSUS SPECIALISM IN PGME

A debate in many countries is whether postgraduate training should be focused on producing generalists or specialists. This debate probably goes back many decades. In 2013 in the United Kingdom Shape of Training, an independent review of the postgraduate medical training, concluded that patients and the public need more doctors who are capable of providing general care in broad specialties across a range of different settings. This is being driven by a growing number of patients with multiple co-morbidities, an ageing

population, health inequities and increasing patient expectations (Shape of Training, 2013). On the other hand, specialization continues internationally to address demands for ever-greater ability in greater depth in ever-expanding fields of medical practice. The Union Européenne des médecins spécialistes has now more than 50 medical specialties (UEMS) and the Association of American Medical Colleges has more than 120 medical specialties and sub-specialties (AAMC). This debate will continue around the world in the twenty-first century, as every country likely needs an appropriate mix of relevant medical expertise to meet the needs of the population effectively.

THE CHALLENGE OF RESIDENT DUTY HOURS

Those involved in postgraduate medical education have long struggled with the competing priorities that surround the issue of residents' work hours: providing each trainee with an adequate amount of clinical, teaching and leadership experience; protecting time for formal teaching and self-study; preserving continuity of patient care and ensuring patient safety; and avoiding excessive fatigue (Weinstein, 2002). As physicians, trainees are part of the workforce and often answer for a large part of the workload after the regular workday. This can become problematic when residents are only providing service, are rarely observed or taught, and have wellness issues related to overwork, stress and sleep deprivation. One of the biggest drivers for re-examining the balance of education and patient care is the effort to reduce duty hours to match what society considers reasonable working hours in other domains (outside of medicine) and to improve patient safety (Imrie et al., 2014). At the same time, there is inconclusive evidence that shortening duty hours has an effect, either positively or negatively, on patient safety, little evidence for an impact on resident education (more time to study versus less patient exposure) and ongoing concerns that the work still needs to be done so substitutes must be found. Regulation of resident duty hours varies worldwide. In the United States, the numbers are still around 80 hours per week with work shifts up to 24 hours. The EU's Working Time Directive affects all workers (including physicians), and limits the working time to 48 hours per week and also limits the length of on-call shifts, although opt-out options have been used.

Table 4.2 Controversies in PGME

Controversy	Challenges
Flexibility in structure	Should all trainees have the same programme and curriculum, or should education be individualized to address learner needs or local context?
Length of training	Is there an 'ideal' duration for postgraduate education? PGME varies from 2 to 10 or more years by discipline and jurisdiction.
Patient safety and quality	What are the patient safety disadvantages of having residents learn by practicing on patients? When should residents be considered safe for autonomous practice within residency? When can residents be supervised 'indirectly'? How can the highest quality of care be maintained when trainees are involved in care?
Curriculum content	Should the formal curriculum focus exclusively on core medical knowledge and expertise, or have a more elaborate and explicit focus (e.g. CanMEDS, roles in Glover-Takahashi et al., 2015 and ACGME competencies)?
Role of research in PGME	Should research training or scholarly work be a mandatory component of PGME?
Education versus service	What is the 'right' balance of patient care versus learning? When is patient care 'not learning'?

"Embarking on a process to improve medical training and align it more closely with the requirements of medical care delivery in the coming years … will require substantial redesign of training programs, not just reduction in working hours."

Drazen & Epstein, 2002

TRAINING CLINICAL SUPERVISORS: FACULTY DEVELOPMENT

Most clinical supervisors are practising physicians who have trained in clinical medicine but do not necessarily have any training in teaching, assessment or supervisory skills. Staff development programmes have addressed many of the needed skills, but, until recently, attending these programmes has not been mandatory and demonstrating mastery and using these skills has not been recognized or rewarded. Over the past decade there has been an increased professionalization of the field, with mandatory teaching skills training and certification or accreditation of clinical supervisors in some constituencies. Faculty development is discussed in more detail in Chapter 40.

The future of PGME

Postgraduate medical education is not a static entity. It is buffeted by the winds of globalization, which appears to manifest as ever-greater international mobility of physicians in training and ever-shrinking number of standards-setting bodies. New designs (such as competency-based medical education), new frameworks of competencies (such as CanMEDS; Frank, Snell & Sherbino, 2015), new selection techniques (such as the MMI), new teaching methods and formats (such as simulation), new assessment strategies (such as the O-Score), all reflect the ongoing innovations of those active in PGME.

Summary

PGME is essential to produce the practising doctors needed by all societies. During residency, trainee physicians experience the majority of their learning and assessment in the workplace – the clinical context. PGME is thus a critical phase of medical training where young doctors develop into mature independent practitioners capable of competently and safely caring for patients. Of all the advances in medical education over the last 100 years, PGME is perhaps the greatest gift of the profession to the world.

References

AAMC: Association of American Medical Colleges. List of AAMC medical specialties and sub-specialties. Available at: www.aamc.org, https://students-residents.aamc.org/attending-medical-school/article/choosing-specialty/. (Accessed 2016).

Ambardekar, A.P., Singh, D., Lockman, J.L., et al., 2016. Pediatric anesthesiology fellow education: is a simulation-based boot camp feasible and valuable? Paediatr. Anaesth. doi:10.1111/pan.12865; [Epub ahead of print].

Cruess, R., McIlroy, J., Cruess, S., et al., 2006. The professionalism mini-evaluation exercise: a preliminary investigation. Acad. Med. 81 (10), S74–S78.

Drazen, J., Epstein, A., 2002. Rethinking medical training — the critical work ahead. N. Engl. J. Med. 347 (16), 1271–1272.

Eraut, M., 2004. Informal learning in the workplace. Stud. Contin. Educ. 26 (2), 247–283.

Frank, J.R., Snell, L., Sherbino, J., 2015. CanMEDS 2015 Competency Framework. Royal College of Physicians and Surgeons of Canada, Ottawa.

Frank, J., Snell, L., Ten Cate, O., et al., 2010. Competency-based medical education: theory to practice. Med. Teach. 32 (8), 638–645.

Glover-Takahashi, S., Abbott, C., Oswald, A., Frank, J., 2015. CanMEDS teaching and assessment tools guide. Royal College of Physicians and Surgeons of Canada, Ottawa.

Hofmeister, M., Lockyer, J., Crutcher, R., 2008. The acceptability of the multiple mini interview for resident selection. Fam. Med. 40 (10), 734–740.

Imrie, K., Dath, D., Bullock, G., et al., 2014. The Resident's dual role as learner and service provider. In: Frank, J.R., Harris, K.A. (Eds.), Competence by design: reshaping Canadian medical education. Royal College of Physicians and Surgeons of Canada, Ottawa, pp. 45–57.

Lave, J., Wenger, E., 1991. Situated learning. Legitimate peripheral participation. Cambridge Univ Press, Cambridge.

Ludmerer, K.M., 2015. Let me heal: the opportunity to preserve excellence in American medicine. Oxford University Press, Oxford, p. 2.

Neher, J., Stevens, N., 2003. The one-minute preceptor: shaping the teaching conversation. Fam. Med. 35 (6), 391–393.

Norcini, J., Blank, L., Duffy, D., Fortna, G., 2003. The mini-CEX: a method for assessing clinical skills. Ann. Intern. Med. 138 (6), 476–481.

Pantaleoni, J.L., Augustine, E.M., Sourkes, B.M., Bachrach, L.K., 2014. Burnout in pediatric residents over a 2-year period: a longitudinal study. Acad. Pediatr. 14 (2), 167–172.

Patterson, F., Knight, A., Dowell, J., et al., 2015. How effective are selection methods in medical education? Med. Educ. 50, 36–60.

RCPSC, 2014. A glossary of medical education terms. Royal College of Physicians and Surgeons of Canada, Ottawa.

Shape of Training, October 2013. Available at: www.shapeoftraining.co.uk. (Accessed 2016).

Snell, L., 2011. The resident as teacher: it's more than just about student learning. J. Grad. Med. Educ. 3 (3), 440–442.

Steinert, Y. Faculty development for postgraduate education – the road Ahead. In: Members of the FMEC PG consortium (Eds.), Future of medical Education in Canada, 2011, p. 3. Available at: https://www.afmc.ca/pdf/fmec/21_Steinert_ Faculty%20Development.pdf. (Accessed 2016).

Sternszus, R., Macdonald, M.E., Steinert, Y., 2015. Resident role modeling: "it just happens". Acad. Med. 91 (3), 427–432.

Swing, S., 2007. The ACGME outcome project: retrospective and prospective. Med. Teach. 29 (7), 648–654.

UEMS: Union Européenne Des Médecins Spécialistes. List of UEMS medical specialties. Available at: www.uems.eu. (Accessed 2016).

Weinstein, D., 2002. Duty hours for resident physicians — tough choices for teaching hospitals. N. Engl. J. Med. 347 (16), 1275–1278.

Wenghofer, E., Klass, D., Abrahamowicz, M., et al., 2009. Doctor's scores on national qualifying examinations predict quality of care in future practice. Med. Educ. 43 (12), 1166–1173.

WFME: World Federation for Medical Education. Postgraduate medical education WFME global standards for quality improvement, the 2015 revision. Available at: http://wfme.org/standards/ pgme/97-final-2015-revision-of-postgraduate-me dical-education-standards/file. (Accessed 26 January 2017).

Wolpaw, T., Wolpaw, D., Papp, K., 2003. SNAPPS: a learner-centered model for outpatient education. Acad. Med. 78 (9), 893–898.

Chapter

5 Continuing professional development

D. Moore

Trends

- Continuing medical education (CME) is increasingly being referred to as continuing professional development (CPD).
- Continuing professional development (CPD) focuses on improving competence and performance to help clinicians provide the best possible care to their patients.
- Opportunities for deliberate practice and expert feedback in learning activities will be a critical part of continuing professional development.

Background

Continuing professional development (CPD) is the means by which clinicians maintain their knowledge and skills related to their professional lives. Currently, CPD is used interchangeably with the term continuing medical education (CME), which obscures the more comprehensive nature of CPD. For years, CME has referred to the formal educational activities that clinicians have attended to keep up to date. The scope of CPD is more comprehensive. It includes not only formal educational activities like CME courses but informal and incidental learning activities as well. Informal learning activities are usually controlled and planned by the learners. A hospital 'huddle' is one example. Incidental learning occurs as the by-product of some other activity and most of the time clinicians do not realize that they have learned something new. More importantly, however, CPD calls for clinicians to engage in a process of monitoring and reflecting on professional performance, identifying opportunities to improve professional practice gaps, engaging in both formal and informal learning activities, and making changes in practice to reduce or eliminate gaps in performance (Campbell et al., 2010).

It is important for course directors and course faculty to understand how clinicians engage in their individual CPD efforts so they would be better able to plan formal CME courses to respond to clinician learning needs. Important findings reported in recent research describing characteristics of effective learning activities can help CME course directors accomplish this. To illustrate how these findings can be applied to learning activities in CPD, this chapter will examine how a fictitious physician learner, Dr Ima Lerner, pursues her CPD.

 "Now that information is ubiquitous, simple information exchange has relatively low value; in its place, shared wisdom and the opportunity to engage in problem-solving in practice-relevant ways have become key."

McMahon, 2016

 Course directors and course faculty should approach their CME course not as an opportunity to provide information about a clinical topic but rather as an opportunity to help clinician participants learn how to use that information in their practices.

How clinicians learn

Dr Lerner is a generalist physician in the community. She has been in practice for about 10 years in a medium-size multi-specialty group. It will be useful to describe how Dr Lerner organizes her CPD efforts in five stages: recognizing an opportunity for improvement; selecting learning as a strategy; engaging in learning; trying out what was learned; and integrating what was learned into practice (Moore 2008; Moore et al., 2009).

RECOGNIZING AN OPPORTUNITY FOR IMPROVEMENT

While in general Dr Lerner feels that she is providing the best possible care to all of her patients, on occasion she might sense that there may be something 'not right' with the outcomes of one group of her patients, those with type 2 diabetes for example. After some reflection, she may begin to feel that there is something different that she should be doing but is not exactly sure what that something should be (Schon, 1983). This emerging realization that there is a difference between what she is doing and what she could be doing makes her uncomfortable, a feeling that is called cognitive dissonance. Like many other clinicians, Dr Lerner wants to do something to address the unpleasant feeling that she may not be doing what is best for her patients. After conversations with several colleagues, she decides to spend some time investigating if there are new approaches to managing patients with type 2 diabetes.

 "The ability to reflect on one's practice (performance) is critical to lifelong self-directed learning."

Kaufman & Mann, 2014

 "The point at which a clinician takes ownership of his or her own learning agenda is a pivotal moment in professional growth. What do I need to learn today?

McMahon, 2016

SEARCHING FOR RESOURCES FOR LEARNING

To investigate approaches to managing patients with type 2 diabetes, she starts a literature search using PubMed. She searches on "type 2 diabetes management" and retrieves more than 16,000 references. Pursuing another option, "comprehensive type 2 diabetes management," she retrieves about 550 references. Realizing that she doesn't have time to sort through all these references and then read the articles she finds, she decides to investigate one of the evidence-based decision support websites. There she discovers several pages of information synthesized from research studies about approaches to managing patients with type 2 diabetes.

She is overwhelmed with the volume of information she has uncovered and decides to talk with one of her more senior colleagues, an endocrinologist, for guidance about her type 2 diabetes patients. He suggests a couple of patient management strategies for her to consider and recommends three articles that have recently been published that he thinks will find their way into the next revision of the diabetes clinical practice guidelines. In addition, he mentioned that as part of a nationwide effort to improve the care of type 2 diabetes, a day-long course on type 2 diabetes sponsored by the national diabetes association would be offered in several locations, including at one of the local hospitals. It would be announced shortly and he suggests that she should consider attending.

Dr Lerner has decided that, in addition to clinical information about managing her patients with type 2 diabetes, she also needs information about shared decision making, and how it might help her understand

why her patients with type 2 diabetes are not progressing as she expects. She feels a sense of relief when she sees that the upcoming diabetes course would cover managing patients with type 2 diabetes *and* shared decision making. The course would be offered in three months. Weighing benefits and costs as well as family and other responsibilities that she has the day that the course is scheduled, she decides that the benefits outweighed the costs and she enrols.

ENGAGING IN LEARNING

Clinicians like Dr Lerner learn informally as well as in formal settings. She has decided, in this case, to participate in a formal course, but she will also engage in a variety of informal learning activities before and after the formal course. She might read some of the articles that were identified in her PubMed search or were summarized on the decision support web page. She might continue her conversations with the endocrinologist and other colleagues. She will continue to attend grand rounds and other regularly scheduled conferences. But she thinks that spending a full day at a course focused on diabetes management will help her address her uneasiness about her type 2 diabetes patients.

Course directors and course faculty become involved in CME activities because they realize that there are new developments in their areas of expertise or they have become aware that patient care that is delivered in their areas of expertise is not as optimal as it could be. Until recently, the goal of course directors and course faculty has been primarily to provide information to help clinicians keep up to date. Information in these updates typically consisted of summaries of a presenter's research, which may or may not have been related to the practice needs of the clinician learners in the audience. It was generally assumed that clinician learners would return to their practices and use this information in caring for their patients. Reports about patients not receiving the best possible care suggest, however, that the expected transfer of this new information was not occurring (Institute of Medicine, 2008).

Now the emphasis in CPD is increasingly on what clinician learners can do with newly learned information in their practices. In part because of concerns about ineffectiveness of the 'update' approach and in part because of changing requirements of accreditation in CPD, the new focus is more and more on developing evidence-based competencies in learners and helping them to use the new competencies in practice to improve the health status of patients (Regnier et al., 2005; Institute of Medicine, 2010).

At the same time, there have been significant discoveries in the learning sciences as well as research in CPD that suggests that learning activities can improve clinician performance and the health of patients if the activities have certain characteristics (Cervero & Gaines, 2015; Davis & Galbraith, 2009; Mayer, 2010;

Bransford et al., 2000; Knox, 2016). Application of these findings in learning activities that clinicians use as part of their continuing professional development will make it more likely that what is learned will be transferred into practice and contribute to the improvement of patient care. Descriptions of these findings follow.

> *"CME activities that are more interactive, use more methods, involve multiple exposures, are longer, and are focused on outcomes that are considered important by physicians lead to more positive outcomes."*
>
> *Cervero & Gaines, 2015*

CONSIDERING PRIOR KNOWLEDGE AND EXPERIENCE OF CLINICIAN PARTICIPANTS

Like most learners, clinician learners enter a learning activity with knowledge, beliefs, attitudes, and ways of doing things that they gained through professional practice, formal courses and informal learning. For a learning activity to be effective, it must build on this prior knowledge and experience and address the gaps between what participants know and do and what they should know and should be doing. Knowing something about the prior knowledge and experience of clinician participants in managing patients with type 2 diabetes, for example, would help course planners begin to understand the difference between what clinician participants know and can do with what they should know and be able to do. In other words, they can begin to understand the professional practice gaps of the clinician participants in managing patients with type 2 diabetes. Many clinician participants enrol in a CME activity with only a vague notion of what their professional practice gaps are. Part of the new role for course directors and course faculty is to help clinician participants recognize more fully what their gaps are.

 Course directors and course faculty should recognize that clinician participants in their formal learning activities may be in the early stages of a CPD process, and they should assist these clinicians in their efforts to articulate their practice-based learning needs.

Many efforts to plan courses for clinicians have used 'needs assessment' surveys asking potential participants about their prior knowledge and expertise. The results of surveys have been too general to help course organizers identify specific content to include in a learning activity. Course organizers were forced to select course content without a genuine understanding of the practice-based learning needs of the potential participants. Self-report surveys do not produce useful data for planning, in part because it is becoming increasingly clear that it is difficult for clinicians (or anyone) to

accurately assess their own performance (Davis et al., 2006).

An alternative to surveys could be to ask clinician participants to work in small groups on authentic case scenarios at the beginning of a learning activity. The scenarios could be designed to challenge them to propose strategies for evaluating and managing simulated patients with type 2 diabetes. A scenario is a patient case with a main storyline designed to bring out a specific learning outcome for a learner. It is a sequence of learning activities that involve complex decision making, problem-solving strategies, intelligent reasoning and critical thinking. A limited amount of information is communicated to learners who must engage in an inquiry learning process to address the issue at the centre of the case (Alinier, 2011). Initially, scenarios can be used to determine the prior knowledge and experience of clinician participants. The results of their work in scenarios could be compared to clinical practice guidelines and/or recent clinical research. This strategy has the potential for identifying professional practice gaps that would create teachable moments for clinician participants predisposing them to learn how to improve their performance. Scenarios could also be sent to clinicians before they arrive at a CME course with a similar effect.

> *"Learning is enhanced when it is relevant, particularly to the solution and understanding of real-life problems and practice."*
>
> *Kaufman & Mann, 2014*

This approach to CPD requires the course director and course faculty to follow a different approach to prepare for the course than it would for a course that was a series of lectures. The type 2 diabetes course would be scenario-based, so a large number of scenarios will be required to reflect the variety of presentations and manifestations of type 2 diabetes. In addition, a certain amount of flexibility has to be built into the scenarios so they can adapt dynamically to the actions or requests of the clinician learners (Alinier, 2011).

FOCUSING ON OUTCOMES IMPORTANT TO CLINICIAN PARTICIPANTS

Recent research suggests that successful learning activities in CPD, those that result in improved clinician performance and enhanced patient health status, focus on outcomes that are considered important to clinician participants (Cervero & Gaines, 2015). The goals of most clinicians for participating in a learning activity are to acquire the knowledge and develop the skills that they feel they need to provide the very best possible care to their patients. For the type 2 diabetes course, these are the outcomes that clinician participants consider important: clinical performance and patient health status. Aligning a course with these clinician learner goals will generate motivation that will initiate and sustain the learning that a clinician pursues. Course directors and course faculty should select topics and content that focus on these outcomes.

It would be ideal if data from the practices of each of the clinician participants were available that would help course directors understand the professional practice gaps of clinician participants as well as help them determine course content. While an increasing number of practices and hospitals are providing physicians with dashboards that summarize their performance in selected key areas (Dowding et al., 2015), these data are not universally available at the present time. Scenarios that are developed to learn about the clinician participants' prior knowledge and experience can help the course director and course faculty understand what the important outcomes are and provide a framework for asking clinician participants about their expectations for the course.

RESPOND POSITIVELY TO THE EXPECTATIONS OF CLINICIAN PARTICIPANTS

Clinicians enrolled in a day-long diabetes course because they expect to acquire the knowledge and develop the skills that they feel they need to provide the very best possible care to their patients. Because the scenario exercises have highlighted gaps in performance that created emerging teachable moments, the course director and course faculty should engage in a discussion with the clinician learners to build on the teachable moments and elicit specific information about what they want to learn. Interactive agenda building is a useful technique to address expectations of the clinician learners and produces an agreement about how the learning activity will meet those expectations (Knox, 2016).

 "There is a good deal of evidence that learning is enhanced when teachers pay attention to the knowledge and beliefs that learners bring to a learning task, use this knowledge as a starting point for new instruction, and monitor students' changing conceptions as instruction proceeds."

Bransford et al., 2000

 Course directors and course faculty should plan their learning activities so they can be adapted to the practice-based learning needs that might emerge during the learning activity.

INTERACTIVITY WITH MULTIPLE METHODS AND MULTIPLE EXPOSURES

Up to this point, the course director and course faculty have been concerned with engaging clinician-participants in activities that will predispose them to learning what they need to know and do to provide the very best possible care to their patients. Next they should be involved in engaging clinician-participants in activities

that enable them to provide the best possible care to their patients. Recent research suggests that interactivity with multiple methods and multiple exposures is associated with effective learning activities in CPD (Cervero & Gaines, 2015; Knox, 2016). Furthermore, recent functional brain imaging studies have suggested that interactive learning tasks carried out in the context of an authentic, problem-based scenario will result in deeper elaborative cognitive processing leading to greater conceptual understanding of the material involved (Dalgarno et al., 2009).

Interactivity and multiple methods in learning activities means providing clinician learners with multiple opportunities to engage with the content and its application in practice with other learners and course faculty. One approach uses a combination of techniques: presentation, example, practise, feedback (Moore et al., 2009), but a rearrangement of the order of these techniques, starting with 'practise' might be more appropriate for inquiry-based learning required for scenario learning.

Practise is generally understood to mean performing an activity or skill repeatedly in order to improve or maintain one's proficiency. The activity or skill could be described in a scenario and scenarios could start each of a series of learning activities to address multiple aspects (exposures) of managing patients with type 2 diabetes. In their assessment of the performance of learners (feedback) in each scenario, course faculty could use chalk-talks (presentation) and case descriptions (examples of best practice) to help learners understand what they did correctly, what was done partially correct and what needs to be added, what was not correct and what was left out.

Course faculty are encouraged to consider scaffolding in designing learning activities for clinician-learners (Reiser & Tabak, 2014). Scaffolding is a process that enables an individual to solve a problem, carry out a task or achieve a goal that would be beyond his or her unassisted efforts. It involves providing assistance to learners on an as-needed basis and fading the assistance as their competence increases. Scaffolding is a metaphor for a structure that is put in place to help learners reach their goals and is removed bit by bit as it is no longer needed, much like a physical scaffold is placed around a building that is under construction and removed as the building nears completion.

 Course directors and course faculty should organize practise and feedback sessions starting with easier scenarios and gradually increasing complexity and decreasing information available for decision making.

To develop mastery in managing patients with type 2 diabetes, clinician learners must acquire component skills, practice integrating them under multiple circumstances, and know when to apply what they have learned. Ultimately the goal of these learning activities is to be able to use what is learned in an educational setting in clinical practice (transfer). Deep conceptual knowledge enables transfer. Deep conceptual knowledge is the combination of declarative knowledge (knowing what to do) and procedural knowledge (knowing how to do it) with conditional knowledge (knowing when to do it and why to do it). Providing clinicians with opportunities to practise using declarative knowledge and procedural in varying settings in a learning activity enables them to develop the conditional knowledge they need for transfer.

LONGER SESSIONS

The multiple educational methods and exposures necessary to develop mastery require longer sessions than are traditionally allocated to sessions in formal CME activities (Cervero & Gaines, 2015). Providing clinician learners with multiple exposures offers an opportunity to practise a developing competence under a variety of circumstances, which contributes to an increasing capability to transfer the competence into practice. Scenarios should be used for this purpose.

Deliberate practice and expert feedback are also important. There are four components to deliberate practice. First, the learner must be motivated to attend to the task to be learned and exert effort to improve performance. Second, the design of the task should take into account the learner's pre-existing knowledge so that the task can be correctly understood after a brief period of instruction. Third, the learner should receive immediate informative feedback and knowledge of results of performance. Fourth, the learner should repeatedly perform the same or similar tasks. Helping clinician learners recognize current competencies and visualize what they need to do to reach desired competencies is the goal of deliberate practice and expert feedback (Ericsson, 2004).

 Course directors and course faculty should reduce the number of topics to be covered in their CME courses and expand the amount of time on one or two topics so learners can experience multiple exposures to the content and have opportunities to practise and receive feedback on their performance.

This will make it more likely that clinicians will use what they are learning in their practices.

SUPPORTIVE LEARNING ENVIRONMENT

For learning activities in CPD to be effective, there must be a supportive learning environment. A supportive learning environment is learner-centred, knowledge-centred, assessment centred, and community-centred (Bransford et al., 2000). A supportive learning environment in CPD is *learner-centred* when the learner is allowed to bring what he or she knows to a learning activity and use it to make connections with what he or she wants to learn. The inquiry nature of the scenario-based approach to learning requires clinician learners like Dr Lerner to draw on what they know, and discussion with other participants in *community-centred* learning environment helps clinician learners articulate what they know and compare what they know to others to identify gaps and fill them through discussion. A *knowledge-centred* learning environment makes resources that a learner needs to learn accessible in appropriate contexts. For example, Dr Lerner might access knowledge online, in materials available in the environment, and from other participants in the community-centred environment who have had relevant experiences. In a supportive learning environment, the purpose of *assessment* is formative, to help learners progress. For example, during discussion Dr Lerner may offer a suggestion for managing a patient with type 2 diabetes that incorrectly applies a strategy from a practice guideline that she accessed online. Feedback from a faculty member or another member of the group could point out the error and help her correct her understanding and strengthen her knowledge. In other cases, feedback could reinforce knowledge that is correct. In a *community-centred* learning environment, learners feel safe to take chances with new learnings and to give and take positive critiques. Groups work will be an important part of learning activities in CPD, and the creation of a supportive learning environment will be important to its success. The willingness of a clinician learner to be engaged in a learning activity is directly related to the supportive emotional, social and intellectual climate that is created in the course.

TRYING OUT WHAT WAS LEARNED

The next stage begins in the course with Dr Lerner feeling less than comfortable with the new knowledge and skills that she has been learning. Dr Lerner begins trying out what she is learning in the course and will continue trying out what she has learned when she returns to her practice. As she progresses through the stage working through scenarios she becomes more skilful and confident. The scenario exercises in the course are an important start for her to try out what she is learning. She is able to experiment, receive feedback from course faculty, and make changes to improve her performance. As she participates in more scenarios, she becomes more confident and comfortable using her newly learned skills and knowledge. The stage is over when she is sufficiently comfortable with her newly learned skills and knowledge and they become second nature.

INCORPORATING WHAT WAS LEARNED

During this final stage, Dr Lerner will integrate what she has learned into her daily routines and it will become a part of what she does during clinical encounters. She will 'reflect on practice' after several 'experiments' (Schon, 1983), and, if the new learning appears to be effective, will move on to incorporating the new knowledge and skills into practice, successfully transferring what was learned into the workplace.

Questions that emerge in this stage for Dr Lerner might include but are not limited to the following: What do I have to do differently in my practice to use what I have learned? How do I make what I have learned a part of my practice? What office routines have to be changed? What new procedures have to be introduced? What training does staff need? What do I have to do for my patients?

If she has not done so already in the previous stage, during this stage, Dr Lerner will have to make sure that office routines and procedures include not only what she has learned but also what she will need to do to implement what she has learned. Most important, she will need to train her staff in what she has learned.

While the cognitive imprint that was created while practising developing skills in scenarios will initially be relatively strong, enabling her to retrieve and apply what she has learned when managing her type 2 diabetes patients, its strength could possibly fade with time and in the context of multiple patients with other complaints. There are several ways that course directors and course faculty could help. Reminders have been suggested to reinforce the strength of the signal from the cognitive imprint. A combination of chart reminders and monthly e-mailed scenarios may be most effective. In some cases, communities of practice have been established that reinforce patient management strategies as well as encourage continuous reflection on their effectiveness (Parboosingh, 2002).

Assessment and evaluation

There are at least three stakeholders who would be interested in knowing if the clinicians who attended the day-long course on type 2 diabetes changed their performance in a way that contributed to improved health status of their patients with type 2 diabetes. They would also like to know if participation in the course was a factor in their behaviour change. The three stakeholders are the leaders of the national diabetes association who supported the course, leadership of medical groups like the one that Dr Lerner belonged to, and the course directors and course faculty.

However, getting data about the effectiveness of the course will be a challenge. Two recent systematic reviews suggested that the evidence for CME effectiveness is limited by weaknesses in the reported validity and reliability of evaluation methods. In a recent study, it was reported that evaluations of CME effects beyond clinician satisfaction were not common (Tian et al., 2007).

Randomized controlled trials (RCT) are considered to be a gold standard in research. But the requirements for rigor in an RCT may be beyond the capabilities of most organizations that want to assess physician learning and impact of their learning (Sullivan, 2011). A quasi-experimental approach might be more feasible. One example of a quasi-experimental design is a one-group pre-post design. While it is a relatively weak design for research, it is an approach that might be the most feasible for evaluating CPD (Shadish et al., 2002). It compares the outcome data of the clinician learners to their baseline data. Occasionally in CPD learning activities, data collection at the second data collection point and beyond is accomplished by a commitment-to-change exercise (Shershneva et al., 2010). In a commitment-to-change exercise, participants in a learning activity are asked to indicate changes they propose to make as a result of what they learned. Requests for data describing the changes that they were able to make are sent to learners periodically. In this way, formative assessment is extended beyond the learning activity.

Summary

This chapter has traced the learning activities of Dr Ima Lerner through five stages of her continuing professional development, demonstrating the interaction between her as a learner and the course director and course faculty. The implications of the changes that are suggested by the findings of recent research in the learning sciences and CPD are profound. Combined with the other changes that are occurring throughout healthcare, the challenges seem almost too daunting to be undertaken. Individuals with responsibilities for helping clinicians with their continuing professional development should take time to reflect and recognize the importance of collaboration. If everything is changing, let's do it together (Shershneva et al., 2008). Something like the Triple Aim of the Institute for Healthcare Improvement (improving the patient experience of care [including quality and satisfaction]; improving the health of populations; and reducing the per capita cost of healthcare) could serve as the organizing principle for a collaborative effort.

References

Alinier, G., 2011. Developing high-fidelity healthcare simulation scenarios: a guide for educators and professionals. Simul. Gaming 42 (1), 9–26.

Bransford, J.D., Brown, A.L., Cocking, R.R., 2000. How people learn: Brain, mind, experience, and school. National Academy Press, Washington DC.

Campbell, C., Silver, I., Sherbino, J., et al., 2010. Competency-based continuing professional development. Med. Teach. 32 (8), 657–662.

Cervero, R.M., Gaines, J.K., 2015. The impact of CME on physician performance and patient health outcomes: an updated synthesis of systematic reviews. J. Contin. Educ. Health Prof. 35 (2), 131–138.

Dalgarno, B., Kennedy, G., Bennett, S., Using brain imaging to explore interactivity and cognition in multiledia learning environments, Paper presented at: 21st Annual Conference of the Australian Computer-Human Interaction Special Interest group (CHISIG) of the Human Factors and Ergonomics Society of Australia, New York, NY 2009, Human Factors and Ergonomics Society of Australia, pp. 405–409.

Davis, D., Galbraith, R., 2009. Continuing medical education effect on practice performance: effectiveness of continuing medical education: American College of chest physicians evidence-based educational guidelines. Chest 135 (3 Suppl.), 42S–48S.

Davis, D.A., Mazmanian, P.E., Fordis, M., et al., 2006. Accuracy of physician self-assessment compared with observed measures of competence: a systematic review. JAMA 296 (9), 1094–1102.

Dowding, D., Randell, R., Gardner, P., et al., 2015. Dashboards for improving patient care: review of the literature. Int. J. Med. Inform. 84 (2), 87–100.

Ericsson, K.A., 2004. Deliberate practice and the acquisition and maintenance of expert performance in medicine and related domains. Acad. Med. 79 (10 Suppl.), S70–S81.

Institute of Medicine (IOM), 2008. Knowing what works in health care: A roadmap for the nation. National Academies Press, Washington, DC.

Institute of Medicine (IOM), 2010. Redesigning Continuing Education in the Health Professions. The National Academies Press, Washington DC.

Kaufman, D.M., Mann, K.V., 2014. Teaching and learning in medical education: How theory can inform practice. In: Swanwick, T. (Ed.), Understanding Medical Education: Evidence, Theory, and Practice. Malden, Wiley Blackwell, Massachusetts, pp. 7–29.

Knox, A.B., 2016. Improving Professional Learning: Twelve Strategies to Enhance Performance. Stylus Publishing, Sterling, Virginia.

Mayer, R.E., 2010. Applying the science of learning to medical education. Med. Educ. 44, 543–549.

McMahon, G.T., 2016. What do I need to learn today? – The evolution of CME. N. Engl. J. Med. 374 (15), 1403–1406.

Moore, D.E. Jr., 2008. How physicians learn and how to design learning experiences for them: An approach based on an interpretive review of the evidence. In: Hager, M. (Ed.), Continuing Education in the Health Professions: Improving Healthcare through Lifelong Learning. Josiah Macy Foundation, New York, pp. 30–62.

Moore, D.E. Jr., Green, J.S., Gallis, H.A., 2009. Achieving desired results and improved outcomes by integrating planning and assessment throughout a learning activity. J. Contin. Educ. Health Prof. 29 (1), 5–18.

Parboosingh, J.T., 2002. Physician communities of practice: where learning and practice are inseparable. J. Contin. Educ. Health Prof. 22 (4), 230–236.

Regnier, K., Kopelow, M., Lane, D., Alden, E., 2005. Accreditation for learning and change: quality and improvement as the outcome. J. Contin. Educ. Health Prof. 25 (3), 174–182.

Reiser, B.J., Tabak, I., 2014. Scaffolding. In: Sawyer, R.K. (Ed.), The Cambridge Handbook of the Learning Sciences. Cambridge University Press, New York, NY, pp. 44–62.

Schon, D., 1983. The Reflective Practitioner: How Professionals Think in Action. Basic Books, New York.

Shadish, W.R., Cook, T.D., Campbell, D.T., 2002. Experimental and Quasi-experimental Designs for Generalized Causal Inference. Houghton-Mifflin, Boston, Massachusetts.

Shershneva, M.B., Mullikin, E.A., Loose, A.S., Olson, C.A., 2008. Learning to collaborate: a case study of performance improvement CME. J. Contin. Educ. Health Prof. 28 (3), 140–147.

Shershneva, M.B., Wang, M.F., Lindeman, G.C., et al., 2010. Commitment to practice change: an evaluator's perspective. Eval. Health Prof. 33 (3), 256–275.

Sullivan, G.M., 2011. Getting off the gold standard: randomized controlled trials and educational research. J Grad Med Educ 3 (3), 285–289.

Tian, J., Atkinson, N.L., Portnoy, B., Gold, R.S., 2007. A systematic review of evaluation in formal continuing medical education. J. Contin. Educ. Health Prof. 27 (1), 16–27.

The hidden curriculum

6

F. W. Hafferty, E. H. Gaufberg

Trends

- The hidden curriculum (HC) is an omnipresent part of all medical learning environments.
- It differentiates between what is formally/intentionally taught versus the range of other lessons students informally and tacitly acquire during training
- It can be both positive and negative
- It cannot be eliminated, but it can be managed
- A major source of HC messaging comes via role modelling
- The HC is a major socializing force and thus plays an important part in professional identity formation.
- The HC plays an important (and largely negative) role in student mistreatment.

 "The real voyage of discovery consists of not in seeking new landscapes but in having new eyes."

Marcel Proust

The hidden curriculum (HC) is a theoretical construct for exploring the continuities and disconnects of educational life. At its most basic level, HC theory highlights the potential for gaps or disconnects between what faculty intend to deliver (the formal curriculum) and what learners take away from those formal lessons; all operating within a system's framework that emphasizes context and the interconnections and interdependencies of system elements. Examples of key influences include pedagogical methods (how content is delivered), the relational context (interactions among faculty and students, including factors such as power and hierarchy), physical context (space, layout, noise) and the context of organizational culture and group values. Building on this conceptual platform, HC theory also recognizes that much of social life, including what happens in educational settings, takes place 'beneath the radar' because the predominance of daily life, educational or otherwise, is routinized and thus taken for granted. Also fundamental to the idea of a HC is

the understanding that becoming a physician involves processes of professional socialization and identity formation within the cultures and related subcultures that make up medicine and medical practice.

 "We (faculty) are teaching far more than we know. Every word we speak, every action we perform, every time we choose not to speak or act, every smile, every curse, every sigh is a lesson in the hidden curriculum."

Gofton & Regehr, 2006

Any attempt to penetrate, decode, and ultimately exert an influence on the HC begins by dissecting the formal curriculum, and thus what is supposed to be going on, at least according to those in power. With this as our foundation, we then can proceed to explore 'what else might be happening'. The space between the official and unofficial, the formal and the informal, the intended and the perceived then becomes our primary workspace. In doing this work, it is important to remember that the HC is not a 'thing' that one finds, fixes, and then files in a 'completed projects' drawer. There always is a hidden counterpart to the formal and intended curriculum. Context always exerts an influence. There always are unseen, unrecognized and un- or under-appreciated factors that influence social life. There always are things that become so routine and taken for granted that they become invisible over time. Purposeful inquiry may uncover and intentionally address pieces of these influences, but no discovery is ever complete and no solution is ever permanent. Finally, the HC system's perspective requires us to acknowledge that any change in context and situation generates a new set of dynamics and thus new sets of influences, which in turn help to construct new (overall) sets of relationships between the formal and hidden dimensions of social life.

Historical context

HC theory has deep conceptual roots within two academic disciplines: sociology and education. Philosopher and educational reformer John Dewey, for example, wrote regarding the importance of 'collateral learning' and the prevailing importance of indirect versus direct classroom instruction in arguing that the incidental learning that accompanies school and classroom life has an even more profound effect on learners than the formal or intended lesson plan. Dewey may not have used the term 'hidden', but he clearly was concerned with the coincidental, unintended, unnoticed and unconscious dimensions of learning.

Sociology, in turn, has had its own set of conceptual precursors, particularly its long tradition of differentiating between the formal and the informal aspects of social life. For example, sociology differentiates between social norms, which often function on an informal level, and laws, which are codified. Moreover, sociology recognizes that there are many instances where norms have a more profound effect on social practices than laws: think of the difference between the posted road or highway speed limit (formal) and the more informal boundaries of acceptable driving speed that govern the actions of both drivers and law enforcement. Joining sociology are the academic literatures of business, management studies, and organizational sciences each with a rich history of differentiating between the formal and informal aspects of work, including the important role of tacit learning in how one learns 'on the job'.

Since the 1990s, there has been a steady stream of articles in medical education literature featuring the HC as a conceptual tool for examining medical training. Topics have included work on professionalism, ethics instruction, faculty development, gender issues, examination policies, identity formation and socialization, summative assessment, reflection, resource allocation, cultural competency, the impact of block rotations on student development, longitudinal training, messages conveyed in case studies, the training of international medical graduates, workforce issues, medical student specialty choice, relations among specialty groups, the HC of scientific research, simulation, and tools to measure the HC. The concept has been used to explore issues across medical specialties ranging from anaesthesiology to surgery, across all levels of medical training from medical school through residency training and onto continuing medical education, and to explore related concepts such as humanism (Martimianakis et al., 2015). The HC also has been used to examine educational issues in over fifty countries.

Definitions and metaphors

 "Lessons from the hidden curriculum are taught implicitly, through role models, institutional leadership, peers, or during the course of practice..."

Fryer-Edwards, 2002

In spite of a rather extensive literature on the HC, and in some cases because of this literature, there can be confusion regarding what does and does not fall under the HC marquee. In this next section, along with subsequent examples, we seek to shed light on this lexiconic muddle.

DEFINITIONS

The formal curriculum is the stated and the intended curriculum. This is what the school or the teacher says is being taught. The formal curriculum has at least two dimensions. The first is that it is formally identified as such: be this in writing (course catalogue, website, course syllabus) or orally by a teacher. A second dimension is intentionality. What does the instructor/school intend to teach or convey to students?

Working 'outward' from the formal, we quickly enter a myriad of distinctions and derivations within the other-than-formal aspects of learning. These dimensions may be tacit, indirect, informal, unintended or otherwise invisible to the participants. What they share in common is that they are neither formally announced nor intended.

Educators often employ a simple dichotomy to differentiate between the formal curriculum and 'everything else' that may be going on within the educational environment. In doing so, some use the term 'hidden' as a master label for anything other than the formal curriculum. Others may use the terms 'hidden' or 'informal' as synonyms. There is nothing intrinsically wrong with such an approach so long as everyone (investigators, subjects and readers) understands that what is being shoehorned into this latter category often can be quite different in terms of structural properties and impact. For example, the null curriculum covers what students learn via what is not taught, highlighted or presented. A literary analogy from a famous Sherlock Homes case is of the behaviour of a dog on the night of a murder.

 Gregory (Scotland Yard detective): "Is there any other point to which you would wish to draw my attention?"
Holmes: "To the curious incident of the dog in the night-time."
Gregory: "The dog did nothing in the night-time."
Holmes: "That was the curious incident."

Sir Arthur Conan Doyle, 1892

While students certainly garner a great deal from what faculty fail to emphasize or do not evaluate/test, this is quite a different type of learning than the more informal rules students tacitly acquire, for example, about how to communicate with a 'difficult patient', how 'best' to present at morning rounds, or how to navigate the various 'workarounds' that are employed in different healthcare settings.

At a basic analytic level, we argue for a basic four (formal, informal, hidden, null) category approach to exploring the HC. In addition to the formal, important learning takes place via the relationships and interactions within the workplace (as one source of the informal curriculum) along with the less visible and/or obvious sources such as organizational culture (as one source of the hidden curriculum). The actual lessons may be similar, but it is important to maintain a conceptual distinction between informal norms that are widely shared and openly recognized versus those influences that are less obvious to or less recognized by participants.

METAPHORS

"There is no question that there is an unseen world. The problem is, how far is it from midtown and how late is it open."

Woody Allen, 1972

While definitional distinctions can be critical for understanding the various types and sources of learning that take place within our learning environments (LEs), these demarcations also can be quite limiting. This is particularly true in the fluid and enigmatic nature of learning: where influences may be hidden at one point in time, formalized at another, yet with these new formal rules gradually slipping beneath conscious reflection and scrutiny over time. For these reasons, using metaphors to crystalize thinking about the HC can be quite liberating in suggesting new ways of thinking about the forces that shape learning. Thus, we might employ the ubiquitous metaphor of the iceberg, with its above-the-surface/visible versus its below-the-water-line/invisible dimensions in reminding ourselves that the less-than-visible aspects of educational life may be more consequential than those that sit above the surface. Alternatively, we might embrace the more enigmatic metaphor of physics with its alternative realities, or the fact that most of the universe is made up of something (dark matter) that is invisible to observers and therefore must be ascertained indirectly. The claim that much of organizational life is shaped by invisible or hidden forces may sound like hyperbole until one realizes how many different areas of science are rooted in a similar contention. After all, we know that most communication is nonverbal, that approximately 80% of mental processing takes place at an unconscious level, and that approximately 80% of effects come from 20% of the causes (e.g. the Pareto 80-20 principle). These realities should at least give us some pause in wondering how much of what our students learn can be attributed solely to our intended curriculum.

Applications: exploring/assessing the hidden curriculum

"...the chief barrier to medical professionalism education is unprofessional conduct by medical educators, which is protected by an established hierarchy of academic authority. Students feel no such protection..."

Brainard & Brislen, 2007

Applying the HC to issues of student learning and faculty development is not an easy or risk-free undertaking. It can involve considerable time and effort, and because it stands in contrast to a 'pure' teaching model (where students are viewed as empty vessels eagerly waiting to be filled by the knowledge, skills, behaviours and values possessed by their faculty), framing issues from a HC perspective may be both disquieting and engender resistance. Nonetheless, by exploring the interface between the formal and the other-than-formal aspects of your own LEs, you may come to more deeply appreciate how the learning taking place within the medical school is shaped by the broader sociocultural environment within which all organizations are located (Hafferty et al., 2015). In this section, we outline practical methods to explore the other-than-formal aspects of LEs. This is an essential step in aligning what we intend to teach with what is actually learned by our trainees.

1. *Getting started:* Learners (faculty and students) should be familiar with the overall conceptual framework as well as key terms (e.g. formal, informal, hidden, null). Being aware of the phenomenon, and ensuring that others in the LE are aware and open to discussion as well, often can be a big part of the solution. Help learners tune in to the unintended learning moments that exist within the educational environment. For example, you might ask students to identify the messages or learning points embedded in common scenarios:

   a. You (the third-year medical student) are expected to do all sorts of nonmedical tasks, such as picking up food for team members.

   b. Your attending physician stays at work until very late most nights. She often misses family events, most recently her partner's birthday. Residents who stay late are lauded as 'heroes' or 'champs'.

   c. Your resident pronounces your 16-year-old patient with cystic fibrosis dead and sits down with you to reflect on the event and to mourn the loss of the patient you cared for together.

   d. Your attending talks about the patient's diagnosis and poor prognosis to the ward team in front of the patient and without including the patient in the conversation or asking if he has any questions.

e. Your grade on a particular rotation is determined largely by your score on a multiple-choice content exam.

f. You observe a morbidly obese patient repeatedly being referred to as a hippopotamus by the intern and resident on your team.

g. You never observe a resident or attending take a sexual history.

Another exercise useful in highlighting the differences between formal and informal curricula is asking learners to identify the 'top ten things I learned in medical school that I wasn't supposed to' (Dosani, 2010). Similarly, both faculty and students can examine their own contribution to the educational environment by asking them to identify and reflect on how they function as role models (peer and otherwise) in various learning environments.

2. *Participant-observer inquiry:* Learners can take on the role of an amateur 'anthropologist of medical culture' (Harvard Macy Faculty, 2011). A brief overview of basic ethnographic methods such as mapping the educational space and objective methods of data collection can be very useful here. Trainees may be asked to describe how people are dressed, the tools they equip themselves with, how they introduce themselves, where they stand or sit when they are in a group, who speaks first and the languages used, or the roles assumed by different members of the healthcare team. Faculty can be asked to do the same exercise. Comparing these two lists can be quite revealing. This method can be used in preclinical and clinical settings. In the pre-clinical setting, one may explore the relative participation (e.g. 'airtime') of faculty versus students in different LEs. In addition, one can examine the use of technology such as laptops or hand-held devices, attendance rates, and late arrivals and the content of pre- and post-class conversations. In clinical settings, such as rounds, a volunteer can time approximately how many minutes are devoted to patients' social/emotional needs versus a range of other topics such as health insurance and other 'business' considerations, the presence of humour, joking or non–patient-related conversations. Asking trainees to write their anthropological observations in the third person, as if they are an outsider assigned to 'look in' to a strange new world, can help with the cultivation of 'HC eyes'.

3. *Share stories from the hidden curriculum.*

   a. Provide scheduled time and space, protected from other responsibilities, for sharing, listening and reflecting on student experiences. The use of triggers from the humanities (art, poetry, literature, film) can provide the learner critical distance and a safe opening to the sharing of personal experiences. Such opportunity for reflection is an important aspect of professional development, and may stem negative effects of the emotional suppression experienced by many medical students, and ultimately may help prevent ethical erosion.

   b. The following writing exercise has proved useful at one medical school (Gaufberg et al., 2010). Post an introduction to the HC concept, students were assigned a brief reflection paper in which they tell a story from the HC and reflect on it. In doing so, students might be asked to take on the above-noted role of participant-observer/ 'anthropologists of medical culture'. These stories can be used to start a discussion. With student permission and/or de-identification, stories may also be used as a form of feedback to faculty and others in educational (grand rounds, workshop) settings, with the opportunity for discussion. Dramatic enactment of the stories in the form of Readers' Theatre can be particularly powerful as a starting place (Bell et al., 2010). On a larger scale, the sharing of humanizing examples from the informal curriculum ('appreciative inquiry') can be an effective means to effect positive institutional change (Suchman et al., 2004).

   c. Have students explore what sociologists refer to as the 'oral culture' of medicine by having students gather and share stories they have heard faculty tell about medical practice and/ or life as a physician. Work to decode the underlying cultural, moral, and normative messages that may be embedded in these stories.

4. *Focus attention and reflect upon workarounds.* Workarounds are the other-than-formal/ unsanctioned ways of getting work done where the official or 'right' way is seen as inefficient, dysfunctional, out of date or otherwise not appropriate. Workarounds can be found in the classroom or in the clinic or wards. Although there are no printed rulebooks for workarounds, initiates soon learn their critical role in getting things done. They also learn that there are right and wrong ways to perform these off-the-books practices. Ask students to come up with one example of a workaround they have engaged in or observed. Ask: "How did you learn the rules of this particular workaround (observation, role

modelling, clues from an insider)?" Encourage students to explore why we even have workarounds, particularly in the face of an ever more highly structured work environment.

5. *Focus on micro-ethical challenges.* Some authors and educators have argued that focusing on day-to-day micro-ethical challenges (Is it okay to 'practise' on patients? What do I do if my resident asks me to falsify a chart? Do I laugh at this dehumanizing joke?) are more developmentally appropriate for medical students than teaching about ethical challenges they will face only as full-fledged clinicians. Micro-ethical challenges often occur within a hierarchy of evaluation in which students believe that the process or outcome of their decisions may have an impact on their grade. Various online forums such as professionalformation.org allow students to share and problem- solve challenges collaboratively.

6. *Turn your attention to the null curriculum.* Review teaching objectives and/or content with an eye towards things that may have been left out. Review your formal curricular offerings and explore how 'missing topics' might communicate messages to both faculty and students about what is and what is not within the scope of the doctor's concern. Correspondingly, what might your patients be concerned about that you fail to discuss or teach? These types of exercises can be particularly difficult. After all, how does one know when something is missing? Nonetheless, decoding what is missing can have a profound impact in reshaping how one does things in the future.

7. *Inventory and take stock of your physical surroundings.* How much and what kind of space does your school devote to clinical learning versus other organizational objectives such as administration or research? A school dominated by lecture rooms but with little space for small-group learning more than likely will stress didactic over interactive learning processes. What about student and faculty awards? Where do you post them, if at all? There is a substantial 'meaning difference' between schools that post awards in highly trafficked areas and those that use a back hallway. In the clinical LE, does the set up favour patient-centred human connection or is the design for the convenience of staff and/ or computer entry? Sometimes physical artefacts can be hiding in plain sight. Over the course of several days, one clinician conscientiously inventoried drug and medical equipment company-branded items as he encountered them during his normal work activities (Hafferty & O'Donnell, 2015). He was dumfounded by the sheer number and density of what he 'newly saw', particularly items that had been 'hiding' in his office.

Student mistreatment: a case study in applying the HC lens

While the list of topics amenable to HC analysis is extensive, we have selected student mistreatment for several reasons. First, in an ideal, healthcare training environment, there is no mistreatment. No medical school formally announces that student *mistreatment* is part of their formal and/or intended curriculum. This singular observation, however obvious, presents us with several interpretive challenges. First, we must be open to the possibility that mistreatment, while not formally claimed, is intended. Second, and even if we eliminate subterfuge, we are left with a range of alternative explanations including the toleration of something (mistreatment) that is neither claimed nor deliberate. Here, our analytic tree further branches into formal versus tacit acceptance, along with the more conventional possibility that what we have is neither formal nor tacit, but rather the presence of fundamental disagreements as to what might constitute *mistreatment* versus other forms of 'treatment' deemed by those with formal control over the LE as necessary in meeting particular pedagogical ends. Thus, a HC approach requires us to be open to the possibility that some pedagogical practice, say the Socratic method (including its range of manifestations), may be deemed desirable by one party (e.g. faculty) while intimidating, disrespectful, bullying or abusive by another (e.g. trainees). Characterizing the latter framings as 'mis-taken' or 'naïve', while certainly the privilege of those in power, misses the HC point. Having faculty dismiss these claims as incorrect or misguided only reinforces the perception. Correspondingly, the claim of mistreatment, even when sincerely perceived, does not make it true. The fact that mistreatment is socially con-structed, and therefore is heavily shaped by context and culture, does not automatically privilege either claim. Nonetheless, and regardless of fact or perception, the HC requires that LEs as contested domains must be remediated. The 'fix' may involve student-targeted education on the structure and purposes of such contested pedagogical practices or it may involve changes in the disputed practices themselves (or some combination of explanation and re-engineering). Whatever the final determination, learner-based percep-tions that they are operating under conditions of mistreatment do not make for a healthy LE.

Claims or counter-claims notwithstanding, one key to a robust HC analysis requires that we go beyond the perception of mistreatment as a dynamic grounded in individual relationships to a consideration that organizations themselves, including their structure and processes, can generate, accentuate and/or perpetuate mistreatment – and do so independent of interpersonal interactions as a causal vehicle. Some may consider an endless cascade of didactic lectures or a parade of scutwork shorn of explanation to be examples of organizational mistreatment. We would concur. In turn, the presence of such structurally based forms of mistreatment, particularly to the degree they exist beneath the radar, will make general accountability and remediation more difficult.

This brings us to a couple of final points on HC decoding. Just as claiming mistreatment does not make it so, the absence of mistreatment claims does not mean that the LE is bereft of mistreatment. Ultimately, a HC approach requires that we obsessively and exhaustively probe the issue at hand. Mistreatment with respect to what? – we must ask. If our answer is mistreatment with respect to 'learning' then we open up a range of interesting challenges including the possibility that many well accepted pedagogical practices, such as high-stakes testing, particular grading policies, or the competition for scarce resources such as status positions (class ranking, chief resident) *may* impede or otherwise distort the formally stated goals of learning. After all, LEs are not supposed to be stress free. Recognizing when and how certain types of stressors are necessary for certain types of learning (particularly, in our case, adult learning) is just as emblematic of a HC approach as deconstructing and remediating practices deemed unwanted or counterproductive.

Finally, any HC biopsy of mistreatment must explore the full range of settings where issues of mistreatment exist within the LE. While there are multiple avenues, we will highlight two here: (1) research/scholarship on mistreatment, and (2) assessments/accreditation of training programs at the undergraduate and graduate medical education levels. In the first example, we may explore how research privileges certain framings of mistreatment while ignoring others – thus legitimizing the former as being 'worthy' of our attention, while delegitimizing the latter as either not worthy of attention or perhaps even something other than mistreatment. In the case of accreditation, how do accrediting bodies hold programmes accountable when it comes to 'mistreatment'? If they frame mistreatment as located only in interpersonal dynamics, for example, then there is every likelihood that this is how programmes themselves, at the administrative level on down, will come to view mistreatment. In turn, faculty, followed by trainees, will be swept along in a cascade of meaning in which organizational sites of mistreatment fall away from consideration and thus remain unaddressed. In terms of power and influence, accrediting bodies can (and do) set the meaning tone for everyone else.

Ultimately, mistreatment is not so much a Justice Potter Stewart "I know it when I see it" phenomenon (e.g. What is pornography?) as it is something one comes to 'know better' when one systematically looks both at its presence and its absence independent of the claims of parties who have an interest in having reality defined in ways favourable to their interests.

Summary

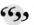 *"The relational processes of the hidden curriculum assure the perpetuation of its content."*

Haidet & Stein, 2006

While no single theme can subsume all of the concepts and framings covered above, there are a few particulars worthy of final comment. First, the HC is a versatile tool. The concept can be applied to a broad range of health education issues. Medical schools 'teach' far more to both faculty and students than they commonly take credit for: or perhaps would want to take credit for. Similarly, faculty and students are perpetually interactive and mutually influential co-participants in creating the normative soup that fuels the formal, informal and hidden curricula of medical education and medical practice. Second, the HC has an incessant and ubiquitous presence within educational settings. There is no LE without a HC. Its impact may be pivotal or relatively insignificant, but it is there nonetheless. Third, and related, the HC is universal. Whatever else links physicians trained in different countries, and whatever constitutes the shared values that allow us to talk about an authentic and international 'medical culture', there is a HC weaving its way through the particulars of any country and its training. Fourth, working with the HC is a reflective act and thus a form of pedagogical reflexivity. It is just as important to critically examine the structure and dynamics of our LEs as it is to deliver curricular content. Fifth, the HC is relational. The HC, like social life, is built in and around, and nourished by, relationships among participants and between participants and the surrounding environment. Sixth, the apprentice-like model that underscores clinical training and the corresponding need to integrate the learner into the workplace, form a LE that is particularly ripe for HC. Finally, and related, there has been a tendency to execute HC reforms by targeting medical students and medical school faculty while ignoring how organizations, institutions, and sociopolitical relations help shape the problematic situations under consideration. While the HC is fundamentally about probing the difference between the stated and the received, it ultimately is about context and about situating some 'piece' within a larger relational whole. Regardless of what things look like 'on the surface', the HC is all about subterrestrial context and its connections.

References

Bell, S.K., Wideroff, M., Gaufberg, E., 2010. Student voices in readers' theater: exploring communication in the hidden curriculum. Patient Educ. Couns. 80 (3), 354–357.

Brainard, A.H., Brislen, H.C., 2007. Viewpoint: learning professionalism: a view from the trenches. Acad. Med. 82 (11), 1010–1014.

Dosani, N., The top 10 things I learned in medical school (but wasn't supposed to!): Plenary Session: The hidden curriculum exposed: perspectives of learners and educators, Canada, May 4, 2010, St. John's Newfoundland.

Fryer-Edwards, K., 2002. Addressing the hidden curriculum in scientific research. Am. J. Bioeth. 2, 58–59.

Gaufberg, E., Batalden, M., Sands, R., Bell, S., 2010. The hidden curriculum: what can we learn from third-year medical student narrative reflections? Acad.Med. 85 (11), 1709–1711.

Gofton, W., Regehr, G., 2006. What we don't know we are teaching: unveiling the hidden curriculum. Clin. Orthop. Relat. Res. 449, 20–27.

Hafferty, F.W., Gaufberg, E.H., O'Donnell, J.F., 2015. The role of the hidden curriculum in "on doctoring" courses. AMA J. Ethics 17, 130–139.

Hafferty, F.W., O'Donnell, J.F. (Eds.), 2015. The Hidden Curriculum in Health Professions Education. University Press of New England (Dartmouth College Press), Lebanon, NH.

Haidet, P., Stein, H.F., 2006. The role of the student-teacher relationship in the formation of physicians: the hidden curriculum as process. J. Gen. Intern. Med. 21 (Suppl. 1), S16–S20.

Harvard Macy Faculty, 2011. Learning to Look: A Hidden Curriculum Exercise. Harvard Macy Institute, Boston, MA.

Martimianakis, M.A., Michalec, B., Lam, J., et al., 2015. Humanism, the hidden curriculum, and educational reform: a scoping review and thematic analysis. Acad. Med. 90, S5–S13.

Suchman, A.L., Williamson, P.R., Litzelman, D.K., et al., 2004. The relationship-centered care initiative discovery team: toward an informal curriculum that teaches professionalism: transforming the social environment of a medical school. J. Gen. Intern. Med. 19 (5 Pt 2), 501–504.

Section 2

Learning situations

Lectures

W. B. Jeffries, K. N. Huggett, J. L. Szarek

Trends

- Improved understanding of lecture as a knowledge construction event
- Increased understanding of encoding and retention of new knowledge
- Recognition of lectures as opportunities for active learning
- Lecture planning accounts for the asynchronous participation of learners who access recorded lectures
- Learning begins before lecture, with application and clarification during assigned lecture time

Lectures in medical teaching

 "LECTURE: a discourse given before an audience upon a given subject, usually for the purpose of instruction."

Oxford English Dictionary

The lecture remains a widespread teaching method in health sciences curricula and remains essentially unchanged over the centuries. The rationale for extensive lecturing is now under scrutiny as the neurobiology of learning becomes better understood, as competing methods are introduced, and as digital technology transforms human communication. The efficacy of lectures is also determined by teacher expertise and learner participation. This chapter provides pathways to understand reasons for lecture success or failure, and methods to prepare optimal lectures and enhance active learning and learning outcomes.

 "A LECTURER is a person who has the bad habit of speaking while someone is sleeping."

Anonymous

Pros and cons of lectures as a primary learning event

Lectures can be an inspiring learning medium, and most students and faculty expect them to be an integral part of knowledge acquisition. It is thus unsurprising that students prefer in-person lectures versus recorded lectures (Bligh, 2000). Lecturing is demonstrably as good as any method in effecting knowledge transfer to learners. Students often prefer lectures because they are usually good guides to summative assessments, and studying lecture notes provides a high yield way to prepare. Svinicki and McKeachie (2013) provides a number of important ways that lectures can be effective (Box 7.1).

Two types of factors interfere with the application of lectures as the primary engine of learning in a health sciences curriculum: individual limitations and pedagogical limitations. Among individual limitations, we have found a wide variance in lecturer presentation skills, confidence, subject knowledge, pedagogical experience and engagement. Deficits in any of these areas limit learning and undermine student enthusiasm and perception of faculty charisma. For the faculty, deficits in these areas can lead to fear, lack of fulfilment and negative teacher ratings. Thus, optimal lecturing is essential and this chapter seeks to address many of these concerns.

Pedagogical limitations of the lecture are harder to overcome. Although the lecture is perceived as an effective and efficient way to transfer information, a growing body of evidence reveals that lectures are suboptimal for development of skills, attitudes and higher levels of knowledge application. We must recognize that although optimal lecturers remain essential for health sciences teaching, other modalities are often superior for the varied outcomes needed for excellent healthcare providers.

 Before preparing a lecture ensure that it is the most appropriate format for the desired outcome. Another modality might be superior.

Learning in a lecture environment

A useful framework to understand knowledge acquisition in a lecture is provided by Constructivist Learning Theory (see Torre et al., 2006 for a review of learning theories related to medical education). In constructivism, learners develop and modify knowledge by

- Presenting up-to-date information
- Summarizing material from a number of sources
- Helping students prepare effectively for active learning by providing an orientation and conceptual framework
- Focusing on key concepts, core principles or ideas

- Vary the visual presentation (include photos, charts, etc.). Don't use small fonts or excessively dim lights. Avoid many visually similar slides in sequence.
- Vary your speaking pace and tone. Monotone deliveries guarantee boredom. Do not read slides; use them as a basis for engaging descriptions and anecdotes.
- Introduce a 'respite' in the lecture. Inactivity blunts attention. Stop lecturing for 1 minute or less and get students on their feet to stretch or briefly exercise.
- Do something unexpected (introduce a patient, perform a demonstration, watch a video, etc.). This resets attention to a higher level, promoting retention.
- Ensure a proper learning environment. Limit distracting noise, conversation and unnecessary use of devices. Improper lighting, seating, air circulation and temperature adversely affect attention. Post-prandial and late afternoon lectures reduce arousal and require extra effort to retain attention.

constructing meaning from new experiences. During a lecture, students must assimilate the presented material by interpreting it, comparing it to their existing knowledge base, creating new meaning (integrated with previously assimilated material) and storing it. Thus in this framework the lecturer's role is to present material to allow the learner to assimilate it through experience. The teacher needs to focus on maintaining learner *attention*, fostering *engagement*, promoting *retention* and projecting effective *organization*.

ATTENTION IN LECTURE

Lectures are ineffective unless the learners pay attention. Unfortunately, during a one-hour lecture attention falls dramatically after only a few minutes and only begins to recover as learners anticipate its conclusion (Bligh, 2000). Factors involved in maintaining student attention include *arousal* and *motivation*. Arousal refers to the overall energy level of learners, whereas motivation refers to energy directed to specific goals (Bligh, 2000). Arousal is maintained through variations in stimulation (presentation style, learning activities, audiovisual material), and environmental factors such as seating, temperature and lighting. A lecturer can increase attention by creating an environment that favours arousal. No more than 10–15 minutes should pass without some active effort (a 'respite') to boost attention (Jeffries, 2014). Box 7.2 includes some ideas on how to accomplish this.

Motivation is important in maintaining attention. The intrinsic motivations of students in the health sciences are both immediate (desire for understanding and engagement, knowledge acquisition for the coming assessment) and far reaching (relevance to their medical careers). Thus it is helpful if students understand the material's importance to the course and its assessments, as well as its relevance to medicine. Clearly outline relevance to course objectives and its assessments to nationally normed comprehensive examinations, and to public health. Nothing increases attention like the phrase 'this will be on the test!'

FOSTERING ENGAGEMENT

Instructor engagement promotes student motivation and attention. Students respond well to a lecturer who connects with the audience. Engage directly with the audience by projecting your knowledge and enthusiasm for the topic. Students respond best to instructors who are organized, professional, and explain the relevance of content to current practice. Students also value the efforts instructors make to link their prior coursework to current lecture content (Onwuegbuzie et al., 2007).

Start each session by introducing yourself, the topic and its relation to the course objectives. The organization of the presentation should be transparent with time built in for questions and summing up. Use presentation space effectively by moving away from the podium when possible to interact directly with learners, make eye contact and gauge interest and enthusiasm. Use audiovisual materials to tell compelling stories, introduce helpful mnemonics and ask provocative questions. To ensure that learners are not confused or disengaged, periodically ask short questions that can be answered via an audience response system or a show of hands. Humour is appreciated and can raise attention, but be careful to be culturally and generationally sensitive! Stories and jokes are more effective when directly in context to the subject at hand; interesting yet extraneous information actually leads to decreased learning of relevant information during lecture (Mayer et al., 2008). End by summing up the salient major points and stay after the session to answer additional questions.

 Arrive early to the session to chat with students, become familiar with the room and its facilities and ensure that the audiovisual materials are working properly.

PROMOTING RETENTION

Retention is the effective encoding of knowledge (through instruction, studying, reflection and creation of meaning) and effective retrieval of that knowledge (which is measured on assessments). We will focus on three practical contributors to retention that are under the lecturer's control: content density and pacing, note taking and retrieval practice.

Mismanagement of content density in a lecture is a common mistake. Attempts to cram 80–90 slides into a one-hour session are doomed to failure. Such lecturers fail to prepare adequately, either by adding too many major topics into the lecture, or including too many extraneous details. Students will have difficulty prioritizing, will gain only superficial knowledge or may abandon attempts to learn the material altogether. Cognitive processing of the information and the creation of an 'internal narrative' by the learner will be impaired.

Content overload leads to pacing errors. Assuming a teacher successfully fosters engagement and promotes attention, material must still be delivered in a way that students can process it from short-term memory into their existing long-term memory (rehearsal) and/or by constructing new meaning. If the pace is too fast, the student will be overwhelmed because of interference, and learning will cease. Conversely, if the pace is too slow, learning may also cease because of decreased arousal with loss of attention. Thus the instructor needs to search for the amount of material that is 'just right'. As a start, plan no more than 2–3 minutes per slide, and build in time for questions and a summary. Pacing is an important consideration when reviewing evaluations to iteratively improve the lecture and course.

 The most common mistake made by lecturers is the inclusion of too much information. Focus on major points with a few salient examples.

Ineffective pacing can also interfere with note taking. Note taking improves retention (Bligh, 2000) and its facilitation provides the instructor with an opportunity to promote learning. Pacing should be slow enough to allow effective note taking. The instructor should closely follow the outline, emphasizing the important points through examples, summaries and reiteration. Handouts encourage note taking by following the lecture organization and providing salient charts, graphs and other materials, while leaving active work for the learner to

---

Box 7.3	**Tips to promote retention**

- Control content density to encompass a few major points.
- Create handout materials that encourage effective note taking.
- Pause after major concepts to allow students to process and formulate questions.
- Embed assessment questions into and/or the end of the lecture.

complete while in class. The instructor should also be cognizant of learner reaction, looking for attitudinal cues from the audience and asking them if further clarification is needed. Pause the presentation following a particularly difficult point to allow students to catch up, reflect and generate questions. This pause can be turned into an active learning exercise, as discussed later in this chapter.

 "Retrieval is not merely a readout of the knowledge stored in one's mind; the act of reconstructing knowledge itself enhances learning."

Karpicke & Blunt, 2011

Neurocognitive studies have shown that in-class assessment can boost retention. A common conception of retention is only as effective storage of information in the memory. However, a less considered component is effective retrieval of that information. Retrieval practice can significantly enhance the learning process through repeated reconstruction of knowledge, producing important learning stimuli (Karpicke & Blunt, 2011). Thus, retrieval practice (e.g. through multiple-choice tests) can be a powerful tool in promoting learning that is superior to other study methods. These findings were foreshadowed by those of Jones (1923, summarized by Bligh, 2000), who found that the decay of knowledge learned in lectures was considerably blunted by immediate testing. Based on these data, we advocate the inclusion of retrieval practice within, or at the end of each lecture. This can be accomplished with short answer examinations on paper or introduced via an audience response system. Box 7.3 summarizes some considerations to promote retention.

Organizing a lecture

Most successful lectures have a transparent organization that helps learners understand expected outcomes. Since optimal organization of a lecture is dictated by the content and context, one should first establish its general purpose. Health science lectures often fall into one of four categories (Jeffries, 2014): 1) presentation of information about a specific subject (e.g. drugs used to lower blood pressure); 2) development of critical thinking skills (e.g. how to interpret plasma electrolyte values); 3) demonstration of a procedure, experiment or clinical approach (e.g. surgical approaches to bowel disease); 4) construction of an argument (e.g. prioritization of patients for treatment with scarce resources).

 All lecture types should include clear and measurable learning objectives that guide the presentation as well as the assessment.

Objectives represent another organizing principle for lectures. The objectives reflect prior student learning and the intended scope of the session. Objectives should specify behaviours that learners could be observed doing as a result of the session (e.g. 'Based on patient laboratory values, identify common electrolyte abnormalities.'). The use of Bloom's taxonomy is helpful both in creating objectives and in gauging their needed complexity (Krathwohl, 2002). The objectives should be specific, but not too numerous.

Once the purpose and objectives are established, organize the lecture based on content and pedagogical efficacy. Brainstorm all content related to the topic with a concept map or other organizing strategy. This will help in four important areas (Jeffries, 2014):

- *Identifying overlaps with other course sessions and previously learned material.* In team-taught courses, determine where your material begins and ends. Avoid undue repetition of previously taught material.
- *Determining the required depth of learning needed.* Many a promising lecture has gone astray by delving too deeply into minutia.
- *Choosing how to organize the material.* This may be already determined in a team-taught course, but the organizational structure must be clear and reflected in handouts.
- *Discovering gaps in your own understanding.* Generate a reading list to cover aspects of the subject not in your area of expertise. Read the relevant chapters in course texts to familiarize yourself with the learner's study materials.

There are many ways to organize the lecture once the above questions have been answered. *Inductive methods* use real-world examples, assembling facts to create a general principle. For example, a story of a viral outbreak could be detailed to introduce theories of epidemiology and public health. *Deductive methods* work the opposite way, discussing general principles followed by examples of their application. In either case, real stories add vividness and clarity to promote understanding and retention. In any case, structure the lecture to deliver major points within the 15-minute attention window. Sum up major points, take questions, and insert lecture respites or learning activities that restore attention before moving to the next major point. Plan to end at least 10 minutes short of the appointed time to allow time for unplanned clarifications and responses to student questions.

Teaching materials

AUDIOVISUALS

Learner understanding is promoted by effective presentation of the underlying outline, clarifying figures and charts, photographs of patient presentation or pathology slides, audience-response questions etc. It is best to mix formats and media to increase attention. If presenting with an electronic format, try these simple guidelines:

- Ensure legibility of text slides when projected, with no more than four to five salient points. Use the largest possible font size (≥18 point). Check that figures are legible and maximum size.
- Text slides should have a light background and dark letters to ensure that room lights can remain on during the presentation.
- Avoid conflicting formats on the same slide.
- Optimal pacing is 2–3 minutes per slide.
- Incorporate instructional elements such as video, demonstration, questions or audience participation to maximize engagement.

AUDIENCE RESPONSE SYSTEM (ARS)

Learners can answer multiple-choice questions during the course of a large-group presentation with an ARS. Systems are available commercially with dedicated devices or services that operate through the learner's computer, tablet or telephone. In the absence of an ARS, provide students with lettered cards that correspond to the question choices. The ARS can instantly calculate answer frequency, recording group data and conferring anonymity on the responders (if desired). The ARS can:

- get ongoing feedback about comprehension. A low frequency of correct answers indicates the need to cover the points again, answering questions along the way.
- provide formative feedback to learners. Students can note areas of weakness for follow-up and extra study.
- provide retrieval practice, especially for important and difficult topics.
- create a summative quiz, when the ARS is programmed to identify each user.
- take class attendance.

LECTURE RECORDINGS

Many institutions record lectures for students to download and use at a later date. Recordings can be audio alone (podcast) with the slides otherwise available, or videocast, which is either the audio synchronized with the slides or a video rendering of the presentation. Some instructors fear that this practice discourages class attendance and impinges on the intellectual property of the lecturer. While we acknowledge these concerns, most lecturers do not have the prerogative to avoid the practice, and in our experience, many students are reviewing the attended lecture and are not using recordings to replace the classroom experience. To promote maximum learning, we present some important considerations to remember when being podcast/videocast.

- *Podcasting.* By recording audio only, learners will have to listen to the lecture and simultaneously review the slides. To ensure students stay oriented, number the slides and periodically state which slide you are discussing. The viewers will not be able to see you point at structures, write on the board etc. Remember to affix your microphone properly and turn it on. Questions from the audience will not be audible and should be repeated before answering.
- *Videocasting.* If a slide is captured from a video camera in the room, there could be a considerable loss of resolution. Thus the aforementioned guidelines for slide legibility are important here. If the system produces only the slides with instructor voice-over, remember that events that happen off screen, such as writing on the board and in-class demonstrations, will not be visible. When pointing at objects on the slides, use the mouse, since a physical or laser pointer will not be visible in the capture.

Active learning in the lecture hall

"Active learning is those [practices] designed at least in part to promote conceptual understanding through interactive engagement of students in heads-on (always) and hands-on (usually) activities which yield immediate feedback through discussion with peers and/or instructors."

Hake, 1998

Active learning is a process in which students are required to *do something*, such as preparative reading, reflective writing, problem solving and/or group discussion. Active learning sessions require preparation by learners and expect higher level learning outcomes versus simple factual recall.

A recent meta-analysis of 225 studies of outcomes in undergraduate science, technology, engineering and mathematics courses demonstrated superior outcomes from active learning methods versus traditional lecture format (Freeman et al., 2014). These compelling data

suggest that active learning methods should supplement or supplant the traditional lecture in the curriculum. Ways to accomplish this include embedding active learning methods into the traditional lecture, and by 'flipping' the lecture to encourage a learner-centreed experience.

"... the evidence is in. The case is closed. Active learning wins."

Maryellen Weimer (Faculty Focus 3, 2015)

EMBEDDED METHODS

Integration of active learning techniques into the lecture hall attempts to transform students from receivers to appliers of knowledge. This creates a powerful impetus for deeper learning and retention. In ordinary lectures, instructors cannot expect learners to progress much beyond remembering and understanding as described in the modified Bloom's taxonomy (Box 7.4), since students generally are experiencing the material for the first time as it is delivered. However, active learning exercises can stimulate application, analysis and evaluation because students are *prepared* with a reading assignment or other learning activity before or during the session. A *modified lecture format* encompasses varying amounts of required preparation (or none) with active learning elements interspersed in the session.

Note check

One can easily introduce active learning with reflective techniques such as note check. Here the lecturer stops and asks participants to review their notes for 1–3 minutes, finding points needing clarification. This provides a break from lecturing with an accompanying arousal boost. It encourages students to quickly review the material, promoting its rehearsal into long-term memory. Note check likewise encourages reflective thinking. Students can be prompted to identify the point of greatest confusion ("the muddiest point" – Angelo & Cross, 1993) to generate class discussions, student written reflections or *impromptu* clarifying explanations.

Box 7.4 Modified Bloom's taxonomy (Krathwohl, 2002)	
Remember	Complexity
Understand	
Apply	
Analyse	
Evaluate	
Create	↓

Low stakes writing assignment

Reflective writing clarifies thinking, improves writing skill and enriches discussion. Thus active learning can be stimulated in class with a low stakes writing assignment (Svinicki & McKeachie, 2013). Students author short explanations of concepts or reflect on a reading assignment. This can trigger subsequent student discussions or higher stakes writing assignments. This format is often called 'one-minute paper' (Angelo & Cross, 1993).

Think-pair-share

There is tremendous potential from group learning activities such as think-pair-share. The lecturer pauses after a salient point and introduces an application question. Participants briefly (1–3 minutes) *think* about the answer individually, relying on lecture information and preparative work. Students then *pair* with their neighbour for discussion. Pairs are then randomly selected to *share* their answer in a large-group discussion. Each pair must be prepared to answer the question if called upon, promoting individual accountability for learning. Correct responses can be summarized by the instructor if conflicting answers are obtained; further discussion can resolve outstanding issues. Think-pair-share can be combined with note check to identify the muddiest points for large-group discussion.

 Learning is improved when students must explain their reasoning to others. Foster this advantage by having students learn in groups.

Buzz groups

Buzz groups are larger cousins of think-pair-share. Buzz groups can be spontaneously formed or preassigned to address tasks or answer questions. For example, students can discuss a case or develop a differential diagnosis and or treatment plan. Students can be afforded time to think on their own or begin group work immediately. Groups report findings to the larger group that can be compiled on the board by the instructor or student volunteers. The best results come when all groups work on the same problem. The lecturer sums up the correct answer and provides any needed clarifying explanations. A variation of this method, called peer learning, was developed by Eric Mazur. In this method, lectures are interspersed with conceptual questions (ConcepTests) completed by individual students. Then student groups reach a consensus on the correct answer with facilitation by the instructor (Fagen et al., 2002).

Games

Classroom learning games can create higher-level learning in a dynamic, fun environment. Games often follow the format of popular entertainment games such as 'Jeopardy'. Free, easy-to-use software that simulates popular games can be found online (e.g. https://www.superteachertools.us). Games involve teams or individuals and can include competitions for prizes. The ARS can be particularly useful. Games introduced during lecture are best placed at the end to minimize disruption and introduce the quiz questions at an optimal time for retrieval practice.

A common criticism of the modified lecture format is that it reduces the time available for the introduction of needed material. This is true as a single think-pair-share exercise can take 5 or 10 minutes. Thus the exercises must be used judiciously if the lecture format is to be retained. However, remember that you are trading factual learning for deep learning. The former likely suffers in the normal attention loss of the lecture format; the latter will bolster retention and learning level. Thus, use active learning exercises for the *most important* concepts, and assign the coverage of displaced facts to the preparation or homework phase.

The flipped classroom

This is a pedagogical model in which the typical lecture and homework elements of a course are reversed (Educause, 2012). The 'homework' consists of preparative material learned *before* the live learning session. In the subsequent large class setting, lecture is replaced with active learning methods. Such methods, such as those above, are combined in sequence to challenge students to achieve higher levels of learning.

A number of studies demonstrate better examination performance relative to historical controls in flipped classrooms. Importantly, in several studies (e.g. Freeman et al., 2011), failure rates decreased up to 60% when using the flipped model. Results of flipped classroom satisfaction studies range from equivocal to favouring the approach. Further research needs to determine which topics and student populations benefit from which types of active learning methods; however, faculty can be assured that the flipped classroom will likely enhance student engagement and performance.

Initial implementation of the flipped classroom requires significant preparation time by the instructor. This decreases in subsequent years. Planning a flipped classroom consists of four steps: determining out-of-class homework, developing the activity, running the session, and evaluation.

OUT-OF-CLASS HOMEWORK

Out-of-class homework can consist of podcasts or videocasts, reading from an assigned text, handouts, or other teaching materials created by the instructor. You could also choose to curate online content (e.g. YouTube, Khan Academy). It is critical to include lesson objectives so that students are ready for class. Homework should be intimately linked to objectives and not overburden the student. Consider reducing in-class contact time to accommodate homework preparation time by the students. This is particularly important if multiple instructors are using a flipped classroom approach and students have several out-of-class assignments to complete. However, reduced contact time is offset by enhanced retention and learning level as whole class periods are dedicated to active learning.

 To hold students accountable to the instructor, themselves and each other for the out-of-class homework, use a readiness assurance test that contributes to their grade.

DEVELOPING THE ACTIVITY

Flipped classroom sessions fail if students do not do preparative homework. Thus, an important consideration is how to hold students accountable to faculty, themselves and each other. A common and easily implemented method is the readiness assurance test (RAT). In the RAT, students answer a few questions that count towards their course grade. Alternatively, students could be asked to submit their muddiest point or to create a memory matrix (Angelo & Cross, 1993) as evidence of homework completion. The former could be used by the instructor during class for class discussion, while the latter could be used by the students during the completion of the activity. Peer evaluation is another method to hold students accountable since group learning depends on everyone being prepared. This can be used instead of or in addition to a RAT.

The activity itself could include a sequence of the embedded activities mentioned above, adaptation of a classroom assessment technique (Angelo & Cross, 1993), or team-based learning. Real-world examples such as patient cases, laboratory data etc., which are sufficiently challenging, provide a context to what the students studied out of class (Jeffries & Huggett, 2014). The common thread in these activities is that students, usually in groups, are given specific application tasks to accomplish and explain their reasoning to their peers and instructor. Regardless of the activity chosen, the activity should challenge students at higher levels of learning, align with the objectives, and, importantly, align with examinations. The activity must fit into allotted class time, including debriefing (see below), so it may be necessary to adjust the activity length after its first use.

RUNNING THE SESSION

Group learning, i.e. sharing and explaining answers with others, creates deeper understanding. Thus, the flipped classroom associates students into small groups within the lecture hall. Small groups are formed spontaneously by convenience or through formal assignment. The latter is preferable since it promotes group accountability; student groups can be maintained for extended periods. Groups should be instructed to explore the logic behind their final answers and alternative responses. Emphasize that mistakes will happen and are part of the learning process. The instructor must carefully monitor the activity timing to reserve a sufficient interval for debriefing. We use a visual indicator (e.g. a placard) that the groups display when finished.

After completing the activity, students should explain their logic to the class to provide immediate respectful feedback. Questions can be answered by the instructor or posed to the groups. In closing the session, emphasize accomplished objectives and acknowledge the hard work of the students.

 Call on students at random rather than asking for volunteers. This promotes accountability among group members.

EVALUATION

Evaluation should include measurements of student learning, students' reactions to the session and faculty peer evaluation. Student learning often is measured with a summative examination. If there are historical performance statistics on an examination used in a class after flipping it, the outcome using the traditional approach can be compared to that in the flipped classes. Such comparisons are useful in assuring ourselves and the administration that the flipped classroom method is not detrimental to student success.

Student and faculty reactions to the session are useful in making adjustments for future sessions. Some examples of statements that may be useful in a student questionnaire are shown in Box 7.5.

Critique of the session by the faculty participants also is useful in making adjustments for future sessions. Immediately after the session, consider whether the pace was appropriate and if the activity was sufficiently challenging. Making adjustments immediately after the session assures that the activity is ready for the next year.

> **Box 7.5   Representative statements to gauge success of a flipped classroom session. Uses a Likert scale from 1 (strongly disagree) to 5 (strongly agree)**
>
> - The pre-work was appropriate to help accomplish the session activity.
> - The session activity was relevant.
> - The session activity was appropriately challenging.
> - The pace of the session was good.
> - Feedback provided during the debriefing session was constructive.

Summary

The lecture is a time-honoured format that remains the most common instructional method in health science education. As more is discovered about the science of learning, the lecture is being adapted to become a more effective learning tool. Keys to promoting learning in the lecture hall include effective organization, maintaining student attention, fostering engagement, and promoting knowledge retention. An important factor in all of these considerations is the density of lecture content, which in turn influences the pace of delivery and note-taking ability. Many studies now show that active learning methods are superior for promoting learning versus passive lecturing. Lecture outcomes can be improved by the introduction of active learning elements or replacing lectures altogether with flipped classroom approaches.

References

Angelo, T.A., Cross, K.P., 1993. Classroom Assessment Techniques: a Handbook for College Teachers. Jossey-Bass, San Francisco.

Bligh, D.A., 2000. What's the Use of Lectures? Jossey-Bass, New York.

Educause Learning Initiative. 7 Things you should know about ... Flipped classroom, 2012. https://net.educause.edu/ir/library/pdf/eli7081.pdf. (Accessed 13 February 2016).

Fagen, A.P., Crouch, C.H., Mazur, E., 2002. Peer Instruction: Results from a Range of Classrooms. Phys. Teach. 40, 206–209.

Freeman, S., Haak, D., Wenderoth, M.P., 2011. Increased course structure improves performance in an introductory biology course. CBE Life Sci. Educ. 10 (2), 175–186.

Freeman, S., Eddy, S.L., McDonough, M., et al., 2014. Active learning increases student performance in science, engineering and mathematics. Proc. Natl. Acad. Sci. U.S.A. 111 (23), 8410–8415.

Hake, R.R., 1998. Interactive-engagement versus traditional methods: a six-thousand-student survey of mechanics test data for introductory physics courses. Am. J. Phys. 66, 64–74.

Jeffries, W.B., 2014. Teaching Large Groups. In: Huggett, K.N., Jeffries, W.B. (Eds.), An Introduction to Medical Teaching. Springer, Dordrecht.

Jeffries, W.B., Huggett, K.N., 2014. Flipping the Classroom. In: Huggett, K.N., Jeffries, W.B. (Eds.), An Introduction to Medical Teaching. Springer, Dordrecht.

Karpicke, J.D., Blunt, J.R., 2011. Retrieval practice produces more learning than elaborate studying with concept mapping. Science 331 (6018), 772–775.

Krathwohl, D.R., 2002. A revision of Bloom's Taxonomy: an overview. Theory Pract. 41 (4), 212–218.

Mayer, R.E., Griffith, E., Jurkowitz, I.T.N., Rothman, D., 2008. Increased interestingness of extraneous details in a multimedia science presentation leads to decreased learning. J. Exp. Psychol. Appl. 14 (4), 329–339.

Onwuegbuzie, A.J., Witcher, A.E., Collins, K.M.T., et al., 2007. Students' perceptions of characteristics of effective college teachers; A validity study of a teaching evaluation form using a mixed-methods analysis. Am. Educ. Res. J. 44 (1), 113–160.

Svinicki, M.D., McKeachie, W.J., 2013. McKeachie's Teaching Tips, fourteenth ed. Wadsworth Publishing, Belmont, CA.

Torre, D.M., Daley, B.J., Sebastian, J.L., Elnicki, D.M., 2006. Overview of current learning theories for medical educators APM perspectives. Am. J. Med. 119 (10), 903–907.

8 Learning in small groups

D. Torre, R. M. Conran, S. J. Durning

Trends

- Increasing emphasis on small-group teaching in both the preclinical and clinical settings
- Growing use of online learning environments and the role of small-group teaching and facilitation
- Increasing the use of self-assessment and peer students evaluations of group teaching

Medical educators can use a number of instructional situations for teaching learners (see Section 2). Small groups represent a teaching situation of growing importance in healthcare education.

Recent studies are beginning to unravel the reasons why small groups have a positive effect on learning performance (van Blankenstein et al., 2011). These studies cite both socio-behavioural and cognitive benefits. Socio-behavioural benefits include promoting learner motivation, social cohesion and authenticity. Cognitive benefits include facilitating elaboration and reflection or recourse to prior knowledge and experiences. For example, social interdependence theory (SIT) (Johnson & Johnson, 2009) provides a theoretical framework for small-group learning. It states that outcomes are defined by your own as well as others' actions. Positive interdependence is a crucial tenet of such theory, which occurs when the individual perceives that his or her own goals can only be achieved if the others in the group achieve their own goals. Therefore, the learner seeks outcomes that are ultimately beneficial to the whole group. Another theoretical framework arguing for the socio-behavioural benefits of small-group teaching is situated learning, which argues that learning is about becoming a member of a community.

Additionally, emotional engagement theories stress that instructional authenticity enables the learner to more meaningfully engage with the learning to enhance learning; small-group teaching enables the potential for more authentic instruction than that provided in the large-group setting.

The reader is encouraged to review the benefits of small-group teaching to maximize potential learning. Furthermore, recent work has shown that learning

situations can be complementary: for example, combining small-group teaching with large-group teaching during lectures (Chapter 7) can facilitate the potential benefits of instruction with each format.

What is a small group?

Small groups are instructional settings that better optimize the instructor-to-learner ratio and foster collaborative learning. Collaborative learning within a small group can be used to clarify concepts, stimulate discussion as well as learn from each other's inquiries and explanations. Small groups can complement large-group learning by having the purpose of clarifying and delve into specific issues that might have emerged from a large-group session, such as a lecture. Additionally, small groups can also help educators integrate material from multiple courses, such as a clinical reasoning small group on chest pain that could integrate anatomy, physiology and pathology concepts into the session.

The size of the small group can vary greatly in healthcare education. Prior studies suggest that groups of five to eight learners may be optimal. However, the number of students in a group should not conform to any set rule.

 The number of students in a small group should not conform to any set rule.

The goal with determining small-group size should focus on effectiveness that will be dependent upon goals and objectives for the session and learner experience/expertise with the content being discussed (i.e. difficulty of the content). For example, if the group is too small or the material is very straightforward to learn, exchange of ideas can be limited, so a balance should be struck in determining the number of students in a small group. The challenge for the healthcare educator is to construct a small-group size that will best facilitate exchange of ideas and concepts for the content being discussed given the learning goals and objectives for the session.

Newble and Cannon (2001) discuss three signature characteristics of small-group teaching: *active participation*, *purposeful activity*, and *face-to-face contact*. We believe that consistently achieving these three characteristics is essential for small-group teaching effectiveness.

 Three signature characteristics of small-group teaching are active participation, purposeful activity, and face-to-face contact.

According to these authors, if the small group lacks *any* of these components, the teaching activity will likely be suboptimal. For example, active participation and purposeful activity are needed for the cognitive benefits of elaboration and reflection. Elaboration and reflection accompanied with face-to-face contact are needed to optimize motivation and emotional engagement with the content. Indeed, the size of the group is less important than fulfilling these three characteristics. For example, effective team-based learning (Chapter 19) allows for larger groups through the formation of smaller 'subgroups' within the teaching setting and can capitalize on these three signature characteristics within each subgroup. Indeed, one of the most often cited reasons for combining lectures with small groups is that it is extremely difficult, if not impossible, to have active participation and purposeful activity in the typical large group lecture setting.

When to use small groups?

The reason(s) for choosing to incorporate small-group teaching into a curriculum should be primarily guided by learning goals and objectives. A secondary reason is the difficulty of the content being presented (which is dependent upon the expertise of the learner with the content). As stated above, if the content presented in the small-group session is too straightforward, the three signature characteristics discussed above are unlikely to be met. Further, since small groups are one of (if not the most) resource-intensive teaching format, the reason(s) for using this format should be carefully considered, weighing the pros and cons of this format with alternatives.

There are many advantages to teaching in small groups, and we have introduced some of the theoretical benefits of this teaching format at the outset of this chapter. Additional benefits include:

1. Small-group instructors can become more familiar with learner's knowledge, skills and experiences with the content being discussed than in larger group teaching settings. Instruction can therefore be more customized or tailored to the learners' needs in small groups. This benefit may be particularly important with complicated material, where learners may have a variety of differences in knowledge, skills and experiences and difficulty with integrating the material to be learned.

2. In small groups, the teacher has more opportunity for individualized feedback, which has been shown to be important, especially for learning complex information.

3. Peer evaluation and self-reflection can add to teacher-directed feedback to enhance the experience for learners.

4. Learners have the opportunity to get to know their classmates and may be more comfortable asking questions during a small-group session than in larger group settings; again this benefit may be particularly relevant when the content to be learned is difficult for the learner (because of their relative level of knowledge of and expertise with the content).

Another potential benefit of small-group teaching is that learners can become familiar with adult learning principles, which are something they will be encouraged to apply for the rest of their professional lives. For example, learners are encouraged to take responsibility for their own learning (self-directed learning or self-regulation, e.g. adequate preparation for the small group, asking questions during the session, follow-up readings after the small-group session has concluded), and learners are encouraged to use problem-solving and reflection skills. In a similar vein, small-group learners have the opportunity to develop important interpersonal and communication skills that they will use in their future practice. Small-group teaching also offers the opportunity for teachers to model professionalism, respect for different opinions, and time management. Finally, small-group teaching promotes engagement between the teacher, learner and content enabling the instructor to reinforce concepts that move beyond recalling content and asking trainees to apply this content in a more meaningful manner than in larger group settings. Therefore, small-group sessions should challenge the learner to apply what is learned in larger settings and/or from textbook readings.

These advantages come at the cost of needing additional faculty for instructional purposes, so medical schools in the United States and elsewhere typically include other teaching formats, such as lectures (face to face or online) and seminars, to introduce content to larger groups and use small-group teaching to reinforce key learning concepts. Finally, recent work from the cognitive-load literature suggests that using small-group sessions for straightforward content can actually increase extraneous (not useful for learning) cognitive-load in learners and potentially impair learning; therefore, careful construction of goals and objectives for the small-group session will help maximize chances of success.

 Careful construction of goals and objectives for the small-group session will help maximize chances of success.

Two additional questions that are relevant to when to use small-group teaching are: What format of small-group teaching? and What type of instructional methods?

WHAT FORMAT OF SMALL-GROUP TEACHING?

A number of small-group teaching formats exist. Formats of small-group teaching include problem-based learning (PBL) (see Chapter 18), case-based learning (CBL), and team-based learning (TBL) (see Chapter 19). This content is beyond the scope of this chapter. The reader is encouraged to review this content in other chapters of this book. A notable distinction between PBL, CBL and TBL is the role of the instructor. In PBL, the instructor is a facilitator; being a subject-matter expert on the content is not required. In CBL, the instructor is a facilitator but also typically provides summative comments at the end of the session, sharing their subject-matter expertise. In TBL, the instructor typically provides both facilitation and subject-matter expertise, the latter often provided through both summative comments and/or pre- and post-session quizzes.

WHAT TYPE OF INSTRUCTIONAL METHODS?

Several instructional methods for small-group teaching exist, and the number of methods involving robust technology is emerging (Box 8.1). Importantly, the most successful methods have clear goals and objectives and are organized around a purposeful activity. In healthcare education, the case-based structured discussion is probably the most common approach. Learners read about and then present a patient case and work through a series of tasks, which could include: asking for additional history and physical examination information, constructing a problem list, generating a differential diagnosis, comparing and contrasting diagnoses, and constructing a treatment plan. In the CBL and TBL formats, time is typically allocated for the small-group

Box 8.1 Instructional methods for small-group setting

- Surrogate patient encounters (i.e. paper cases, DVD cases, standardized patients)
- Actual patients
- Journal articles (e.g. thought-provoking reading material)
- Internet-based materials (e.g. Wiki, blog, discussion board)
- Role plays
- Multiple-choice or open-ended questions
- A pre-structured, partially completed - instructional unit of material

instructor to clarify important teaching points and answer additional questions. In the PBL method, emphasis is placed on asking questions, and the teacher may or may not provide summary or conclusion remarks. There are also instructional models, such as the 'one-minute preceptor', which can be particularly effective in clinical teaching of small groups (Neher et al., 1992). In this model, the teacher probes for understanding and then evaluates or comes to an educational diagnosis of the learner and provides next steps for improvement. One other model or technique that can be useful in teaching small groups in the clinical setting is SNAPPS (Wolpaw et al., 2009). In this technique, the teacher asks leaners to summarize findings, narrow and analyze the differential, while leaners can probe and ask questions to the preceptor, and then select a topic for self-study. This technique, like the one minute preceptor, can be most helpful in both the ambulatory or inpatient clinical setting with small groups of students (three to four).

One other instructional method that could promote small-group learning is concept mapping. The construction of a concept map by a small group of learners fosters interactions, promotes communication, creates sharing of knowledge and ultimately allows the group to critique and learn from each other in an active and meaningful way. Such strategy can be used in classrooms or in the setting of online learning.

How to effectively conduct a small-group teaching session

PREPARING FOR THE SMALL-GROUP SESSION

Preparing for the small-group teaching session shares many similarities to preparing for other teaching sessions, like larger group teaching sessions. First, determine the learning objectives for the session. Become familiar with students' experience (if any) with the content being discussed from other aspects of the curriculum. Know what 'success looks like' for the session.

 Know what 'success looks like' for the small group session.

This can be done by completing the statement, 'By the end of the session, learners will be able to...', keeping in mind that small-group sessions are an optimal place to ask learners to demonstrate higher-order skills, such as, problem solving, reflection, and clinical reasoning. The reader is encouraged to review materials (Huggett, 2010) on constructing goals and objectives. Second, know your audience (the learners) and the curriculum. For example, what has been the learners' prior experience with the content to be discussed in the small-group session in the curriculum? What topic or concept(s) might be particularly challenging for the learners? Third, become familiar with the structure of the small-group teaching session to include time for the session, instructional materials, and number of sessions. Think about the activities and methods needed to achieve success. For example, is a review of a pertinent case from the last session or beginning the session with one or more multiple-choice or open-ended questions needed? Fourth, it can also be very helpful to develop an instructional 'agenda' for the small-group teaching session. This optimally will be provided by the course or clerkship director (e.g. key teaching points and students' strengths or difficulties with the content from other aspects of the course). We believe that providing instructors with key teaching points, particularly for CBL and TBL, is important to maximize effectiveness of the session. These teaching points can also be used for examination purposes and should reflect what is essential: key elements for discussion in the session. We do not, however, believe that these key teaching points should require most or all of the time scheduled for the small-group session. Indeed, providing teachers with a comprehensive or highly time-consuming list for discussion can lead to mini-lectures and/or stifling discussion.

LEADING THE SMALL-GROUP SESSION

Experienced small-group instructors recognize that their teaching style and the dynamics of the group are important elements. The time that the instructor spends preparing in advance should improve the organization and flow of the session. The attitude and behaviour (both verbal and nonverbal) of the instructor is one of, if not the most critical element for small-group teaching success (Jaques, 2003). In the actual session, the focus should be on the *learner*.

We believe that an effective approach is to introduce your role at the first session, and let learners know how and when they can reach you outside of the session if they have additional questions or concerns. Each small group can be different based on the dynamics of the group members and the content being covered, so careful attention to the group dynamics as well as your own teaching strengths and weaknesses is important for success. Emphasizing the learner-centred approach is necessary for effective small-group sessions. In this approach, the teacher seeks understanding and provides frequent feedback to help the individual learner and the group to improve.

CONDITIONS FOR AN EFFECTIVE SESSION

The beginning of the small-group session is very important. In effective sessions, the instructor will typically set the learning climate, state the goals and objectives, and provide some basic 'ground rules', which outline what is acceptable and unacceptable behaviour (e.g. arriving late or holding 'sidebar' conversations). Ground rules are important because successful small

groups rarely occur simply because there is the meeting of a talented teacher with highly motivated learners. Discuss expectations for preparation, participation and evaluation. This is important, as studies suggest that when learners are aware of evaluation criteria, they are likely to be more willing to participate. Try to generate a learning environment that is cooperative rather than competitive, as the latter can lead to lack of participation by all but the most dominant members. A cooperative as opposed to a competitive learning environment can be particularly challenging to balance: evaluating learners while fostering a cooperative learning environment.

 "The secret of education is respecting the pupil."
Ralph Waldo Emerson

Some ways to improve this balance include making small-group session grades formative, using an evaluation system that sets learners up for success, and/or holding multiple small-group sessions with learners (e.g. they receive a grade at the very end versus after each session).

In the adult learning model, the teacher as lecturer is replaced with the teacher as facilitator. We believe that in a highly effective small-group session it may at times be difficult to distinguish the teacher from the learners. For instructors brought up in the lecture format of teaching and learning, small-group teaching can be a difficult skill set to acquire. Some teachers, who are highly effective in large-group settings (e.g. lectures) are not skilled at small-group teaching and will resort to mini-lectures if not provided with training in small-group teaching. Faculty development needs should be identified and addressed.

 Do not assume that a teacher's success in large-group teaching will equate to effective small-group teaching.

For example, highly effective lecturers may be uncomfortable with silence, unexpected discussion directions or how to convey key teaching points without using the podium with PowerPoint slides. Some general guidelines or tips for the small group teacher are given in Box 8.2.

We believe that small-group instructors need to understand group dynamics to be successful in this teaching format, particularly when the session is going in a less than optimal fashion. Scholtes et al., (2000) describe stages that groups often undergo that can help the small-group teacher. These four stages are outlined below and, notably, characteristics of an effective small-group teacher at each stage are listed in parentheses.

Forming: group members feel excitement and anticipation; some experience anxiety (develop relationships and establish rules)

Box 8.2 **Tips for a successful small-group session**

Define the problem and purposes of the session

Coordinate statements: clarify and relate statements versus lecturing

Seek information (request facts from learners) and opinions

Give information (fill in gaps in group knowledge)

Test feasibility (challenge practicality and correctness of suggested solutions)

Expect silence, lack of knowledge and uncertainty

Facilitate a positive learning environment

Give students positive feedback and don't ask 'read my mind' questions

Don't provide too much information (don't lecture and encourage students to follow up on questions raised during the session to enhance their learning)

Probe thinking process: try to think out loud with providing explanations to help students with complex tasks like clinical reasoning; ask students to explain their underlying thought process as well as the concepts they are applying, assumptions they are making and approach to the problem

Encourage participation of all group members (and prevent monopolization of the session by one or two students)

Practice higher-order skills (interpretation, reflection, synthesis, transfer)

Think out loud (students can benefit from hearing thoughts and feelings of others)

Stress the value of diversity of opinions and respect for peers

Facilitate learner interaction (enhance understanding, promoting teamwork)

Stress how a question can be addressed from many different perspectives

Review and reinforce teaching goals and objectives

Keep time constraints (time management skills)

Provide regular and timely feedback

Create learning material and tasks that emphasize sharing of information and group's communication

Create opportunities for informal interaction among members of the group (e.g. social gathering)

Storming: resistance to tasks or expressed concerns about too much work; arguments (aid resolution of issues)

Norming: demonstrate acceptance of others in group; cohesion; fosters discussion and feedback (promote collaboration)

Performing: group's ability to work through problems; understanding of strengths and weaknesses of group members (monitor progress and provide feedback)

Evaluating (assessing) the small-group session

Evaluation of the small-group session involves two components, *evaluation of small-group members* and *evaluation of the teacher*. The former is important to emphasize that the activity is a meaningful part of the curriculum, and the latter is important to help the instructor become even more effective in this role. Both foster communication skills (team member versus leader) that ultimately can affect patient care. From a programme evaluation perspective, small-group evaluation, in large part, reflects the adequacy of the learning environment (infrastructure, resources, and personnel).

Evaluation of small-group teaching and participation

It is important to make criteria for participation explicit to the learner. This may actually foster their participation. When possible, invite small-group learners to participate in determining criteria so they feel responsible for their learning and success of the group. Examples of criteria are available elsewhere. In establishing criteria for small-group evaluation, it is important to allow flexibility for small-group teacher style, provide clear guidelines that both teachers and learners can understand, and not set up a summative environment as this may detract from learner's participation. Students' self-assessment evaluation coupled with evaluation of their peers, teacher's evaluation from students and peer-teaching evaluations can all be useful tools to gather information about group teaching.

1. Students' self-assessment, and in particular students' evaluation of their peers in the group, may be helpful to avoid social loafing, thus enhancing individual accountability and responsibility. Social loafing is the reduction of individual effort when working with others, ultimately hindering achievement of the group's goals. Evaluation of small-group learning can be accomplished by assessing the group's ability to solve a clinical or educational problem, complete a project or create an instructional course. For

example, the teacher may provide a group with a clinical vignette of a patient with difficulty breathing and expect the group to generate a differential diagnosis of the problem coupled with an explanation of why each diagnosis is likely or unlikely. The ability of the group to search, analyze, process and synthesize information to arrive at a correct diagnosis may constitute a measurable learning outcome.

2. Teacher's evaluation: formal questionnaires and surveys may be given to students to evaluate the effectiveness of each teacher in the small-group setting, with a focus on his or her ability to act as a facilitator, role model and developer of instruction for the group.

3. Peer faculty evaluation is a particularly helpful and formative, yet often an underutilized evaluation strategy. Data can be collected through direct observation of teaching with a structured evaluation form or videotape review of a prior teaching session. Importantly, direct observation by peers should seek to obtain adequate sampling (view the teacher on multiple occasions) to ensure reliability of the data. Yet such formative evaluation strategy needs to be non-judgemental, immediate and delivered in a non-threatening way.

Also, evaluation data needs to be collected in an accurate and timely manner, and timing is an important issue as one does not want to collect such data too far after the actual teaching event.

Ultimately, providing small-group teachers with acknowledgments of excellence, such as teaching awards, can help motivate teachers, while promoting a climate of continual improvement. The reader is encouraged to view resources regarding this topic, which is beyond the scope of this chapter.

Encouraging faculty participation should be the goal of any academic institution. Faculty (instructors) can benefit in several ways. Most important is enhancing their own communication skills that ultimately enhance patient care. Encouraging faculty participation also serves as a means to expose learners to the various specialties in medicine. Exposure to different clinical specialties (e.g. internal medicine and surgery) of instructors may affect learner's career choices. Faculty participation also provides the learner with a potential mentor based on a mutual rapport that can continue throughout the curriculum. Institutional support through monetary bonuses, faculty appointments, continuing medical education credit and academic awards can also enhance involvement. In addition to the above, institutions may benefit from small-group

teaching as a recruitment tool to recruit faculty who seek opportunities for student interaction and to document active learning as an accreditation criterion.

Summary

Small-group teaching can be a highly effective educational method. Benefits of this method can be maximized by carefully considering the goals and objectives of the session, by providing materials in which the learners can meaningfully engage in the content, having awareness of small-group teaching benefits, and incorporating a system of learner as well as teacher evaluation and feedback that is clear and explicit. The attitude of the teacher and rapport developed with the learner is also critical for success. Knowledge of some of the theoretical frameworks of small group learning coupled with the practice of a few effective techniques can greatly enhance teaching effectiveness in the small-group setting.

Further information

Huggett, K.N., 2010. Teaching in small groups. In: Jeffries, W.B., Huggett, K. (Eds.), An Introduction to Medical Teaching. Springer, London, pp. 27–39.

Jaques, D., 2003. Teaching small groups. BMJ 326, 492–494.

Johnson, D.W., Johnson, R.T., 2009. An educational psychology success story: social interdependence theory and cooperative learning. Educ. Res. 38 (5), 365–379.

Neher, J.O., Gordon, K.C., Meyer, B., Stevens, N., 1992. A five-step "microskills" model of clinical teaching. J. Am. Board Fam. Pract. 5, 419–424.

Newble, D.I., Cannon, R.A. (Eds.), 2001. A Handbook for Medical Teachers, forth ed. Kluwer Academic Publishers, The Netherlands.

Scholtes, P.R., Joiner, B.L., Joiner, B.J., 2000. The TEAM Handbook. Oriel, Inc, Madison, WI.

van Blankenstein, F.M., Dolmans, D.H.J.M., van der Vleuten, C.P.M., Schmidt, H.G., 2011. Which cognitive processes support learning during small-group discussion? The role of providing explanations and listening to others. Instr. Sci. 39 (2), 189–204.

Wolpaw, T.P., Papp, K.K., Bordage, G., 2009. Using SNAPPS to facilitate the expression of clinical reasoning and uncertainties: a randomized comparison group trial. Acad. Med. 84 (4), 517–524.

9 Learning with patients: inpatient and outpatient

J. A. Dent, S. Ramani

Trends

- Bedside teaching provides a unique opportunity for clinical tutors to role-model a holistic approach to patient care.
- Educational strategies provide a road map for maximizing the usefulness of this resource for student learning.
- Ambulatory care teaching is worthy of further development and investment by medical schools and teaching hospitals.
- New approaches to clinical assessment and staff development should be adopted to maximize the learning opportunities provided by inpatients and outpatients.

Introduction

Clinical teaching at the bedside is the essence of medical school experience. Students are motivated by the stimulus of patient contact, they learn to apply the theoretical concepts learned during preclinical years and discover the humanism of medicine; the art that goes with the science.

 "To study the phenomena of disease without books is to sail an uncharted sea, whilst to study books without patients is not to go to sea at all."

Sir William Osler

But the traditional, consultant-led ward round, which epitomises the view of bedside teaching, has not been without its shortcomings. Students may feel academically unprepared or inexperienced in the learning style required in an unfamiliar environment. Perceived inappropriate comments, unpredictable starts, cancellations and a chaotic work environment may discourage students and decrease the value of the experience. Advances in medical treatment and changing patterns

of healthcare delivery have led towards increased ambulatory and community care such that today's teaching hospitals may paradoxically have fewer patients appropriate for bedside teaching than previously. For the purposes of this chapter, we define bedside teaching as one that occurs whenever patients are present: hospital wards, ambulatory teaching, clinical conferences and simulation centres where students practise patient-care skills.

 "More medicine is now practiced in the ambulatory setting making the in-patient arena less representative of the actual practice of medicine and a less desirable place for students to glean the fundamentals of clinical care and problem solving than in the past."

Fincher & Albritton, 1993

Despite these challenges, bedside teaching provides optimal opportunities for the demonstration and observation of physical examination, communication skills, interpersonal skills and for role modelling a holistic approach to patient care. Not surprisingly, this form of teaching is rated as one of the most valuable methods of clinical teaching. Yet, bedside teaching has been declining in medical schools since the early 1960s (Peters & Ten Cate, 2014). While time constraints are often reported as a major barrier, it also appears that clinical acumen is now perceived as being of secondary importance to clinical imaging and extensive investigations (Ramani & Orlander, 2013).

The 'learning triad'

Traditional clinical teaching brings together the 'learning triad' of patient, student and clinician/tutor in a particular clinical environment. When all works well, this provides an ideal situation for effective student learning. Direct contact with patients is essential for the development of clinical reasoning, communication skills, professional attitudes and empathy, but preparation is required from each party involved.

"Skills such as professionalism, humanism and patient communication are best taught at the bedside, and proficiency in clinical skills may eventually decrease the overreliance on investigations."

Ramani & Orlander, 2013

PATIENTS

Before the session, patients should be invited to participate and have the opportunity to decline to participate without feeling coerced. Some institutions may require formal documentation of informed consent. Patients should be adequately briefed about the goals of the session and who the participants will be.

During the session, patients should be actively engaged in the discussion and feel welcome to participate. Depending on the model of ward teaching used, a variety of patients will be required for varying lengths of time but remember that consideration should be given to their needs and the possibility that other healthcare staff and visitors may also need to see them. Usually patients enjoy the experience and feel they have contributed to student learning.

Afterwards, patients may be asked to give some simple feedback to students. Don't forget to thank patients for taking part and to clarify any confusions that may have been created.

STUDENTS

It is best if students have had some prior experience with simulated patients in supervised learning venues where they have practised physical examination and communication skills. Between two and five students is probably the optimal number for bedside teaching. Students should comply with the medical school's directives on appropriate appearance and behaviour and, if unaccompanied by a clinical tutor, should introduce themselves to staff and patients clearly stating the purpose of their visit.

During the teaching session, students may feel intimidated by the unfamiliar environment, the proximity of other healthcare staff and putting personal questions to patients. They may be unsure of their knowledge base or clinical abilities and fearful of consultant criticism. As a result, some may avoid participation, while others monopolize conversations with patients and tutors. Tutors need to look out for these behaviours, provide a non-threatening learning environment, allay anxieties and ensure that all students have the opportunity to participate.

Afterwards, remember to debrief the students, provide time for questions, and clarify any misunderstandings.

TUTORS

Tutors for bedside teaching in all clinical settings may be consultant staff, junior hospital doctors, nurses or student peers. Preparation is critical to a successful bedside teaching session and may include enhancing clinical skills, establishing educational goals, orienting patients ahead of time and being prepared to deal with unpredictable incidents that may arise (Cox, 1993).

 The seven roles of a clinician/teacher useful for achieving good clinical teaching:
* medical expert
* communicator
* collaborator
* manager
* advocate
* scholar
* professional.

Appropriate knowledge

Experienced clinical teachers are soon able to assess both the patient's diagnosis and requirements as well as the students' level of understanding. This ability to link clinical reasoning with instructional reasoning enables them to quickly adapt the clinical teaching session to the needs of the students.

Six domains of knowledge have been described, which an effective clinical tutor will apply (Irby, 1992):
* Knowledge of medicine: integrating the patient's clinical problem to background knowledge of basic sciences, clinical sciences and clinical experience
* Knowledge of patients: a familiarity with disease and illness from experience of previous patients
* Knowledge of the context: an awareness of patients in their social context and their stage of treatment
* Knowledge of learners: an understanding of the students' present stage in the course and of the curriculum requirements for that stage
* Knowledge of the general principles of teaching, including:
  - getting students involved in the learning process by indicating its relevance
  - asking questions, perhaps by using the patient as an example of a problem-solving approach to the condition
  - keeping students' attention by indicating the relevance of the topic to another learning situation
  - relating the case being presented to broader aspects of the curriculum
  - meeting individual needs by responding to specific questions and providing personal tuition

- being realistic and selective so that relevant cases are chosen
- providing feedback by critiquing case reports, presentations or examination technique
• Knowledge of case-based teaching scripts: the ability to demonstrate the patient as representative of a certain clinical problem. The specifics of the case are used but added to from other knowledge and experiences in order to make further generalised comments about the condition.

Appropriate skills

If demonstrating clinical tasks to students in the ward or ambulatory setting, tutors should be competent in performing them in whatever uniform approach has been taught in the clinical skills centre. They should avoid demonstrating inappropriate 'shortcuts' to junior students. Validated shortcuts can be taught to more senior students with detailed explanation of their appropriate use.

Appropriate attitudes

Whether they appreciate its significance or not, tutors are powerful role models for students, so it is most important that they demonstrate appropriate knowledge, skills and attitudes (Cruess et al., 2008).

 "The essential feature is enthusiasm on the part of the teacher."

Rees, 1987

Any tutor responsible for scheduled clinical teaching, in the wards, clinics, clinical conferences or simulation centres, must arrive punctually, introduce themselves to the students and demonstrate an enthusiastic approach to the session. A negative impression at this stage will have an immediate negative effect on the students' attitude and on the value of the session. Tutors should show a professional approach to the patients and interact appropriately with them and the students.

Afterwards, try to reflect on the teaching event and identify any parts you could have done better.

Educational strategies for bedside teaching

Though models for effective bedside teaching have been described specifically for ward-based and ambulatory teaching, many of these educational principles and strategies can be adapted for different clinical settings. Some established models are described in this section.

Strategies for inpatients

COX'S CYCLE

A linked two-cycle model has been described (Cox, 1993) to maximize the students' learning from each patient contact.

The 'experience cycle', involves student preparation and briefing to ensure that they are aware of what they are going to see and the opportunities available for learning. Before beginning, students should be briefed so that they understand the purpose of the session and the goals to be achieved. Any warnings about the patient conditions to be seen should be given and checks made on students' level of initial understanding. This is followed by the clinical experience of interacting with their patient, which may include history taking and physical examination, discussing the illness and thinking about management.

After leaving the patient, the experience cycle concludes with debriefing when the information gathered is reviewed and interpreted and any misperceptions or misunderstandings clarified. The experience cycle maximizes the value of the time spent with the patient.

The 'explanation cycle' begins with reflection when students are encouraged to consider their recent clinical interaction in the light of previous experiences. Explication continues with the understanding of the clinical experiences at different levels according to the students' stage of learning and its integration into their previous learning experiences. Finally, a working knowledge is synthesised, which prepares the students for seeing a subsequent patient (Fig. 9.1).

 Twelve tips to improve bedside teaching (Ramani, 2003):
  1. Preparation: revise your own skills, the learners' needs and the curriculum.
  2. Planning: construct a road map of the activities and objectives of the session.
  3. Orientation: orientate the learners to your plans for the session.
  4. Introduction: introduce everyone present including the patient!
  5. Interaction: role-model a doctor–patient interaction.
  6. Observation: watch how the students are proceeding.
  7. Instruction: provide instruction.
  8. Summary: tell the students what they have been taught.
  9. Debriefing: time for questions and clarifications.
  10. Feedback: allow time to give positive and constructive feedback to students.
  11. Reflection: evaluate from your perspective what went well and what was less successful.
  12. Preparation: prepare for your next bedside teaching session.

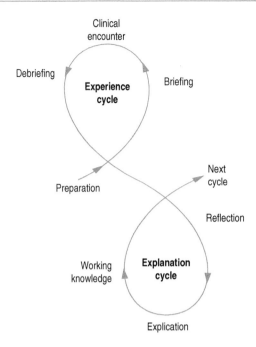

Clinical
encounter

Debriefing

**Experience
cycle**

Briefing

Preparation

Next
cycle

Reflection

Working
knowledge

**Explanation
cycle**

Explication

Fig. 9.1 Experience and explanation cycles.

(redrawn from Cox, 1993, with modifications).

MIPLAN

Stickrath and colleagues described a three-part model for efficient bedside teaching (Stickrath et al., 2013):

- M: meeting between teacher and learners to get acquainted, set goals, clarify expectations
- I: five teaching behaviours at the bedside:
    - introductions: introducing the team to patients and orienting them to the agenda
    - in the moment: focused listening
    - inspection: observation of patient and engagement of entire team
    - interruptions: minimizing them
    - independent thought: encouraging clinical reasoning.
- PLAN: algorithm for teaching after bedside presentations
    - patient care: clarification of clinical findings, role-modelling
    - learners' questions: responding to questions
    - attending's agenda: teaching points, referring to relevant literature
    - next steps: debriefing, feedback, questions for further learning.

Strategies for outpatients

A structured approach is the key to maximizing the learning opportunities available to students in any ambulatory care venue (Dent, 2005). Two key models, SNAPPS and microskills for students are described below.

LEARNER-CENTRED APPROACH

Students present cases to their tutor in a structured way under the heading SNAPPS, which encourages a question and answer approach (Wolpaw et al., 2003).
Summarise the history and physical findings
Narrow down the differential diagnosis
Analyze the diagnosis by comparing possibilities
Probe the preceptor with questions
Plan patient management
Select a case issue for self-directed learning

MICROSKILLS FOR STUDENTS

Lipsky and colleagues describe how students can take the initiative both before and after the outpatient event to facilitate their own learning (Lipsky et al., 1999).

 Twelve tips for students to improve their learning in the ambulatory setting:
1. Orientate to the objectives of the session
2. Share their stage of clinical experience with the tutor
3. Orientate to the clinical location
4. Read around the clinical conditions to be seen
5. Review case notes or summaries provided
6. Be prepared to propose a diagnosis and management plan
7. Explain their reasons for these decisions
8. Seek self-assessment opportunities
9. Seek feedback time from the tutor
10. Generalize the learning experience
11. Reflect on their learning
12. Identify future learning issues

Based on Lipsky et al, 1999

Educational strategies applicable to all clinical settings

OUTCOME-BASED EDUCATION

Though many of the educational objectives of the clinical curriculum are experienced to different extents by students in individual ward-based or ambulatory clinical rotations, combined they span the complete spectrum of desired outcomes (Fig. 9.2), for example:
- Clinical skills: history taking and physical examination
- Communication skills

- Clinical reasoning
- Practical procedures: venepuncture, etc.
- Patient investigation and management: requesting laboratory investigations
- Data interpretation and retrieval
- Professional skills
- Transferable skills
- Attitude and ethics

See Chapter 15 *Outcome-based education.*

All these aspects can be seen in the context of the patient as an individual rather than in the purely theoretical context presented in lectures. Students should be encouraged to plan private study time to practise clinical skills further.

TIME-EFFICIENT STRATEGIES FOR LEARNING AND PERFORMANCE

Irby and Wilkerson describe strategies for teaching when time is limited (Irby & Wilkerson, 2008) (Box 9.1).

STRUCTURED LOGBOOKS

A structured logbook can help students to organise the content of their ambulatory care and inpatient sessions to easily identify the educational opportunities available. It should direct students on how to continue

their learning after the event. The EPITOMISE logbook, based on the learning outcomes of the Scottish Doctor, has been used to focus student learning by asking them to document their experiences under each learning outcome point and reflect on what further learning needs they can now identify and meet (Dent & Davis, 1995). The variety of patients with clinical

---

Box 9.1 Teaching strategies for clinical teachers

Planning
- Direct/orientate learners
- Create a positive learning environment
- Pre-select patients
- Prime/brief learners

Teaching
- Teach from clinical cases
- Use questions to diagnose learners
- Ask advanced learners to participate in teaching
- Use 'illness scripts' and 'teaching scripts'

Evaluating and reflecting
- Evaluate learners
- Provide feedback
- Promote self-assessment and self-directed learning

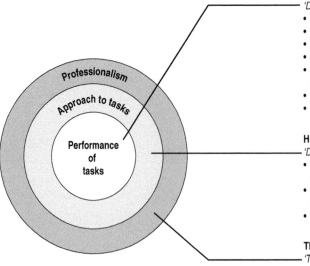

What a doctor is able to do
'Doing the right thing'
- Competence in clinical skills
- Competence in practical procedures
- Competence in investigating a patient
- Competence in patient management
- Competence in health promotion and disease prevention
- Competence in communication
- Competence in handling and retrieval of information

How the doctor approaches their practice
'Doing the thing right'
- With understanding of basic, clinical and social sciences and underlying principles
- With appropriate attitudes, ethical stance and legal responsibilities
- With appropriate decision making, clinical reasoning and judgement

The doctor as a professional
'The right person doing it'
- An understanding of the doctor's role in the health service
- An aptitude for personal development and a demonstration of appropriate transferable skills

Fig. 9.2 The 12 learning outcomes of the Scottish Doctor (Simpson et al, 2002).

problems suitable for students will inevitably vary in all real clinical settings and clinical teaching, particularly in inpatient settings, tends to be opportunistic. Logbooks may thus be used to assess the range of clinical conditions seen and identify omissions in student experience, but their primary role should be to help students reflect on their clinical experiences and provide a focus for periodic tutor-review, mentoring and feedback.

TASK-BASED LEARNING

A list of tasks to be performed or procedures to be observed and carried out is usually a course requirement in ward-based and ambulatory rotations. Students should be given this list and their proficiency in any of these tasks can be scored in their clinical record book. These tasks may include:

- Participate in consultation with the attending staff.
- Interview and examine patients.
- Review a number of new radiographs with the radiologist.
- Observe specific inpatient and outpatient procedures performed by junior doctors or consultants.
  Additional tasks for future learning can then be built around each.

PROBLEM-BASED LEARNING

The patient's presenting complaint can be used as the focus of a problem-based learning exercise in which basic sciences and clinical sciences can be integrated. If feasible, patients can be invited to attend these conferences and interact directly with students. The presence of patients always adds great educational value to all sessions.

STUDY GUIDES

A prescribed list of conditions to be seen in the ward or ambulatory settings may be laid out in the study guide with the learning points to be achieved documented for each.

CASE STUDIES

'Focus scripts' described by Peltier and colleagues (Peltier et al., 2007) are used to facilitate the learning of history taking and physical examination skills. Similarly, using the patient journey as a model, students may be directed to follow a patient through a series of ambulatory care experiences from the outpatient department, through clinical investigations and preoperative assessment to the day-surgery unit and follow-up clinic (Hanna & Dent, 2006). This strategy can also be applied effectively to the ward-based environment.

Hospital ward opportunities – models for managing learning in the ward

APPRENTICESHIP/SHADOWING A JUNIOR DOCTOR MODEL

Shadowing a junior doctor for several weeks on the unit where they will subsequently be working has become a required part of the final-year programme for medical students in the United Kingdom. Opportunities are plentiful for junior doctors to model task-based learning and professionalism.

GRAND ROUNDS

Popular in some countries, this consultant-led ward round or conference room presentation usually includes senior clinicians, trainees, junior doctors and other healthcare professionals.

BUSINESS WARD ROUND

This is a challenging activity for both clinicians and students. Little time is available for formal teaching, observing student performance or providing feedback. It may be necessary for the clinician to explain decisions being made in a variety of levels of complexity depending on the experience or seniority of others on the ward round. There may be little time for direct student teaching, but time-efficient teaching strategies described above would be effective in this setting.

TEACHING WARD ROUND

In this specially scheduled teaching event, students see a small number of selected patients who provide opportunities to elicit physical signs and hear aspects of the case history. At the bedside the tutor can lead the session in different ways:

- *Demonstrator model.* The clinical tutor demonstrates aspects of the case history and physical examination to the students.
- *Tutor model.* The clinical tutor stands to the side and critiques each student in turn as they interview the patient and carry out physical examination.
- *Observer model.* The clinical tutor observes a single student or pair of students in a longer portion of history taking or examination, providing feedback to them all at the end as they discuss their findings and clinical interpretation.
- *Report-back model.* Students interview and examine patients without supervision and subsequently report back to the tutor elsewhere to present the case and receive feedback on content and delivery.

CLINICAL CONFERENCE

Diagnostic and management problems are discussed by the group of healthcare professionals. Students have the opportunity to observe the multifaceted management of difficult cases and the spectrum of professional input that may be required.

TRAINING WARD

A purpose-made training ward has been found to provide students with a useful opportunity to develop skills and knowledge in relation to patient management and interprofessional teamwork (Reeves et al., 2002).

Ambulatory care opportunities

WHEN SHOULD AMBULATORY CARE TEACHING BE PROVIDED?

As hospital wards may no longer have patients with common clinical problems who are sufficiently well to see students, ambulatory care can offer a wide range of suitable clinical opportunities for undergraduates at all stages of learning. Less experienced students who are still developing their communication and examination skills can practise these in the dedicated teaching environment of the ambulatory care teaching centre (ACTC), which provides a stepping-stone from practising with simulated patients and manikins in the clinical skills centre to meeting real patients in the busy environment of everyday outpatient department.

In later clinical years, when students have more extensive clinical experience, placement in routine clinics may be more appropriate. In these circumstances, students can often learn as apprentices as part of the clinical team.

TRADITIONAL VENUES

Having one student joining a clinician in their clinic can be a relatively straightforward experience, but a variety of models can be used depending on their experience.

Sitting-in model

One-to-one teaching is much appreciated by students who can observe the patient consultation by sitting with the clinician as they learn to interact confidently with the clinician and patients, but they may not have the chance to see patients independently. Less confident students may feel vulnerable in this setting and need encouragement to participate but more senior students may be able to function more fully.

Apprenticeship/parallel consultation model

A small number of senior students may be able to interview the patient either alone or under supervision. This involves active student–patient interaction, which reinforces learning. Some students may feel intimidated when performing under observation, but if a separate room is available they can interview and examine a patient without constraints before later presenting the case to the tutor. Walters and colleagues found that the overall consultation time was not increased when rural GPs supervised medical students in this model (Walters et al., 2008).

Report-back model

Students see patients without supervision and at an appointed time present them to the clinician. Students have time and space to interview and examine their patient at their own pace. Meanwhile, the clinician will have been able to see other patients attending the clinic independently.

 Decide which model you are going to use in your clinic depending on how many rooms are available for you to use and how many members of staff are available to help with the clinic. Don't be afraid to change models during the clinic to vary the session for the students and yourself.

Other models may be useful if a larger group is attending your clinic.

Grandstand model

Frequently, students are crowded into the consulting room attempting to observe and hear the consultation. Interaction with both patient and clinician is limited, and patients may feel threatened by the large audience. The clinician's interaction with the patient may also be inhibited. The use of a study guide or logbook to direct independent learning may be helpful for students here.

Breakout model

Students sit in with the clinician and observe a whole consultation with a patient. They then take it in turns, individually or in pairs, to take the patients to another room to go over parts of the interview or examination again at their own pace.

Supervising model

If several rooms are available, the students may be divided into smaller groups to see selected patients independently in a separate room. After a suitable time, the clinician can go to each room in turn to hear the students' report on their interview. The students have time and space to interview and examine their patient at their own pace and benefit from individual feedback on their performance.

ADDITIONAL VENUES

Teaching opportunities with outpatients may also be found in clinical investigations units, the radiology unit, the day surgery unit, a dialysis unit as well as in clinic waiting areas and with other healthcare professionals.

INNOVATIVE VENUES

Ambulatory care teaching centre (ACTC)

This specific teaching area provides a structured programme for teaching with ambulatory patients. An ambulatory care teaching centre (Dent et al., 2001) can give students the opportunity to meet selected patients with problems relevant to their stage of learning and timetabled clinical tutors who are not being required to provide patient care at the same time. Unlike a routine outpatient clinic this protected environment helps students to feel comfortable to practise focused interview or examination skills free from embarrassment or time constraints.

Clinicians with an interest in teaching can be asked to take special teaching sessions in the ACTC, often with the help of patients invited to attend from a 'bank' of patient volunteers. Students can rotate between different tutors who can supervise different activities such as history taking, physical examination or procedural skills.

Supplementary resources such as summarised case notes for the patients invited, laboratory reports, radiographs or revision material from basic sciences all help students to integrate their learning. A supply of video recordings to illustrate history taking and clinical examination technique provide a useful backup resource.

Integrated ambulatory care programme

In the University of Otago, Dunedin, an ambulatory care teaching resource has been created to provide fourth-year students with the opportunity to see a variety of invited patients illustrating clinical conditions in particular organ systems. Students appreciated the dedicated and structured teaching time in a learner-friendly environment (Latta et al., 2013).

 Developing a teaching programme in ambulatory care requires:
the identification of available venues
development of innovative teaching venues
the cooperation of enthusiastic staff
a structured approach to teaching and learning
a staff development programme
establishing a patient 'bank'
team-based approach to teaching (consultants, nurses, allied healthcare professionals, etc.)

Assessment of bedside learning

Assessment of bedside skills may be carried out through review of written material (Denton et al., 2006).

* Tutor review of a logbook or e-logbook can be done by the tutor in isolation but is more

valuable for formative assessment if carried out together with the student.

* A checklist can be used to monitor tasks accomplished during the session, but descriptors should be used to guide the assessor to evaluate the level of student competency achieved more precisely.
* Reflective diaries are valuable for student revision and reflection and also to identify any omissions in their learning.

Alternatively, students' clinical skills can be formally assessed (see Chapter 35, *Performance assessment*), but this may be more difficult given the time constraints of the inpatient and ambulatory care settings.

* Mini CEX (Norcini et al., 2003). Multiple short, focused assessments of clinical skills followed by feedback are carried out by a variety of assessors during the attachment.
* Direct observation of procedural skills (DOPS) (Norcini & Burch, 2007). The student's or trainee's ability to carry out a wide range of procedures can be closely assessed using a structured score sheet followed by feedback.
* Microskills for students (Lipsky et al., 1999). Students take the initiative to seek self-assessment opportunities and feedback throughout the clinical session.

Staff development

 Seven factors of effective teaching:
* knowledge
* organisation and clarity
* enthusiasm
* group instructional skills
* clinical supervision skills
* clinical competence
* modelling professional characteristics.

Irby et al., 1991

All those involved in clinical teaching bring a different perspective to patient care, which is valuable for student learning. Sometimes they will have received no specific preparation for the teaching session, and may not know how any particular session fits into the totality of the students' clinical experience at a particular stage of the course. Tutors' individual approaches to clinical examination will also differ as examination technique may not be standardised within the medical school. While it may be of benefit for more confident students to observe a variety of different approaches to clinical skills, weaker ones will find this lack of consistency confusing. Ideally, tutors should be briefed so that they are familiar with the approach to physical examination taught in the clinical skills centre and with the levels

Table 9.1 Training clinicians for their teaching role

Tasks of a clinical teacher (doing the right thing)	Approach to teaching (doing the thing right)	Teacher as a professional (the right person doing it)
Time efficient teaching Inpatient teaching Outpatient teaching Teaching at the bedside Work-based assessment of learners in the clinical setting Providing feedback	Showing enthusiasm for teaching and towards learners Understanding learning principles relevant to clinical teaching Using appropriate teaching strategies for different levels of learners Knowing and applying principles of effective feedback Modelling good, professional behaviour including evidence-based patient care Grasping the unexpected teaching moment	Soliciting feedback on teaching Self-reflection on teaching strengths and weaknesses Seeking professional development in teaching Mentoring and seeking mentoring Engaging in educational scholarship

of expertise required of students at the various stages of the medical course.

Formal staff development sessions may be required to help colleagues unfamiliar with the medical school curriculum, student learning needs, or with clinical teaching in the context of providing patient care. Simple instructional booklets can be used for on-the-spot instruction and advice (Dent & Davis, 2008).

The importance of training clinicians for their teaching role has been repeatedly emphasised. Ramani and Leinster (Ramani & Leinster, 2008) have particularly applied this model for teachers in the clinical environment (Table 9.1).

Summary

The ward setting, traditionally the bastion of clinical learning experiences, is no longer the dominant venue for clinical teaching as inpatients are now fewer in number and more often acutely ill. Transferring the emphasis of teaching to the ambulatory care setting opens a number of previously underutilised venues for student–patient interaction, namely 'bedside teaching'. The educational objectives to be achieved are different in ward-based and ambulatory teaching, but are synergistic and complement each other.

A teaching programme optimally combining ward-based and ambulatory care can be facilitated by:
- the identification of all available clinical venues in combination with case-based conferences
- developing new and innovative teaching venues, such as a simulated ward or ambulatory care teaching centre
- a structured approach to teaching and learning
- developing a volunteer patient 'bank' for teaching exercises
- a staff development programme
- establishment of a team-based approach to clinical teaching utilizing staff from a variety of healthcare disciplines.

Ward-based and ambulatory-based teaching offer unique opportunities for student learning, but each setting comes with its own set of challenges. To attain maximum benefit from all clinical venues, patients, students and tutors must each be appropriately prepared and the educational objectives must be understood. Various strategies can be used in both the planning and organisation of clinical teaching, and a variety of models to manage student–patient interaction in various settings can offer maximum advantage. Finally, a variety of teaching styles can be utilized to provide the widest spectrum of learning opportunities for the students.

 "A good consultant is accessible, approachable and friendly, with the power of a god, the patience of a saint and the sense of humour of an undergraduate."

Lowry, 1987

References

Cox, K., 1993. Planning bedside teaching–2. Preparation before entering the wards. Med. J. Aust. 158 (5), 355–495.

Cruess, S.R., Cruess, R.L., Steinert, Y., 2008. Role modelling–making the most of a powerful teaching strategy. BMJ 336 (7646), 718–721.

Dent, J.A., 2005. AMEE Guide No 26: clinical teaching in ambulatory care settings: making the most of learning opportunities with outpatients. Med. Teach. 2794, 302–315.

Dent, J.A., Angell-Preece, H.M., Ball, H.M., Ker, J.S., 2001. Using the Ambulatory Care Teaching Centre to develop opportunities for integrated learning. Med. Teach. 23 (2), 171–175.

Dent, J.A., Davis, M.H., 1995. Role of ambulatory care for student-patient interaction: the EPITOME model. Med. Educ. 29 (1), 58–60.

Dent, J.A., Davis, M.H., 2008. "Getting Started..." A Practical Guide for Clinical Tutors. University of Dundee, Centre for Medical Education, Dundee.

Denton, G.D., Demott, C., Pangaro, L.N., Hemmer, P.A., 2006. Narrative review: use of student-generated logbooks in undergraduate medical education. Teach. Learn. Med. 18 (2), 153–164.

Hanna, A., Dent, J.A., 2006. Developing teaching opportunities in a day surgery unit. Clin. Teach. 3 (3), 180–184.

Irby, D.M., Ramsay, P.G., Gillmore, G.M., Schaad, D., 1991. Characteristics of effective clinical teachers of ambulatory care medicine. Acad. Med. 66 (1), 54–55.

Irby, D.M., 1992. How attending physicians make instructional decisions when conducting teaching rounds. Acad. Med. 67 (10), 630–638.

Irby, D.M., Wilkerson, L., 2008. Teaching when time is limited. BMJ 336 (7640), 384–387.

Latta, L., Tordoff, D., Manning, P., Dent, J., 2013. Enhancing clinical skill development through an Ambulatory Medicine Teaching Programme: an evaluation study. Med. Teach. 35 (8), 648–654.

Lipsky, M., Taylor, C., Schnuth, R., 1999. Microskills for students: twelve tips for improving learning in the ambulatory setting. Med. Teach. 21 (5), 469–472.

Norcini, J., Burch, V., 2007. Workplace-based assessment as an educational tool: AMEE Guide No. 31. Med. Teach. 29 (9), 855–871.

Norcini, J.J., Blank, L.L., Duffy, F.D., Fortna, G.S., 2003. The mini-CEX: a method for assessing clinical skills. Ann. Intern. Med. 138 (6), 476–481.

Peltier, D., Regan-Smith, M., Wofford, J., et al., 2007. Teaching focused histories and physical exams in ambulatory care: a multi-institutional randomized trial. Teach. Learn. Med. 19 (3), 244–250.

Peters, M., Ten Cate, O., 2014. Bedside teaching in medical education: a literature review. Perspect Med. Educ. 3 (2), 76–88.

Ramani, S., 2003. Twelve tips to improve bedside teaching. Med. Teach. 25 (2), 112–115.

Ramani, S., Leinster, S., 2008. AMEE Guide no. 34: teaching in the clinical environment. Med. Teach. 30 (4), 347–364.

Ramani, S., Orlander, J.D., 2013. Human dimensions in bedside teaching: focus group discussions of teachers and learners. Teach. Learn. Med. 25 (4), 312–318.

Reeves, S., Freeth, D., Mccrorie, P., Perry, D., 2002. It teaches you what to expect in future ...': interprofessional learning on a training ward for medical, nursing, occupational therapy and physiotherapy students. Med. Educ. 36 (4), 337–344.

Simpson, J.G., Furnace, J., Crosby, J., et al., 2002. The Scottish doctor - leaning outcomes for the medical undergraduate in Scotland: a foundation for competent and reflective practitioners. Med. Teach. 14, 136–143.

Stickrath, C., Aagaard, E., Anderson, M., 2013. MiPLAN: a learner-centered model for bedside teaching in today's academic medical centers. Acad. Med. 88 (3), 322–327.

Walters, L., Worley, P., Prideaux, D., Lange, K., 2008. Do consultations in rural general practice take more time when practitioners are precepting medical students? Med. Educ. 42 (1), 69–73.

Wolpaw, T.M., Wolpaw, D.R., Papp, K.K., 2003. SNAPPS: a learner-centered model for outpatient education. Acad. Med. 78 (9), 893–898.

Learning in the community

I. D. Couper, P. S. Worley

Trends

- Care of undifferentiated patients, typically found at community level, is a basis for learning of clinical reasoning and integration of theory into clinical practice.
- Context is critical. Multiple contexts are needed, including community contexts, to prepare graduates for practice. Implementation of community-based medical education (CBME) will also vary significantly over different contexts.
- Early exposure to communities provides a constructive foundation for learning.
- Longitudinal exposure to the same community, over the course of an academic year or an entire degree programme, has been found to be beneficial as it enables meaningful and motivating pedagogic relationships between students, patients and clinicians.
- Community engagement – reciprocal involvement with communities – is a critical element of social accountability.
- A 'symbiotic' approach of collaboration between stakeholders enhances CBME.
- CBME is enhanced if the focus of a curriculum is on learning rather than teaching.

Introduction

Medical schools are searching for new sites in which to prepare the next generation of doctors. This is being driven by the need for global scaling up of health professions education, creating pressure on tertiary academic hospitals that have limited capacity to absorb students, and the challenges faced in producing fit-for-purpose, high-quality medical graduates who can practise competently at all levels of the healthcare system. One solution, for many schools, is community-based medical education (CBME).

What is community-based medical education?

CBME refers to medical education that is conducted outside a tertiary or large secondary level hospital.

Community-oriented medical education, on the other hand, describes curricula that are based on addressing the health needs of the local community and preparing graduates to work in that community. More recently, the term 'community-engaged medical education' has been used to describe the combination of both community-oriented and community-based medical education where, in addition, members of the community are actively involved in policy development, implementation and evaluation of the medical education programme (Strasser et al., 2015).

It may be argued that tertiary hospitals are also 'in the community'. Globally, the health system has developed tertiary centres to cater for the high-technology elements of healthcare efficiently and to a high standard. This has resulted in a system that is primarily accountable internally, through processes of audit and peer review. It is not accountable to any one local community, as patients are admitted from many different communities, often over significant distances. CBME focuses on the local care provided to patients both before the decision to refer to a tertiary hospital and after the decision to discharge the patient from such care. Patients in these settings often have undifferentiated problems and/or are being seen for multiple problems concurrently.

When discussing CBME in primary care, it is important to understand the difference between the uses of the terms 'primary care' and 'primary healthcare'. The former refers to the first point of contact for members of the community with the health system and will usually not require a referral. Primary healthcare (PHC) concerns a philosophy of healthcare that emphasizes the need to address the priority health problems in the community by providing promotive, preventive, curative, rehabilitative and palliative services. Accordingly, PHC proposes broad-based approaches to health through collaboration between sectors and advocates strong participation of 'consumers' in healthcare planning. Most CBME curricula are based on a PHC philosophy and are conducted in a primary care setting, but it is possible for neither of these two elements to be present, for example, in a rotation based in the private clinic of a psychiatrist with the primary aim of learning advanced psychotherapy.

Common settings for CBME include:

- general practice/family medicine clinic
- village/community health centres
- specialist, consulting clinics
- patients' homes
- schools
- factories
- farms
- community fairs
- shopping centres.

Goals of CBME

 "CBE provides students with opportunities to become increasingly involved in health issues and, as their competency grows, to plan and provide care. CBE is about engaging in a creative way with communities in the context of real health problems while at the same time learning essential attitudes and skills applicable in both hospital and community settings."

Mennin & Mennin, 2006

There are a wide range of mechanisms involved in affording different kinds of community-related learning experiences (Ellaway et al., 2016). The setting and structure of CBME are principally determined by the aims of the particular component of the curriculum to be delivered. The goals of most CBME programmes focus on preparing students to work in rural or under-served areas and/or to equip them for practice of high-quality primary care. However, there are a wide range of goals that can be achieved, which can be divided into preclinical and clinical aims.

PRECLINICAL AIMS

CBME has been used to advantage for learning in such diverse areas as epidemiology, preventative health, public health principles, community development, the social impact of illness, the PHC approach, the healthcare team and understanding how patients interact with the healthcare system. It is also commonly used for learning basic clinical skills, especially communication skills, and for learning a variety of professional development skills through the mentorship of primary care doctors.

These latter aims could also be learned in a tertiary hospital with no particular disadvantage but are often taught in the community because the faculty members who have a special interest in these areas, and have been delegated with the responsibility for teaching them, are often primary care practitioners.

CLINICAL AIMS

The curricular aims of clinical CBME courses largely fall into four categories, three of which are typically associated with ambulatory care in the context of the hospital being the primary locus for training and a fourth that has the community as the primary locus.

To learn about general practice/ family medicine

A primary care, general practice or family medicine rotation is the most common clinical CBME attachment and appears in most contemporary medical curricula. It occurs either in a short, discrete block of time or in a continuity rotation of perhaps a full or half day per week for a semester, a year or more. There are advantages and disadvantages with both models (Table 10.1).

Whichever structure is chosen, it is essential to have a well-planned orientation to the rotation, the practice and the community. This may also involve intensive instruction in relevant clinical skills and in the structure of healthcare delivery in the local community, especially if this is the first such exposure for students. Many additional useful tasks may be linked to these rotations, such as doing home visits, developing an ecomap of local resources or health facilities available to patients, meeting with community-based organizations or support groups, and visits to other health workers in the area. An opportunity to debrief and reflect on their experiences is also helpful to consolidate students' learning and conduct course evaluation. These suggestions are relevant to both undergraduate and postgraduate learning.

To learn about a particular specialty other than general practice/family medicine

There are a number of good examples of this type of CBME. At the University of Pretoria in South Africa, students spend part of a seven-week community-based rotation specifically developing obstetric skills. In addition to such undergraduate models, postgraduate training programmes in disciplines traditionally taught in hospitals, for example, paediatrics, psychiatry and internal medicine, are creating CBME learning experiences as they seek to prepare their residents appropriately for current and future practice. In a further example, from the United Kingdom, community-situated hospitals have been redeveloped as ambulatory rural diagnostic and treatment centres (RDTCs). In these facilities a wide range of healthcare activities take place on an ambulatory basis. These centres can provide students with ideal opportunities to experience outpatient consultations, clinical investigations and day case therapy and surgery. A 4-week structured clinical attachment in the RDTC can provide new learning

Table 10.1 Community-based medical education (CBME) in general practice/primary care

Type of CBME	Advantages	Disadvantages
Discrete block	Immersion experience	Requires accommodation for student
	Allows student to focus entirely on general practice	Large variation in student experience at different times of the year
	Easy to timetable	School and public holidays impact have significant negative impact
	Intense mentorship relationship	Adverse effect on practice income or consulting time
	Often has a regenerative feeling for the student: 'a change is as good as a holiday'	Can be tiring for the preceptor
	Possibility of using rural and remote practices	
	Easy to conduct evaluation and assessment before and afterwards	
Continuity rotation	Can follow specific patients over time	May be conflicts with activities in the 'feeder' rotation
	Can see seasonal differences in practice	Available sites limited by recurring transport costs and time
	Usually no student accommodation required	May be seen by student as less important than the concurrent hospital-based discipline
	Can integrate learning with another hospital-based discipline	Preceptor may lose interest, leave, get unwell over the extended time period
	Student can develop a specific role in the practice over time	Evaluation often contaminated by variable concurrent learning in hospital
	Impact on practice income may be less apparent as only one session per week	
	May appear less tiring to the preceptor as effort is spread over a longer period	

opportunities focused on ambulatory and community care (Dent et al., 2001; Dent et al., 2007).

To learn about primary care

In this model, the tertiary hospital is still the primary learning area, but community sites are used to fill in the gaps in the curriculum because of a mismatch between curriculum goals and what is achievable in the hospital context. Important areas covered may be in relation to learning about primary healthcare, community-based practice, team-based care and working with communities. The primary care context can be used to integrate learning from a range of disciplines, for integrating clinical practice and public health, and for interprofessional and multidisciplinary learning.

The Integrated Primary Care (IPC) block at the University of the Witwatersrand, Johannesburg is an example of this. Students complete a 6-week rotation in primary care clinics and community hospitals, applying the knowledge and skills acquired from the major specialties (from internal medicine to public health)

to undifferentiated patients, their families and communities, in an integrated programme that is jointly managed and examined by representatives from the major disciplines, and are orientated to the importance of primary healthcare.

To learn multiple disciplines concurrently

In this case, the whole curriculum is based on community practice, whether this is for one year or for the entire period of training. This might be the orientation of a whole medical school, such as Walter Sisulu University in South Africa, University of Wollongong in Australia, Ateneo de Zamboanga University in the Philippines, and the Northern Ontario School of Medicine in Canada, or an option for a subgroup of students, such as the Flinders Parallel Rural Community Curriculum (PRCC) at Flinders University in Australia, a model followed by many Australian medical schools.

This concept takes advantage of the broad patient base in primary care and has been implemented in both urban and rural settings. There are two principal reasons for why rural settings are particularly popular.

They relate to educational opportunities and health policy agendas.

Rural practice, in most countries, has a broader range of patients, involves fewer referrals, and the clinicians are more likely to have significant roles in primary care, emergency medicine, obstetrics and inpatient care. Thus, it is relatively simple for the rural preceptor to give students access to continuity of care through initial diagnosis, investigation, initial management (including as an inpatient) and ongoing care of a range of patients.

Extended rotations of this type have also been shown to be associated with a high number of students choosing a career in rural practice, and thus have been supported financially by governments as a significant long-term strategy with regard to the rural medical workforce. Evaluation of the Flinders experience has shown that students in CBME perform better in examinations than their hospital-based peers and develop the skills and personal qualities required to practise in areas of need (Worley et al., 2004; Couper & Worley, 2010). Experiences in Africa also support CBME providing "contextual learning that addresses workforce scarcity by enabling trainees to acquire the competencies and values needed to provide care in local communities" (Mariam et al., 2014).

Based on the Flinders experience, the contrasts between this extended form of CBME and multiple tertiary hospital rotations, combining inpatient and ambulatory outpatient experience, are summarized in Table 10.2.

Practical principles for successful CBME

Although advocates of CBME will talk in passionate terms about its advantages, experienced innovators will rightly point out that success is not guaranteed. It is certainly possible to have poor quality CBME, and even in successful programmes, the issues of sustainability over time and quality control over numerous sites are important challenges that need to be recognized at the outset. For example, the main challenges identified in CBME programmes in Africa centred around four areas: shortage of staff, both in absolute numbers and in terms of interest; infrastructure and logistics; student numbers and attitudes; and inflexible or unclear curricula (Mariam et al., 2014). All of these need to be addressed.

Previous analysis of the literature on CBME, combined with the authors' experience in CBME development and management, has led to the recognition of four key relationships that are crucial to success (Worley, 2002).

THE CLINICIAN–PATIENT RELATIONSHIP

Enabling the student to participate, in a meaningful way, in the clinician–patient interaction is a key to medical education in any context. Although the primary care system emphasizes the importance of the doctor–patient relationship, successfully integrating the student

Table 10.2 Comparison of extended CBME and tertiary rotations

Education factors	Sequential tertiary rotations	Extended CBME
Illness spectrum	Highly filtered case-mix; all of high severity and complexity	Greater access to common conditions; many different levels of severity and complexity
Contact with patients	Cross-sectional; snapshot of patients at similar points in their illness	Longitudinal; see improvement/relapse/further decision making over time
Role in patient care	Passive; students feel 'in the way'; as soon as the students have learnt the specific functioning of one team, they move to another ward and discipline with new supervisors and expectations	Active; valued extended time in a single setting with the same supervisor enables safe participation to increase over the year
Student attitude	Regard time on ward as 'study'	Regard time in practice as 'work'
Access to subspecialist expertise	Face to face, easy to organize	By planned visits, internet resources, or video-conferenced tutorials
Professional development	See supervising clinicians only in clinical context and role	See supervising clinicians in clinical and social/family contexts and roles
Delegation of teaching	Specialist supervisors delegate significant amount of teaching to junior medical staff	Primary care practitioner supervisors delegate some teaching to resident and visiting specialists
Modelling for future practice	Learning in a high-technology, high-cost environment	Learning in a low-technology, low-cost environment

into this privileged interaction requires explicit attention in CBME. It is not automatic and requires permission, planning and that the student is prepared well beforehand. It also requires attention being paid to establishing effective working relationships with non-doctor clinicians, who in many contexts, particularly in Africa, are the primary clinical supervisors of medical students.

As clinical CBME usually occurs in pressurized, first-line consulting rooms, in practices or in clinics, it is more likely to be successful and sustainable if it can be structured in a way that enhances, rather than detracts from, the clinician's work and the patient's satisfaction with the care provided. Patient consent is a key first step. This is easier to manage if student teaching is seen as a 'norm' within the clinic, rather than an unusual occurrence. That is, the clinic is branded as a teaching site where it is expected that students will be part of the healthcare team.

Evaluations of patient satisfaction with student participation in such community settings have been extremely positive. In particular, there appears to be a certain 'status' attached by patients to their carer being an affiliated university teacher, a recognition of the importance of training the next generation of doctors well, and an appreciation of the extra time and interest a student may give to a patient. In the context of rural CBME, patients may see this as their opportunity to recruit a potential future doctor to their region.

Teaching takes time, and it is important to structure this teaching to have the least negative impact on the number of patients that can be seen. If this is not the case, the clinician may decide to discontinue involvement, require significant financial compensation or encourage purely passive observation by the student. All these are undesirable. Experience with extended CBME programmes indicates that it may even be possible to increase practice capacity by involving the students in useful components of the patient care (Walters et al., 2008). It appears that this capacity increases as the student's time in a particular practice increases. At the same time, the student's role in contributing to patient care must not be abused; students need time to learn from each patient they see.

How can students become integrated in a meaningful and helpful way? The following practical suggestions have been found to be useful:

- Ensure there is a separate consulting room available for student use.

- Modify the appointment schedule, without reducing the total number of patients, so that patients are booked in simultaneous pairs, one for the student and one for the doctor. The doctor sees his or her patient first, then moves to the other room to see the student's patient.

- Encourage patients seen by the student to return when the student is consulting.

- Provide a quiet student study area in the health facility with Internet access.
- Arrange a system for the student to be contacted for after-hours or emergency calls.
- Allow students choice in their practice sites.
- Involve the host facility or practice in student selection and matching.
- Provide training and academic recognition for local supervisors.
- Employ an administrator to timetable and coordinate the multiple learning sites/sessions for each student.
- Encourage academic staff to work clinically in the community selected for teaching.

It is recognized that these suggestions are easier to achieve in a resource-rich environment, but they provide useful principles for all CBME programmes, and many can be implemented with a minimum of resources. There are many tools that can be used as adjuncts to consulting-room learning. These might include logbooks, self- and peer-assessment tasks, skills lists and specific activity requirements, such as home visits, working with other professionals, accompanying patients who are referred and attending support groups or local health service meetings. The basis for the success of these is student-directed learning, where students have flexibility to meet their own needs, measured against clear objectives. This is not simply a cost-effective strategy for resource-constrained environments, but a highly effective way of learning. Appointing appropriate mentors is also critical to success.

 "Rurally based students saw double the number of common medical conditions and assisted in, or performed, six times as many procedures as city-based students, with the result that the majority of the students were sure they had a better educational experience than their city counterparts."

Worley et al., 2000

THE UNIVERSITY–HEALTH SERVICE RELATIONSHIP

In many tertiary centres today there is considerable tension between the research and education agenda of the university and the clinical service targets of the health service. In CBME contexts, the challenge is to enable the presence of medical students to enhance the objectives of both organizations and create a symbiotic relationship between the two.

How can this be achieved? What does the health service gain?

Bringing medical education to a health service can be seen as recognition of the quality of that service. A university presence may also bring with it expectations and expertise in audit, quality control and peer review that improve patient care and further validate this perceived higher status as a teaching centre. The presence of students can be a powerful motivator for local health service staff, many of whom describe a new sense of meaning in their work as a result of students' presence.

Students can also be given tasks that contribute to the health service beyond patient care. Health service managers should be consulted, and should see students as being able to assist them in meeting some of their goals. Health facility audits, quality improvement projects, creation of facility ecomaps and resource lists, and similar student activities, conducted with the support and guidance of health facility managers, can assist health service development and ensure that students are seen to be useful by these managers, not only by clinicians. Beyond that, these activities can be critical in developing students' ability both to contribute to and critique the performance of the health system in the context of a local community and a multiprofessional team, which are essential ingredients of twenty-first century medical education (Frenk et al., 2010). It is helpful to have a formal agreement between the university and the health service that outlines how the parties will balance service delivery, teaching requirements, and meeting community needs.

How does the university benefit?

In addition to the health service providing access to valuable clinical education opportunities for the university, the community setting can open up new avenues of clinical and health service research and with this the funds to undertake this work jointly. This perspective may be important when innovators seek to encourage tertiary academics to participate in community-based programmes.

There can be benefit to both organizations from shared resources. For example, students and staff in community settings require access to the latest and widest information sources available to supplement their clinical experiences. This may be through internet and university library access, tutorials from visiting academics, specifically developed electronic materials or video-conferenced educational sessions. These same resources can be put to good use by the health service. This may lead to joint funding of the infrastructure required.

Shared ownership of curriculum development and student selection enhances commitment from clinicians and the community. This increases the likelihood that students will develop a deeper understanding of the contribution of social and environmental factors to causation and prevention of ill-health (Dreyer et al., 2015).

THE GOVERNMENT–COMMUNITY RELATIONSHIP

Gaining an appreciation of the health needs of communities, and methods to address these through local initiative and government policy, are important aspects of most modern medical programmes. CBME can provide excellent opportunities for such learning. This includes understanding the tensions that often exist between national government policy and local community perceptions of health service priorities.

A further key notion that underpins successful CBME is the creation of a university presence in a local community that brings together national policy and local community needs. The first mechanism for this is through targeted research. Medical students, especially as part of their preclinical learning, can engage in locally driven research that can lead to changes in local understanding and practice. Examples of this may include understanding the occupational health risks of vineyard workers, or factors that improve the local uptake of chemically impregnated mosquito nets. This research may also provide data that enable access to further government funding sources.

Second, students are 'sensitised' to the health needs of underserved populations through participation in community development. This may involve local implementation of national priorities such as immunization, sanitation, food hygiene practices, antenatal care and agricultural safety. This is best undertaken whilst living in the community concerned.

Third, the effectiveness of CBME as a local medical recruitment tool is a powerful synergy of local workforce needs with national workforce policy. This can be both a means to access additional educational funding from national sources and a motivator for continued community participation. This is not, however, inevitable. It will only be effective if the student experience is a positive one. It will be facilitated if both the local community and the potential government funders have a sense of ownership and engagement with the CBME programme and have formal roles within it. This may be attained through an advisory committee, student selection, social introductions to community groups, support for student accommodation or transport subsidies

In light of these potential benefits, it is important for universities to be diligent in collecting appropriate workforce data and maintaining a longitudinal database of their students' career paths. If students gain a sense of 'belonging' and appreciation from 'their' community, and an understanding of the relevant government policy agendas, they can become passionate and articulate advocates for the community and see immediate results from their learning at a population level.

Many medical schools are now recognizing this government–community relationship as they attempt to deliver socially accountable medical education. The Training for Health Equity Network (THEnet, www.thenetcommunity.org) is a small group of innovative medical schools that are committed to this approach and have developed an evaluation framework to guide its implementation (see Chapter 48 on *The Medical*

Teacher and Social Accountability). Community-based medical education, as an effective long-term workforce redistribution strategy, can provide a point of synergy between a local community's priorities and government policy.

THE PERSONAL–PROFESSIONAL RELATIONSHIP

The final relationship to consider in making the most of CBME is the tension that often exists between the personal values and priorities of the individual physician and the expectations of the profession. Education in primary care settings can result in students spending a relatively large amount of time with one supervisor. This can lead to the development of an effective mentor relationship that can assist the student in analysing their own personal values in the light of professional norms, but it requires vulnerability on behalf of both supervisor and student for this to happen. A well-developed mentor relationship may persist after the student leaves and prove influential in future career decisions.

Many clinical educators are concerned at the attrition of humanistic values that occurs in traditional medical school training. The continuity that extended CBME provides has been shown to mitigate against this attrition and enhance important values such as empathy and altruism. The Consortium for Longitudinal Integrated Clerkships (CLIC, www.clicmeded.com) is a network of medical schools that are committed to this continuity approach to medical education, which is being implemented using a variety of different approaches around the world (Worley et al., 2016).

CBME is also an excellent opportunity for students to observe the role of clinicians outside the clinic, both in terms of further professional responsibilities, such as community health education, and in terms of how being a doctor impacts on their family and social life in that community. This is best learned if the student is a resident in the community. It is crucial to find accommodation for students that will support the experience as being a positive one. In this regard, curriculum planners should pay attention to the growing number of students who have partners and children. A community experience may be used by the whole family to determine the benefits and disadvantages of living and working in such a community after graduation, but this requires significant additional expense.

Sen Gupta et al. (2009) articulate three essential requirements for CBME to succeed: student accommodation and teaching space, committed clinical teachers, and appropriate case load. One additional factor that is important to be aware of is student safety. This may entail educating students about issues of safe travel, carefully managing physical risks to students in communities where violence is a significant issue, managing the risk to the student of exposure to communicable diseases such as HIV, and assisting students to deal with relative isolation, cultural change and, for some, living away from home for the first time. Students must have clarity on insurance policies in terms of the extent of coverage and the responsibility expected from them. Students also, from time to time, become unwell, or have family or social crises. They need to have access to assistance independent of their teacher/assessor. Such resources should be arranged before any need arises, and students should have written and verbal explanation of the arrangements.

CBME academic and administrative staff who support the personal and professional development of their students will find that the students not only gain cognitive and psychomotor knowledge and skills during their attachment but also have the opportunity to gain affective skills and find themselves changed by the experience.

Summary

Community-based medical education is an increasingly popular tool in the medical educator's toolbox. Its use reflects the growing importance of community-based practice in the twenty-first century health system. There are many forms of CBME allied to the various curricular aims it is intended to deliver, and curricula are increasingly being developed on the basis of clear medical education research.

Moving medical education from tertiary centres into the community involves institutional change and requires proactive leadership and significant resources. CBME is not a cheaper alternative to traditional medical education. Teaching in the community may require additional time and person-power because of the low student–teacher ratio and the costs of supporting students at a distance, such as accommodation, travel for students and academic staff, and information and communication technology. Whatever form CBME takes, it is important to evaluate it by seeking feedback from patients, staff and students. The results may be pleasantly surprising (Dent et al., 2001) and will help to refine the programme for future use.

Whilst it is clear that further research is urgently required, it is hoped that the principles outlined in this chapter can help innovators to avoid major pitfalls and increase the likelihood of positive feedback from all the stakeholders involved. Successful change involves rethinking problems as opportunities and having the creativity to find practical solutions. Organizations such as the Network: Towards Unity for Health, THEnet and CLIC can provide a forum for exchange of ideas and support for change agents. Become aware of the CBME initiatives worldwide through the Network's and CLIC's regular international conferences: you will be inspired and invigorated.

Pay as much attention to the students' learning of 'heart' knowledge as you do to their 'head' knowledge.

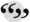 *"As medical education policy advisers and leaders in the USA and beyond seek to grow the physician workforce in ways that are cost-effective and sustainable, provide clinical training more appropriate to common community needs, and balance the distribution of newly trained physicians toward areas both clinically and geographically underserved, it is clear they are favouring the model and associated merits of community-based/distributive medical education."*

Farnsworth et al., 2012

References

Couper, I.D., Worley, P.S., 2010. Meeting the challenges of training more medical students: lessons from Flinders University's distributed medical education program. Medical Journal of Australia 193 (1), 34–36.

Dent, J.A., Angell-Preece, H.M., Ball, H.M.-L., Ker, J.S., 2001. Using the ambulatory care teaching centre to develop opportunities for integrated learning. Med. Teach. 23 (2), 171–175.

Dent, J., Skene, S., Nathwani, D., et al., 2007. Design, implementation and evaluation of a medical education programme using the ambulatory diagnostic and treatment centre. Med. Teach. 29 (4), 341–345.

Dreyer, A., Couper, I., Bailey, R., et al., 2015. Identifying approaches and tools for evaluating community-based medical education programmes in Africa. Afr. J. Health Prof. Educ. 7 (1 Suppl. 1), 134–139.

Ellaway, R.H., O'Gorman, L., Strasser, R., et al., 2016. A critical hybrid realist-outcomes systematic review of relationships between medical education programmes and communities: BEME Guide No. 35. Med. Teach. 38 (3), 229–245.

Farnsworth, T.J., et al., 2012. Community-based distributive medical education: advantaging society. Med. Educ. Online 17, 8432.

Frenk, J., Chen, L., Bhutta, Z.A., et al., 2010. Health professionals for a new century: transforming education to strengthen health systems in an interdependent world. Lancet 376 (9756), 1923–1958.

Mariam, D.H., Sagay, A.S., Arubaku, W., et al., 2014. Community-based education programs in Africa: faculty experience within the Medical Education Partnership Initiative (MEPI) network. Acad. Med. 89 (8 Suppl.), S50–S54.

Mennin, S., Mennin, R., 2006. Community Based Medical Education. Clin. Teach. 392, 90–96.

Sen Gupta, T.K., Murray, R.B., Beaton, N.S., et al., 2009. A tale of three hospitals: solving learning and workforce needs together. Med. J. Aust. 191 (2), 105–109.

Strasser, R., Worley, P., Cristobal, F., et al., 2015. Putting Communities in the Driving Seat: the Realities of Community Engaged Medical Education. Acad. Med. 90 (11), 1466–1470.

Walters, L., Worley, P., Prideaux, D., Lange, K., 2008. Do consultations in general practice take more time when practitioners are precepting medical students? Med. Educ. 42 (1), 69–73.

Worley, P.S., Prideaux, D.J., Strasser, R.P., et al., 2000. Why we should teach undergraduate medical students in rural communities. Med. J. Aust. 172 (12), 615–617.

Worley, P., 2002. Relationships: a new way to analyse community-based medical education? (Part one). Educ. Health 15 (2), 117–128.

Worley, P., Esterman, A., Prideaux, D., 2004. Cohort study of examination performance of undergraduate medical students learning in community settings. BMJ 328 (7433), 207–209.

Worley, P., Couper, I., Strasser, R., et al., 2016. A typology of longitudinal integrated clerkships. Med. Educ. 50 (9), 922–932.

Further reading

Hays, R., 2007. Community-oriented medical education. Teach. Teach. Educ. 23 (3), 286–293.

Hunt, J.B., Bonham, C., Jones, L., 2011. Understanding the goals of service learning and community-based medical education: a systematic review. Acad. Med. 86 (2), 246–251.

Maley, M., Worley, P., Dent, J., 2009. Using rural and remote settings in the undergraduate medical curriculum: AMEE Guide No. 47. Med. Teach. 31 (11), 969–983.

11 Learning in rural and remote locations

J. Rourke, L. Rourke

Trends

- Recognition that rural medical practices can provide an excellent learning environment for medical students and vocational trainees/residents.
- Inclusion of some rural learning experiences for all students in an increasing number of medical schools.
- Development of longitudinal in-depth rural learning experiences at innovative medical schools for students and vocational trainees/residents.

 Learning in rural/remote locations can be an outstanding and sometimes life changing experience.

Introduction

The rural/remote location is an ideal setting for practical community-based education where medical learners can develop knowledge, skills and attitudes that are useful in any medical practice setting. In this chapter, 'medical learners' refers to students and vocational trainees/residents.

As discovering the joys and challenges of rural/remote practice can lead some medical learners to choose rural/remote practice as a career, and as medical schools expand and address their social responsibility to train physicians for practice in locations and in fields where they are most needed, more medical learners at different stages of their education are experiencing training in a *distributed medical education* model using rural locations (Curran & Rourke, 2004; Rourke et al., 2005; Eley et al., 2008; Norris et al., 2009; Maley et al., 2010; Rourke, 2010; Wong et al., 2010; Rourke, 2011; Crampton et al., 2013; Bosco & Oandasan, 2015). This includes longitudinal integrated clinical clerkships (LICs) that embed the main clinical learning in rural medical practice with rural doctors as the main teachers (see Chapter12 *Learning in longitudinal integrated clerkships*).

There is substantial literature that shows that medical learners in rural settings, at a variety of learning stages, *do as well as or better than* urban learners on medical examinations and other measures of performance, and also have high student satisfaction and perception of a positive learning atmosphere (Bianchi, et al., 2008; Crampton, et al., 2013; Denz-Penhey & Murdoch, 2010; Hirsh et al., 2012; Power et al., 2006; Schauer & Schieve, 2006; Waters et al., 2006; Barrett, et al., 2011). Although more research is needed, this may counteract the documented ethics erosion in medical students during the clinical years (Norris et al., 2009; Poncelet, et al., 2009).

This rural training trend provides the opportunity for rural general practitioners/family physicians, consultants and other rural healthcare professionals to become more involved as medical teachers (sometimes called preceptors in the medical literature). Many rural physicians are *enthusiastic natural teachers* with broad clinical skills, developed by managing a wide variety of patient care challenges within strong community–patient–physician relationships. They experience value in being a preceptor, especially their own resultant professional enrichment as well as the rewards of the medical teacher/learner relationship.

A needs analysis study, however, found that "the majority of rural preceptors had no clear understanding of how what they taught fitted into the overall curriculum, their role as a clinical teacher had not been clearly defined ... and that undergraduate students had little understanding of what they needed to learn during their attachment" (Baker, et al., 2003). These challenges may be addressed with clearer communication between the programme and the rural preceptor.

 Consistently positive rural/remote teaching and learning experiences combine good planning and excellent learning settings with interested learners and enthusiastic teachers.

This chapter is organized according to the following practical framework (Rourke & Rourke, 1996):
- before the learner arrives
- the first day
- during the rotation
- assessment and wrap-up.

Before the learner arrives

Good planning and preparation prior to the arrival of the medical learner are essential to set the stage for a successful rural learning/teaching experience.

Preceptor preparation, programme support, a well-prepared physician's office and staff, engaged colleagues, helpful hospital and healthcare organizations, and community partnerships are vital components to have in place for a successful rural clinical experience. Clear communication is essential at every step of the way.

PROGRAM SUPPORT AND PRECEPTOR PREPARATION

Teaching medical learners is like medical practice: no matter how much experience one has, there is always more to learn.

Successful teaching and learning in the rural setting require extensive support and communication with the programme responsible for the learners. Ideally, rural medical teachers are part of a *rural medical education network* with faculty development to cultivate their teaching skills. Well-functioning programmes also provide extensive faculty development that brings together the regional rural medical teachers for information sharing, planning and faculty development sessions. Interactive collegial workshops focused on teaching in a rural setting can be particularly helpful and enjoyable learning opportunities for rural physicians.

In many areas worldwide, rural doctor associations have taken the lead in providing workshops and developing resource materials. As well, some medical organizations and university faculties of medicine have begun to provide faculty development and continuing medical education (CME) via distance learning, on-the-road learning, and other innovative formats that are ideal for rural medical teachers (Bosco & Oandasan, 2015; Chater et al., 2014; Delver et al., 2014; McCarthy et al., 2016; Rourke, 2011; Wong, et al., 2010).

Information technology that provides access to the medical school's teaching and clinical resources should be made available to those at the rural site. Rural medical learners and teachers should be able to participate in relevant distance learning–supported educational opportunities and clinical rounds.

Programme support should include site development visits to the rural practice so that expectations, issues and concerns can be dealt with face to face and in a collegial constructive manner.

There needs to be a clear understanding of the learner's, the rural medical teacher's and the programme's roles and responsibilities.

Many rural medical teachers accept a number of learners, which means that they are working with a range of learner knowledge, skills, objectives, and programme expectations. Programmes should give medical learners and their rural teachers clear information that outlines the programme's *learning objectives and expected/required evaluation.*

In addition, the programme should provide the rural medical teacher with a letter or other indication that the learner is in good standing. Any major outstanding concerns or issues should be communicated to the rural medical teacher prior to the learner's arrival, especially if they could add an undue element of risk to patient safety and the rural teacher's medical practice.

Programme financial support for learner travel, accommodation, information technology and other expenses should be clearly established before the rotation.

Rural medical teachers are an invaluable teaching resource and need to be recognized in a positive fashion, both academically and financially. In the past, financial support for rural medical teachers has often been severely lacking. Programmes need to realize that teaching in the often busy rural clinical setting requires a significant time commitment, often at the expense of monetary remuneration and personal time.

A WELL-PREPARED PHYSICIAN'S OFFICE AND STAFF

Positive and supportive office staff members are key to a happy and successful practice. Similarly, their engagement is just as vital to the rural learning and teaching experience.

When incorporating a learner into a practice, it is very helpful *to involve the staff* in planning how best to use the office space, organize scheduling and handle communication with patients. Ideally, there will be enough examining rooms to accommodate the learner(s) as well as a separate review and study space equipped with high-speed Internet access.

It is very important that all involved understand the skill level, roles and responsibilities of the learner and how to best integrate their involvement into the care of patients and other office activities. The staff can contribute significantly to a positive teaching and learning experience by helping to select and introduce the most appropriate patients for the learner and by responding positively to questions from both patients and the learner. Staff and patients can be an invaluable source of feedback regarding their experience with the learner.

Preparing a learner's manual can consolidate the practice preparation and planning and is an invaluable guide to prepare and orient learners.

Useful features of a learner's manual include information about the community and area including climate, travel information, community resources and social and recreational opportunities; accommodation arrangements; a description of the practice including schedules, location and key personnel; related community and hospital learning activities with other physician colleagues and allied health personnel; and copies of office, electronic medical record, hospital and other protocols for learners.

Ideally, the learner's manual will be made available on the web with links to a variety of relevant resources for the learner to review prior to arrival.

MAIN PRECEPTOR/RURAL MEDICAL TEACHER AND ENGAGED COLLEAGUES

It is important that there is a main preceptor/rural medical teacher with responsibility for the organization, orientation, supervision and evaluation of the learner, and for ongoing communication with the programme.

The coordinating role of the rural teacher becomes even more essential with longer rural placements.

In the past, learners on rural rotations were often placed with solo rural physicians. Increasingly in the twenty-first century, rural physicians work with a small number of close colleagues, either in a group practice or in a shared patient care/call coverage arrangement within a community or hospital setting. In this setting, there may be one or several rural physicians who will periodically take on the main preceptor/medical teacher role.

Involvement of other colleagues provides a broader rural experience by utilizing different teachers' knowledge, skills and attitudes. This also provides the opportunity for experienced rural teachers to help their colleagues in also becoming medical teachers. Care needs to be taken in the choice and role of colleagues to ensure a positive learning experience.

HELPFUL HOSPITAL AND HEALTHCARE ORGANIZATIONS

Hospital-based care is a much more active component of practice for many rural general practitioners/family physicians than for their urban colleagues. Similarly, rural specialist consultants may provide a much broader generalist approach to care than their urban colleagues. This can significantly broaden and enhance the learning opportunities for learners on rural rotations.

Compared to many urban locations, physicians and allied healthcare professionals in a rural community are often easily accessible to each other, particularly if they work in close proximity at the rural community hospital. Thus it can be an ideal model of a collegial interdisciplinary team providing care in practice. Team members can also provide valuable learning opportunities and feedback for the rural medical learner.

Before the rotation begins, the rural medical teacher should establish appropriate protocols with the approval of the hospital medical advisory committee to outline the level of activities and supervision for learners at different stages of education. A supportive hospital administration and staff and regional healthcare organization along with the training programme can be very helpful with enabling this process.

COMMUNITY PARTNERSHIPS

Rural communities increasingly see the value of rural medical learners as potential future recruits to help stabilize their long-term physician workforce.

There is increasing evidence of the positive effect of rural placements, especially those with longitudinal continuity, on community engagement for learners, preceptors, and the community (Crampton, et al., 2013; Denz-Penhey & Murdoch, 2010, Hirsh et al., 2012). Many rural communities are exceptional places to live and work, and are often located in areas where urban dwellers go for their holidays. Communities can facilitate the rural medical learner's welcome and involvement in social and recreational activities and thus spark the learner's interest in future practice in a rural setting. Positive community engagement reduces the potential for rural medical learners' sense of isolation and shifts some of the organizational burden away from the rural medical teacher.

Ongoing communication with all involved participants – training programme, office staff, colleagues, hospital, healthcare organizations and community – prior to each learner's arrival will pave the way for a positive learning experience.

The first day

The main preceptor/rural medical teacher should set aside a block of time on the first day to welcome and orient the learner.

The first day is critical in establishing a positive impression and setting out clear roles and expectations. Dedicated time should be scheduled on the first day or shortly thereafter for the rural preceptor and learner to establish mutual expectations, roles and responsibilities (often termed contracting). Ideally, the learner will have individual goals in addition to the expectations of the programme. Equally important is discussing potential problems, concerns or anticipated absences of the learner. The physician's office staff, hospital staff and community members should play a key role in the orientation as well. A letter/notice introducing the learner that is displayed in the reception area and examining rooms and signed by the preceptor can help connect the learner and patients. Patient care responsibilities should start slowly and be gradually increased to help avoid the whirlwind of information and responsibilities that can overwhelm a learner at the start of a rural rotation.

During the rotation

 As much of the learning is centred around patient care, the rural medical teacher has a dual role, providing both patient care and teaching effectively and efficiently.

Adding a learner to the patient care process will require a well-planned and flexible schedule to both accommodate patient care needs and optimize the learning/teaching experience. Time is required for review and discussion throughout and at the end of the day. Patients, staff, physicians and learners all appreciate good scheduling. Time-efficient strategies for clinical teaching are described elsewhere in this book.

 Six attributes of community preceptors/rural medical teachers who were scored highly by medical students:
1. Welcoming learners as legitimate participants in a community of practice
2. Creating a central role for learners in patient care and teaching
3. Regularly engaging learners in self-reflection to monitor their progress
4. Helping learners discover learning opportunities in routine patient encounters
5. Using feedback to shape rather than evaluate learner performance
6. Creating an environment where learners feel comfortable practising new skills with patients.

Adapted from Manyon et al., 2003

A learner's role and contribution to patient care will be dependent on their level of education and knowledge, skills and attitudes. As the learner demonstrates competence and commitment to care, their level of responsibility can be increased within the range expected for their educational level in keeping with the concept of *graded responsibility*. The learner should be involved in the follow-up care of patients they have assessed, as *continuity of care* is a vital component of rural patient care, learning and teaching. This may include a variety of settings such as the physician's office, the hospital, the nursing home and the patient's home. It can also involve following patients through specialist/consultant and allied healthcare investigations and treatments, especially in longitudinal integrated clerkships.

The rural patient care setting is ideal for *case-based discussion and learning using a patient-centred approach* (Stewart et al., 2014).

 The CanMEDS roles describe seven aspects of the ideal physician: medical expert, communicator, collaborator, leader/manager, health advocate, scholar and professional. (Frank, et al., 2015). These CanMEDS roles have been modified for Family Medicine (Tannenbaum et al., 2009).

Learners in a rural setting can see how these CanMEDS roles are integrated in the medical practice on a daily basis (Box 11.1).

It is advisable to set aside dedicated time for *discussion of broader issues* such as the doctor–patient relationship and social relationships in small communities. Learners can observe how professionalism and compartmentalization allow rural teachers to combine, yet keep separate, patient care responsibilities and social relationships in rural communities. It is necessary to maintain objectivity and appropriate standard of care for all patients. The awareness of how to set appropriate and flexible personal/professional boundaries, how to maintain work–life balance, and how to foster resilience are valued skills in all settings, both rural and urban (Rourke & Rourke, 2014).

Many rural medical teachers are also involved in *local leadership roles*. Rural communities, as smaller microcosms, often provide opportunities for rural physicians to 'make a difference', not only in individual patient's lives but in the local health system, the community, and beyond. Ideally, the learner will not only witness this advocacy and leadership, but will participate in it as well.

 Rural medical teachers should never underestimate the role modelling and mentorship they provide to their learners.

Satisfaction of the rural medical teacher with their professional and personal life is almost always apparent to the learner. This can be challenging when rural teaching locations have a shortage of physicians and the medical teachers have heavier-than-optimal clinical loads. Similarly, the level of collegiality between rural medical teachers and their family physician, consultant and allied healthcare colleagues is evident.

 Enthusiasm or disillusion with rural practice or living can significantly affect a learner's view of rural practice and influence future career plans.

Learners can also make an excellent contribution to learning/teaching by leading discussions and preparing presentations on topics of interest or importance to the learner, physicians, staff, other health professionals, patients and/or community.

> **Box 11.1   CanMEDS roles can be adapted into rural learning objectives**
>
> **Medical expert/clinical decision maker: 'Know and do the right thing.'**
>
> Identify the knowledge and skills required for a rural/community-based practice and note how they differ from urban practice.
>
> Identify limitations and demonstrate use of referral resources appropriately.
>
> Demonstrate diagnostic and therapeutic skills for ethical and effective evidence-based patient care within the context and limitations of the rural/community environment.
>
> Identify peer review, audit, and other methods of assessing one's practice and rural/community patient care.
>
> **Communicator:** 'Communication is the key to success.'
>
> Identify particular healthcare challenges and difficulties from a rural/community patient's cultural and geographic context.
>
> Demonstrate good interviewing and communication skills with patients.
>
> Demonstrate effective communication with all members of the rural/community healthcare team as member, coordinator and leader.
>
> **Collaborator:** 'Work with others.'
>
> Identify and use local community resources, programmes and distant referral resource and clinical-support networks.
>
> Demonstrate collaboration with local family physicians, consultants, allied health professionals and tertiary care subspecialists.
>
> Identify when and how to effectively transfer patients from smaller referring centres to tertiary care centres.
>
> **Leader/Manager:** 'Be an effective leader.'
>
> Engage with others to develop high-quality rural health care systems.
>
> Identify and develop effective practice appropriate for the rural community.
>
> Identify benefits and risks of investigations and treatments available locally, regionally and at tertiary care centres.
>
> **Health advocate:** 'You can make a difference in your community!'
>
> Identify existing, potential and needed resources to meet the unique needs of your patients and community.
>
> Advocate for accessible and appropriate rural healthcare for your patients and your community.
>
> Become involved in community determinants of health issues.
>
> **Scholar:** 'Yes, you can be a scholar in the country.'
>
> Develop self-directed, life-long learning strategies including use of distance education to maintain up-to-date and competent skills relevant to a rural/community setting.
>
> Develop/participate in community-based health research.
>
> **Professional/personal:** 'Remember yourself, your partner, and your children.'
>
> Identify and experience the joys and challenges of rural/community medical practice and life.
>
> Develop strategies to balance personal, family and professional needs and demands, foster resilience, and avoid burnout.
>
> Demonstrate a positive attitude and working relationships with patients, staff, administration and colleagues.
>
> Modified from Rourke & Frank, 2005 and Frank et al 2015

OBSERVATION/DEMONSTRATION/FEEDBACK

 There is no substitute for the direct observation of the learner, the direct demonstration of clinical skills by the teacher and the provision of effective feedback.

Direct observation at the start of the rotation can help provide the medical teacher with a clear understanding of the learner's knowledge, skills and attitudes, criteria that are vital to determining the level of responsibility that the learner can be given. Direct observation helps the learner and teacher identify both areas of strength and areas for improvement and can avoid the all too easy over- or underestimation of a learner's abilities and needs. The one-on-one learning/teaching in rural practice provides the ideal setting for immediate assessment and rapid advancement of learning. Daily informal discussions, encouragement and advice should be part of the fabric of the rural rotation.

Both learner and teacher can monitor progress by repeated direct observation. Some programmes provide video equipment to aid in the process of direct observation. This can be a very valuable teaching tool but does require additional consideration with regard to patient privacy, acceptance and consent.

As with advanced skill development processes for musicians, athletes and others, demonstration of procedures and techniques by the teacher, and/or

Box 11.2 Modified Pendleton's rules for direct observation and/or videotape review

1. **Clarify**

   Ask for clarification of information and feelings as necessary.

2. **Good points first**

   Ask the learner what they did well.

   Tell the learner what you observed that was done well.

3. **Areas to improve**

   Ask the learner to identify what they had difficulty with and what could be improved.

   Provide specific suggestions for improvement.

4. **Constructive summary**

   Mutually develop a constructive summary.

Adapted from Pendleton et al., 1984.

through simulation, followed by the opportunity for deliberate practise can accelerate procedural skills development and mastery in medical learners.

Providing effective feedback is a core skill for medical teachers and often requires significant faculty development.

 "Identify feedback, because it is often not recognized as such by the learner."

Osmun & Parr, 2011

 The most helpful and appreciated feedback is frequent, timely, specific and constructive.

Modified Pendleton's rules provide a useful framework that can be easily used in the rural setting (Pendleton et al., 1984) (Box 11.2).

Providing feedback to and assessment of the rural learner may pose *unique opportunities and challenges*. The rural setting, with its close teacher–learner relationship and low number of learners, often provides the opportunity for in-depth understanding and identification of strengths and weaknesses that may be more difficult to identify in a larger training milieu. Good feedback that addresses these concerns is important for the learner's future progress. Giving negative feedback, however, can be particularly difficult in this setting for several reasons: fewer local teaching colleagues for support, distant programme support, and social connections between the rural teacher and learner. As with professional–personal patient boundaries, this situation requires skill on the part of the rural teacher, including the ability to compartmentalize, and awareness of the power differential between the teacher and learner. In these instances, programme support to the rural teacher is vital.

Assessment and wrap-up

In addition to the frequent informal feedback provided throughout the rotation, specific times for more formal assessment should be set aside throughout and at the end of the rural rotation. Ideally, assessments are linked to the objectives for the rotation. The CanMEDS roles for physicians provide a broad framework for learning objectives and evaluation that can be functionally adapted to emphasize the broad and important knowledge, skills and attitudes required for exemplary rural practice (see Box 11.1).

Rural medical education assessments should have multiple inputs and be multidirectional. Patients, staff and other physicians and health professionals involved with the learner can provide valuable multisource feedback for both formative and summative assessments (Davis et al., 2006).

Rural medical teachers should understand the difference between '*formative*' and '*summative*' assessment. Formative assessment is ongoing and designed to teach and form future learning. Summative assessment is an evaluation of the learner and occurs at the end of the rotation.

 A mid-rotation formative assessment provides the opportunity for the learner and main preceptor to discuss progress, problems and planning for the remainder of the rotation.

A mid-rotation formative assessment helps set the stage so that the end of rotation summative assessment does not come as a surprise. If a learner is showing signs of major difficulty by the mid-term assessment, the programme should be notified and involved in planning how best to address this for the remainder of the rotation or in remedial alternatives. Learners in longitudinal integrated clinical clerkships require multiple regularly scheduled progress assessments that can be considered multiple mid-rotation assessments that are vital to shaping their learning journey.

The summative end of rotation assessment should be done with the learner before they leave the rotation. Any major concerns should be clearly outlined and discussed. The requisite paper or electronic forms should be sent immediately to the programme so that they can help shape the learner's future training.

In addition to the assessment of the learner by the medical teacher, the medical teacher should be evaluated by the learner. Learners are often reluctant to give direct negative feedback when providing assessments of a preceptor or a specific rotation, with concerns that it may affect future training or employment options. For this reason learner assessments of a training location and preceptors are often anonymized, and information is provided back to the medical teacher only when three or more learner assessments have been received. In addition to evaluating the medical teacher, the assessment should also include other aspects of the rural experience including accommodation, social/community interactions, and information technology and programme support.

Troubled and troubling learners

Learners are not immune from illnesses and emotional stresses. These problems can be aggravated by a rural rotation that places the learner in a new location with new expectations and roles far away from the support of close friends and family. Learners belonging to minority groups may have difficulty finding people with similar interests, experiences or cultural norms in the rural community (Steinert & Walsh, 2006). Despite the best of intentions, the close one-on-one nature of the rural rotation can potentially lead to conflict between the learner and medical teacher, staff or others. When isolation is a significant problem, consideration should be given to placing two learners at the same site. This approach also provides leadership and teaching opportunities for the learners themselves, particularly if they are at different stages in their education.

The teacher and programme should be prepared to help learners with illnesses and stresses by arranging timely and appropriate medical care and counselling as required. While it is important that the rural medical teacher be empathic and supportive, they should if possible *avoid assuming the role of personal physician or counsellor for the learner*. This blurring of boundaries may compromise the medical care or counselling needed by the learner, as well as the teaching/learning rotation and subsequent evaluation. When a learner is ill, arrangements may need to be made for time off. Occasionally the illness has the potential to interfere with the learner's competence in providing patient care. Particularly with psychiatric illness, the potential for suicide must not be ignored.

 In all cases of ill, troubled or troubling learners, involvement of physician colleagues and programme support personnel is vital.

Summary

Rural and remote locations are becoming an increasingly important setting for medical education. Good planning and effective communication before the learner arrives, on the first day, during the rotation and at assessment and wrap-up can help ensure the success of rural learning experiences.

Before the learner arrives, good preparation involving the rural medical teacher, office and staff, colleagues, hospital and community and programme organization and support sets the stage for success.

Welcome and orientation on the first day followed closely by contracting regarding programme and individual learner goals, concerns, expectations, roles and responsibilities, and early direct observation of the learner establishes a strong foundation for progress through the rotation.

During the rotation, learning is facilitated by appropriate scheduling with case-based time-efficient strategies for clinical teaching including demonstration, observation and feedback. The rural and remote medical setting can also show a wide scope of medical care in various settings, interprofessional team care, role modelling and mentorship, and community leadership and involvement with personal/professional boundaries, balance and resilience. The CanMEDS roles for physicians provide a broad framework to apply in the teaching setting. Faculty development can be a key to acquiring effective skills in providing feedback.

Assessment should be informal and formal, formative and summative, linked to the rotation objectives, and multisource and multidirectional. In cases of ill, troubled or troubling learners, additional support should always be sought.

It takes courage to welcome learners into one's rural practice and become a rural medical teacher, but the benefits are many. We have found that learners have stimulated us to demonstrate excellent medical care and to stay up to date. Learners have enriched our lives and those of our staff, our colleagues, our children and our community. It is a great joy to watch learners advancing in knowledge, skills and attitudes, while appreciating the joys and challenges of rural practice and rural life enroute to becoming exemplary physicians, both rural and urban, and themselves medical teachers for future learners.

Acknowledgements

We would like to acknowledge the tremendous contribution of our teachers, learners, colleagues, staff and patients to our teaching and learning over the years.

References

Baker, P.G., Dalton, L., Walker, J., 2003. Rural general practitioner preceptors – how can effective undergraduate teaching be supported or improved? Rural Remote Health 3 (1), 107.

Barrett, F.A., Lipsky, S., Lutfiyya, M.N., 2011. The impact of rural training experiences on medical students: a critical review. Acad Med 86, 259–263.

Bianchi, F., Stobbe, K., Eva, K., 2008. Comparing academic performance of medical students in distributed learning sites: the McMaster experience. Med. Teach. 30 (1), 67–71.

Bosco, C., Oandasan, I., 2015. Review of family medicine within rural and remote Canada: education, practice, and policy. The College of Family Physicians of Canada, Ontario.

Chater, A.B., Rourke, J., Couper, I.D., et al. (Eds.), 2014. WONCA Rural Medical Education Guidebook. World Organization of Family Doctors

(WONCA) Working Party on Rural Practice. Available at: www.globalfamilydoctor.com.

Crampton, P.E., McLachlan, J.C., Illing, J.C., 2013. A systematic literature review of undergraduate clinical placements in underserved areas. Med. Educ. 47 (10), 969–978.

Curran, V., Rourke, J., 2004. The role of medical education in the recruitment and retention of rural physicians. Med. Teach. 26 (3), 265–272.

Davis, D.A., Mazmanian, P.E., Fordis, M., et al., 2006. Accuracy of physician self-assessment compared with observed measures of competence: a systematic review. JAMA 296 (9), 1094–1102.

Delver, H., Jackson, W., Lee, S., Palacios, M., 2014. FM POD: an evidence-based blended teaching skills program for rural preceptors. Fam. Med. 46 (5), 369–377.

Denz-Penhey, H., Murdoch, J.C., 2010. Is small beautiful? Student performance and perceptions of their experience at larger and smaller sites in rural and remote longitudinal integrated clerkships in the Rural Clinical School of Western Australia. Rural Remote Health 10 (3), 1–7.

Eley, D.S., Young, L., Wilkinson, D., et al., 2008. Coping with increasing numbers of medical students in rural clinical schools: options and opportunities. Med J Aust. 188 (11), 669–671.

Frank, J.R., Snell, L., Sherbino, J. (Eds.), 2015. Can-MEDS 2015 Physician Competency Framework. Royal College of Physicians and Surgeons of Canada, Ontario.

Hirsh, D., Gaufberg, E., Ogur, B., et al., 2012. Educational outcomes of the Harvard Medical School–Cambridge integrated clerkship: a way forward for medical education. Acad Med 87 (5), 643–650.

Maley, M., Worley, P., Dent, J., 2010. Using rural and remote settings in the undergraduate medical curriculum. AMEE Guide 47. Med. Teach. 31 (11), 969–983.

Manyon, A., Shipengrover, J., McGuigan, D., et al., 2003. Defining differences in the instructional styles of community preceptors. Fam. Med. 35 (3), 181–186.

McCarthy, P., Bethune, C., Fitzgerald, S., et al., 2016. Curriculum development of 6for6: Longitudinal research skills program for rural and remote family physicians. Can. Fam. Physician 62 (2), e89–e95.

Norris, T.E., Schaad, D.C., DeWitt, D., et al., 2009. Longitudinal integrated clerkships for medical students: an innovation adopted by medical schools in Australia, Canada, South Africa, and the United States. Acad Med 84 (7), 902–907.

Osmun, W.E., Parr, J., 2011. The occasional teacher. Part 4: feedback and evaluation. Can. J. Rural Med. 16 (3), 96.

Pendleton, D., Schofield, T., Tate, P., Havelock, P., 1984. An approach to learning and teaching. The consultation: an approach to learning and teaching. Oxford University Press, Oxford, pp. 68–72.

Poncelet, A.N., Hauer, K.E., O'Brien, B., 2009. The longitudinal integrated clerkship. Virtual Mentor 11 (11), 864–869.

Power, D.V., Harris, I.B., Swentko, W., et al., 2006. Comparing rural-trained medical students with their peers: performance in a primary care OSCE. Teach. Learn. Med. 18 (3), 196–202.

Rourke, J., 2010. How can medical schools contribute to the education, recruitment and retention of rural physicians in their region? Bull World Health Organ 88 (5), 395–396.

Rourke, J., 2011. Key challenges in rural medical education. Int J Child Health Hum Dev 4 (1), 9–14.

Rourke, J., Frank, J.R., 2005. Implementing the CanMEDS physician roles in rural specialist education: the multi-specialty community training network. Educ. for Health 18 (3), 368–378. Joint issue with Rural and Remote Health 5:406.

Rourke, J., Rourke, L.L., 1996. Practical tips for rural family physicians teaching residents. Can. J. Rural Med. 1 (2), 63–69.

Rourke, J.T.B., Incitti, F., Rourke, L.L., Kennard, M., 2005. Relationship between practice location of Ontario family physicians and their rural background or amount of rural medical education experience. Can. J. Rural Med. 10 (4), 231–239.

Rourke, L., Rourke, J., 2014. Boundaries and balance: managing relationships in rural practice. In: Chater, A.B., Rourke, J., Couper, I.D., Strasser, R.P., Reid, S., et al. (Eds.), WONCA Rural Medical Education Guidebook. World Organization of Family Doctors (WONCA) Working Party on Rural Practice. Available at: http://www.globalfamilydoctor.com/groups/WorkingParties/RuralPractice/ruralguidebook.aspx. (Accessed 7 January 2017).

Schauer, R.W., Schieve, D., 2006. Performance of medical students in a nontraditional rural clinical programme, 1998–99 through 2003–04. Acad Med 81 (7), 603–607.

Steinert, Y., Walsh, A. (Eds.), 2006. A faculty development program for teachers of international medical graduates. The Association of Faculties of Medicine of Canada Ottawa, Ontario. Available at: https://afmc.ca/timg/default_en.htm. (Accessed 7 January 2017).

Stewart, M., Brown, J.B., Weston, W.W., et al., 2014. Patient-centered medicine: transforming the clinical method, 3rd ed. Radcliffe Publishing Ltd, Oxford.

Tannenbaum, D., Konkin, J., Parsons, E., et al., 2009. CanMEDS-family medicine: a framework of competencies in family medicine. College of Family physicians of Canada. Working Group on Curriculum Review. Available at: http://www.cfpc.ca/ProjectAssets/Templates/Resource.aspx?id=3031. (Accessed 7 January 2017).

Waters, B., Hughes, J., Forbes, K., Wilkinson, D., 2006. Comparative academic performance of medical students in rural and urban clinical settings. Med. Educ. 40 (2), 117–120.

Wong, G., Greenhalgh, T., Pawson, R., 2010. Internet-based medical education: a realist review of what works, for whom and in what circumstances. BMC Med. Educ. 10 (1), 12.

12 Learning in longitudinal integrated clerkships

D. Hirsh, L. K. Walters

Trends

- LICs are growing rapidly in developed countries in rural community and urban academic hospital settings.
- Educational leaders create LICs to align educational delivery with clinical delivery.
- LICs address four imperatives: connecting educational structures to the sciences of learning, stemming ethical erosion, improving health systems, and meeting societal needs.
- LICs provide 'educational continuity' through the continuities of patient care, faculty supervision, and the clinical curriculum.
- In LICs, students' commitment and sense of duty drive their learning.

Introduction

Educational, health system, and governmental leaders are re-envisioning health professions education. These leaders are guided by powerful learner, patient, institutional and societal imperatives (Frenk et al., 2010). The current processes and outcomes of medical education are inviting critical questions: What is the ultimate aim of medical education, and whom should it serve? (Hirsh & Worley, 2013) Who decides?

Practical questions about the design of clinical medical education stand out. How can medical education best foster learning and retention of science? What are the best ways to 'translate' learned science into evidence-based practice? What is the developmental trajectory of medical learners? How can medical education support and drive humanism, empathy, cultural competency, curiosity and inquiry? How can medical education improve the quality and cost of care, patient safety, access, equity, social accountability and community engagement? What pedagogic methods and educational structures best meet learner, teacher, patient, institutional and societal needs?

From the time of the first known longitudinal integrated clerkship (LIC) in 1971 to the present, LIC,

leaders have sought to address the core questions and imperatives facing medical education and care delivery by prototyping new structures of educational delivery. The creators of LIC models intend specifically for structures of clinical education to benefit learners maximally, while addressing clinical delivery, health system and populations' needs.

Central to the LIC movement is the notion that transformation of the processes and outputs of clinical education should benefit and advance the processes and outputs of clinical delivery. LIC planners are clear that the model itself is not the goal – progress in education and care delivery is the goal. LICs should thus be understood as means, not ends. LICs are enactments of educational principles to serve individual (learner, teacher, patient), organizational (office practice, institution), and community (collective, geographical and cultural) ends (Greenhill & Walters, 2014). University and health system leaders who advocate for LICs seek explicitly that the model itself drive continuous quality improvement of education and care delivery alike.

 "Educational and care delivery transformation must progress together and inexorably."

To characterize how such beliefs led to actual plans and products, this chapter will review the definition, history, rationale and structures of LICs, summarize data and literature about these models, and set forth future visions.

Definition

The link from these foundational values to the LIC definition are manifest in the framework of educational continuity (Hirsh et al., 2007) and the power of relationships as formative forces of education and caregiving (Worley et al., 2006). The definition of these 'first generation' LICs arose from a consensus conference following the international Consortium of Longitudinal Integrated Clerkships meeting in Cambridge, Massachusetts (USA) in 2007. At that time, educational scholars and LIC leaders from the known programmes characterized LICs by considering all LIC-like programmes described in the medical literature. Accordingly, LICs are defined as the central element of clinical education whereby medical students:

1. participate in the comprehensive care of patients over time

2. engage in continuing learning relationships with these patients' clinicians

3. meet the majority of the year's core clinical competencies, across multiple disciplines simultaneously through these experiences. (Walters et al., 2012).

Importantly, the consensus definition does not dictate a length of an LIC only the 'majority' of the year's core clinical competencies. The leaders at the consensus conference assumed that most core clinical years last for at least 1 year. Thereby, the expectation arose that LICs would all proceed for no less than half an academic year. This concept had educational grounding. The length expectation arose from conceptualizing how much experience a learner needs to be oriented to, affected by, and able to contribute to a learning and practice environment. Extensive experience across a wide array of programmes and time, suggest a minimum of 6 months appears right, but the minimum and maximum 'dose' of an LIC remains an area of intense interest.

Reviewing the history of and rationale for LICs will help connect this definition to the animated models, their outcomes, and future visions.

History

In 1971, the Government of Minnesota (USA) determined that the state's medical school was not adequately fulfilling the state's workforce needs. Too few graduates were choosing to work in rural areas, and too few were choosing the specialty disciplines that would serve the population health needs. Primary care in general and family medicine in particular were in short supply, and the state sought a remedy. In response, educational leaders developed the Rural Physician Associate Program (RPAP) to address this charge, and did so by challenging several longstanding notions about how medical education delivery should commence.

RPAP:

1. eschewed traditional block rotations (TBRs) in the core clinical (third) year of US medical school in favour of a single multidisciplinary immersive experience

2. situated medical students outside the major academic teaching hospital in ambulatory office venues

3. dispersed medical students to live and learn in small communities, some far outside the major metropolitan area; enlisted clinicians as educators rather than employed academic physicians with research duties

4. situated students in family medicine rather than in the traditional specialties

5. ensured students engaged a diverse array of acutely and chronically ill patients along with patients in need of preventive services.

The RPAP model succeeded. Learner outcomes and workforce outcomes clearly demonstrated that the programme achieved the university's and the state government's goals (Verby et al., 1991). Other dispersed rural medical student education programmes followed in Washington, Michigan, Hawaii, South Dakota and North Dakota. Several programmes were parts of major research-oriented universities. Along with 40 years of data from RPAP, these programmes' outcomes were impressive and met student, institutional and community goals.

The first known urban LIC was outside North America. In 1993, educators created the Cambridge Community-based Clinical Course in Cambridge, England. This programme again demonstrated the feasibility and success of the LIC concept at a research-oriented university. Like its predecessors, the programme showed excellent programmatic outcomes for non-rotational, ambulatory training in the community, in this case, an urban community.

Building on Cambridge's UK success, and connecting to the rural mandate of the early LICs in the USA, Flinders University in Australia developed its LIC in 1997. That model, known as Parallel Rural Community Curriculum (PRCC), paved the path of LICs in Australia and became an engine of LIC research. Indeed, PRCC outcomes directly supported a critical governmental workforce mandate in Australia, the creation of the Rural Clinical Schools funding. Unsurprisingly, now nearly half of all schools across that nation are running LICs. Some, such as the University of Wollongong in New South Wales, offer the LIC to their entire class.

The rapid growth of LICs appears to trace to the development of the model in two urban academic schools in the USA. In 2004, Harvard Medical School launched the Cambridge Integrated Clerkship (CIC) in Cambridge, Massachusetts. Like its namesake in England, the model thrived, but unlike the original LICs in the United States and the United Kingdom, this programme relied on specialist clinicians. The CIC's goals did not relate to workforce but to advancing student's clinical and scientific learning and professionalism. Robust data and a series of publications outlined the model's principles, structure and results and further propelled the LIC movement (Hirsh et al., 2012; Ogur & Hirsh, 2009; Ogur et al., 2007; Hirsh et al., 2007). Subsequently, a collective of educational leaders and executives dedicated to advancing clinical medical education formed the international Consortium of Longitudinal Integrates Clerkships (CLIC) organization.

Following Cambridge (USA), another breakthrough arose when the University of California San Francisco (UCSF) created the first LIC situated in a highly sub-specialized, research intensive, quaternary medical centre. That programme, Parnassus Integrated Student Clinical Experiences (PISCES), extended the model's venues and reach, demonstrating success in the most sub-specialized clinical settings (Poncelet et al., 2011). PISCES also advanced the LIC research agenda, and multiple publications further characterized the model's processes and outcomes.

Thereafter, Columbia University, the University of North Carolina, Duke University, and universities in Alberta, British Columbia and Ontario, alongside other well regarded institutions in North America, applied LIC pedagogy to new settings and with new institutional goals. Many new LIC programmes integrated health system goals into the model – simultaneously providing high-level clinical education alongside management, leadership, and clinical delivery redesign training.

Northern Ontario School of Medicine became the first school in North America to use the LIC design for all of their students. Other new medical schools followed. Medical schools are also scaling and expanding LICs within their institutions; for example, the University of South Dakota has expanded the LIC to their entire class; the University of Minnesota has created urban LICs and specialty-enhanced LICs (e.g. to advance paediatric training), and UCSF has created an LIC at Kaiser Permanente, a large health system renowned for clinical delivery transformation and quality. UCSF has also expanded their quaternary hospital LIC and added a rural programme. Worldwide, LICs are growing rapidly with more than a doubling of the number of known institutions creating LICs since 2009.

Rationale

LICs arise in the context of serious concerns facing educational, clinical, health system and governmental leaders. LICs also arise after a time of significant progress in the sciences of learning and during an era demanding improved healthcare delivery. Consequently, four imperatives underpin the 'case for change' driving educational transformation in general and LIC transformation specifically: learning, professional, health system and societal imperatives.

LEARNING IMPERATIVES

This imperative argues that the sciences of learning should inform our education structures. Beyond pedagogy, the actual 'structure' of the education matters. Alongside the numerous fields of study describing the formative power of relationships to foster knowledge, skill and professional formation, empirical science demonstrates educational structures and practices that best support learning and retention (Rohrer & Pashler, 2010). Two domains of empirical study stand out for the weight of evidence and their connection to clinical education redesign: spacing and interleaving learning.

Spacing learning over time improves retention. *Spacing* refers to serially revisiting learning (content or skills, for example) with time between to consolidate, reflect upon, and even, 'necessarily forget' learned material. Spacing learning drives the 'longitudinal' concept of LICs. *Interleaving* refers to studying multiple discrete areas simultaneously. Imagine, for example, learning multiple languages at once, or the familiar situation of taking several different academic courses at once. Interleaving, like spacing, increases retention of learned material in the longer term. The interleaving effect provides benefits independent of and complimentary to the spacing effect. Interleaving drives the 'integration' concept in LICs.

Taken together, concepts from relational, social and workplace learning, alongside the sciences of longitudinal (spacing) and integrated (interleaved) learning led to the principle of educational continuity (Hirsh et al., 2007) that underpins LICs. Educational continuity in the clinical context sets up a series of 'sub-continuities': continuity of the care (of patients and populations), of supervision (by faculty and the interprofessional team), of the curriculum, and with peers. Importantly, this framework also fosters a continuity of learners' idealism – the core human values that drive their personal and professional growth.

With educational continuity (Fig. 12.1), students learn, revisit, and relearn concepts or skills and have important formative experiences over time (spacing). This model also affords opportunities for engaging multiple concepts simultaneously (interleaving). Iterative multisource feedback alongside iterative self and group reflection occur over time as well. The factor of time changes the nature of relationships as an educational force. With time and the relational continuity the model affords, students have different engagement with 'faculty' than short and more anonymous encounters allow (Walters et al., 2011). A student's 'faculty' consists of peers, the physician faculty, and all the others with whom the student has workplace and learning relationships. The trajectory of each student will differ, and continuity of the educational environment should allow for both standardization and individualization (Cooke et al., 2010).

 "With educational continuity, faculty have extended time with their students. Faculty say, 'The time together matters—it means I am teaching 'my' student and not just 'a' student.'"

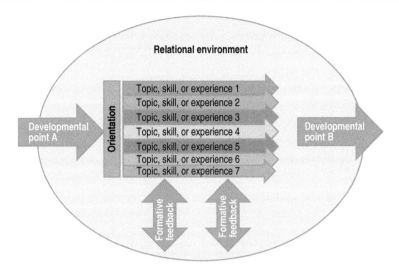

Fig. 12.1 Educational continuity.

PROFESSIONAL IMPERATIVES

Educational structures should attend deliberately to the hidden curricular influences (see Chapter 6) that can undermine learning and professional development or that adversely affect student wellbeing (Hirsh, 2014; Hirsh et al., 2012). Structural, tacit, and overt forms of objectifying or diminishing learners, patients, co-workers, and populations threaten learning and professional practice in overt ways and subtle ways. Students receive a powerful message if they are demeaned, but also when they are relegated to anonymity or to passive or insignificant roles. LIC leaders seek to address the hidden curriculum and reconstitute medical education such that: 1) the most able and professional teachers, clinicians, and scientists oversee students' learning and growth; and 2) learning occurs in educational structures that support students' development through meaningful, engaged, and authentic roles in caregiving(Hirsh & Worley, 2013; Hirsh et al., 2012).

HEALTH SYSTEM IMPERATIVES

Health systems, from individual teachers and clinicians to offices and institutions as a whole, need to change the educational formulation from 'student as burden' (or bystander) to 'student as benefit'. With the affordance of relationships and time, students should improve patient care – the quality, safety, access, efficiency and just delivery. Students may complete longitudinal projects for the office in which they work, may serve as health advocates as they 'walk in their patients shoes' across the venues of care, and may unearth and serve to improve office or health system processes. Along with quality and safety, health system imperatives also demand satisfying patients, providing access, and attracting patients to care. Healthcare

imperatives argue for education that improves care and care delivery to individuals and populations, in real time, as a consequence of the educational model.

The LIC design also benefits medical schools that are expanding enrolment to address physician workforce shortages. LICs create opportunities to place students in smaller communities that cannot support TBRs. Opening new venues for teaching and learning creates 'mission-driven' growth and connects health system imperatives to societal imperatives.

SOCIETAL IMPERATIVES

This imperative argues that medical education models should attend to workforce and community needs. LIC leaders advocate for education that is socially accountable and community engaged. LIC leaders seek to address under-served regions (e.g. urban, rural, remote), under-served disciplines and specialties (whether surgical/technical, specialist, primary care or psychosocial), and under-served populations (that may exist in under-served and well-served regions alike). LIC leaders seek to create structures of medical education that address the 'outputs' of our educational system.

Model types

With the rapid expansion of LICs, researchers are defining LIC typologies. Multiple ongoing research projects should help clarify what defines LICs versus LIC-like programmes. Typological clarity should help drive research that characterizes what works (e.g. which LIC elements foster what learning and professional impacts), for whom, in what context and why. More clarity will also extend understanding of the patient, faculty, office/institutional, and community impacts of LICs and other educational transformations. As educational leaders invent 'second generation' LICs and as the literature awaits research typologies, two current LIC model types uphold the 2007 international CLIC consensus definition: the generalist models and the multi-specialty 'streams' models.

GENERALIST MODEL LICS

In the generalist model LICs, the programme situates students in general practitioner or family medicine offices. In these settings, the rich diversity of clinical experiences meets all scholastic objectives. Students' principal preceptors are generalists who ensure the students' authentic and meaningful roles in care as they build a 'cohort' of patients to follow longitudinally. Specialty experiences typically precede the LIC time, follow the LIC time, or both. In addition, students in the rural areas meet the specialists who 'come to town' to provide clinical service and lead case-based small-group teaching sessions.

In this model, the students are active, relevant members of the healthcare delivery team and develop critical skills to serve the patients and populations in real time. To date, most generalist model LICs reside in suburban, rural and remote settings, but the model may exist in any centre with adequate generalist resources. Because the students are often dispersed into the community and immersed in the generalist practice, some leaders refer to generalist model LICs as 'dispersed-immersed' models.

 Generalist faculty explain, "Students have meaningful roles in care as 'the curriculum walks in the door.'"

MULTI-SPECIALTY 'STREAMS' MODEL LICS

The multispecialty LICs at Harvard and UCSF use a different structure. In the multi-specialty models, the students attend multiple ambulatory specialty clinics in the same week, seeing their individual specialty preceptor's patients. With their preceptors, the students build their 'cohort' of patients in each of these disciplines simultaneously.

In the multi-specialty stream LICs, like in the generalist LICs, faculty and students together build the students' patient cohort by considering multiple factors: 1) curricular goals (to create a diverse patient panel representative of the core conditions the curriculum seeks the student to engage); 2) patient needs (chronically ill, critically ill, and disenfranchised patients who benefit from student longitudinal involvement); 3) practicality (patients whom the student can actually follow); and 4) patient consent. Faculty and students consent patients verbally, explain the programme, and set expectations.

In the multi-specialty streams model, like the generalist model, the students may follow the patients across venues to other specialists. The specialty streams chosen, the size of the student cohort in each discipline, and the amount of time dedicated each week or fortnight depends on each school's objectives. The published literature about the Harvard and UCSF models outlines the weekly schedule (Ogur et al., 2007; Poncelet et al., 2011).

The generalist model and multi-specialty streams model LICs create similar affordances that may account for their similar outcomes. In each model the student has ongoing educational continuity and relationships with their:

- patients, peers, and preceptors
- office and institutional environment and the interprofessional co-workers therein
- courses' core themes
- community.

LICs' relational continuity supports students' personal and professional development differently than can occur in time-limited, discontinuous TBRs. LIC data demonstrate students' clinical excellence *and* students upholding their ideals and the ideals of the profession.

Strengths of LICs

FOR INDIVIDUAL STUDENTS, DOCTORS, AND PATIENTS

Multiple studies demonstrate the value of LICs for individual students (Walters et al., 2012). Students perform at least as well and often better on examinations compared to students in TBRs. Studies demonstrate these results repeatedly, across disciplines, over time, and on both content and clinical examinations (including national board exams in USA and Canada and on internal examinations in Australia and other countries) (Walters et al., 2012).

Clinical teachers report that LIC students are more work-ready than their peers trained in TBRs (Walters et al., 2012). LIC students express greater confidence in high-order clinical skills including: dealing with uncertainty, reflective practice, being self-directed, working with diverse populations, and understanding the healthcare system (Walters et al., 2012). LIC programmes facilitate a developmental learning trajectory of knowledge and skill through iterative feedback, and this continuity supports activities tailored to individual student's needs. Close oversight by experienced clinicians in practice supports robust assessment across the array of students' competencies. The LIC structure of oversight and time should support learner progression based upon faculty entrustment (Hirsh et al., 2014).

Doctors involved in LIC programmes describe finding their professional lives as clinical teachers more satisfying (Walters et al., 2011). As the student–preceptor relationship develops, clinicians value the contribution of medical students, report high levels of satisfaction with precepting and take increased ownership of student learning (Walters et al., 2011). Clinical teachers see LIC students move from peripheral roles (e.g. sharing information and providing support to patients) to having a more central doctor-like role (e.g. taking responsibility for explaining management to patients). Rural general practitioners describe strong interest in participating in LICs because they perceive a greater capacity to recruit into their discipline through more meaningful engagement with student learning than they gain from short-term placements (Walters et al., 2012). Urban specialists also espouse this value.

Patients who develop longitudinal relationships with LIC students benefit from the trust and mutual respect that develops over time. Students facilitate communication of important information across the health system and create a positive impact on their patients' wellbeing through their emotional support (Ogur & Hirsh, 2009). Patients perceive they have greater access to care from students in urban LICs; they note students are easier to reach and take more time to answer questions. Patients report that students improved the quality of their care through education about the disease and therapy.

 LIC faculty note that patients ask, "Can I have my own personal medical student?"

FOR ORGANISATIONS

Hospitals and their patients benefit from students serving as guides and 'interpreters' of the health system who can compensate for shortcomings in the system (Ogur & Hirsh, 2009). Late in the year, LIC students can see 'extra' patients and thereby increase provider volume. Between visits students call patients to check in and help foster adherence to care plans. Students can extend care to the home. Benefits arise from students in meaningful roles who, because of time and relationships, extend the reach and oversight of the care team.

Engaging in LICs provides individual practices many affordances: the status of partnering with a medical school, recruitment of residents and faculty, succession planning, enhanced access to information technology (and to students' command of it), the inspiration and capacity to commence research and quality improvement activities, opportunities to engage clinicians in academic roles beyond traditional clinical practice, and in some programmes, financial support for teaching and clinic infrastructure (Walters et al., 2012). In small hospitals with limited previous student placements, LICs have driven organizational change,

and new journal clubs and clinical quality improvement processes (Walters et al., 2012). Clinicians involved in LICs report that they appreciate the culture of learning, the educational community of practice and the increased interprofessional work (Greenhill & Walters, 2014). The longitudinal and immersive nature of the LIC students' engagement enhances these benefits (Hogenbirk et al., 2015).

FOR COMMUNITIES

For medical schools and universities with a social accountability mandate, LIC transformation drives meaningful community engagement. Through institutional involvement with community members, leaders, and policymakers educational planning and care delivery planning may be co-designed and mutually beneficial. In some cases, economic development and increased social capacity follows, such as formal arrangements for renting housing, and employing people as standardized patients (Greenhill & Walters, 2014).

Whole universities use LICs specifically to engage communities and offer population health benefits. In communities where social determinants of health significantly influence health equity, LIC students are more likely than their peers to report incorporating primary healthcare concepts into their clinical practice (Walters et al., 2012). Students who undertake LICs demonstrate significant public orientation and many choose to contribute to the community in which they study (Walters et al., 2012). At follow-up 4 to 6 years after their clerkships, twice as many LIC graduates report participating in social justice and health advocacy (50%) compared to their TBR graduate peers (23%) (Gaufberg et al., 2014).

Communities benefit when student skills more closely meet community desires for their physicians. Studies demonstrate LIC students increased their patient-centred skills, developed better clinical communication, and developed deeper understanding of the psychosocial component of illness (Walters et al., 2012). LIC students' stronger patient-centred attitudes endured into and beyond residency compared with peers from TBRs (Gaufberg et al., 2014).

Community involvement beyond the healthcare arena facilitates a sense of citizenship in students and generates a sense of prestige in communities that host LIC students. Patients in a rural setting note that students enrich the community. When it is a programme goal, situating LIC students to live and work in rural areas positively influences rural career choice in primary care and beyond. Longer LIC placements may have greater impact on recruitment to rural practice. LICs also appear to drive specialist retention in under-served areas and under-served disciplines, and have been powerfully successful for urban and rural and primary and specialty mandates alike (Hirsh et al., 2012; Walters et al., 2012).

Challenges of LICs

FOR THE INDIVIDUAL STUDENTS AND FACULTY

Learning experiences are not always comfortable, and LIC students often need reassurance about their trajectory. For example, even as data repeatedly confirm LIC students' breadth of clinical experience (experiences exceeding peers in TBRs), LIC students may *perceive* gaps in their clinical exposure. If gaps do exist, the longitudinal design allows students' logs to guide additional patient experiences. Programme leaders may also need to remind students that the LIC fits as a part of the curriculum (with future hospital-based experiences forthcoming thereafter).

Students may feel stress and uncertainty, and may struggle, when facing unpredictable clinical opportunities and when engaging multiple disciplines simultaneously. For students, LIC leaders should review the trajectory of LIC learning and the benefits of interleaving. Leaders can teach explicitly about the merits of 'desirable difficulty' in learning and of 'disorientating dilemmas' (à la transformative learning theory). LIC leaders should make students aware that they are likely to experience this 'conscious incompetence' (Greenhill et al., 2015). Intentional and proper faculty support, peer support, and connections to 'near-peer' LIC graduates all help to contextualize LIC students' experiences (Greenhill et al., 2015).

Balancing patient and learner needs requires attention, and course planners should provide dedicated faculty development in this domain. Even as research suggests patients are happy for increased involvement of students, faculty must manage consent and confidentiality intentionally, especially for disenfranchised and vulnerable patients. Small settings may make guarding students' confidentiality more complex as well.

Faculty sometimes experience tension between the demands of clinical service and the commitment to teaching. Fortunately, this tension is reported to be less in LICs. In the LIC model, clinicians do not need to serially reinitiate with a new learner several times each year and clinicians and their students build collaborative working relationships over time. With students' increasing clinical capacity and familiarity with the setting, the patients' and the team's needs, the non-transience of LIC students progressively creates a legitimate contribution to the clinical outputs and no decrease in faculty 'throughput' (Walters et al., 2012; Walters, 2014). Context specific orientation for students and faculty development also serve this goal.

FOR ORGANISATIONS

In some ambulatory practices, effective precepting involves reorganizing clinic processes to accommodate LIC students. Parallel consulting enables efficient use of clinic infrastructure and patient booking systems to enable LIC students to see patients on their own, prior to the supervising doctor joining the consult (Walters, 2014). The continuity of the student in the clinic enables student consulting sessions, rostering, and student assessment to be incorporated into routine operational duties of the medical practice.

LICs require careful administrative organisation for timetabling students' access to specialist theatre and consulting sessions. Initially, vertical integration with the medical curriculum and horizontal integration of placements and teaching sessions take strategic planning, operational care, and patience. Effective leadership of LICs and strong administrative capacity are essential for LICs programmes to reach their transformative potential.

FOR COMMUNITIES

Communities hosting students in LICs believe that they make important contributions to medical education and they may expect in return to have a secure, high quality medical workforce in their community in the future. This perception creates a weighty responsibility for institutional and programmatic leaders and individual students to meet. Even as LICs readily achieve student and medical school goals, institutional leaders must support the development of realistic community stakeholder expectations.

Future visions

LICs have redefined educational practice. Evidence of the impact of LICs on individual students, clinicians, and patients is well advanced (Walters et al., 2012). Medical education and care delivery will benefit by scholars moving away from 'justification research' of what appears to be a resolved question (LICs are at least as effective and in many domains more effective than the TBRs) to investigating the processes and reasons for the LIC results (Walters et al., 2012). Exploratory and explanatory research using realist evaluation frameworks should seek to describe more fully what works, for whom, in which context, and why. This vision calls leaders to extend our understanding of clinical education within and beyond medicine (Hirsh & Worley, 2013).

Summary

LICs support learning through relational continuity (Hirsh et al., 2007) and through spacing and interleaving learning. In LICs, students' authentic and meaningful roles drive their learning and their care. Medical students are fundamentally changed by the LIC experience, and many emerge transformed at a very human and personal level. So, too, are the students' teachers and patients.

In generalist models and multi-specialty models, and across multiple care delivery contexts, LICs are thriving. For decades, the medical education literature has demonstrated the LIC model's success and reach. LICs are an educational force providing powerful benefits for learners and teachers, for patients and practices, and for hospitals and the community. Nonetheless, medical educators should not enshrine historical, current, or next generation LIC models. LIC leaders believe that clinical education delivery should advance inexorably, continually adapting new educational prototypes to best create the future doctors our society needs.

References

Cooke, M., Irby, D.M., O'Brien, B., 2010. Educating Physicians: A Call for Reform of Medical School and Residency. Jossey-Bass, Carnegie Foundation for Advancement of Teaching, San Francisco.

Frenk, J., Chen, L., Bhutta, Z.A., et al., 2010. Health professionals for a new century: transforming education to strengthen health systems in an interdependent world. Lancet 376 (9756), 1923–1958.

Greenhill, J., Walters, L., 2014. Longitudinal Integrated Clerkships. Acad. Med. 89 (3), 526.

Greenhill, J., Fielke, K., Richards, J., et al., 2015. Towards an understanding of medical student resilience in longitudinal integrated clerkships. BMC Med. Educ. 15 (137). Available at: http://bmcmededuc.biomedcentral.com/articles/10.1186/s12909-015-0404-4. (Accessed 17 January 2017).

Gaufberg, E., Hirsh, D., Krupat, E., et al., 2014. Into the Future: Patient- Centeredness Endures in Longitudinal Integrated Clerkship Graduates. Med. Educ. 48 (6), 572–582.

Hirsh, D., 2014. Longitudinal integrated clerkships: embracing the hidden curriculum, stemming ethical erosion, transforming medical education. In: Hafferty, F.W., ODonnell, J. (Eds.), The Hidden Curriculum in Health Professions Education. Dartmouth College Press, Hanover.

Hirsh, D.A., Holmboe, E.S., Ten Cate, O., 2014. Time to trust: longitudinal integrated clerkships and entrustable professional activities. Acad. Med. 89 (2), 201–204.

Hirsh, D., Worley, P., 2013. Better learning, better doctors, better community: how transforming clinical education can help repair society. Med. Educ. 47 (9), 942–949.

Hirsh, D., Gaufberg, E., Ogur, B., et al., 2012. Educational outcomes of the harvard medical school-cambridge integrated clerkship: a way forward for medical education. Acad. Med. 87 (5), 1–8.

Hirsh, D., Ogur, B., Thibault, G., Cox, M., 2007. New models of clinical clerkships: "continuity" as an organizing principle for clinical education reform. N. Engl. J. Med. 356 (8), 858–866.

Hogenbirk, J., Robinson, D., Hill, M., et al., 2015. The economic contribution of the Northern Ontario School of Medicine to communities participating in distributed medical education. Can. J. Rural Med. 20 (1), 25–32.

Ogur, B., Hirsh, D., 2009. Learning through longitudinal patient care - narratives from the harvard medical school - cambridge integrated clerkship. Acad. Med. 84 (7), 844–850.

Ogur, B., Hirsh, D., Krupat, E., Bor, D., 2007. The harvard medical school-cambridge integrated clerkship: an innovative model of clinical education. Acad. Med. 82 (4), 397–404.

Poncelet, A.N., Bokser, S., Calton, B., et al., 2011. Development of a longitudinal integrated clerkship at an academic medical centre. Med. Educ. Online 16, 5939.

Rohrer, D., Pashler, H., 2010. Recent research on human learning challenges conventional instructional strategies. Educ. Res. 39 (5), 406–412.

Verby, J.E., Newell, J.P., Andresen, S.A., Swentko, W., 1991. Changing the medical school curriculum to improve access to primary care. JAMA 266 (1), 110–113.

Walters, L., Prideaux, D., Worley, P., Greenhill, J., 2011. Demonstrating the value of longitudinal integrated placements for general practice preceptors. Med. Educ. 45 (5), 455–463.

Walters, L., Greenhill, J., Richards, J., et al., 2012. Outcomes of longitudinal integrated clinical placements for students, clinicians and society. Med. Educ. 46 (11), 1028–1041.

Walters, L., 2014. Parallel consulting in community-based medical education. In: Chater AB RJ, Couper ID, Strasser RP eds. *Wonca Rural Medical Education Guidebook World Organisation of Family Doctors: Wonca Working Party on Rural Practice*. Available from www.globalfamilydoctor.com. (Accessed 14 January 2017).

Worley, P., Prideaux, D., Strasser, R., et al., 2006. Empirical evidence for symbiotic medical education: a comparative analysis of community and tertiary-based programmes. Med. Educ. 40 (2), 109–116.

Learning in a simulated environment

R. Kneebone, D. Nestel, F. Bello

Trends

- Simulation is a means, not an end.
- Simulation must be authentic, reflecting and resonating at some level with the realities of the clinical world.
- Simulation consists of selection, abstraction, re-presentation and intensification.
- Simulation does not need to be complex or expensive in order to be effective.
- Simulation technology will continue to advance rapidly, opening up further opportunities for simulation-based training.
- Simulation can integrate 'communication' (clinical teams and simulated patients) with 'procedural' skills (technology).

Introduction

Simulation has come of age. Decades of debate about whether or not simulation 'works' have changed into discussions about how to embed and implement it. An initial preoccupation with high technology and a focus on anaesthesia and the interventional specialties has broadened to include simulation at every level of clinical education. This reflects changing patterns of clinical practice and a shift from earlier models of clinical apprenticeship. The question is no longer *if* we should use simulation, but *how*.

Yet confusion remains, and learning through simulation is often perceived as a specialized domain requiring dedicated facilities and complex equipment. Simulation is often framed as an end in itself, detaching technical procedures from their clinical context and presenting them as something that can be practised in isolation. Terms such as 'simulation centre' and 'skills centre' make simulation itself the focus, rather than addressing what is to be simulated and why. This historical association with expensive static facilities and high technology can mask the widespread usefulness of simulation at

much simpler levels. Although such practise is invaluable, simulation must remain an adjunct to learning with real patients in the company of colleagues, not a substitute.

Unhelpful distinctions between 'technical' and 'non-technical' skills compartmentalize educational practice. This chapter resists such notions of separation, arguing instead for an integration of approaches and resources and asserting that simulation – like lectures, seminars, bedside teaching or any other educational approach – is a means rather than an end. Running alongside clinical practice, simulation offers a parallel resource to support learners as their clinical experience grows and develops.

 Like other educational methods, simulation can support students in preparing them to learn *in* and *from* clinical practice.

This chapter is for the general medical reader rather than the simulation specialist. It is not aimed primarily at those undertaking highly specialized training for advanced surgical and anaesthetic procedures. It sets out to give an accessible account of current developments, focusing on the learning rather than the environment of the chapter title. Simulation, we argue, can happen anywhere – not just in simulation centres.

A challenge is for clinicians and educators to take back control and democratize simulation, whether or not they have access to costly specialised facilities. We therefore start by going back to basics, asking what are the clinical and educational challenges to which simulation can offer solutions (Kneebone, 2010).

Background

We define simulation as a process where principles of design are used to integrate clinical care with education. The central focus is what takes place between two people – a clinician and a patient, or a teacher and a learner – held together in a relationship of care. Knowledge and skill must be applied within a context of trust, integrity and professionalism, and simulation must reflect this human relationship.

The acquisition of expertise requires sustained deliberate practise with the intention to improve, underpinned by feedback and critique in a supportive environment conducive to learning. The ability to pause, restart and replay a clinical encounter provides invaluable opportunities to apply educational principles to the clinical setting. It is also important for learners to experience failure, and to recognize when they are approaching (or crossing) the limits of their competence. Such ideals often conflict with the constraints and dangers of the clinical setting.

Simulation offers a solution to some of these challenges, identifying aspects of clinical care (with all the dangers and complexities that implies) and transplanting those to a safe setting where the educational needs of learners are treated as prime and where no real patient can suffer harm.

 Simulation offers learners the opportunity to rehearse elements of clinical care in patient-safe environments and to receive feedback intended to develop future practice.

We therefore argue that simulation is not an end in itself, but rather a means to support learning. In recent years the emphasis has moved from practising so-called 'technical' skills on isolated models to a more comprehensive vision that encompasses the complex human context of unique individuals working together. This needs to take into account what educational theory can tell us about how people learn, especially under conditions of pressure and stress.

Earlier discussions centred on practical issues such as the provision of simulators or the detailed recreation of clinical settings. The debate now is how to embed simulation most appropriately within the world of clinical practice, ensuring a proper balance between technicist and humanist perspectives. We cannot think of patients as depersonalized bodies and procedures as tasks performed according to a formula. Each encounter with a patient or colleague is unique.

This chapter challenges the notion that simulation requires costly static facilities. Developments such as 'in situ' simulation blur the edges between clinical care and education, by taking simulation into clinical settings. Our own developments of hybrid, distributed and sequential simulation (described below) offer further possibilities. More recently still, simulation has been used as a means of sharing the closed practices of healthcare with patients and those who care for them and with publics and society at large.

Simulation as design

Simulation can be thought of as a verb rather than a noun – an activity or method rather than a place or an array of physical simulators. Viewed as an activity, simulation is much more flexible than is commonly perceived and can be adapted, modified and shaped according to individual circumstances and needs. To do this, a conceptual framework is necessary.

Framed as an active process, simulation involves the following elements:

Selection from the complex world of what is to be examined, taught and learned. This requires dialogue between 'clinician,' 'educator' and 'patient' perspectives. For example, learning a bedside procedure (such as inserting a urinary catheter in a distressed elderly man with acute retention of urine following an operation) might be identified as a learning need.

Abstraction of the selection, removing it from its originary setting. This requires analysis of the key objectives in terms of clinician–patient interaction (including fine motor skills) and clinical learning. In the example above, inserting the catheter requires a combination of procedural skill (inserting the catheter accurately and safely) and interpersonal sensitivity (reassuring a distressed patient while working with a clinical colleague).

Re-presentation of the abstracted selection. This provides the opportunity to carry out the task in question, performing the practical procedure on a model while engaging with the patient as a person. This may take place within a dedicated centre or in alternative venues, allowing selected aspects of clinical practice to be addressed within a safe yet realistic simulated setting. Such settings take the needs of clinicians, patients, learners and educators into account in designing apt environments for learning that balance challenge and support.

Intensification is an outcome of this process. By stripping away what is inessential (such as distractions from other patients on a ward or other elements of real-world complexity), learners are freed up to focus on their individual learning needs at that moment.

 A conceptual framework for designing simulations is comprised of selection, abstraction, re-presentation and intensification.

Simulated patients

The next section outlines the pivotal role of simulated patients (SPs) in capturing the essence of clinical practice and implementing the 're-presentation' described above. At the core of healthcare practice is the communication between patients and healthcare professionals. Kneebone (2014) describes how this relationship of care is mediated by voice:

"[Voice]…is a complex concept that can be read in both literal and metaphorical terms. From this perspective, voice – extended to include

facial expression, gesture, touch, even clinical interventions – is medicine's primary medium of connection. Making sense of voice involves the ability to transmit and receive simultaneously, continually modulating one in response to the other."

It is through this notion of voice, that SPs make their contribution to medical and health professional education – as a proxy for real patients in this relationship of care.

Simulated patient methodology and trends in medical education

Since the 1960s there have been reports of SPs in medical and later in health professions education. The first documented accounts of SP work are attributed to Barrows (Wallace, 2006) a neurologist and innovative educator in the United States. Barrows experimented with teaching well people to demonstrate clinical signs in order to prepare medical students for clerkships. However, he was concerned with more than the clinical signs, coaching SPs to present the gestalt of the patient. Skilled clinicians were unable to detect that SPs were not 'real'. Although there was initial resistance by his peers, Barrows persisted and there is now a sophisticated global SP industry. In the United States and Canada, there are well established specialist roles of SP educators, whose key responsibility is to manage SP programmes that service medical and other health professions curricula, especially for assessments. While maintaining their specialist role, many SP educators are aligning their work with simulation practitioners who work with manikins, task trainers or other simulators.

Fundamental concepts in simulated patient methodology

Although SPs are now described as well people trained to portray a patient in a healthcare scenario and to offer feedback to learners on how they were received or experienced (Nestel & Bearman, 2015), their range of practices varies tremendously. SP methodology refers to scholarship associated with SP-based practices for educational and/or research purposes. In this chapter, we use the 'P' in 'SP' to refer to patients but it could quite easily refer to other participants such as relatives, bystanders, healthcare professionals or others in scenarios. We also use the term *simulated* rather than *standardized* (a common North American usage) to reflect our values about relationships of care and their portrayal by SPs.

An effective relationship is one in which the continual modulation of voice leads to respectful understanding. A tension in contemporary SP methodology is reconciling the standardization of SP portrayals required for objective structured clinical examinations (OSCEs) with the representation of the complexity of real clinician–patient relationships. Indeed, we value individual variation as a particular strength of SP methodology, capturing the uncertainties and unpredictability of clinical practice. This affords learners the opportunity to be immersed in SP-based scenarios, to reflect on what occurred and to share insights from SPs.

Discourses of clinical competence

International trends in medical education have influenced SP practices, especially the focus on medical competence and its shifting discourses as described by Hodges (2012). In SP methodology, the *performance* discourse is illustrated by providing the opportunity for learners to demonstrate their ability to perform a clinical skill with an SP (e.g. history-taking, explaining a procedure). In the *psychometric* discourse of competence, all behaviours are considered to be measurable and as such translatable to numbers. Standardization and SP-based stations in OSCEs offer an obvious example. This has probably had the most profound impact on SP methodology, leading to the term 'standardized' patient as used in the United States and Canada. Standardization often reduces exchanges within the OSCE station to overly simplistic cues and responses that do not reflect real relationships but privilege specific clinical actions. This is a move away from Barrow's original concept. A more recent discourse of competence as *reflection*, is represented by learners making meaning of clinical encounters through feedback from SPs. This feedback is intended to shape learners' future practices. A shift to a *production* discourse of competence focuses on quality outcomes illustrated by a current project of the US-based Association of Standardized Patient Educators (ASPE) in developing standards for SP practices. Each of these discourses of competence has varying degrees of presence in contemporary SP practices. It is important to reflect on these discourses as they significantly influence the ways in which SPs approach their work. Finally, Bearman and Nestel (2015) note an emerging *complexity* discourse of SP methodology, a theme developed in this chapter.

Scope of SP practice

SPs can contribute to a wide range of patient-based healthcare scenarios and be coached to describe symptoms and demonstrate signs, supporting the development of communication, professionalism and patient safety. Participation in SP-based scenarios enables learners to experience these core components of clinical practice in a patient-safe environment. Commonly, scenarios focus on exchanges between learners and SPs in clinical tasks such as history-taking, negotiating management plans, sharing information and much more. Specific clinical characteristics of illnesses and diseases can be portrayed, including acute and chronic conditions affecting any body system and age of patient.

Because SPs look, sound and behave as real patients, they can contribute to the development of clinical reasoning, physical examination, investigative, procedural, operative and therapeutic skills through appropriate scenarios. Recent developments focus on interprofessional collaborative practice, placing SPs at the centre of team-based simulations. Although SPs usually work in simulated environments, they sometimes work in real clinical ('in situ') settings. An obvious advantage here is the authenticity of the environment, reflecting the setting in which the learners are or will be expected to practise. A variation on in situ simulations are incognito or unannounced SPs, where the SP is functioning as a mystery shopper might in retail, but here the SP works in a clinical setting and makes judgements of learner performance and clinical processes in the workplace.

Hybrid simulations

The potential of SPs continues to expand. Mastering procedural skills within an authentic context of clinical challenge is a case in point. Our group has pioneered the concept of hybrid simulation, in which a simulator is placed beside an SP to enable procedural, operative and investigative skills to be practised and consolidated (Kneebone & Nestel, 2010; Kneebone et al., 2002). For example, a suture pad strapped to the arm of an SP to enable a learner to practise wound closure, a simulator arm positioned on an SP for learners to practise establishing an intravenous line, a virtual reality simulator placed at the end of an examination couch with the SP lying on their side with legs drawn up for learners to practise flexible sigmoidoscopy. Drapes, other props, make-up and moulage products create an illusion of seamlessness between the simulator and the SP.

We developed this approach to support learners in the challenges of integrating the complex sets of skills required for safe and effective care. Hybrid simulations facilitate this integration, and are suited to most clinical events in which the patient is conscious. Many manufacturers now develop simulators to accommodate hybrid simulations. Other examples include stethoscopes that play pre-recorded auscultatory sounds when appropriately positioned on an SP's chest or abdomen. Such developments continue to expand the scope of practice of SPs.

Patients' voices

Although these are exciting advances, much SP-based work is framed from clinician perspectives and the needs of the curriculum rather than presenting authentic patients' voices. Scenarios are often seen as "a mirror for the teachers' preconceptions rather than as an authentic reflection of a patient encounter" (Nestel and Kneebone, 2010). It is common for clinicians to determine learning goals, design scenarios and direct feedback that inadvertently overlook patients' perspectives and experiences (Kassab et al., 2011). Even the way we have described the hybrid simulations above privileges clinical tasks over patients' experiences. SP methodology offers unique opportunities to access the complexity of clinical practice, to explore the relationship of care and to examine the voices of learners and SPs in a particular place and time.

 Simulated patients are proxies for real patients – that is, portraying and offering feedback from patients' (not clinicians') perspectives.

When empowered, SPs can make a unique contribution by speaking for patients rather than clinicians (Powell et al., 2016). Strategies include *patient* participation in all stages of SP methodology, from establishing learning goals to evaluation, and in selection, abstraction, re-presentation and intensification. Co-construction of scenarios by clinicians, learners and patients may ensure that all perspectives are valued in the process of learning about relationships of care. Although it may be impracticable to do this every time, it must happen often enough to ensure that learners learn what patients value.

Another strategy is to base scenarios on real patients' histories, an approach that is usually 'filtered' through clinicians' perspectives (Weldon et al., 2015). Inviting real patients to work with SPs is a seemingly obvious, but underutilized strategy (Powell et al., 2016). Of course, there are limitations with this approach. These include the willingness, ability and suitability of real patients to participate (one important reason for involving SPs in the first place), the impact on a real patient of an actor portraying their experience (a potentially confronting experience) and the sharing of personal information (issues of confidentiality). Locating the teaching of clinical skills as part of a broader arc of patient care (including discharge planning, say, or other follow-up care) offers more patient-centred approaches to learning.

Qualities of simulated patients

A spectrum of SP practices ranges from simple to complex, and this expanded scope of practice requires high levels of expertise. The demands on the SP in a scenario are varied, but usually require the ability to remain in role while responding appropriately to cues offered by the learner. SPs need to be able to recall what they noticed about what the learner was offering, what they themselves transmitted in response and why – all key constituents of feedback. Added to this is the emotional load of role portrayal, of many repetitions of a scenario, of working with a facilitator, and offering what is often trenchant feedback to learners. The SP will be expected to report on more than the words and gestures exchanged, but the way in which the learner used the environment or artefacts in the setting – the placement of medical notes, the positioning of chairs, the handling of medical equipment and more. Specialist language may be required to get at the essence of the relationship of care.

The role of the SP is extremely complex. A dramatic arts background offers a solid foundation, especially in managing the emotional work of role portrayal, while a deep understanding of educational principles is also essential. Performance and educational experience are required for successful work at the complex end of the spectrum of SP practices.

Supporting simulated patients in role portrayal and feedback

Two main types of support for SPs are required – in portraying roles (re-presentation) and in offering feedback (intensification). For role portrayal, commencing with character development rather than the clinical event is one way of focusing attention on the patient as an individual (Nestel et al., 2015). SPs are encouraged to focus on embodying the person whom they will be portraying – of considering who that person is outside the clinical encounter. Only after this is achieved does the training shift to placing the person as a patient in a clinical context. Scenarios usually incorporate a written briefing document or SP role that guides preparation and rehearsal. There may be safety issues to be considered in teaching SPs to portray clinical signs and for working in hybrid simulations. Where SPs are being prepared for OSCEs, training needs to focus on establishing the parameters for appropriate responses.

There are many approaches to managing feedback for learners and each requires support. It is beyond the scope of this chapter to outline these in detail. Here we consider verbal feedback immediately after a simulation. Facilitator-led feedback should have an invitational quality, which empowers SPs to share their experiences. Observers (e.g. other learners) may experience the scenario differently to the learner and the SP. Being a participant within the scenario offers a different experience to looking in from the outside. Acknowledging and respecting this difference privileges the relationship of care.

SPs usually step out of role to offer feedback. They speak from their experience within the scenario, drawing on their in-the-moment decisions. Learner and SP relationships offer a different dynamic to that which learners have with real patients. Although learners often report forgetting that they are in a simulation soon

after it commences, the fact remains that it is a simulation. The power balance can shift in either direction and in part depends on the commitment of all participants in the scenario to use the experience as a learning opportunity.

Simply providing the opportunity for learners to practise skills in scenarios is insufficient. Feedback (e.g. spoken, audiovisual, rating forms) from multiple perspectives (e.g. clinicians, peers and SPs), together with reflection by which the learner makes meaning for future practice is critical. This is the forum for the *voices* described above to be explored. It is important to share scholarly research on what comprises patient-centred care and associated clinician behaviours. However, SPs must be encouraged to make meaning of this research relative to their own experiences, the roles they portray and the settings in which they work.

 By using the conceptual framework described above, simulated patients can contribute to all phases of simulation design and therefore make truly patient originating offerings to learners.

A key feature of simulation is that scenarios may be paused and the evolving clinician–patient relationship discussed. The learner can reflect on their progress with the SP and identify suggestions for development – a continual modulation of the participants' voices. When the scenario is resumed, new ideas can be tested out. Time can also be compressed or expanded to enable access to particular elements of the relationship (see Sequential simulation below).

There is a growing recognition of the pressures experienced by SPs as their work becomes more complex. SPs may endure significant stress during simulations and feedback and should be given the opportunity to 'de-role' – an explicit strategy to ensure that they have completely stepped out of role at the end of each session.

Simulation technology

The discussion now moves to the other key element in simulation – technology. Simulation technology has benefitted from advances in materials science, virtual reality (VR) computing, mobile devices and advanced human–computer interfaces. Whilst there is no doubt that it can play an important facilitating role in the simulation as design process described above, there is also a real danger of technology dominating the simulation discourse. It is, therefore, crucial to acknowledge that the educational value of simulation technology lies not on how technically advanced or sophisticated it is, but on how well it can support the learning outcomes of a particular educational encounter. Thus, clear vision and a good understanding of the affordances and limitations of a specific simulation technology is essential to make good use of its potential, ensure a balanced partnership between pedagogy and technology, and avoid the simulation agenda being driven by the naturally vested interests of simulator and simulation technology companies.

A key use of simulation technology is to enable the re-presentation of the abstracted selection in the simulation as design process (see above), through the development of simulators, defined here as apparatus designed for rehearsing selected aspects of clinical practice. We recognize three main types of simulators: physical models, VR simulators and hybrid simulators.

 Simulation technology benefits from rapid advances in many other areas, but its true value must be defined as how well it can support the intended learning outcomes.

PHYSICAL MODELS

Physical or benchtop models are widely used at undergraduate and early postgraduate levels of training (Bradley, 2006). Also known as part-task trainers, they tend to focus on specific skills, examinations or procedures, allowing novices to practise them repeatedly. Made from a variety of plastic, silicon and other materials, they aim to resemble the look and feel of real life tissues and organs, offering direct handling of instruments and interaction with real materials. Clinical procedures simulated include venepuncture, cannulation, urinary catheterization, basic suturing, bowel and vascular anastomosis, hernia repair, as well as other commonly performed surgical tasks and physical examinations.

Recent advances in materials science and cross-fertilization between model makers, artists and medical educators have resulted in extremely realistic, visually and tactile as well as functionally complex bespoke benchtop models. Physical models are relatively cheap in comparison to the other types of simulators. However, major drawbacks include fixed anatomy, wear and tear and lack of facilities for formative and summative assessment. The majority of these models also tend to be used in isolation separate from their clinical context, which can lead to a reductionist approach to learning.

VIRTUAL REALITY SIMULATORS

VR is well-established as a teaching tool in a variety of non-medical domains such as aviation, the military and the nuclear power industry (Krummel, 1998). For example, the use of VR simulators in aviation is recognized as a major contributor to a nearly 50% reduction in the rate of human error–related airline crashes since the 1970s (Levin, 2004).

The last twenty years have seen VR technology used to recreate a wide range of surgical procedures with an increasing level of realism, allowing learners to interact with a high-fidelity computer-based simulator (Olasky et al., 2015). Minimal access interventions are particularly suited as manipulating objects at a distance with suitable instruments, while watching a 2D screen, already reflects standard practice in minimal access surgery. Such simulators consist of a suitable human–computer interface resembling the instruments used, a screen to display the virtual environment, and a computer to run the simulation. Learners may choose procedures with varying levels of difficulty; performance metrics (e.g. time taken, economy of movement, errors made) and the procedure itself can be recorded automatically. Feedback based on these metrics is normally provided after the procedure, with or without a tutor's input.

Several generations of VR simulators have been developed. In the late 1990s, the first generation focused on training basic skills by performing isolated tasks (e.g. pick and place, navigation) using abstract scenes and 2D representations of geometric solids (e.g. MIST-VR). The early 2000s witnessed the second generation focusing also on basic skills, but attempted to achieve this by using more realistic procedural tasks (e.g. LapSim). In the mid-2000s, the third generation allowed entire procedures to be simulated, introducing a degree of anatomical variability to create a range of difficulty levels, moving beyond psychomotor skill and beginning to include decision making (e.g. LapMentor). The current fourth generation reflects progress in computer graphics, design, interfacing and visualisation, as well as enhanced ergonomics, improved content and curriculum management, and better integration with simulated clinical settings (e.g. VIST-LAB). One of its aims is to offer patient-specific simulation that allows specialists to plan and rehearse challenging cases before an actual operation. Whilst minimal access interventions continue to dominate, the range of surgical and non-surgical specialities supported has increased significantly (e.g. dentistry, endoscopy, orthopaedics, neuro, urology, gynaecology, ophthalmology).

Cost and the need for ongoing specialised support is one of the major drawbacks of VR simulators. Their design and development demands considerable resources, whilst their wider adoption requires tackling a range of practical, administrative, educational and financial challenges (Olasky et al., 2015).

Hybrid simulators

In this section we draw a terminological distinction (based on usage in the literature) between hybrid simula*tors* and the broader concept of hybrid simula*tion* (outlined above). Hybrid simulators are a combination of a physical model with customized software and electronics/mechatronics, offering a range of interactive settings that support learning. They lend themselves well to supporting hybrid simulation through their use with SPs and have the potential for also supporting team training, moving beyond practising isolated technical skills and recreating the context of clinical practice.

Hybrid simulators include full-body manikins able to provide tactile, auditory and visual stimuli (e.g. Laerdal SimMan, CAE METIman). Such simulators present a range of pathophysiological variables and can respond to the administration of drugs, as well as give immediate feedback to a range of interventions. Manikins are routinely used for anaesthetic training and are becoming increasingly common in other domains. They may be used within a dedicated educational facility, but also in the field. Full-body simulation allows for both basic procedural practise, as well as immersive scenarios offering an opportunity to practise and reflect on critical diagnostic, management skills, communication, organization, and multitasking.

Hybrid simulators also cover endoscopy, endovascular and urological interventions (e.g. EndoVR, EndoSIM, VIST-C, URO MENTOR), combining an authentic interface (endoscope, catheters/guidewires, cystoscope) with a realistic VR display. Such simulators are able to mimic a range of diagnostic and therapeutic interventions, at different levels of difficulty, allowing novice and intermediate learners to gain the basics of manipulative skill through repeated practise. Decision making is enhanced by the display of vital signs, haemodynamic wave tracings, and patient responses that appropriately reflect relevant physiology. Performance metrics are captured and presented after each procedure. A range of pathological conditions and technical challenge levels is also offered.

As technology continues to advance, hybrid simulators and VR simulators are converging, offering a wider range of functionality, larger selection of procedures, more sophisticated interfacing, photo-realistic graphics rendering, and a more holistic integration within immersive scenarios.

 Simulators range from simple benchtop models to highly complex full-body manikins and virtual reality computing systems.

Current and future trends

Simulation-related technology has advanced dramatically since the first recognized medical simulators. Large increases in computational power are accompanied by substantial progress in graphics, optics, sensor technology, touch-enabled human–computer-interfaces, mobile technology and materials science. Unified software development platforms that facilitate rapid prototyping and beta testing, as well as reutilization of software components are emerging. All of these, coupled with the wide availability and cost effectiveness of 3D printing, relentless progress in the fields of medical imaging, instrumentation, diagnosis and intervention,

are resulting in a new paradigm where simulation technology is required and able to support, in a coherent and coordinated manner, training and practice across all stages of healthcare. Consultation, specialist diagnosis, pre-operative planning, intra-operative guidance, post-operative recovery, discharge, reintegration into and care in the community can all now be taken into account.

Further improvements in the realism and functionality of physical models can be expected, with *smart* benchtop models incorporating sensor and actuating technologies to provide real-time feedback, reproduce physiological behaviour, and support more complex interactions. Integration between physical models and advanced software simulations will continue, blurring the boundaries between simulator types. At the same time, software development will converge towards more powerful, unified development platforms borrowed from the gaming industry. This will set the scene for a more cost-effective VR simulation development model based around a 'simulation app store', where simulation users download simulator apps that can then be tailored and executed on a common smart simulation platform, which in turn will result in more flexible and affordable simulators.

 Further advances in simulation technology are expected to make simulation more affordable and more widely available.

Simulation in the twenty-first century

The discussions above have outlined two distinct approaches to simulation. Historically, these have evolved along separate lines. We argue that much can be gained by aligning these traditions. In addition to our work on the concept of hybrid simulation described above, the following examples highlight such possibilities.

Distributed simulation creates 'realistic enough' clinical environments that are portable and relatively low cost (Kneebone et al., 2010; Kassab et al., 2011). Physical contexts of care are provided by lightweight backdrops, often presented within an inflatable enclosure to delineate a consulting room, ward, operating theatre or intensive care unit. A sense of authenticity is created by clinicians working together to enact pathways of care, which they carry out in real life, using actual clinical equipment to treat the 'patient' (represented by SPs, physical models or hybrid simulation). This 'minimal necessary complexity' allows the most appropriate level of detail for the purpose at hand to be selected, adjusting this as appropriate for selected participants.

Sequential simulation moves beyond single episodes to portray sequences of care, highlighting connections between elements in a clinical pathway (Powell et al.,

2016; Weldon et al., 2015). By concatenating a series of 'scenes' (for example a patient at home, in their community physician's consulting room, in an ambulance, a hospital ward, operating theatre or intensive care unit), a clinical trajectory of days or weeks can been condensed into half an hour or less. In addition to addressing skills within a given section of the healthcare system, this allows transitions between phases of care to be rehearsed and examined.

The combination of distributed and sequential simulation opens opportunities for clinicians to engage with patients, their carers and the general public (Kneebone et al., in review). By inviting non-clinicians to watch, take part in and interrogate pathways of care through simulation, healthcare professionals can widen their perspectives and gain valuable insights (Tang et al., 2013).

Integrated procedural performance instrument (IPPI) overcomes some of the limitations of OSCE-style assessment (such as an unduly formulaic approach based on learning prescribed procedures) by incorporating unpredictability within clinical scenarios (Kneebone et al., 2006). A series of stations integrates humanist and technicist challenges (such as siting an intravenous line in a patient with visual disability, or giving an injection to an angry and abusive patient). Structured feedback from SPs and clinician observers acts as an aid to self-critique and reflection by learners.

Summary

Simulation is central to contemporary clinical education and its role is set to expand. Yet simulation is often equated with costly, high-tech facilities dominated by a profitable industry. This chapter challenges assumptions about the need for cost, complexity and specialist expertise. In many cases, simulation is an activity that can be carried out anywhere and does not depend upon elaborate or expensive facilities.

Of course in many cases sophisticated facilities are essential. Simulation and its technologies have a crucial role in allowing invasive procedural skills to be practised and assessed. As science and clinical care become ever more sophisticated, the need for specialized techniques to be practised in safety becomes increasingly evident. It is essential that emerging techniques are accompanied by the means of learning to perform them safely and well. Technological advances offer huge potential, especially in addressing the learning of 'unsighted' procedures mediated by touch, such as rectal or vaginal examination. The rapid development of haptic simulation holds the promise of new approaches to multi-sensory learning.

Yet an emphasis on high technology for a specialized few can hide the benefits of simulation for the many. This chapter argues that much may be achieved by simple means – by using existing resources imaginatively,
by thinking laterally and by resisting pressures from the commercial world to equate value with cost. The role of SPs in creating the human framework of care is crucial. The examples from the authors' work show that surprisingly much may be achieved with surprisingly little.

By framing simulation as an educational approach rather than a fixed product – a means of learning, not an end in itself – we can harness the creativity of patients, clinicians and all those who teach and learn. By doing so we can ensure that the relationship of care – in education as much as in clinical practice – remains at the centre of everything we do.

References

Bearman, M., Nestel, D., 2015. The future of simulated patient methodology. In: Nestel, D., Bearman, M. (Eds.), Simulated Patient Methodology: Theory, Evidence and Practice. Wiley Blackwell, West Sussex.

Bradley, P., 2006. The history of simulation in medical education and possible future directions. Med. Educ. 40 (3), 254–262.

Hodges, B., 2012. The Shifting Discourses of Simulation. In: Hodges, B., Lingard, L. (Eds.), The Question of Competence: Reconsidering Medical Education in the Twenty-First Century. Cornell University Press, New York, pp. 14–41.

Kassab, E., Tun, J.K., Arora, S., et al., 2011. "Blowing up the Barriers" in surgical training: exploring and validating the concept of distributed simulation. Ann. Surg. 254 (6), 1059–1065.

Kneebone, R., 2010. Simulation, safety and surgery. Qual. Saf. Health Care 19 (Suppl. 3), i47–i52.

Kneebone, R., 2014. Escaping Babel: the surgical voice. Lancet 384 (9949), 1179–1180.

Kneebone, R., Arora, S., King, D., et al., 2010. Distributed simulation – accessible immersive training. Med. Teach. 32 (1), 65–70.

Kneebone, R., Kidd, J., Nestel, D., et al., 2002. An innovative model for teaching and learning clinical procedures. Med. Educ. 36 (7), 628–634.

Kneebone, R., Nestel, D., 2010. Learning and teaching clinical procedures. In: Dornan, S.E. (Ed.), Medical Education: Theory and Practice. Elsevier.

Kneebone, R., Nestel, D., Yadollahi, F., et al., 2006. Assessing procedural skills in context: exploring the feasibility of an Integrated Procedural Performance Instrument (IPPI). Med. Educ. 40 (11), 1105–1114.

Kneebone, R., Weldon, S., Bello, F., Engaging patients and clinicians through simulation: rebalancing the dynamics of care. Advances in Simulation, In review.

Krummel, T., 1998. Surgical simulation and virtual reality: the coming revolution. Ann. Surg. 228, 635–637.

Levin, A., Fewer crashes caused by pilots, in *USA Today (Online)*. 2004). USA Today (Online), March 2nd, p 2. p. 2.

Nestel, D., Bearman, M., 2015. Introduction to simulated patient methodology. In: Nestel, D., Bearman, M. (Eds.), Simulated Patient Methodology: Theory, Evidence and Practice. Wiley Blackwell, West Sussex.

Nestel, D., Fleishman, C., Bearman, M., 2015. Preparation: Developing scenarios and training for role portrayal. In: Nestel, D., Bearman, M. (Eds.), Simulated Patient Methodology: Theory, Evidence and Practice. Wiley Blackwell, West Sussex, pp. 63–70.

Nestel, D., Kneebone, R., 2010. Authentic patient perspectives in simulations for procedural and surgical skills. Acad. Med. 85 (5), 889–893.

Olasky, J., Sankaranarayanan, G., Seymour, N., et al., 2015. Identifying Opportunities for Virtual Reality Simulation in Surgical Education: A Review of the Proceedings from the Innovation, Design, and Emerging Alliances in Surgery (IDEAS) Conference: VR Surgery. Surg. Innov. 22 (5), 514–521.

Powell, P., Sorefan, Z., Hamilton, S., et al., 2016. Exploring the potential of sequential simulation. Clin Teach 13 (2), 112–118.

Tang, J., Maroothynaden, J., Bello, F., Kneebone, R., 2013. Public engagement through shared immersion: participating in the processes of research. Sci. Commun. 35 (5), 654–666.

Wallace, P., 2006. Coaching Standardized Patients for Use in Assessment of Clinical Competence. Springer, US.

Weldon, S.M., Ralhan, S., Paice, E., et al., 2015. Sequential Simulation (SqS): an innovative approach to educating GP receptionists about integrated care via a patient journey–a mixed methods approach. BMC Fam. Pract. 16 (1), 109.

Further reading and resources

Dudley, F., 2012. The Simulated Patient Handbook: A Comprehensive Guide for Facilitators and Simulated Patients. Radcliffe Publishing Ltd, London.

Nestel, D., Bearman, M. (Eds.), 2015. Simulated Patient Methodology: Theory, Evidence and Practice. Wiley Blackwell, West Sussex.

Victorian Simulated Patient Network www.vspn .edu.au.

Association of Standardized Patient Educators www. aspeducators.org. (Accessed 9 January 2017).

Distance education

J. Grant, A. Zachariah

Trends

- Medical education is already a distributed learning system, using a variety of hospital and community settings for learning. Distance learning is a quality assured, managed extension of these current practices.

- As more community-oriented schools are established, distance learning will become an important way of managing learning and ensuring equivalent educational opportunities across all locations.

- Distance learning methods for postgraduate and specialty training can effectively support trainees working throughout the healthcare system.

Before you begin ...

In this chapter, we hope to show you that distance learning is a very rich educational approach, well-suited to learning medicine. A central core of any distance learning programme is a specially written workbook that requires the learner to be actively engaged in thinking and processing new knowledge. All the wide variety of learning experiences that a medical student has should be organized around the workbook.

So we present this chapter as a small example of a distance learning workbook. It gives you the opportunity to experience distance learning, see how a distance learning course is constructed, undertake different types of exercises and get feedback on your learning.

So let's begin!

INTRODUCTION TO THE COURSE

Welcome to this short course on distance learning in medicine! It consists of a *workbook* that should take you about 1 hour to study.

As medical schools increasingly place students in community settings (Strasser, 2016) and postgraduate trainees are dispersed across urban and remote communities (Cleland et al., 2012), distance learning is one of the most needed and appropriate modes of medical education. If we think about medical education, we realize that our students and postgraduate trainees are widely distributed throughout the healthcare system. So both learning and teaching are distributed. Lea and Nicholl (2002) refer to "the fading boundaries between traditional higher education and distance education contexts and the breaking down of distinctions between formal and informal sites of learning".

So distance learning is perhaps just a logical development of many current practices in medical education.

Learning activities

In this course you will find a number of brief exercises called 'learning activities'. These are one of the most important parts of learning at a distance. They give you the opportunity to think about, use, apply and understand more fully the content being presented. And each gives you feedback on your responses, which is essential to productive learning (Hattie & Timperley, 2007).

Objectives

After completion of this course, you should be able to:

- define 'distance learning' and consider its advantages and disadvantages
- outline how distance education courses may be designed for clinical medicine
- identify the media and learning experiences that can be blended into a distance learning course for medicine
- describe the structure of a distance learning text and the design of learning activities
- describe how students learning at a distance can receive feedback
- describe how distance learning courses are developed
- describe the meaning of a wrap-around course and how this may be used in medical education
- discuss quality assurance in distance learning.

Contents

Planning study time is a key skill for students learning at a distance. Table 14.1 will help you plan your study time now.

Table 14.1

Table of contents	Time for study	Page
1. WHAT IS DISTANCE LEARNING?	3 minutes	p. 103
Activity 1. What methods can be used to help a medical student or doctor learn at a distance?	3 minutes	p. 103
Activity 2. Advantages and disadvantages of distance learning in medical education	2 minutes	p. 103
2. TECHNOLOGY AND DISTANCE LEARNING	3 minutes	p. 104
Activity 3. Technology and print in distance learning	3 minutes	p. 104
3. THE STRUCTURE OF A DISTANCE LEARNING TEXT	3 minutes	p. 105
Activity 4. Features of distance learning texts	5 minutes	p. 105
Activity 5. Design of learning activities	5 minutes	p. 105
4. PROVIDING STUDENTS WITH FEEDBACK ON LEARNING	2 minutes	p. 107
5. BLENDING DIFFERENT ELEMENTS OF THE COURSE	4 minutes	p. 107
6. MANAGING CLINICAL ATTACHMENTS BY DISTANCE LEARNING	3 minutes	p. 108

Table 14.1 continued

Table of contents	Time for study	Page
Activity 6. What are the principles of designing clinical experience on a distance learning course?	3 minutes	p. 108
7. THE STUDENT'S LEARNING EXPERIENCE	3 minutes	p. 109
8. MANAGING DISTANCE LEARNING	3 minutes	p. 109
9. DEVELOPMENT OF DISTANCE LEARNING COURSES	5 minutes	p. 110
10.QUALITY ASSURANCE IN DISTANCE LEARNING	3 minutes	p. 111
Activity 7. Quality assurance in distance learning	5 minutes	p. 111
11.CONCLUSION	2 minutes	p. 111
ESTIMATED TOTAL STUDY TIME FOR THIS WORKBOOK: 1 hour		

WHAT IS DISTANCE LEARNING?

Let's think about the various methods that are available to help people who are learning medicine at a distance (Table 14.2). Try the following activity, then read the feedback (Table 14.3).

Table 14.2 Activity 1

What methods can be used to help a medical student or doctor learn at a distance?	Allow 3 minutes
Please jot down here your ideas about what methods can be used to help students and doctors learning at a distance. Do this before reading the feedback that follows!	

Table 14.3 Feedback. A number of people have tried the activity. They listed the following methods. Compare what you said with their list.

Printed workbooks	DVDs	Email
Learning packages	Video conferencing	Face-to-face tutorials
Guided texts	CDs	Web-based resources
Online library resources	Telephone tutorials and feedback	Computer conferencing
Telemedicine	Television	Radio programmes
Community/clinical work	Online teaching	E-learning courses
Readers and textbooks	Residential meetings/skills labs	Student discussion groups (live, online)
Virtual and simulated environments, e.g. virtual microscope	Tutor-marked assignments and feedback	Assessments: computer-based, paper-based, practical

This activity shows that distance learning is made up of a wide variety of experiences, blended together to make one well-planned course. It is clear that distance learning has many of the same components as traditional learning. The only difference is that in distance learning, these are all carefully planned, blended, managed and quality assured.

Given this, how shall we define distance learning? Grant (2008) defines 'distance learning' as:

Individual study of specially prepared learning materials, usually print and sometimes e-learning, supplemented by integrated learning resources, other learning experiences, including face-to-face teaching and practical experience, feedback on learning and student support.

Distance learning provides a rich, planned experience for learners, quality assured, flexible and cost effective.

So now, consider the advantages and disadvantages of distance learning for medical education by trying Activity 2 (Table 14.4) and then reading the feedback (Table 14.5).

Table 14.4 Activity 2

Advantages and disadvantages of distance learning in medical education	Allow 2 minutes
What do you think are the advantages and disadvantages of using distance education in medical teaching? Jot down your thoughts in the following space.	
Advantages	Disadvantages

Table 14.5 Feedback

Advantages	Disadvantages
Makes quality-assured teaching available to all	Clinical skills development requires integrated face-to-face teaching
Is particularly useful for physicians who are working full time or have limited time available. Is an excellent method for knowledge development	Distance education courses require supervision of clinical experience and careful planning to ensure an appropriate blend of learning opportunities within limited time
Can reach out to doctors in remote locations and those who have not had the opportunity for postgraduate study	Distance learning takes initial skilled effort to design and produce
Can be cost-effective and uses teachers' time efficiently	

TECHNOLOGY AND DISTANCE LEARNING

Although many people equate e-learning and distance learning, you can see from Activity 1 that technology offers just one way of learning. It should be used when the curriculum demands it, and when it is feasible and cost-effective. Technology is simply another medium alongside all the others. The next activity (Table 14.6) asks you to think about this.

Table 14.6 Activity 3

Technology and print in distance learning		Allow 3 minutes	
Complete the following chart to help you analyze the relative strengths and weaknesses of technology and print for distance learning.			
Technology		Print	
Strengths	Weaknesses	Strengths	Weaknesses

Feedback

Technology

You might have said that technology offers rich, interactive visual images, immediate feedback, better illustrations, student–teacher communication and a more modern feel.

But you might have noted that technology is expensive to produce, requires access to hardware, broadband and regular electricity, is not portable, requires typing skills, does not easily allow scribbling, highlighting and note-taking, is more difficult to flick backwards and forwards, is harder on the eyes and tends to imply entertainment rather than learning. Other concerns are technical problems, a perceived lack of sense of community and time constraints (Song et al., 2004).

Print

Print is limited in visual presentation, seems more old-fashioned, is less flexible in giving feedback and offers no interpersonal communication.

But print is cost-effective, is easily updated, is flexible to use, requires no equipment or back-up, allows note-taking and highlighting, requires no technical skills, is portable and flexible and is the most familiar medium for learning. Teachers can reach out to students who do not have regular Internet. Busy practising physicians can keep the text in hand and do small activities whenever they have time.

THE STRUCTURE OF A DISTANCE LEARNING TEXT

You will remember that the definition of distance learning given previously on page 103 emphasizes that materials must be 'specially prepared'. The next two activities (Tables 14.7 to 14.9) ask you to think about what this means.

Table 14.7 Activity 4

Features of distance learning texts	Allow 5 minutes
Look through this chapter. Note down any features that make it different from a usual book chapter. Say what you think the function of each feature is in terms of helping the distance learner.	
Feature	Function

Table 14.8 Feedback. You might have noticed the following:

Clear aims, instructions, timings	Ensures learners are clear about the task and can plan their time
Conversational style	Simulates a tutorial atmosphere
Short sections	So that the learner has a sense of progress and will not skip sections
Clear page layout	So that the learner does not get lost in a variety of boxes and options
In-text activities with timings	Ensures that the learner is active, thinking and applying learning within an appropriate amount of time
Feedback	So that the learner knows if he or she is on track and to offer new information

Table 14.9 Activity 5

Design of learning activities   Allow 5 minutes
Read the following activity taken from the module on 'Respiratory problems and HIV infection' from the Fellowship in HIV Medicine course at Christian Medical College (CMC), Vellore. The student would have studied a text beforehand. Then answer the two questions that follow.
Pneumonia
The following exercise will help you learn the approach to a patient with HIV infection and pneumonia.
A 30-year-old woman diagnosed with HIV infection 5 years ago presents with acute-onset fever with chills, cough and purulent blood-tinged sputum of 3 days duration. She complains of sharp pain on the right side of the chest, which increases with deep breaths.
On examination: she appears ill and toxic, pulse rate 130/min, respiratory rate 26/min, temperature 103°F. She has flaring of alae nasi. Oral candidiasis present. Impaired resonance over axillary and infrascapular areas on the right side, bronchial breathing and increased vocal resonance over the same areas.
1. What is your clinical diagnosis?
2. What is the likely organism causing this infection?
3. Does this patient require admission?
4. What tests will you order immediately?
5. What treatment will you start?
Now answer these questions:
a. What are the design features of the above activity that foster clinical learning?
b. What other types and designs of activities might be appropriate for a clinical course?

Whether the medium is print or technology, these design features are essential to supporting and retaining the interest and understanding of the learner. Distance learning texts must be written to encourage the learner to keep studying, give a sense of progress, stimulate active learning, give feedback and offer 'a tutorial in print' (Rowntree, 1982). Distance learning texts for medicine may be written to teach the basic sciences, or the application of clinical sciences by, for example, simulating a ward round, providing clinical information, asking and answering questions, encouraging reflection and emphasizing learning points.

Now let's turn to the design of learning activities that stimulate active learning and a sense of achievement and give feedback to the student.

FEEDBACK

a. Features in the design of this activity which facilitate learning in medicine:
  - The activity provides appropriate clinical information for a common clinical problem and simulates learning at the bedside
  - The questions focus on the important learning objectives relating to this clinical problem
  - The student studies relevant information beforehand and then applies it through the activity

- Clear timings are given
- The purpose of the exercise is clear.

b. Distance learning activities appropriate for a clinical course:

- Providing clinical, microbiology and X-ray images
- Sequencing case information in time as the case evolves
- Writing prescriptions
- Designing patient information sheets
- Preparing a local guideline
- Filling in blanks, matching items, extended matching activities
- Labelling diagrams.

Distance learning modules can be completely self-contained, where all the resources are provided in the module. Modules also may be designed as 'wrap-around' materials that complement a prescribed text. Such a module requires clear instructions regarding navigating through the prescribed text and attention to timing. In general, the wrap-around text would present activities and commentary to prepare students for readings from the text and then to help them to use or reflect on that reading.

 Which approach you choose will depend on the texts that are available, for example, the distance learning modules for the Christian Medical College (CMC) Fellowship in HIV Medicine course were completely self-contained, because of the absence of good texts in HIV care for the Indian setting. However, for another course for new junior doctors, we have developed wrap-around modules that complement standard undergraduate textbooks.

PROVIDING STUDENTS WITH FEEDBACK ON LEARNING

Students need to know how well they are progressing and understanding, so feedback on learning is essential in distance learning, as it is for all learning. This is achieved in a number of ways, some of which you have already experienced here. Feedback to the student is deliberately offered in:

- in-text activities
- tutor-marked assignments
- tutorials
- student groups
- online support
- supervision of related practical and clinical work
- assessments.

If you reflect on your own education, you might wonder whether you received such consistent and deliberate comments and guidance!

BLENDING DIFFERENT ELEMENTS OF THE COURSE

The activities so far have shown that distance education is made up of a rich variety of learning activities. It is much more than a delivery medium. But this richness poses the challenge of integrating and blending the resources and experiences without losing the student along an insufficiently signposted path. In this, distance learning is a special case of the blended learning that is seen in traditional education.

 Blended learning is a coherent design approach that openly assesses and integrates the strengths of face-to-face and online learning to address worthwhile educational goals. Garrison & Vaughan, 2008

The key to success is simple:

- Provide all learning resources so that they are available at the time the student needs them. Avoid, for example, asking the student to access patient records if they are likely to be studying in their room at night!
- Use one central learning guide: this can be, for example, the distance learning course in print, or a curriculum map in print or on a PDA (hand-held computer) associated with a timetable and learning resources.
- In the central guidance, give clear instructions on what resources to access or activities to undertake and ensure that the student returns from these to the central guidance.
- Use clear icons alongside the text to indicate the type of resource to be accessed. For example:

 The student is directed to certain pages of supplied material and then asked to return to the workbook.

 Next, the student is directed to the relevant section of a CD to watch an interview with a patient.

 Finally, the student would be referred to the patient's notes provided and asked to read their history.

MANAGING CLINICAL ATTACHMENTS BY DISTANCE LEARNING

Clinical attachments everywhere can be supported by distance learning. This might involve:

- a *distance learning workbook* with supporting materials
- a paper or computer-based *curriculum map* of content to be covered
- a reflective *portfolio* submitted online to a mentor or peer group for comment
- structured *preparatory and reflective exercises* and projects linked to clinical experience
- *formative assessments*
- ongoing *clinical assessments* with feedback linked to the curriculum map
- *quality control* of the clinical attachment, to include support to teachers.

To think about this more, try the next learning activity (Table 14.10).

Table 14.10 Activity 6

What are the principles of designing clinical experience on a distance learning course?	**Allow 3 minutes**

Consider here what principles you might follow in designing distance learning materials to support students on clinical attachments.

Feedback

We think that the following elements are important:

- The clinical learning objectives should be clear
- The student requires exposure to common clinical problems
- Adequacy of the exposure and level of skill development should be monitored through case records, log books and formative assessments
- The student should take the appropriate level of clinical responsibility necessary for their learning
- The course should make maximum use of the clinical experience available
- The distance learning guidance should prepare students for the clinical experience and enable them to reflect on it. The clinical teacher or supervisor should be aware of the distance learning component and support the students appropriately.

In some courses, clinical contacts are planned centrally. For the CMC Fellowship in HIV Medicine course, students have three clinical contact periods, totalling 5 weeks, at the central training institute, spread over the year. These are designed for progressive skills development and increasing responsibility. The students also improve their skills through clinical care projects at their local institutions. In other courses, clinical work may be planned carefully at the students' institutions or elsewhere supervised by local trained tutors. A portfolio or map of the clinical experience may assist the student.

THE STUDENT'S LEARNING EXPERIENCE

A wide variety of experiences are available to the distance learning student, just as they are to students in conventional programmes. A difference between the two will be the central learning guide, which might be the organizing vehicle for:

- studying specially prepared course materials
- undertaking learning activities and checking understanding
- referring to web-based or CD-ROM resources
- online conferencing with peers
- participating in asynchronous online tutorial groups
- participating in synchronous online 'expert' events
- telephone or web-based tutorials
- working within a virtual clinical environment
- exercises to prepare for and reflect on clinical work
- submitting electronic tutor-marked assignments, receiving and discussing feedback
- discussion with a mentor about progress and integration of course components.

These activities might look suspiciously like a conventional course. But the main difference is the degree of organization, the central distance learning text, the style of those materials and the amount of planned support and feedback that the student receives. Distance learning should be an enhanced educational experience because every detail, including support for teachers, is carefully planned and managed.

MANAGING DISTANCE LEARNING

It will be clear by now that a distance learning course is carefully planned and highly managed. Ensuring that all the parts of the course are working and being presented and used in time; that all students are progressing properly; and that teachers are supported and students are active requires a learning management system (LMS). This can be paper-based, but is often a centralized, computer-based system, offering the following functions:

- student registration
- student records
- teacher records, including appraisals and feedback
- timetables
- learning resources
- assessments
- assessment records
- messaging
- records of communications with students and teachers
- evaluation and monitoring data.

Most of these functions can also be offered by an efficient office, if reliable technology is not available. Whatever system is used, whether high- or low-tech, the lesson is the same: management systems that track course development and implementation, student progress and teacher activity are fundamental to success in distance learning (Grant, 2015).

DEVELOPMENT OF DISTANCE LEARNING COURSES (TABLE 14.11)

Table 14.11   Distance learning courses require very careful preparation and development. They should all go through the following stages.

Needs assessment	Determines what content is required at what level
Feasibility study	The course design must fit the available funding, staffing, infrastructure and opportunities for teaching and learning
Multidisciplinary course team	The development team should have experts in distance learning, content experts, assessment experts and an administrator
Three drafts with piloting at draft two	To ensure that the student's journey through the course is as effective as possible, courses should go through stages of outlining the content of each element of the course, then a first draft, which is discussed by the course team, and a second draft, which is worked through by 'pretend' students to test timing and clarity, and reviewed by an external content expert, before preparing the third and final draft
Planning clinical experience	Careful planning of clinical experience at a local centre or main training centre
	Development of appropriate portfolios, log books and case records to record clinical exposure
Preparation and support of tutors	Teachers should be trained in supporting students in relation to: • course content and structure • giving written and verbal feedback • clinical supervision • project guidance • e-mentoring • spotting students in difficulties • student assessment
Preparation and support for students	All students require initial information about: • course structure and content • how to access and use the course elements and resources • organization of time • communication with other students and teachers' sources of support • the assessment system • what feedback to expect • responsibilities as learners
Preparing assessment methods	Preparation of guidelines for all assessments, project work and final examination. Setting the pass standards.
Evaluation and monitoring methods	Appropriate methods of gathering information are essential for trouble shooting and improvement
Maintenance course team for monitoring and updating	Once the course is up and running, a team is required to monitor its implementation, the activities of tutors and progress of students, to oversee the reliability and validity of the assessments and to decide when updating is required

QUALITY ASSURANCE IN DISTANCE LEARNING

Quality assurance is fundamental to the success of any distance learning course. Try the next activity (Table 14.12).

Table 14.12 Activity 7

Quality assurance in distance learning	Allow 5 minutes
This activity will help you to review everything that you have learned in this course, as well as addressing a very important issue: quality.	
Look back over this course and see if you can spot all the elements of distance learning design and development that form part of the quality assurance strategy.	

Feedback

You might have noticed the following quality assurance activities.

During course development:

* Needs assessment and feasibility study
* Careful course design and development to ensure relevance and usefulness
* Team feedback to authors
* Testing course materials in draft
* Trying out activities to collect material for feedback
* External assessment of the course.

Of tutors:

* Preparation of local tutors
* Ongoing monitoring and support for tutors.

For learners:

* Preparation of learners
* Support and feedback for learners locally and centrally.

Of the course:

* Evaluation and monitoring the course in use, tutor activity, student progress, assessment process and results
* Updating as required.

CONCLUSION

In this short distance learning course, we have tried to provide you with some insight into the potential of developing distance learning for medical education. This would not be too far from the blended learning that already occurs. Distance learning may be used for a small undergraduate clinical posting, for a complete postgraduate training programme or even for a whole medical school course. The example of the CMC HIV course has shown that distance education can not only train doctors but also strengthen clinical services at the community level.

Whatever media you use, however, the same rules of development and design apply, as you have learned in this course. We hope you have enjoyed it.

References

Cleland, J., Johnston, P.W., Walker, L., Needham, G., 2012. Attracting healthcare professionals to remote and rural medicine: learning from doctors in training in the north of Scotland. Med. Teach. 34 (7), e476–e482.

Garrison, D.R., Vaughan, N.D., 2008. Blended Learning in Higher Education: Framework, Principles, and Guidelines. Jossey-Bass, San Francisco.

Grant, J., 2008. Using open and distance learning to develop clinical reasoning skills. In: Higgs, J., Jones, M.A., Loftus, S., Christensen, N. (Eds.), Clinical Reasoning in the Health Professions. Elsevier, New York.

Grant, J., 2015. Distance learning in medical education. In: Bhuiyan, P.S., Rege, N.N., Supe, A. (Eds.), The Art of Teaching Medical Students. Elsevier, New Delhi.

Hattie, J., Timperley, H., 2007. The power of feedback. Rev. Educ. Res. 77 (1), 81–112.

Lea, M., Nicoll, K. (Eds.), 2002. Distributed learning: Social and cultural approaches to learning. Routledge, London.

Rowntree, D., 1982. Educational Technology in Curriculum Development. Harper & Row., London.

Song, L., Singleton, E.S., Hill, J.R., Myung, H.K., 2004. Improving Online learning: student perceptions of useful and challenging characteristics. Internet High. Educ. 7 (1), 59–70.

Strasser, R., 2016. Students learning medicine in general practice in Canada and Australia. Aust. Fam. Physician 45 (1-2), 22–25.

Further reading

Lentell, H., Perraton, H. (Eds.), 2003. Policy for Open and Distance Learning: World Review of Distance Education and Open Learning, vol. 4. Routledge, Abingdon.

Mills, R., Tait, A. (Eds.), 2002. Rethinking Learner Support in Distance Education: Change and Continuity in an International Context. Routledge, Abingdon.

Salmon, G., 2004. *E-moderating*. The Key to Online Teaching and Learning. Routledge, Abingdon.

Section 3

Educational strategies and technologies

Outcome-based education

E. S. Holmboe, R. M. Harden

Trends

- Adoption of outcome-based medical education has accelerated, in part because of growing and changing health and healthcare needs of patients and populations.
- The establishment of outcome- (competency-) based education is now a key feature in curriculum planning.
- Milestones and entrustable professional activities (EPAs) are increasingly used to facilitate the implementation of outcomes-based education.

A move from process to product

The seeds of the outcome-based moment were actually planted some time ago. McGaghie and colleagues argued in a World Health Organisation publication for an outcome-based approach to medical education (McGaghie & Lipson, 1978). In the years that followed, policy makers began to recognize the pernicious quality and safety problems within the healthcare system culminating in a number of landmark reports by the end of the twentieth century (IOM, 2001; Frenk et al., 2010). Over the last 20 years there has been a dramatic change, with consideration of the competencies and abilities expected of a doctor high on the agenda. Indeed, it can be argued that the move to outcome-based education has been the most significant development in medical education in the past one or two decades: more important than the changes in educational strategies, such as problem-based learning; in instructional methods, such as the use of new learning technologies; and in approaches to assessment, including the use of portfolios. All of these are important. They are, however, a means to an end: what matters are the abilities gained by the doctor as a result of the educational experience.

One of the most effective ways a teacher can facilitate students' learning is to discuss the expected learning outcomes with them on day one of the course.

A vision of the type of doctor to be graduated and the associated learning outcomes are the first two of the 10 questions to be answered in the development of a curriculum as described in Chapter 2. Only when these have been specified can we consider the content of the curriculum, the teaching and learning methods, the educational strategies and the approach to student assessment to be adopted (Fig. 15.1).

There has been a change in emphasis from process, where what matters is the education approach, to the product, where the abilities and attitudes of the graduates are of key importance. This is the essence of outcome-based education (OBE). The use made of simulators and e-learning, team-based and interprofessional approaches to the curriculum and assessment techniques such as the OSCE and the Mini-CEX are important and are addressed in other chapters in this book. Their contribution to the education programme, however, must be guided by the expected learning outcomes.

 "A good archer is not known by his arrows but by his aim."

Thomas Fuller

The trend towards OBE

OBE is now at the cutting edge of curriculum development internationally. The United Kingdom's General Medical Council (GMC) guidelines for medical schools, *Tomorrow's Doctors*, changed from an emphasis in 1993 on issues such as integration, problem-based learning and the abuse of lectures, to guidelines in 2003 and 2009 that highlighted the expected learning outcomes to be achieved on completion of the undergraduate course.

 "In line with current educational theory and research we [the UK's General Medical Council] have adopted an outcomes-based model. This sets out what is to be achieved and assessed at the end of the medical course."

Rubin & Franchi-Christopher, 2002

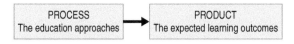

Fig. 15.1 In OBE there is a move from an emphasis on process to an emphasis on product.

The 2013 and 2014 AMEE conferences saw continued increases in the number of presentations on the topic from multiple researchers and educators around the world. The 4th Asia Pacific Medical Education Conference (APMEC) in Singapore had OBE as its theme.

The Association of American Medical Colleges (AAMC) has also taken a further step into outcome-based education with the launch in 2014 of the Core Entrustable Professional Activities for Entering Residency (CEPAERs) initiative (Englander, 2014). This initiative was partly in response to continued frustration of residency programme directors that too many medical schools' graduates are insufficiently prepared for residency. In Canada, the CanMEDS recommendations from the Royal College of Physicians and Surgeons of Canada and in the United States, the Accreditation Council for Graduate Medical Education (ACGME) areas of competence set out the expected learning outcomes in postgraduate education. Finally, AMEE and the International Competency-based Medical Education (ICBME) consortium sponsored an international summit in 2016 to take stock of progress and ongoing innovation regarding CBME and OBE. Finally, the rise of milestones and entrustable professional activities is a clear signal the world has moved from OBE principles and philosophy to wide spread implementation.

 "Education must be based on the health needs of the populations served… Competency-based education (CBE) is an approach to preparing physicians for practice that is fundamentally oriented to graduate outcome abilities and organized around competencies derived from an analysis of societal and patient needs."

Carraccio et al., 2015

Why the move to OBE?

OBE is not some passing fad that lacks an educational underpinning. While there has been some opposition to the approach, there are sound reasons for the position OBE now has at the forefront of education thinking. Here are some of the arguments for adopting OBE.

ATTENTION TO QUALITY OF CARE AND NEGLECTED AREAS OF COMPETENCE

Multiple reports from the World Health Organization (WHO), Organization for Economic Cooperation and Development (OECD), the Commonwealth Fund

(CMWF) among others have reported on persistent gaps in quality and safety across the globe (Mossialos et al., 2015). Substantial and unwarranted variation in healthcare delivery plagues all health systems. In addition, the Institute of Medicine (IOM) report and adverse events and near-miss reporting in the United Kingdom have documented high rates of preventable medical errors (IOM, 2001; Shaw et al., 2005). This has understandably led policy makers to look to the medical education enterprise as part of the solution by better preparing health professionals for twenty-first-century practice.

Consideration of the expected learning outcomes for an educational programme leads to a questioning of the validity of what is currently taught, and thus possible omissions or neglected areas can be identified. These can include communication skills, clinical reasoning, decision making, self-assessment, quality and safety improvement skills, interprofessional teamwork, creativity, patient safety and social responsibility: all important abilities for the practising doctor. The need to specify the abilities expected of our students on graduation and the delivery of a course of studies to achieve this is a message with which it is difficult to disagree (Crosson et al., 2011).

THE PROBLEM OF INFORMATION OVERLOAD

Advances in medicine and the medical sciences, with the doubling of knowledge every 2 years, poses a significant problem for the medical curriculum. While the length of the course has remained relatively constant, what the student might be expected to learn has expanded hugely. No longer can we say to students, "I cannot say precisely what I want you to learn from the course; just do your own thing." We need to specify more clearly from the wide range of possibilities what it is we expect the student to learn.

ASSESSMENT OF THE LEARNER'S PROGRESS AND THE CONTINUUM OF EDUCATION

The need for a more seamless transition between the undergraduate, postgraduate and continuing phases of education is now accepted. Implicit in this is a clear statement of the learning outcomes expected of the student or trainee, for example the required communication skills, prescribing skills or mastery of practical procedures, at the end of each stage before they move on to the next phase of their training. Clarity is also necessary with regard to the required achievements by learners as they progress through each phase of the training programme including the 4, 5 or 6 years of the undergraduate curriculum. It is useful to chart a student's progress towards each of the learning outcomes (Fig. 15.2).

Learning outcomes provide a vocabulary to support the planning of the continuum of medical education across the different phases.

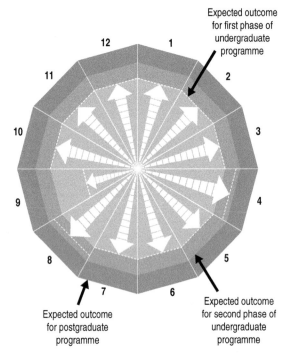

Expected outcome
for first phase of
undergraduate
programme

Expected outcome
for postgraduate
programme

Expected outcome
for second phase of
undergraduate
programme

Fig. 15.2 A representation of progress by a first-phase student in relation to each of 12 learning outcome domains. The expected progress for each outcome is indicated by the inner target for the first phase of the programme, by the middle target for the second phase of the curriculum and by the outer target for postgraduate training. (with permission from Harden RM: Learning outcomes as a tool to assess progression, *Medical Teacher* 29(7):678–682, 2007)

The student's progress in each of the outcome domains can be looked at from different perspectives (Harden, 2007):

• Increased breadth, e.g. extension to new topics or different practice contexts
• Increased difficulty, e.g. more advanced or in-depth consideration
• Increased utility and application to medical practice, e.g. a move from theory to practice and integration of what is learned into the work of a doctor
• Increased proficiency, e.g. more efficient performance with fewer errors and less need for supervision.

STUDENT-CENTRED AND INDIVIDUALIZED LEARNING

 "When we talk about individualisation … we mean the ability of educational programs to adjust to meet students' and residents' learning needs and offer educational experiences that acknowledge differences in background, preparation, and rate

of mastering concepts and skills, in contrast to the current one-size-fits-all approach."
Cooke et al., 2010

As described in Chapters 2 and 44, there is a move to student-centred education and independent learning. A clear understanding of the required learning outcomes by the teacher and student is necessary if the student is expected to take more responsibility for his or her own learning. Standardization of learning outcomes and individualization of the learning process was one of four goals for medical education identified in the Carnegie Foundation for the Advancement of Teaching Report, Educating Physicians (Cooke et al., 2010). Clearly stated learning outcomes, Cooke and colleagues suggest, contribute to increased efficiency of education, tailoring the education to the needs of the individual learner and possibly reducing the duration of training time for a trainee. Student centeredness also requires attention to helping learners engage in the regulation of their learning with a keen focus on goal setting, feedback seeking behaviours, self-motivation and self-monitoring of their learning.

ACCOUNTABILITY

The different stakeholders, including students, teachers, the profession, the public and government, now expect a clear statement of exit learning outcomes against which an education programme can be judged. No longer is it appropriate to see the programme as some form of 'Magical Mystery Tour' where the endpoint of training is uncertain. This is even more important at a time of financial constraint where resources may be limited.

 "There needs to be a clear definition of the end point of training and the competences which will need to be achieved."
Calman, 2000

A clear statement of learning outcomes is essential to support the current emphasis on academic standards and the accreditation of the education programme of a school. Learning outcomes are also important in the recognition of excellence in education in a medical school through programmes such as the ASPIRE-to-excellence initiative (www.aspire-to-excellence.org).

Implementation of OBE

LEARNING OUTCOMES AND INSTRUCTIONAL OBJECTIVES

In OBE the learning outcomes are identified, made explicit and communicated to all concerned. Recognition of the need to provide the learner with information about the end point and direction of travel is not new. In the 1960s, promoting the use of instructional objectives, Mager asked, if one doesn't know where one is going, how can one decide how to get there? Learning outcomes differ from instructional objectives, and five important differences can be recognized (Harden, 2002):

- Learning outcomes, if set out appropriately, are intuitive and user-friendly. They can be used easily in curriculum planning, in teaching and learning and in assessment.
- Learning outcomes are broad statements and are usually designed round a framework of 8–12 higher-order outcomes.
- The outcomes recognize the authentic interaction and integration in clinical practice of knowledge, skills and attitudes and the artificiality of separating these.
- Learning outcomes represent what is achieved and assessed at the end of a course of study and not only the aspirations or what is intended to be achieved.
- A design-down approach encourages ownership of the outcomes by teachers and students.

OUTCOME FRAMEWORKS

Learning outcomes are commonly presented as an agreed-upon set of domains within a framework that describes the larger picture of the abilities expected of a doctor. The move to competency-based education has much in common with outcome-based education, and competency frameworks may be similar to outcome frameworks (Albanese et al., 2008). The Dundee three-circle model (Fig. 15.3) as adopted in the Scottish Doctor is an example of an outcome framework. It covers the following:

1. *In the inner circle (doing the right thing)*: the technical competencies – what a doctor should be able to do, as classified in seven domains, e.g. communication skills and practical skills and procedures.
2. *In the middle circle (doing the thing right)*: the intellectual, emotional and analytical competencies – how the doctor approaches his or her practice. This includes an understanding of basic and clinical sciences, appropriate attitudes and appropriate judgement and decision making.
3. *In the outer circle (the right person doing it)*: the personal intelligences – the doctor as a professional including the role of the doctor and the doctor's personal development.

The Global Minimum Essential Requirements (GMER) specification used a similar framework (Schwarz & Wojtczak, 2002). The ACGME defined six general competencies thought to be common to physicians training in all specialties (Leach, 2004). These are related to the Scottish Doctor outcomes in Fig. 15.4. The CanMEDS framework, recently updated and revised, is based on the six physician roles: medical expert, communicator, collaborator, leader, health advocate, scholar and professional (Frank et al.,, 2015). Each principal domain in an outcome or competency framework can be specified in more detail.

SELECTING OR PREPARING AN OUTCOME FRAMEWORK

When a set of learning outcomes is developed for the first time, there are the following possibilities with regard to the use of a framework:

- An existing framework, as described above, can be adopted.

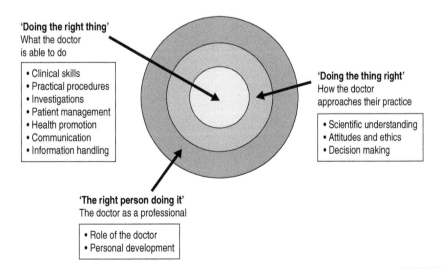

Fig. 15.3 The Dundee three-circle framework as adopted in the Scottish Doctor with 12 learning outcome domains. (from Scottish Deans' Medical Curriculum Group: *The Scottish Doctor*, 2008. AMEE, Dundee)

The Scottish Doctor Learning Outcomes			ACGME Outcome Project					
			a Patient Care	b Medical Knowledge	c Practice-based Learning and Improvement	d Interpersonal and Communication Skills	e Professionalism	f System-Based Practice
A	1	Clinical Skills						
	2	Practical Procedures						
	3	Patient Investigation						
	4	Patient Management						
	5	Health Promotion and Disease Prevention						
	6	Communication						
	7	Information Handling						
B	8	Scientific Basis						
	9	Attitude and Ethics						
	10	Decision Making						
C	11	Role of Doctor in Health System						
	12	Personal Development						

Fig. 15.4 The ACGME and the Scottish Doctor learning outcomes.

Box 15.1 Criteria for an outcome/ competency framework

- The framework is clear, unambiguous and intuitive to the users.
- It reflects accepted and defined areas of competence.
- The vision and mission of the programme are reflected in the domains chosen.
- It is manageable in terms of the number of outcome domains (usually 6–12).
- It supports the development of enabling outcomes in each of the domains.
- The relationship between different outcomes is indicated.

- An existing framework can be modified to suit the specific needs of the education programme.
- A new framework can be developed. Any new framework should be checked against the criteria for an outcome framework as described in Box 15.1.

Implementing OBE

An important step in implementing OBE is to determine what framework you will use to implement OBE. As described above, a number of countries have chosen to use a competency model to operationalize OBE. Competencies can be a valuable mechanism to describe the overarching outcomes. However, implementing competencies has proved challenging. This led to the development initially of parallel concepts, milestones and entrustable professional activities. Milestones provide narrative descriptors of the competencies and sub-competencies along a developmental continuum with varying degrees of granularity. Simply stated, milestones describe performance levels learners are expected to demonstrate for skills, knowledge and behaviours in the pertinent clinical competency domains. They lay out a framework of observable behaviours and other attributes associated with learners' development as physicians (Fig. 15.5). The ACGME now requires use of milestones as part of accreditation in the United States (Holmboe et al., 2015).

EPAs were originally conceptualized in the Netherlands and were first applied in physician assistant and obstetrics/gynaecology training. As defined by Ten Cate recently:

> *"EPAs are units of professional practice, defined as tasks or responsibilities that trainees are entrusted to perform unsupervised once they have attained sufficient specific competence. EPAs are independently executable, observable, and measurable in their process and outcome, and, therefore, suitable for entrustment decisions."*
>
> Ten Cate et al., 2016

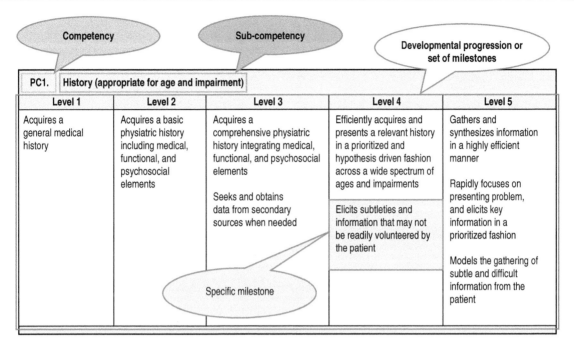

Fig. 15.5 Example template for the creation of the ACGME specialty milestones describing five developmental stages for postgraduate training programmes. (with permission from ACGME)

It is the activity that is 'entrusted' to the learner and EPAs should represent the core of the profession. Simply defined, EPAs describe what we expect a particular specialist to be able to do without supervision upon graduation from residency and fellowship. EPAs have become increasingly popular among a number of specialties in a number of countries as an approach to define more holistic outcomes for training programmes, using milestones as 'building blocks' to create EPAs that define the core activities of a specialty. Both milestones and EPAs can guide both assessment programmes and curriculum (Ten Cate et al., 2015).

AN OUTCOME-BASED CURRICULUM

In OBE decisions about teaching and learning methods, curriculum content, educational strategies, assessment, the educational environment and even student selection should be based on the specified learning outcomes (Harden et al., 1999a) (Fig. 15.6). To date, much of the attention in OBE has focused on the specification of learning outcomes and less on the implementation of an OBE approach in practice. There are two requirements for OBE. The first is that learning outcomes are clearly defined and presented. The second is that decisions relating to the curriculum are based on the learning outcomes specified. One can infer that a programme is outcome-based only if both conditions are met (Spady, 1994). Do not use learning outcomes as a window dressing for your courses or teaching

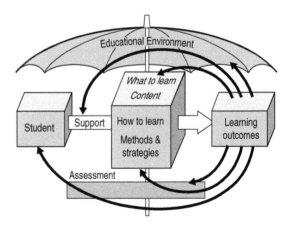

Fig. 15.6 A model for the curriculum emphasizing the importance of educational outcomes in curriculum planning. (with permission from Harden et al.,: An introduction to outcome-based education, *Medical Teacher* 21(1):7–14, 1999a)

programme. The learning outcomes need to inform the decisions you take as a teacher or trainee.

An outcome-based design sequence should be adopted in which the first step is the specification of the exit learning outcomes for the curriculum. The next step is to derive the outcomes for the different phases of the curriculum from these exit outcomes.

A blueprint should then be developed relating each learning outcome for the phase to the learning opportunities and to the assessment. A combination of competencies, milestones and EPAs can help in these initial steps. The process is repeated for the courses within each phase, the units within each course and the learning activities within each unit. In this 'design-down' process, the outcomes for the phases, courses, units and learning activities should be aligned with and contribute to the exit outcomes.

"Teachers should be informed of and have easy access to written learning outcomes for their courses so that they can plan their teaching strategies and methods."

Subha Ramani, 2006

In OBE there also has to be an acknowledgement that it is the teacher's responsibility to ensure that all students master the learning outcomes, and how this is achieved may vary from student to student.

Myths about OBE

If there is a problem with OBE, it does not rest with the principle but with how it is implemented in practice.

There are a number of misconceptions or misunderstandings about OBE:

- Some teachers are concerned that OBE is concerned with detail and that the big picture may be missed. While this may have been true with the objectives movement in the 1960s, OBE is concerned with broad parameters for competence and meta-competence (Harden et al., 1999b; Frank et al., 2010).
- Some teachers see OBE as a threat, bringing loss of their freedom or autonomy. On the contrary, OBE does not dictate teaching methods: the existence of an agreed-upon set of outcomes empowers teachers to develop their own programme that they believe will help the student to achieve the required learning outcomes.

"There is a fine line between the competency framework that emancipates learners and that which prevents their 'expansive learning'."

Dornan, 2010

- Others believe that OBE ignores trends in medical education and the move to student-centred learning. On the contrary, in OBE students are 'active agents' empowered to take more, not less, responsibility for their own learning. In OBE, teacher and learners can engage in a co-production relationship around curriculum and assessment (Holmboe & Batalden, 2015).

- Some teachers are concerned that OBE is about minimum competence. This need not be the situation. Learning outcomes can be specified at different levels of mastery as demonstrated in the Brown abilities (Smith & Dollase, 1999). In addition, milestones in use in several educational systems explicitly define aspirational levels of performance and development.

Summary

OBE is a key development and a response to current challenges facing medical education that offers many advantages. A statement of learning outcomes, often through competencies, milestones and EPAs, provides a language or vocabulary that helps to chart the progress of students through the different phases of education and to identify a learning programme to meet their personal needs.

Only when the end point of the journey is determined can the best way to get there be decided.

Learning outcomes should be specified using an appropriate outcome framework. An existing framework can be adopted or modified or a new framework created. Using the learning framework, outcomes should be developed for each course and learning experience. Decisions about the curriculum content, teaching methods, educational strategies and assessment should be related to the agreed learning outcomes.

References

Albanese, M.A., Mejicano, G., Mullan, P., et al., 2008. Defining characteristics of educational competencies. Med. Educ. 42 (3), 248–255.

Calman, K.C., 2000. Postgraduate specialist training and continuing professional development. Med. Teach. 22 (5), 448–451.

Carraccio, C., Englander, R., Van Melle, E., et al.; International Competency-Based Medical Education Collaborators, 2015. Advancing Competency-Based Medical Education: A Charter for Clinician-Educators. Acad. Med. [Epub ahead of print].

Cooke, M., Irby, D.M., O'Brien, B.C., 2010. Educating Physicians: A Call for Reform of Medical Schools and Residency. Jossey-Bass, San Francisco.

Crosson, F.J., Leu, J., Roemer, B.M., Ross, M.N., 2011. Gaps In residency training should be addressed to better prepare doctors for a twenty-first-century delivery system. Health Aff. 30 (11), 1–7.

Englander, R., Core Entrustable Professional Activities for Entering Residency. Association of American Medical Colleges. 2014.

Frank, J.R., Snell, L.S., Cate, O.T., et al., 2010. Competency-based medical education: theory to practice. Med. Teach. 32 (8), 638–645.

Frank, J.R., Snell, L., Sherbino, J., 2015. CanMEDS 2015 Physician Competency Framework. Royal College of Physicians and Surgeons of Canada, Ottawa.

Frenk, J., Chen, L., Bhutta, Z.A., et al., 2010. Health professionals for a new century: transforming education to strengthen health systems in an interdependent world. Lancet 376 (9756), 1923–1958.

Harden, R.M., 2002. Learning outcomes and instructional objectives: is there a difference? Med. Teach. 24 (2), 151–155.

Harden, R.M., 2007. Learning outcomes as a tool to assess progression. Med. Teach. 29 (7), 678–682.

Harden, R.M., Crosby, J.R., Davis, M.H., 1999a. An introduction to outcome-based education. Med. Teach. 21 (1), 7–14.

Harden, R.M., Crosby, J.R., Davis, M.H., Friedman, M., 1999b. From competency to meta-competency: a model for the specification of learning outcomes. Med. Teach. 21 (6), 546–552.

Holmboe, E.S., Batalden, P., 2015. Achieving the desired transformation: thoughts on next steps for outcomes-based medical education. Acad. Med. 90 (9), 1215–1223.

Holmboe, E.S., Yamazaki, K., Edgar, L., et al., 2015. Reflections on the first 2 years of milestone implementation. J. Grad. Med. Educ. 7 (3), 506–511.

Institute of Medicine, 2001. Crossing the Quality Chasm: A New Health System for the Twenty-first Century. National Academies Press, Washington, DC.

Leach, D.C., 2004. A model for GME: shifting from process to outcomes. A progress report from the Accreditation Council for Graduate Medical Education. Med. Educ. 38 (1), 12–14.

McGaghie, W.C., Lipson, L., Competency-based curriculum development in medical education: An introduction: World Health Organization Geneva. 1978.

Mossialos, E., Wenzl, M., Osborn, R., Anderson, C., 2015. International profiles of health care systems, 2014: Australia, Canada, Denmark, England, France, Germany, Italy, Japan, The Netherlands, New Zealand, Norway, Singapore, Sweden, Switzerland, and the United States. The Commonwealth Fund: New York. (Retrieved August 11, 2015). Available from: www.commonwealthfund.org/publications/fund-reports/2015/jan/international-profiles-2014.

Schwarz, M.R., Wojtczak, A., 2002. Global minimum essential requirements: a road towards competency-oriented medical education. Med. Teach. 24 (2), 125–129.

Shaw, R., Drever, F., Hughes, H., et al., 2005. Adverse events and near miss reporting in the NHS. Qual. Saf. Health Care 14 (4), 279–283.

Smith, S.R., Dollase, R., 1999. Planning, implementing and evaluating a competency-based curriculum. Med. Teach. 21 (1), 15–22.

Spady, W.G., 1994. Outcome-Based Education: Critical Issues and Answers. The American Association of School Administrators, Arlington, VA.

Ten Cate, O., Chen, H.C., Hoff, R.G., et al., 2015. Curriculum development for the workplace using Entrustable Professional Activities (EPAs): AMEE Guide No. 99. Med. Teach. 37 (11), 983–1002.

Ten Cate, O., Hart, D., Ankel, F., et al.; International Competency-Based Medical Education Collaborators, 2016. Entrustment Decision Making in Clinical Training. Acad. Med. 91 (2), 191–198.

Integrated learning

R. C. Bandaranayake

Trends

- Continuing emphasis on integrated learning in the undergraduate medical curriculum
- Increasing attempts to introduce work-integrated learning, particularly in community and hospital settings
- Increasing opportunities for medical students to undertake interprofessional learning in conjunction with other health professions students

Introduction

Over the last two decades many national and international bodies concerned with undergraduate medical education have exhorted medical schools to adopt practices in the curriculum that promote the integration of learning. The Australian Medical Council in 1998, the Gulf Cooperation Council Medical Colleges Deans' Committee in 2001, the World Federation for Medical Education in 2003, the General Medical Council in the United Kingdom in 2009 and the Liaison Committee on Medical Education for medical schools in the United States and Canada in 2010 emphasized the need for the integration of learning in the guidelines and standards promulgated for the improvement of medical education.

 "The curriculum will be structured to provide a balance of learning opportunities and to integrate the learning of basic and clinical sciences, enabling students to link theory and practice."

General Medical Council, 2009

This chapter focuses on providing guidance to the undergraduate medical teacher on how to bring about this desirable practice in the students whose learning is entrusted to them. Following the definition of terms related to integration and different types of integrated learning, the rationale for this practice and strategies

for practical implementation in the classroom are dealt with. The chapter concludes with an examination of some barriers to integrated learning and the critical role played by the student assessment system in fostering it.

Some definitions

Integration is defined, in Webster's Encyclopaedia, as "combining or coordinating separate elements so as to provide a harmonious interrelated whole". It is important for the medical teacher to realize that 'part' (element) and 'whole' are relative, as the *whole* in one sense may be *part* of a larger 'whole'. For example, several parts, such as the convoluted tubules and loop of Henle, constitute the nephron, a part of the kidney; the kidney is part of a larger whole, the urinary system, which in turn is part of an even larger whole, the human body. The essential criterion for integration is the linking of the different parts in a way that the whole functions properly. Any system consists of inter-related components linked to each other to ensure the proper functioning of the system. The nephron is a 'system' and its parts must be linked to each other for it to function, just as the several parts of the urinary system must be linked for it to carry out its important functions. The mere summation of the different parts without linking would not produce an integrated whole. *Integrated learning*, then, is the ability of the learner to link the various 'parts' he or she encounters in one or more learning experiences in a way that is both meaningful (related to previous learning) and relevant (related to perceptions of future application) (Bandaranayake, 2011).

 "It does not always follow that several units add up to unity. In fact, a subject made up of units tends, from the viewpoint of the student, to fall into a pattern of discrete, separate and unrelated experiences".

Capehart, 1958

Integration of learning must take place in the mind of each learner, as what is meaningful or relevant to one learner may not be so for another. The teacher's role is to foster integrated learning by facilitating the formation of such links by the student. *Integrated teaching* is facilitating integrative behaviour in the student by various methods, to be considered later in this chapter. As teachers, our aim should to be to develop individuals who integrate for themselves, rather than merely accept the integrations made by others.

 The teacher should foster integrated learning by facilitating the formation of links between concepts and units of study by the student.

The terms 'horizontal integration' and 'vertical integration' have been used in different senses by various writers. In this chapter horizontal integration refers to the linking of concepts, principles and factual information across disciplines learnt at a given level in such a way that the learner understands phenomena in a holistic manner; vertical integration refers to linking across disciplines conventionally taught at different levels of the curriculum. Thus linking of normal structure and function would be horizontal integration, while linking normal structure and function to deviations from the normal and their clinical effects would be vertical integration. 'Problem-based integration' is one method of achieving both horizontal and vertical integration by engaging students in solving clinical or community problems in order to acquire the learning that is required to solve these problems.

A more recently introduced concept is that of 'work-integrated learning'. This refers to the opportunities afforded to students to learn from actually participating in the work they envisage doing in the future, including clinical and community placements. 'Community-based integration' is similar in that students learn by being based in a community and participating in the health-related activities of the community. 'Multi-professional integration' refers to learning experiences arranged for students from two or more health professions together in order to prepare them to act cooperatively and collaboratively in providing healthcare to patients and communities.

Rationale for integrated learning

Two main approaches to learning have been identified: a surface approach associated with the passive acquisition of knowledge, and a deep approach associated with understanding of what is learnt. The deep approach to learning is obviously more appropriate for the education of the health professional, who is called upon to apply the learning acquired to novel situations that may be encountered in practice. Such application can only be achieved if basic facts and principles are understood. Understanding is prerequisite to the search for links among elements. Thus integrated learning is intimately related to deep learning.

Integrated learning is also complementary to creative thinking, as creativity is a function of identifying links between seemingly unrelated elements. A student who is learning about jaundice for the first time may, through understanding, be able to explain the pathogenesis of haemolytic jaundice. With creative thinking he or she may then be able to apply that understanding to explain obstructive jaundice by linking it to his or her knowledge of the anatomical arrangement of the biliary tree.

Vertically integrated learning increases intrinsic motivation as the learner relates his or her learning to future practice. It also enhances long-term memory as the learner immediately applies newly acquired facts and concepts to clinical and community situations. Professional practice requires the practitioner to link learning from different sources and disciplines. Thus, integrated learning prepares the future practitioner better than conventional discipline-based learning.

Integrated learning reduces the amount of repetition in the curriculum. When both structure and function of a given organ are studied together, rather than at separate times, the need does not exist for each to be repeated when the other is studied. This is particularly important as knowledge grows exponentially and curricular time is limited to accommodate this expanding body of knowledge. Learning to integrate knowledge provides the self-directed learner with a method of learning that helps them cope with this knowledge growth even after they graduate from medical school.

Learning that takes place in an environment that resembles as closely as possible that in which the learner applies the learning is more likely to be seen as relevant and is retained longer. This is the rationale for strategies such as community-based integration and work-integrated learning.

 "Emphasizing the relevance of classroom knowledge to personal concerns enables the students to make increasingly significant personal integration."
Mayhew, 1958

Strategies for integrated learning

Ever since the pioneering effort at curriculum integration in the medical school at Case Western Reserve in 1952, many curricula have changed from a conventional discipline-based curriculum to an integrated organ-systems-based curriculum, particularly in the pre-clinical phase. In many of these schools the management of that part of the curriculum has shifted from the hands of departments to interdisciplinary committees, often based on body organ systems. Such organizational and structural changes in the management and implementation of the curriculum have made it easier for the medical teacher to facilitate integrated learning in medical students, as well as for the medical student to learn in an integrated manner. However, organizational changes per se are not a guarantee that students undertake, or teachers facilitate, integrated learning. It is still possible for a disciplinary expert in a so-called integrated curriculum to teach his or her discipline without an exposition of how that discipline links with other disciplines. It is also possible for the student in such a curriculum to undertake self-study discipline-wise, particularly when confronted with a discipline-based examination system.

On the other hand, teachers within a discipline-based curriculum can still facilitate integrated learning in students by showing students how their discipline links with others. For example, Nagaiah et al. (2014) describe a case-based learning strategy to motivate first-year medical students to learn biochemistry in a vertically integrated manner. Zhang & Fenderson (2014) describe how cadaver dissection in anatomy provides opportunities for pre-clinical students to document and discuss with peers any pathological findings encountered, in order to develop their integrated learning skills. The basic science teacher can emphasize links even within his or her own discipline, such as between embryological development and adult structure in the case of anatomy. As mentioned earlier, part and whole are relative terms, and disciplinary teachers should at the least facilitate linking within their own disciplines. The closer one gets to the 'wholeness' on which the practitioner bases his or her practice in real life, the more integrated is the learning.

 Even within a discipline-based curriculum, the teacher should facilitate integrated learning in students by showing them how his or her discipline links with others.

Irrespective of the type of curriculum, the teacher's role is to facilitate the linking of elements taught, at the same time or at different times, by him or her, or by others, as long as they add up to a meaningful whole. The teacher has an important role to play in facilitating integrated learning (Bandaranayake, 2013). Firstly, he or she must correct students' conception of learning as accumulation of knowledge, but encourage them to look for links among the component parts of a topic or unit of study in such a way that they could apply this learning to real-world problems. The teacher can act as a role model in this respect by providing examples of how links can be established between their and other teachers' contributions. Secondly, teachers can facilitate integrated learning through appropriate course design. Teachers who are intent on content coverage do not provide adequate opportunities for students to identify their own links in self-study. Lectures with some unanswered questions, problem-solving exercises based on what students have just learnt and assignments that call upon their skills in application are potent means of encouraging students to identify and develop links among the elements.

 "The teacher who exemplifies integrating behaviour in his classroom, may be successful in having his students adopt this behaviour as a desirable goal toward which to strive."

Krathwohl, 1958

 Encourage students to develop links among elements during self-study by posing unanswered questions in lectures and setting problem-solving exercises, and assignments requiring them to apply what they have just learned.

The development of concept maps is an effective way of exercising students' skills of integrated learning. A concept map is a diagrammatic representation of the links between the elements in a particular content area. Students can be encouraged to draw such concept maps in self-study. The mental activity involved in developing relationships among the elements results in effective learning. Prideaux & Ash (2013) have extended this idea further to help teachers design integrated courses by placing key concepts in the centre, with related content around it, so that students can see the relationships between the different elements of a course.

The importance of context in enhancing integrated learning has been emphasized earlier. The physical context in which learning occurs, such as clinical or community settings, determines the extent to which students are able to retrieve what is learnt when required to do so in practice. The concept of context specificity refers to the similarity of the context in which learning takes place to the one in which such learning is applied (Regehr & Norman, 1996). This similarity influences the learner's ability to retrieve the learning when called upon to apply it. In a previous publication (Bandaranayake, 2011), the importance of the 'psychological environment' in which learning takes place has been pointed out. The psychological environment refers to the mental context in which learning takes place. If this context is similar, or as close as possible, to the mental context in which that learning is applied, retrieval of learning is facilitated. The mental context in which learning is applied by the practitioner is one of problem solving. The daily routine of the doctor can be seen as a series of problem-solving exercises. If the medical student learns in an environment of problem solving retrieval is facilitated. This is one reason why problem-based learning (PBL) is an effective way of promoting integrated learning.

 "A factor that enhances integration in problem-based learning is that students are placed in a similar 'psychological environment' to that in which they would apply their learning in future professional life."

Bandaranayake, 2011

In most medical schools PBL is practised in the pre-clinical phase of the curriculum, while problem solving is the main learning strategy in the clinical phase. One reason for this is the logistical difficulty of having a uniform set of experiences for all students in the clinical phase because of the variety of clerkship rotations that they pursue in the teaching hospital. Harden et al. (2000) have pointed out the tensions between integration, including PBL, and clinical attachments. Interdisciplinary clinical clerkships are practically difficult to mount, except in limited areas, such as neurology grand rounds between neurosurgery and neurology teams.

Medical schools have adopted various strategies to overcome these tensions while keeping the fundamental and inevitable nature of clinical clerkships intact. One is the judicious use of case-based learning (CBL), as practised in the Gulf Medical University in Ajman in the United Arab Emirates (Thomas & Ashok Raj, 2012). Following organ-systems integration in the pre-clinical phase of the curriculum, students from all the clerkships in the hospital meet in small groups in the afternoon to discuss specially constructed scenarios on a given theme (e.g. chest pain), with the aim of developing their diagnostic skills. This is followed by a large-group resource session, where experts jointly undertake an exposition of the theme, to further consolidate their diagnostic skills.

Harden et al. (2000) advocate the use of task-based learning (TBL), where more responsibility is given to students to integrate their learning by dealing with clinical tasks, each of which meets the criteria of importance, relevance, and the potential for linking with the basic sciences and for developing generic clinical competencies. An example of such a task is the management of a patient with abdominal pain. The students have the opportunity to view this task from the perspective of different clinical attachments.

Some schools resort to community-based clinical attachments to encourage integrated learning in the clinical years. An extreme example of this is the rural community curriculum at the School of Medicine, Flinders University in Adelaide, Australia, where students spend a whole year of clinical studies in rural general practices and rural hospitals (Prideaux & Ash, 2013).

In the real world of healthcare, teams function as an integral unit with an acute awareness of each other's role. The focus of multi-professional integration is to familiarize each member of the team with their respective roles in the delivery of healthcare, and to develop skills in working together. The environment in which such multi-professional learning takes place should reflect the reality of the situation in which healthcare is delivered. Teachers from the different health professions should be prepared adequately and developed as teaching teams if multi-professional integration is to be successful. Furthermore, the objectives and content of the multi-professional teaching sessions should be such that they are of relevance to all members of the team.

 When planning multi-professional learning the teacher should create an environment and learning tasks that reflect the reality of the situation in which the relevant healthcare is delivered by the various health professionals.

Barriers to integrated learning

It has been shown above that even the departmental structure of the medical school or the discipline-based organization of the curriculum should not preclude attempts to foster integrated learning in students. There is no doubt, however, that the 'territorial' mentality of some disciplinary teachers is the major deterrent to integration. In their attempts to promote their own discipline, such teachers seem to forget or ignore the primary aim of most medical schools, which is to produce basic doctors. Instead they teach as though they aim to produce graduates of their own ilk. Through a series of experiences in assisting schools to change disciplinary curricula into integrated ones, the author has concluded that the crucial ingredients for successful change are the development of ownership of the change, of skills in implementing integrated teaching activities and of assessing students in an integrated manner (Bandaranayake, 2011). As long as curriculum decision making is left in the hands of individuals or departments with such a territorial mentality, attempts at integration would be thwarted. An interdisciplinary decision-making body is essential for an integrated curriculum to succeed. Nevertheless, teachers who recognize the value of integrated learning can undertake teaching within their own spheres to produce integrating learners. Ultimately what is important is not whether the curriculum is integrated but that the learners develop integrating skills that would stand them in good stead in future practice. In the face of resistance to change, the concerned teacher can adopt an appropriate level of integrated teaching, as depicted in Harden's 'integration ladder' (Fig. 16.1; Harden, 2000).

 "The task is not that of communicating to the individual an integrated view of all knowledge; it is rather that of developing individuals who will seek to do this for themselves."

Dressel, 1958

 The teacher should adopt that level of integrated teaching appropriate to the teaching situation he or she finds himself or herself in, irrespective of the organizational or curricular structure of the medical school.

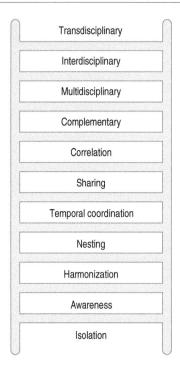

Transdisciplinary

Interdisciplinary

Multidisciplinary

Complementary

Correlation

Sharing

Temporal coordination

Nesting

Harmonization

Awareness

Isolation

Fig. 16.1 The integration ladder (Harden, 2000).

The 'Ba-Ma' model, proposed in the Bologna Declaration of 1999 for medical education in Europe, specifies a three-stage degree sequence at bachelor's, master's and doctorate levels, and has been viewed by some as going against the grain of integration between the basic and clinical sciences (Cumming, 2010). Cumming argues that this criticism can be overcome by retaining the primarily medical nature of each stage and ensuring that horizontal and vertical integration are promoted in the teaching, learning and assessment processes. Again, it is not necessarily the structure of education that determines the degree of integration, but the nature of educational activities undertaken by both teachers and students.

Integrated student assessment

Integrated teaching followed by discipline-based student assessment procedures is unlikely to produce integrating learners. The important role played by student assessment in driving learning is often not recognized by schools that profess to implement integrated curricula. In some instances, bureaucratic procedures, such as an insistence by higher authorities on discipline-based scores in final examinations, act as a barrier to integrated learning by students. In a few instances, schools have had to abandon their attempts at integration because of such procedures.

In preparing for examinations students are conditioned by the nature of examinations that they or their predecessors have been subjected to. If the examinations are discipline-based, so will their preparation for such examinations, defeating the goal of producing integrating learners. If students are exposed to the basic medical sciences in an integrated manner, the assessment items should test whether they are able to link concepts from these sciences; if application of the sciences to clinical situations is valued, test items should test their ability to apply rather than recall or reproduce factual information; if problem solving is an objective, they should be confronted with appropriate problems in the assessment process.

 If integrated learning is to be promoted, a test paper should not merely be a collection of test items from different disciplines; rather, individual test items should test whether students are able to link concepts from different disciplines through understanding, application or problem solving.

The construction of integrated test items mandates the formation of interdisciplinary teams for their creation. Teachers have to be given adequate time for test item construction and improvement through discussion. The development of banks of integrated test items would go a long way to making the work involved more manageable in the long run.

Integrated test items could be both free- and fixed-response. Stations for objective structured practical (OSPE) and clinical examinations (OSCE) could also be constructed in an integrated manner by interdisciplinary teams. The disadvantage of poor sampling in the long case clinical examination, which resulted in its gradual demise in many medical school assessment systems in spite of its integrative capacity, can be partly overcome by the use of such techniques as the direct observation clinical encounter examination (DOCEE), similar to an OSCE with a reduced number of stations but with increased time at each. An example of an integrated OSPE/OSCE station is given below. Examples of other types of integrated test items can be found in Bandaranayake (2011).

Example of an integrated OSCE/OSPE station (reproduced from Bandaranayake, 2011, p. 86)

Part A. Examine the pathological specimen provided.

1. Name the organ from which this specimen was taken.

2. Describe the macroscopic appearance of the specimen, pointing out particularly its abnormal features.

3. State your diagnostic conclusion from the specimen, justifying your conclusion from the specimen's abnormal features.

4. Write the main clinical symptoms and signs you would expect this patient to have shown before his death.

Part B. The histopathological slide provided was taken from a biopsy of the organ.

5. Write the histological features seen that either support or do not support your diagnosis.

This station links macroscopic pathology, histopathology and clinical features.

Summary

The critical factor in integrated learning is the ability to link concepts from different but related fields. The teacher's aim should be to produce learners who are able to undertake their own integrations, rather than to always present them with already integrated material. The teacher can demonstrate how such integration can be achieved through appropriate examples, and set assignments that call upon the students' integrative capacity. While it is easier to develop integrating learners in a curriculum that is integrated in its structure and organization, integrated learning can be promoted by teachers even in a discipline-based curriculum within their limited spheres of responsibility. The important place of integrated student assessment procedures in producing integrating learners is emphasized.

References

Bandaranayake, R.C., 2011. The Integrated Medical Curriculum. Radcliffe, London, p. 2, 53, 83-86, 111-124.

Bandaranayake, R.C., 2013. Study skills. In: Walsh, K. (Ed.), Oxford Textbook of Medical Education. Oxford University Press, Oxford, pp. 250–251.

Capehart, B.E., 1958. Illustrative courses and programs in selected secondary schools. In: Henry, N.B. (Ed.), The Integration of Educational Experiences, 57th Yearbook of the National Society for the Study of Education, Part III. University of Chicago Press., Chicago, IL, Chapter X, p. 199.

Cumming, A., 2010. The Bologna process, medical education and integrated learning. Med. Teach. 32 (4), 316–318.

Dressel, P.L., 1958. The meaning and significance of integration. In: Henry, N.B. (Ed.), The Integration of Educational Experiences, op. cit. Chapter I p. 5.

General Medical Council, 2009. Tomorrow's Doctors: Outcomes and Standards for Undergraduate Medical Education. General Medical Council, London. Section 101.

Harden, R.M., 2000. The integration ladder: a tool for curriculum planning and evaluation. Med. Educ. 34 (7), 551–557.

Harden, R.M., Crosby, J., Davies, M.H., et al., 2000. Task-based learning: the answer to integration and problem-based learning in the clinical years. Med. Educ. 34 (5), 391–397.

Krathwohl, D.R., 1958. The psychological bases for integration. In: Henry, N.B. (Ed.), The Integration of Educational Experiences, op. cit. Chapter III p. 54.

Mayhew, L.B., 1958. Illustrative courses and programs in colleges and universities. In: Henry, N.B. (Ed.), The Integration of Educational Experiences, op. cit. Chapter XI p. 222.

Nagaiah, B.H., Gowda, V.B.S., Jeyachristy, S.A., Maung, T.M., 2014. Motivating first year medical students to learn biochemistry by case based learning. Int. J. Biochem. Res. 5 (7), 461–464.

Prideaux, D., Ash, J.K., 2013. Integrated learning. In: Dent, J.A., Harden, R.M. (Eds.), A Practical Guide for Medical Teachers, fourth ed. Elsevier, London, pp. 183–189.

Regehr, G., Norman, G.R., 1996. Issues in cognitive psychology; implications for professional education. Acad. Med. 71 (9), 988–1001.

Thomas, I.N., Ashok Raj, G., 2012. Implementing a learner centered curriculum using a novel educational strategy in the hospital. Med. Sci. Educ. (IAMSE) 22 (45), 313.

Zhang, G., Fenderson, B.A., 2014. Pathology encountered during cadaver dissection provides an opportunity for integrated learning and critical thinking. Austin J. Anat. 1 (5), 1027–1029.

Chapter

17 Interprofessional education

J. E. Thistlethwaite, P. H. Vlasses

Trends

- Interprofessional education involving health and social care professional students and practitioners from other health care professions is becoming more common globally.
- Medical school faculty development is increasingly focused on interprofessional education capabilities.
- Interprofessional learning outcomes and competencies are now included in licensing and accreditation standards in many countries.

Definitions

The adjective 'interprofessional' describes a strategy in which learners and practitioners learn and work together for a common goal at any stage of education and training. It implies dialogue and negotiation, consensus and compromise, as well as mutual understanding and respect. The World Health Organization, drawing on the work of CAIPE (the Centre for the Advancement of Interprofessional Education), defines interprofessional education (IPE) as: "when students from two or more professions learn about, from and with each other to enable effective collaboration and improve health outcomes" and interprofessional collaborative practice (IPCP) as: "when multiple health workers from different professional backgrounds work together with patients, families, carers, and communities to deliver the highest quality of care" (WHO, 2010). Collaboration, and therefore collaborative practice, as a goal of IPE is now becoming a commonly used term, along with teamwork.

 The prepositions 'from', 'with' and 'about' in the definition of IPE are important and necessary as they imply that interprofessional learning should be interactive and equitable.

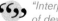 *"Interprofessional collaboration is 'the process of developing and maintaining effective*

interprofessional working relationships with learners, practitioners, patients/clients/families and communities to enable optimal health outcomes.'"

The Canadian Interprofessional Health Collaborative, 2010

History

IPE dates back over fifty years. Activities involving diverse health professional students learning together have been described in Australia, the United Kingdom and the United States amongst other countries since the 1960s (Barr, 2014). The U.S. Institute of Medicine first called for interprofessional education in the health professions in 1972 and reiterated the need in its subsequent reports. A common feature of the early initiatives is the lack of sustainability due to non-recurrent funding and loss of the interprofessional champion within a particular institution, highlighting the need for embedding IPE into curricula and academic succession planning.

The rationale for IPE

Health and social care delivery is increasingly becoming a collaborative process involving well-defined teams or looser alliances of health professionals. Such collaboration is necessary as medical knowledge increases, practitioners specialize in narrower fields and patients move between primary, secondary and tertiary care sectors. In addition, the population is ageing and there is a higher prevalence of chronic and complex conditions. It is rare that one professional can meet the needs and expectations of each patient, family and community. Policy drivers also include the patient safety agenda and public inquiries into adverse patient outcomes that frequently result from poor communication between health and social care professionals (Thistlethwaite, 2012).

That health professions education needs to keep pace with changes in practice was emphasized in 2010 by the Lancet Commission, a group of world leaders, which developed a shared vision for the future of education. While there has been some criticism of this paper, as it did not recognize what was already being achieved in IPE, it did correctly stress the need for medical education to become more involved in the interprofessional movement. It also suggested strategies to break down the professional silos of contemporary training and to better prepare graduates for team-based care delivery through team-based learning (Frenk et al., 2010). In the same year the World Health Organization published its framework for action, advocating for IPE as part of a global health agenda (WHO, 2010).

 "…we call for a new round of more agile and rapid adaptation of core competencies based on transnational, multiprofessional, and long-term perspectives to serve the needs of individuals and populations."

Frenk et al., 2010, p. 1954

Curriculum development

While we acknowledge that the logistics of developing and delivering effective IPE can be complex, we also recognize that difficulties are frequently put forward as a reason for stifling innovation. Successful curriculum development involves an interprofessional approach: harnessing the enthusiasm and motivation of educators and clinicians across faculties, schools, disciplines and clinical locations. A useful model for planning an interprofessional curricular approach is the four-dimensional (4D) framework (Lee et al., 2013) (Table 17.1).

The first dimension is identifying future healthcare practice needs and using these as the rationale for change, taking into account global health imperatives, educational reforms and theories, as well as local conditions and accreditation body requirements. Regarding

Table 17.1 The four-dimensional (4-D) curriculum development framework for IPE (adapted from Lee et al., 2013)

Dimension	Description
1. Identifying future health care needs	Curriculum takes into account global health and education reforms, and local needs
2. Defining and understanding competencies for practice	The desired outcomes of IPE for changing health service delivery; expertise required
3. Teaching, learning and assessment	Appropriate methods and activities to align with dimensions 1 & 2
4. Supporting institution delivery	Takes into account local institutional logistics that shape curriculum design

the last, lack of accreditation requirements for IPE for many years was used as an excuse to not address IPE in health professions curricula. However, accreditors in a number of countries including the United States and Australia and across health professions have added specific standards regarding interprofessional competencies and standards (examples in Table 17.2). The standards for each profession often use different language for similar concepts, and work is needed to agree a set of competencies or learning outcomes in common across all professions. This could be based on one of the existing frameworks mentioned below.

 " 'In an effort to strengthen ties across health professions and better provide integrated healthcare for the public good, several of the nation's [USA] leading accrediting agencies have announced the formation of Health Professions Accreditors Collaborative (HPAC). Members of HPAC include the:
- *Accreditation Council for Pharmacy Education (ACPE)*
- *Commission on Collegiate Nursing Education (CCNE)*
- *Commission on Dental Accreditation (CODA)*
- *Commission on Osteopathic College Accreditation (COCA)*
- *Council on Education for Public Health (CEPH)*
- *Liaison Committee for Medical Education (LCME)*

HPAC members are committed to discussing important developments in interprofessional education (IPE) and exploring opportunities to engage in collaborative projects. HPAC will communicate with stakeholders around issues in IPE with the common goal to better prepare students to engage in interprofessional collaborative practice."

Press release, HPAC, 2014

Once a planning team is identified, dimension two involves their understanding and defining the competencies required for interprofessional practice by all learners within their institution or setting. These should take into account the professional accreditation standards set for pre-qualification or post-qualification continuing professional development (CPD) programmes. The most frequently defined learning outcomes fall into six main areas: teamwork; communication; understanding of roles and responsibilities; ethical issues; the patient; and learning/reflection (Thistlethwaite & Moran 2010). For dimension three, appropriate and relevant learning activities as well as assessments need to be aligned with outcomes or competencies. The feasibility of such activities is dependent on careful consideration being given to: the number of learners and their professions; which activities are mandatory and which elective;

Table 17.2   Examples of accreditation standards for medical education

Country	Body	Year	Standards
Australia	AMC	2012	4.8 Describe and respect the roles and expertise of other health care professionals; demonstrate ability to learn and work effectively as a member of an IP team
UK	GMC	2009	22. Learn effectively within a multiprofessional team Work with colleagues in ways that best serve the interests of patients, passing on information and handing over care, demonstrating flexibility, adaptability and a problem solving approach
US/Canada	LCME	2013	7.9. Interprofessional Collaborative Skills: to function collaboratively on health care teams that include health professionals from other disciplines as they provide coordinated services to patients. Curricular experiences include practitioners and/or students from the other health professions

AMC – Australian Medical Council
GMC – General Medical Council
LCME – Liaison Council for Medical Education

the timing (early, late or throughout the course); the number of hours; location (e.g. classroom, clinic, ward, simulation laboratory); the type and timing of assessments; facilitators and their training; timetable coordination; and budget.

 "Frameworks for IPE include those of IPEC (the Interprofessional Education Collaborative), the CIHC (the Canadian Interprofessional Health Collaborative) and the Curtin Interprofessional Capability Framework."

Thistlethwaite et al., 2014

Learning activities

Dimension three focuses on delivery: learning and teaching activities, and assessment. The common curriculum model involves students from different health and social care professions spending one or more weeks learning together full-time on a defined topic. For this to be interprofessional, the learning should be interactive and not didactic; the interprofessional learning activities need to be explicit. The interprofessional spiral curriculum exposes students to IPE at an early stage in their training through group work, case studies and online modules, with subsequent immersion in clinical and simulation experiences in the later years. All health professional students undertake clinical rotations: by mapping such attachments, it should be possible to bring students together to provide team-based experiences that are as authentic as possible. In addition, it may be possible to develop training wards based on the Swedish model, longitudinal integrated clerkships (LICs), which have interprofessional opportunities, and student-run interprofessional clinics (SRCs). There is as yet no consensus as to how long a clinical rotation should be to enable a learner to feel part of a local team or community of practice (Thistlethwaite, 2015).

 All health professional students undergo clinical attachments at various points in their training – by mapping such attachments it should be possible to bring the professions together at some point to provide as authentic team-based experiences as possible.

Adult learning theory recommends that learning experiences should be relevant to the learner. Thus students should have the opportunity to engage in authentic clinical and team-based tasks. A major issue, however, is that of the hidden curriculum: what students learn from observation, institutional cultures and role models. Some students may not observe interprofessional teamwork in action during their clinical placements because such teamwork is not explicit, does not look like the models they have learnt about, or does not exist. This lack of experience may lead students to question the very nature of interprofessionalism and IPE. After any interprofessional activity students need to be debriefed about what they have seen and learnt, be given time to discuss the type or lack of teamwork they have observed, and be encouraged to consider how teamwork and collaborative practice may be fostered in the environments in which they have been placed.

 Educators need to ensure that students are exposed to interprofessional practice during their programmes; they may attend multidisciplinary team meetings in hospital or primary care, work within operating theatres, be attached to well-functioning clinics or be supported in student-run clinics.

Assessment

 As IPE is an interactive, collaborative learning process, assessment is ideally team based.

When educators define competencies that should be achieved, they also need to develop robust and feasible assessment methods to measure those competencies. The assessment of teamwork may be a challenge as it should be undertaken during observation of learners working in teams and carrying out teamwork tasks, either during simulation or in clinical and professional settings. Assessment may involve such team-based activities as projects and presentations, simulations involving multiple professionals, team-based objective structured clinical evaluation (T-OSCE) stations and the preparation of patient care plans. Educators need to decide whether the task is a collective responsibility, with all students in a team receiving the same mark, or whether individuals are assessed on individual team performance, perhaps involving peer marking. However, as students may work infrequently in defined interprofessional teams, observation of their teamwork as a work-based assessment may be difficult. A team may be formed specifically for the purpose of assessment, for example for a simulation or T-OSCE. This type of 'teamwork' is similar to clinical tasks such as the response to a cardiac arrest with a team forming in response to an incident, however clinical teams in other settings take time to form and gel and thus to perform optimally.

 "The alignment of outcomes, activities and assessment follows from constructivist learning theory and instructional design, ensuring learning is student-centered with meaning derived from the learning experience."

Biggs & Tang, 2007

Other considerations include: timing; weighting of any summative assessment in terms of whether it is graded, or pass/fail only; which professions are involved; whether assessors need to be of the same profession as each learner; what type of faculty development is required to observe, give feedback and assess; and the impact of the assessment on the learners.

Summative is more problematic than formative assessment, as professional accreditation or licensing bodies usually have different requirements in terms of grading and types of examinations and may insist that students are assessed by members of the same profession. Portfolios, with reflective components and with students' collected evidence of achieving outcomes, are a useful option but there may be issues relating to reliability and feasibility. Multisource feedback (MSF) forms may also be included, with students asking for feedback on performance from a number of different health professionals and patients with whom they come into contact. MSF is also a valuable method for assessment of post-qualification clinicians.

 When planning interprofessional activities remember to build in an evaluation and/or research plan and consider whether ethical approval is required if there is an intention to disseminate the results.

 "The reason for evaluation is to 'provide accountability for health and social care resources to those who provide or control them – regional/ national authorities, research and service funders, consumers and foundations'."

Reeves et al., 2010

Post-qualification

Continuing professional development (CPD) has traditionally been focused at the level of the individual healthcare practitioner. More recently, the value of CPD involving health practitioner teams learning together and focusing jointly on quality and safety gaps in healthcare has been identified as a strategic resource. For example, in the United States, a unique accreditation model has been developed to incentivize and facilitate team-based continuing professional development (http://jointaccreditation.org/).

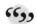 **Joint Accreditation for Continuing Interprofessional Education™**

"Joint Accreditation: promotes interprofessional continuing education (IPCE) activities specifically designed to improve interprofessional collaborative practice (IPCP) in health care delivery; establishes the standards for education providers to deliver continuing education planned 'by the healthcare team for the healthcare team'; offers organizations the opportunity to be simultaneously accredited to provide medicine, pharmacy, and nursing continuing education activities through a single, unified application process and set of accreditation standards. This distinction is awarded by the Accreditation Council for Continuing Medical Education (ACCME), the Accreditation Council for Pharmacy Education (ACPE) and the American Nurses Credentialing Center (ANCC)"

Vlasses, 2015

Impact and effectiveness of IPE

To date, research on IPE has focused on participants' attitudes and learning before and after specified IPE courses, simulations, and experiences in practice. A small and growing literature indicates evidence of the effectiveness of IPE. A diverse collection of methods and tools are used to assess and evaluate IPE learners and programmes; these are often used without an explicit programme-evaluation framework (Blue et al., 2015).

One test of the effectiveness of IPE is whether it leads to IPCP and, ultimately, whether IPCP improves patient care. Cochrane Collaboration reviews suggest that practice-based IPCP interventions can improve healthcare processes and outcomes, but because of limitations owing to the small number of studies, sample sizes, problems with conceptualizing and measuring collaboration, and heterogeneity of interventions and settings, it is difficult to draw generalizable inferences about the key elements of IPCP and its effectiveness. After determining that no existing models sufficiently incorporate all of the necessary components to guide future research on the impact of interprofessional education on collaborative practice and patient outcomes, the Institute of Medicine (IOM) has developed a conceptual model that includes the education-to-practice continuum, a broad array of learning, health, and system outcomes, and major enabling and interfering factors (IOM, 2015).

Faculty development for IPE

Faculty members in the health professions who were trained and practice in a more traditional, siloed model of care need targeted IPE faculty development to be effective educators in team-based models of care. The attributes required for optimal interprofessional facilitations, drawn from a number of sources, are listed in Box 17.1. TeamSTEPPS is an evidence-based framework to optimize team performance across the healthcare delivery system that many faculty development programmes in North America have incorporated (http://www.ahrq.gov/professionals/education/curriculum-tools/teamstepps/instructor/essentials/pocketguide.html#frame). The University of Toronto has developed excellent resources to support faculty IPE development (http://www.ipe.utoronto.ca/continuing-professional-development).

Overcoming challenges

Over the years, there have been many challenges and barriers to the development of effective IPE and IPCP. These factors include:

- Resistance to change/Where's the evidence?
- Lack of leadership (administrative and faculty)
- Crowded curricula
- Cost factors and few incentives
- Separation of professional programmes within a campus and across universities
- Lack of accreditation expectations
- Treating IPE as an 'add on' rather than a change in curricular philosophy.

Supporting institutional delivery is the final dimension of the 4D-framework. In organizations where these challenges have, or are being overcome, some common factors are observed such as commitment of the university and health system leadership to IPE and IPCP; motivated champions; collaborative interprofessional curriculum development and oversight and adequate resources. In addition we advocate for recognition of interprofessional teaching, scholarship and research in faculty promotion and tenure guidelines with incentives to undertake faculty development to enhance interprofessional leadership.

 " 'It was an encouraging feeling to have the support, camaraderie and cooperation of the other students and preceptors in the community, and it gave us the opportunity to experience both learning and teaching roles with each other. It made me aware of some of the misconceptions existing between professions and the limitations of our own profession."

Medical student, WHO, 2010

Summary

The changing nature of modern health and social care delivery, with an increasing emphasis on collaboration between practitioners, is the stimulus for greater awareness and development of IPE. There is growing evidence for the effectiveness of learning and working together. It is important that interprofessional learning outcomes are explicit and align with activities and assessment. Post-qualification learning is best carried out in established teams for relevance. Faculty development is crucial for success. As further research is needed in this field, rigorous evaluation should be planned for and research questions considered. Successful IPE is challenging but also rewarding, and helps us share values and experience with other colleagues.

Box 17.1   The attributes of an effective interprofessional facilitator

- Competencies relating to teamwork theory and team building
- Experience of working in a healthcare team – ideally interprofessional rather than multiprofessional
- Experience of collaborative practice and the ability to promote this within the workplace
- Knowledge of others' professional roles and responsibilities
- Awareness of boundary issues and the issues regarding blurring of professional roles
- An understanding of the process of professional socialization and how this might impact on interprofessional interactions
- Skills in negotiation and conflict resolution
- Knowledge of the evidence for IPE

References

Barr, H., 2014. Leading the way. In: Forman, D., Jones, M., Thistlethwaite, J.E. (Eds.), Leadership Development for Interprofessional Education and Collaborative Practice. Palgrave, Basingstoke, pp. 15–25.

Biggs, J.B., Tang, C., 2007. Teaching for Quality Learning at University: What the Student Does, 3rd ed. McGraw-Hill/Society for Research in Higher Education and Open University, Maidenhead.

Blue, A.V., Chesluk, B.J., Conforti, L.N., Holmboe, E.S., 2015. Assessment and evaluation in interprofessional education: exploring the field. J. Allied Health 44 (2), 73–82.

Canadian Interprofessional Health Collaborative. A national interprofessional competency framework, 2010. Available at: http://www.cihc.ca/files/CIHC_IPCompetencies_Feb1210.pdf. (Accessed 1 January 2017).

Frenk, J., Chen, L., Butta, Z.A., et al., 2010. Health professionals for a new century: transforming education to strengthen health systems in an interdependent world. Lancet 376 (9756), 1923–1958.

HPAC. New Health Professions Accreditors Collaborative Forms to Stimulate Interprofessional Engagement. Available at http://acpe-accredit.org/pdf/HPAC_PressRelease12152014.pdf. (Accessed 1 January 2017).

IOM (Institute of Medicine), 2015. Measuring the Impact of Interprofessional Education on Collaborative Practice and Patient Outcomes. The National Academies Press, Washington, DC.

Lee, A., Steketee, C., Rogers, G., Moran, M., 2013. Towards a theoretical framework for curriculum development in health professional education. Focus Health Prof. Educ. 14 (3), 70–83.

Reeves, S., Lewin, S., Espin, S., Zwarenstein, M., 2010. Interprofessional Teamwork for Health and Social Care. Blackwell Publishing, Oxford.

Thistlethwaite, J.E., 2012. Interprofessional education: a review of context, learning and the research agenda. Med. Educ. 46 (1), 58–70.

Thistlethwaite, J.E., 2015. Assessment of interprofessional teamwork: an international perspective. In: Forman, D., Jones, M., Thistlethwaite, J.E. (Eds.), Leadership Development for Interprofessional Education and Collaborative Practice. Palgrave, Basingstoke, pp. 135–152.

Thistlethwaite, J.E., Forman, D., Rogers, G., et al., 2014. Interprofessional education competencies and frameworks in health: a comparative analysis. Acad. Med. 89 (6), 869–875.

Thistlethwaite, J.E., Moran, M., 2010. Learning outcomes for interprofessional education (IPE): literature review and synthesis. J. Interprof. Care 24 (5), 503–513.

Vlasses, P.H. Leadership Interviews, 2015. Available at http://jointaccreditation.org/videos. (Accessed 1 January 2017).

World Health Organization (WHO), 2010. Framework for Action on Interprofessional Education and Collaborative Practice. WHO, Geneva.

Problem-based learning

M. S. Wilkes, M. Srinivasan

Trends

- Problem-based Learning is a well-accepted, small-group teaching format that was developed to promote active learning, problem solving, teamwork, and life-long learning.

- Educators no longer feel constrained to use a single, rigidly defined method of active small-group learning, and now choose the instructional method best suited to their learner's needs, developmental stage, and context/content.

- Educators now have large 'toolbox' available, with multiple tools to engage learners.
  Other engagement options include case-based learning, team-based learning, diagnostic reasoning seminars, standardized patient interactions, procedural simulation, teamwork simulations, and hybrid techniques that utilize informatics and small-group learning.

Perspectives in problem-based learning

PROBLEM-BASED LEARNING FORMAT

 "PBL methodology aims to provide learners with real-world experience in problem solving."

In its purest form, PBL is a student-centred approach to learning, which relies upon carefully constructed problems (typically, clinical challenges) that serve as a stimulus for small groups of learners to engage in self-directed inquiry. During the PBL sessions, learners solve the problem together in teams – integrating knowledge, theory and practice in the process. The PBL problem-solving technique process is organized, requiring that all team members contribute.

 "In PBL, learners work in teams to independently seek information and solve problems."

Over the past half century, PBL has been used around the world in various stages of education – from elementary schools to technical schools to graduate schools. In medicine there is great variability of how PBL is integrated into education, and variability about what constitutes PBL. PBL may be used only in certain classes, only in certain years of medical school, or it may serve as the delivery model for the entire core curriculum of a medical school. Hybrid models of PBL merge PBL with case-based learning (CBL) or simulation-based training.

Creating PBL courses: a systems perspective

 "PBL is an ineffective way of imparting high volume of information. PBL is an outstanding way to encouraging problem solving and teamwork."

In most countries, total curricular time of medical training is fixed, with limits on total student contact/ study time per week. Established lecture-based courses that wish to transition to PBL formats typically cut direct contact hours by about 40% to allow students time to learn curricular content independently. In-class time focuses on problem solving and student-lead discussion. When introducing a new PBL course, difficult negotiations are often required to determine what other curricular elements are 'cut' to allow for PBL sessions. Of course, planning is easier when PBL courses are electives (therefore, not subject to specific hours restrictions) or are part of a new school of medicine.

Substantial staff time is required for the development and implementation of the PBL curricula. Educators should be provided sufficient incentive (pay and time) to develop the curriculum, conduct faculty development, implement the course and evaluate outcomes. At least one faculty member is required for a PBL small group of 6–10 students. Given the low faculty–student ratio and the need for sustainability, a senior institutional champion should help secure resources and the participation of the required number of faculty. Faculty development is crucial to ensure that the faculty understand how to facilitate small groups (and when necessary to intervene), how to promote a safe learning environment during the sessions, understand the content at a general level, and appreciate the PBL approach to assessment of the students. Time for faculty development should be built into the PBL course.

 Consider whether PBL is the right instructional format for the educational learning objective.

Once curricular time and resources have been secured, PBL curriculum may be created following a standard curriculum development process, such as David Kern's six-step model. After appropriate needs assessment and stakeholder analysis, the educators should establish competencies, learning objectives and milestones to be achieved during the PBL course. Careful attention is required to ensure that PBL is the correct educational strategy to meet the learning objectives. Stakeholder input is critical at this stage, to ensure that learner, educator and organizational needs are met.

 "Learning the process of independent learning is as important as the outcome of learning, as this vital for life-long learning."

Early on educators should identify which PBL outcomes they will evaluate. *Process* PBL outcomes might include assessment of overall teamwork and individual contribution to the team/learning climate, and approach to independent learning. *Performance* PBL outcomes might include assessment of the approach taken to develop a solution to the PBL challenge, or learner self-perception of skills in problem solving, motivation, or the specific content covered. Clarity of content and outcomes is crucial to shape the development and assessment of the curriculum.

Writing PBL cases

Before actually writing the PBL case, it is necessary to determine the expected learning outcomes. Attention should be given to other activities occurring in the curriculum, to help build depth and reinforce learning around the PBL objectives. Many schools are happy to share their educational materials, including PBL cases, with appropriate attribution, making it unnecessary to recreate the wheel.

 The PBL problem or prompt should be 'just right' – not too easy (boring) or too challenging (frustrating).

A well-constructed PBL problem drives a team-directed, self-managing group towards problem resolution in an organized manner of inquiry. The problems should be at the right developmental level – not too easy (which leads to boredom) or too challenging (which leads to frustration). Here, it is important to remember that learners are being asked to create their own contextual framework, rather than being given a pre-formed approach. As such, learning and synthesizing content will take longer, even when building upon an existing body of knowledge. Triggers for medical PBL problems may include any relevant source (news stories, policy white papers, clinical problems with data/images/growth charts, real or standardized patient interactions, video clips, movie clips, photographs, laboratory/experimental data, and more).

For instance, when writing a clinical or foundational science case for early pre-clinical students, educators might use a video clip of a straightforward problem, such as an adult with a cough, or use a simulated patient to play the mother of a child who presents with asthma. Depending upon time limitations, it may be realistic to weave other issues into the case (e.g. clinical, societal, epidemiologic, ethical, legal or behavioural issues).

Cases may unfold in stages, simulating the passage of time that occurs in clinical scenarios. For instance, in part one of a paper case, a mother may bring her child into an outpatient clinic with specific concerns that the child is not following a standard growth curve. Learners would learn the causes of failure to thrive, and develop their own approach to this problem. As the case unfolds over time, additional clinical (or historical) information may be presented – allowing for a 'deeper dive' into such concepts as disparities in healthcare and links between economics, living situation, gender, and health. Learners should have access to resources necessary to solve the problem (online resources, access to experts, videos, clinical data, radiographs, and more).

For each step in the unfolding PBL case, the authors should develop trigger questions and activities to focus group activities. Depending on learner developmental level, questions may be more or less specific.

- "What are the major causes of growth delay in young children?" (novice)
- "How would you interpret this growth chart?" (intermediate)
- "How likely are false positives and false negatives for this result?" (intermediate)
- "What diagnostic test(s) would you order at this point and why?" (advanced)
- "What are critical physical exam findings that would increase or decrease your decision to intervene?" (advanced)

Once developed, cases should be reviewed by content experts for accuracy and relevancy. Using a plan–do–study–act approach, educators should revise the cases based on feedback from faculty and learners.

Running PBL small groups

Typically, PBL teams are composed of 6–10 learners. A team that is too large will not allow for participation by all learners. A team that is too small may not have enough people to address the learning objectives, or have sufficiently divergent viewpoints to ensure a robust discussion. Learner groups may be composed of only medical students, or may be interdisciplinary (nursing, pharmacy, veterinary, social work, dentistry etc.), depending on the course objectives and collaborative environment.

The classic approach to PBL is rigidly organized. On a rotating basis, small groups assign roles to students: 'chair' or 'moderator', a 'scribe' a 'web searcher' and participants. The group moderator is responsible for leading the group through the learning process, managing the discussion, ensuring everyone has a chance of participation, ensuring that no one dominates the discussion, minding time, and keeping the group focused. The scribe records assignments, resources used, and points made by the group members, and the web searcher is responsible for identifying high-quality resources. All others participate actively, and take on specific tasks to help the group address the case.

Classically, a PBL session uses this time-honoured approach:

1. Present the case (classically on paper, but sometimes video, audio, patient data, or a letter/phone call from a patient)
2. Define the problem, key questions and an approach to inquiry
3. Divide into learning issues/tasks and collect information
4. Self-directed learning ('private study')
5. Report back to group to share learning
6. Generate hypotheses
7. Integrate knowledge
8. Evaluate group process and learning.

Once the team defines the problem on their own, they typically brainstorm about how to approach the problem. What is known by the group? What is unknown? What are potential approaches to address the problem? The team then creates potential solutions and generates hypothesis. The moderator ensures everyone's voice is heard, and encourages follow-up questions/inquiry. During the process, the scribe organizes and structures the problem/issues for the group. The group formulates their own learning objectives, and assigns specific learning objectives to individuals. After a period of private study that might range from 20 minutes to several days, the group meets to collect and discuss their results. In a high-performing group, this discussion is deep and vibrant – and individuals draw upon each other's strengths and ask each other clarifying questions. They refine their hypothesis, test alternate hypothesis, and come to conclusion about their best responses to the question. A poorly performing team may need some redirection from an observant faculty, who will ask stimulating questions to get the group back on track.

 Give sufficient time to solve the PBL problem.

If this learning format is unfamiliar to learners, they will need training in PBL small-group facilitation – either by watching a PBL session in advance (live/recorded), watching a PBL tutorial about the process, and/or by receiving instruction and feedback in class by the PBL faculty tutor.

Faculty as tutor

In PBL, faculty are referred to as 'tutors', and take on a unique role. The tutor is NOT expected to be a content expert, but rather a small-group facilitator whose goal is to keep the group on task. For instance, if the group strays from the assignment or becomes stuck, the tutor will prompt them to consider alternative possibilities. The tutor is responsible for ensuring that the group maintains a positive learning environment. For instance, the tutor should have developed skills to manage disruptors, passive members, or intragroup conflicts – only if the group cannot manage these independently. Conventional PBL curriculum requires that the tutor generally remains silent, watching group dynamics, and intervening only if there are problems with group dynamics. In a well-functioning PBL group, the tutor might not need to be present for most of the case, until the final discussion.

 In PBL sessions, students take the lead and explore the topic. Faculty should only clarify misconceptions if the student/group is very confused.

The tutor may stimulate curiosity by asking Socratic questions, such as "What is your approach to... so far?" or "What might you be missing?" and "How would your approach change if the patient was from a different culture?" If learners ask the tutor content-specific questions, tutors are encouraged to reflect the questions back to the team, and encourage the team to develop creative approaches to problem solving. Tutors are encouraged not to intervene when learners go 'off-track' because, according to the core tenants of PBL, such divergences are a form of exploration and allow learners to self-correct, to gain insight and to self-regulate.

 Faculty should reflect back questions to students, rather than answer the question themselves.

Tutoring in this format is uncomfortable for many faculty, who are used to being content experts, and sharing their viewpoints and perspectives. They are used to correcting misperceptions, and may be inexperienced in small-group facilitation. It may also be frustrating for students who do not understand why a faculty member who knows the answer will not provide guidance or correct faulty data. Thus, faculty training in this methodology and in small-group facilitation is critical – including learning to trust learners to develop solutions to the problem. In this regard, 'silence' is often the best teaching tool.

Evaluating PBL session outcomes

Typically, PBL assessment includes subjective evaluation of group processes by tutors and/or peers, rather than standardized or written test performance. Learner outcomes include learner participation, role completion, self-assessment of motivation or self-efficacy. Team outcomes may include degree of teamwork, management of conflict, utilization of resources, approach to the clinical problem, final case decision, or project presentation. Tutor outcomes may be assessed by learners (or self-assessed by faculty), including creating a safe learning environment, facilitation when necessary, non-interference in the group process, and appropriate guidance consistent with the goals of the course. If tutors are charged with 'grading' or evaluating the small group's final decisions regarding the problem (versus just assessing group process), case authors should develop a specific scoring guide or matrix for learner evaluation.

PBL controversies

Advocates of pure PBL argue that PBL echoes real life. In clinical practice, answers are not always available, and ambiguity is a normal part of learning. Faculty are initially reluctant to trust young learners to solve problems independently. There is general agreement that when learners are properly prepared with realistic expectations, they enjoy PBL sessions, and find them clinically relevant and engaging. Learners report that well-done PBL sessions drive towards integration of learning topics, particularly foundational science and clinical practice. Using Tuckman's (1965) model of small-group processes, well-functioning groups (performing) become self-regulatory. There is less data to support claims that PBL enhances clinical problem solving, improves motivation, or better prepares students for national assessment examinations. There are also concerns about the uniformity of learning and about the uniformity of learner assessment following PBL. Like other resource-intensive small-group teaching methods, educators must demonstrate why the expenditures of time and resources justify the PBL curricular investment.

Outcomes of PBL courses

Over the past half century, PBL, or a variation of it, has been attempted by schools around the world, with varying outcomes. Some of the variability in outcomes may result from the experience of the curriculum planners, some from students' age, experience, and preparation, some from institutional investment/underinvestment, and some from the assessment methods. Self-report by many students suggest a preference for this learning method over traditional didactics, and there is data to suggest improvement in self-reported teamwork, leadership and problem-solving skills. Since the emphasis of the curriculum is on problem solving, and not knowledge acquisition, PBL groups generally perform as well as (but not better than) groups learning the same material in a traditional lecture/discussion format. Successful PBL participation may better prepare students for clinical work that requires teamwork and problem solving. PBL participants do not perform better on multiple-choice or standardized written tests, indicating that PBL is not a superior learning format for content taught on national exams. Anecdotally, students have reported that they learn less overall content in a PBL course, and have to study exam-related content on their own (cram schools or board review books). They also report relying on sources of information (readings, web searches, videos) for which they do not have the perspective to evaluate the credibility. When students discuss the case with colleagues outside of their group there is often angst about which group was correct and what data or references were more accurate.

Reasons to consider using a PBL approach

Theoretically, small-group learning in general and PBL in particular, has many advantages over traditional didactic curricula.

1. PBL is widely used around the world, in multiple disciplines, and is generally well-accepted by learners, faculty and institutions.

2. PBL cases may mimic the open nature of clinical inquiry in real-life settings, building tolerance for ambiguity and developing approaches for unanswered questions.

3. Templates and prototype cases are available from a variety of sources (such as MedEd Portal, and from individual universities) easing the transition from a traditional curriculum to PBL small-group curriculum.

4. Students prefer active learning to passive learning formats, including PBL.

5. Well-run PBL groups evolve into self-directed, self-managing accountable teams, building learner collaborative skill sets.

6. If implemented and supported well, PBL students may become curious, motivated, lifelong learners.

7. PBL addresses issues crucial to lifelong learning (team work, finding information, being an effective communicator, and the integration of information to solve problems).

General disadvantages of small-group learning

While PBL has the above advantages, it also has significant limitations. General limitations are similar across all small-group teaching methods. For instance, small-group teaching methods require substantial faculty contact time (often with a large number of trained faculty), commitment from faculty and students to the process, a greater tolerance for variability in learning, and a need for new assessment measures. Change is never easy – for either students or faculty. Shifting curricula from a traditional didactic to small group learning format requires trust, faculty time, faculty expertise (content/methods), and tutor/student training in the format. Small-group learning is resource intensive, and challenging for untrained individual faculty without institutional support. Implementing small-group courses requires a realignment of faculty rewards and incentives. Teaching recognition is no longer based on the 'sage on the stage', but rather on engagement and participation with small groups of learners. Learner assessment needs careful reconsideration, as the outcomes move from exclusively knowledge to a combination of knowledge, skills, attitudes, teamwork and behaviours.

Specific disadvantages of PBL as a learning format

PBL sessions may not be structured for optimal decision making as they ask learners to construct meaning independently from data without providing guidance on optimal directions, credible references, nor guides to decision making. As such, the PBL learning process is inherently exploratory, and therefore inefficient. These inefficiencies highlight the downstream consequences of PBL as an educational methodology, for learners and for tutors.

Issues with PBL as an educational methodology

MATCHING LEARNING OBJECTIVES WITH EDUCATIONAL METHODOLOGY

The optimal structure of educational tasks should focus on the essential activities to meet session learning objectives. Depending on how the learning objectives

of a session or course are defined, independently seeking and synthesizing information sources may be purposeful or may be inefficient. In addition, advances in understanding the decision-making process and cognitive errors have sharpened our understanding of clinical reasoning. Learners may approach clinical problems using different strategies – using both fast mental processes (mental shortcuts [heuristics] and pattern recognition) and more deliberate, analytic techniques. Some strategies include deductive reasoning or top-to-bottom logic (starting with a given general premise that is assumed to be true and then drawing conclusions), inductive reasoning or bottom-up reasoning (exploring premises and attempting to draw conclusions), and abductive reasoning (creating and testing hypothesis to explain observations). If efficient learning or information application are main learning objectives, PBL may not be the best instruction method, and other instructional methodologies should be considered.

EXTRANEOUS LOAD

Medicine has a moderately well-defined body of knowledge, which often includes best practices in approaching problems. Pure PBL enthusiasts require learners to seek all information on their own, and construct their own meaning – without being provided curated information/frameworks that might enhance their learning. Given the 'hunt and gather' unstructured nature of these PBL sessions, learners spend long periods of time sorting through unfiltered information usually on the Internet but also from other sources such as textbooks. This inefficiency is often frustrating to students, can be extremely time consuming, and may result in erroneous information.

Alternatively, a related teaching format is called case-based learning, and directly reduces extrinsic task load. The CBL case may be identical to the PBL case, but despite being a small-group exercise the methodology is very different. In CBL cases, faculty provide students information that is curated ahead of time ("Here are some high quality sources of information you might consider."), and may assign readings to individuals before the sessions. Sometimes information can be primary data (a study or policy paper) but other times students might be provided a series of videotaped answers to questions posed to a content expert on the specific topic of the patient in the case. Some argue that pre-class preparation can shift the use of team time from discovery to application, thus allowing time for a deeper discussion of the issues at hand. Students come into the PBL sessions without much preparation, whereas in CBL they come prepared to discuss the topic. Faculty often play a more active and engaged role.

VARIABLE SESSION EXPERIENCES

While the discovery process is important, it is not usual for small groups to reach different conclusions based on their interpretation of different sources of information. Subsequently, students find it frustrating to hear colleagues from other groups discussing their conclusions to a case. Students are left with uncertainty as what is the better solution and what is the 'correct' answer on an assessment exercise.

SCAFFOLDING

Scaffolding refers to providing learners appropriate guidance so that they can achieve competency with assistance from a more knowledgeable individual/group – without frustration. PBL is a fine approach to use if the course/session goal is to stimulate curiosity, encourage teamwork and problem solve. However, as mentioned in classic PBL, faculty are prohibited from guiding the student's learning to any significant degree. Thus, expert faculty's expertise is not utilized. Students also voice concern that they are not given guidance about how much detail to learn, and what content to focus on. Further, depending upon their developmental stage, learners may need help interpreting data such as laboratory, radiologic or pathology reports. Overall, this lack of scaffolding may lead to frustration and delays in acquiring clinical reasoning skills, especially early on in training.

RESOURCE USE

Having expert faculty in the room without the ability to utilize their expertise may be a waste of valuable resources. Many PBL sessions could probably run just a well with non-medical staff trained in small-group facilitation. To better utilize faculty expertise, the CBL format encourages faculty to provide some perspective/experience, after eliciting perspectives and insights from the group and to challenge misperceptions early on.

Issues with students

SMALL-GROUP DYSFUNCTION

In many groups, the ideal Tuckman small-group development process (forming, storming, norming, performing, adjourning) may not occur. Groups may fight, may not support each other, have members who undermine each other, or may not have the skills or maturity to collaborate. Skilled facilitators are necessary to help guide the group back to functionality, or reform the group. While true group dysfunction may be a rare occurrence, handling it requires skill and expertise.

STUDENT PREPARATION

Students who come to a PBL-laden curriculum typically have had didactic education and need to be retrained on how to work in groups, how to engage in independent learning, and most importantly what is required to pass examinations. As such, students usually need

training in PBL techniques, and reorientation of expectations to fully engage in PBL sessions.

EVALUATION AND OUTCOMES

Since the focus on PBL is teamwork, problem solving, synthesis, application and deductive/abductive reasoning, acquisition of specific content is often not emphasized. Students in PBL-driven curriculums are often left on their own to learn and understand course content. Also, 'success' in the small group is often difficult to define, and providing detailed, constructive feedback to students (or faculty) is often ignored or not done well. Evaluation modalities may focus on the individual learners.

Issues with tutors

Tutors require special training and education both on facilitation and on providing effective, honest feedback. There is great variability between groups, not only in terms of outcomes of learning but in the role played by the tutor. In sessions, some tutors follow strict rules that limit engagement, while others being far more active, leading to variability in the educational experience of the learner. Still other faculty are resistant to the ideas of small-group teaching using the classic refrain, "we never did it this way… and we turned out just fine!".

Active learning beyond the PBL format – expanding the educator toolbox

All modalities of teaching and learning may have a place in medical education, including lectures/demonstrations. PBL was one of the first well-described active learning formats, beyond traditional lab work and scientific experimentation. Over the past 50 years, many have experimented with alternative formats to promote active learning specific to their goals. These multi-modal approaches to curriculum delivery have expanded the educator toolbox, and increased the flexibility of educators to reach their goals (Fig. 18.1).

Newer small-group active techniques include case-based learning, team-based learning, case conferences for diagnostic reasoning and clinical decision making, simulation training, and teamwork training. Case-based learning (such as, 'doctoring' formats) may use standardized patients working off carefully crafted scripts to ensure that specific clinical issues are raised and addressed in a safe environment, where mistakes that students inevitably make will not hurt real patients. There may also be some role for the use of 'real patients' who present with real physical findings. The inclusion of non-physician teachers (particularly psychologists, as well as nurses and social workers) can augment

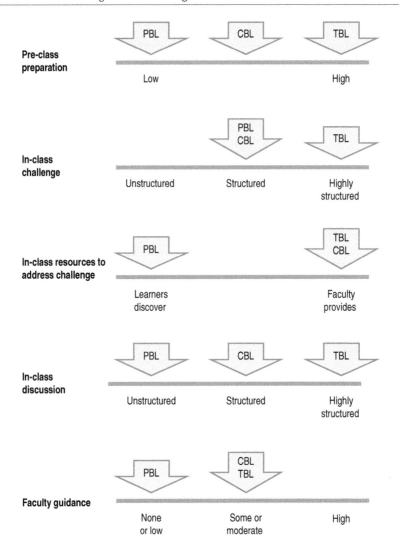

Fig. 18.1 Comparison of problem-based learning, cased-based learning and team-based learning.

learning and open the perspective of medical students and residents. Similarly, there may be an important role to be played by laypeople, as observers, commentators, and even as faculty. Another approach, team-based learning (TBL), ensures that learners come having prepared their content and are ready to engage. Even the evaluation structure empowers the group to work with accountability, while creating friendly competition between groups. While all small-group and active-learning formats have the option of creating longitudinal challenge and projects, longitudinal-group projects are central feature of team-based learning. In addition, all small-group learning formats can play a much larger role in promoting and monitoring student wellness, self-care, and resiliency. Table 18.1 outlines a few active learning modalities appropriate for small-group learning.

Summary

Problem-based learning is one of many approaches to small-group, self-directed learning that enhances teamwork and problem-solving skills in medical education. Regardless of small-group method used, many areas are ripe for active development. Some of these areas include making teaching material more stimulating, enhanced use of technology (e.g. web-based interactive programmes, simulation tools, portfolios to allow for reflection, action planning, and timely faculty feedback etc.), and improving assessment skills and instruments.

Movement towards a self-directed small-group learning experience requires more than new instructional design. It often requires culture change including the philosophy behind the selection of medical students, the provision of far greater resources, support for

Table 18.1   Educator toolbox: small-group active learning modalities

	Brief description	**Advantages**	**Disadvantages**
Problem-based learning	Small groupswork together on a single problem as a self-directed group, finding new information, and solving the problem together. Problem is typically a real/simulated/paper/video patient case. The faculty keeps the group on track, encourages autonomy, and may ask a few probing questions. Curricula involves one or multiple PBL cases.	Stimulates curiosity Encourages teamwork Forces application of information Build life-long learning skills Builds leadership Encourages deep understanding Preferred by learners over traditional didactic curriculum All students participate actively	Inefficient learning Does not correct mistakes of learners Does not utilize faculty expertise Does not cover too much material in total curriculum Subjective outcome evaluation No improvement of standardized test scores Must train faculty and learners in format Need many facilitators Learning is not uniform across groups
Case-based learning	Individuals in small group are given curated information ahead of time and come to group prepared to address a clinical problem. Problem presented in class is typically a real/simulated/paper/video patient case. Faculty more strongly probe and provide guidance. Curricula involves multiple CBL cases and cases often cover content that is multidimensional (bioscience, ethics, epidemiology, behavioural, communication skills, etc.).	Efficient learning Curated information Stimulates curiosity Encourages discussion and application Forces application of information Corrects misconceptions in real time Encouraged deep understanding Preferred by learners over PBL All students participate actively	Does not cover too much material in total curriculum Subjective outcome evaluation No improvement of standardized test scores Must train faculty in format Need many facilitators
Team-based learning	Individuals are given curated information ahead of time, and quizzed individually on the material. Individuals work in teams on the same quiz information. Teams present their information at the same time to the class, and argue for points. Faculty provides a mini-lecture about the topic, teams are then given a more substantive application assignment that lasts over several sessions, and solutions are presented at the same time.	Efficient learning Does not cover too much material in curriculum All learners' scores improve on standardized testing, including high and low performers Outcomes are clearly evaluated – group scores reflect each Improvement in standardized test scores Faculty expertise utilized Need few facilitators All students participate actively	Needs lots of faculty time to develop curriculum, quizzes, and larger project creation Must train faculty in format May or may not stimulate teamwork and problem solving depending on how the project is set up

course faculty, and altered incentives for medical school faculty. In addition, medical school administrations must commit to ensure that the larger curriculum does not subvert small-group teaching. PBL, as a well-tested small-group instructional method, will continue to have a place in medical education, especially in promoting lifelong learning skills.

Reference

Tuckman, B., 1965. Developmental sequence in small groups. Psychol. Bull. 63, 384–399.

Further reading

Barrows, H.S., 1996. Problem Based Learning in Medicine and Beyond: A Brief Overview. New Directions for Teaching and Learning. No 80. Jossey-Bass., pp. p2–p12.

Belland, B.R., French, B.F., Ertmer, P.A., 2009. Validity and problem-based learning research: a review of instruments used to assess intended learning outcomes. IJPBL. 3, 1, 59–89.

Hmelo-Silver, C.E., Barrows, H.S., 2006. Goals and strategies of a problem-based learning faciliator. IJPBL. 1 (1), 21–39.

Freeman, S., Eddy, S.L., McDonough, L., et al., 2014. Active learning increases student performance in science, engineering, and mathematics. Proc. Natl. Acad. Sci. U.S.A. 111 (23), 8410–8415.

Hoffman, K., Hosokawa, M., Blake, R., et al., 2006. Problem-based learning outcomes: ten years of experience at the University of Missouri-Columbia School of Medicine. Acad. Med. 81, 617–625.

Khanova, J., Roth, M.T., Rodgers, J.E., McLaughlin, J.E., 2015. Student experiences across multiple flipped classrooms in a single curriculum. Med. Educ. 49, 1038–1048.

Prince, K.J.A.H., van Mameren, H., Hylkema, N., et al., 2003. Does problem based learning lead to deficiencies in basic science knowledge? An empiric case on anatomy. Med. Educ. 37, 15–21.

Srinivasan, M., Wilkes, M.S., Stevenson, F., et al., 2007. Comparing problem-based learning with case-based learning: effects of a major curricular shift at two institutions. Acad. Med. 82 (1), 74–82.

Wilkes, M.S., Usatine, R., Slavin, S., Hoffman, J.R., 1998. Doctoring: University of California, Los Angeles. Acad. Med. 73 (1), 32–40.

Wood, D.F., 2003. ABC of learning and teaching in medicine: problem based learning. BMJ 326, 328–330.

Wilkes, M.S., Hoffman, J.R., Slavin, S.J., et al., 2013. The next generation of doctoring. Acad. Med. 88 (4), 438–441.

Team-based learning

D. Parmelee, A. Hyderi, L. K. Michaelsen

Trends

- TBL is a clearly defined, effective approach to 'flipping the classroom'.
- Learners have individual and team accountability for mastering content, making specific, collaborative decisions, and contributing to their peers' education.
- The instructor, a content expert, poses questions, stimulates debate, and clarifies only when necessary.
- TBL assures knowledge mastery, authentic application of knowledge, development of effective teamwork, and self-directed learning.

What is team-based learning?

Team-based learning (TBL) is an active learning instructional strategy that provides students with opportunities to apply conceptual knowledge through a sequence of events that includes individual work, teamwork and immediate feedback. It is very much learner-centred, and engages students with the kinds of problems they will encounter in clinical practice. It also promotes the development of professional competencies in interpersonal skills, teamwork and peer feedback (Michaelsen et al., 2008a).

The evidence for its academic effectiveness is growing, with an emerging track record for improving academic outcomes (Huggins & Stamatel, 2015; Haidet et al., 2014; McCormack & Garvan, 2014; Lubeck et al., 2013; Mennenga, 2013; Thomas & Bowen, 2011). TBL was first developed to maintain a focus on applying course concepts in the business school domain even though the teaching occurred in large classes.

How does TBL work?

Team-based learning's sequence of steps are forward thinking, guiding students into thinking progressively, gaining the ability to look beyond the 'now' and constantly asking, "What's next?" TBL sequences the

learning process (Michaelsen et al., 2008b) for the students through the following steps (Fig. 19.1).

STUDENTS' PERSPECTIVE

TBL recurring steps

Step 1 – advance assignment

Out-of-class/individual

Students receive a list of learning activities, accompanied by a set of learning goals that include those that are higher order as they are reflective of the Team Application (tAPP) problems, and those that are more foundational as they are reflective of the readiness assurance tests. Students study materials in preparation for the TBL session. Learning activities may include readings, videos, labs, tutorials, lectures, etc. Additionally, several medical schools have begun to implement an advance organizer that provides the students with the higher-order learning objectives associated with the tAPP problems, or provides the cases for the tAPP problems and then as part of the advance assignment asks them generate their own self-directed learning goals that would help them achieve the higher-order learning objectives and/or help answer the case. This advance organizer can have students list which resources they utilized for their self-study, and this list can be evaluated by the faculty after the in-class components for their quality and strength of evidence.

Step 2 – iRAT – individual readiness assurance test

In-class/individual

Each student completes a set (10–20) of multiple-choice questions that focus on the concepts they need to master in order to be able to solve the Team Application (tAPP) problems.

Step 3 – tRAT – team readiness assurance test

In-class/team

This is the same set of questions that each student has answered individually! But now the team must

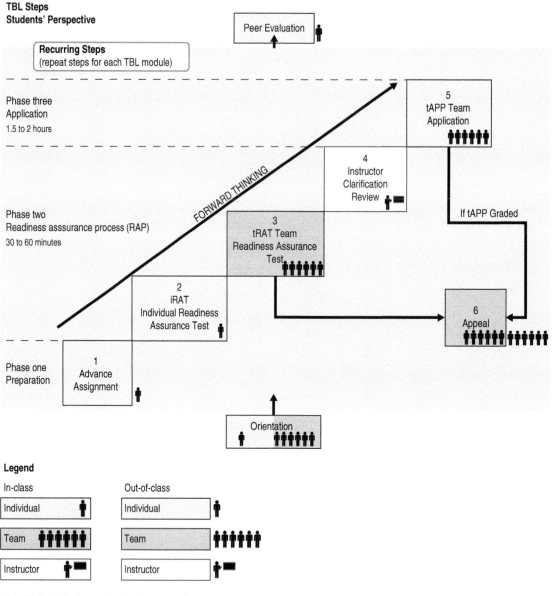

Fig. 19.1 TBL steps: students' perspective.

answer them through a consensus-building discussion. There must be a mechanism so that the team knows, as immediately as possible, whether or not they have selected the correct answers for two very different reasons. One is because immediate feedback is key to content learning. Immediate feedback also enables teams to discover the relationship between members' actions and the quality of the resulting outcomes so they can improve their decision-making processes.

Step 4 – instructor clarification review

In-class/instructor

Students get clarification from the instructor on the concepts they have been struggling with during the tRAT. At the end of the Clarification Review, students should feel confident that they are adequately prepared to solve more complex problems for the next TBL step: the Team Application.

Step 5 – team application – tAPP

In-class/team

This is the most important step! Students, in teams, are presented with a scenario/vignette that is similar to the type of problem with which they will be grappling in their careers. They are challenged to make interpretations, calculations, predictions, analyses and syntheses of given information and make a specific choice from a range of options. Teams then simultaneously post their choices and then participate in a discussion in which they are asked explain or defend their choice to the rest of the class.

The tAPP's structure follows the 4 Ss:

- **Significant problem:** Problems represent the type of situation that the students are about to face in the workplace or are foundational to the next level of study. Though students are encouraged to locate the best sources online or other sources at hand to develop their answers as they would in the 'real world', the greatest learning occurs through their discussion and debate.
- **Same problem:** Every team works on the same problem at the same time. Ideally, different teams will select different options for solutions.
- **Specific choice:** Each team must make a specific choice through their intra-team discussion. They should never be asked to produce a lengthy document. Teams should be able to display their choices easily so that all teams can see them.
- **Simultaneous report:** When it is time for teams to display their specific choices to a particular question, they do so at the same time. This way, everyone gets immediate feedback on where they might stand in the posting and they are then accountable to explain and defend their decision.

Step 3A and/or 6 – appeal

In-class/out-of-class/team

A team may request that the instructor consider an alternate answer to the one designated as 'best'. The team must provide either a clear and usable re-write of the question if they think it was poorly worded or a rationale with references as to why their choice was as good as the 'best' chosen by the instructor. Only a team that takes the steps to write an Appeal is eligible to receive credit for a particular question.

TBL nonrecurring steps
Orientation

Out-of-class/in-class/individual/team

Students read a brief article about TBL in preparation for the Orientation session, or the course syllabus as the first Advance Assignment. In class, students take an iRAT individually, followed by a tRAT in teams and then the tAPP.

Peer evaluation

Out-of-class/individual

Each student must evaluate each of his or her teammates on their contributions to the team's success and their own learning. It should be done anonymously, but team members are encouraged to speak directly to one another in providing feedback.

What does a TBL session look like?

If you visit a classroom while there is ongoing TBL, you will be impressed by the amount of body movement and talking. No student will be snoozing or reading the news. It is noisy because, for most of the time frame, the students are discussing, debating, even arguing within their teams as they achieve consensus on the questions so they will have answers they will be able to defend. There is a great deal of peer–peer teaching as members of a team ensure that they all 'get on the same page' with what they know and don't know.

If you start class on time with the iRAT, all students will be in class early. The room will be silent as they answer the set of questions, then when time is called, they will burst into discussion about the questions.

Students use the Immediate Feedback Assessment Technique (IF-AT) form to answer the tRAT questions. The IF-AT is a multiple-choice answer form with a thin opaque film covering the answer options. Instead of using a pencil to fill in a circle, students scratch off the answer as if scratching a lottery ticket. If the answer is correct, a star appears somewhere within the rectangle indicating the correct answer. Students earn partial credit for a second attempt and learn the correct response for each question while taking the tRAT. If they do not get it right the first time, they will immediately re-engage on that question and make another selection, but not without careful consideration since the stakes are higher. More information about the IF-AT form is available at the Epstein Educational Enterprises website (http://www.epsteineducation.com/).

Once all teams have completed the tRAT using the IF-AT form, there should be time for a whole-class discussion of one or two of the questions that the class should select (remember, by now, a lot of peer teaching has occurred as well as immediate feedback). The instructor either makes decisions on the spot about whether or not to accept more than one answer or defers to the Appeal process. The instructor takes the time to assure that all key concepts tested in the RATs are understood by the whole class. The instructor may provide a brief, focused presentation (Instructor Clarification Review) on key concepts in preparation for the tAPP.

Moving onto the tAPP, the case or problems for this phase can be in envelopes at each team location, displayed on screens in the classroom or posted on a website. Once members of a team feel that they are ready to discuss, they do so. Each team discovers its own process to make the best decisions on the options provided in the questions. The instructor calls time and requests the simultaneous response posting of team choices: methods used for posting answers include large colour-coded laminated cards with the options A, B, C, etc., and Audience Response System 'clickers'.

Next, the instructor probes for why a team has made a specific choice and why not another one. Once there has been sufficient but not excessive presentation of differing positions, the instructor states why he or she likes one or another better. The instructor may concur that two of the choices are equal depending upon how one interprets the data. If this component counts for a grade, then Appeals are invited for those teams that disagree with the final in-class answer(s).

What are the ingredients for a successful TBL module?

 Selecting learning activities can be a challenge for those in medical education since the lecture-based pedagogy has been the mainstay for so many years. TBL can eliminate lectures that are primarily 'information transmitting', for the content can be assigned from a text, PowerPoint with notes or even a multimedia online tutorial. Or students can be given the 'case' of the Application Exercise to clarify what they already know and learn what they feel they do not know in order to be able to address questions that it will generate in class.

A great deal of thought and planning goes into a successful TBL module. First and foremost, one evaluates the context in which one is teaching (the situational factors) and creates a course design that meets the course goals. We recommend starting with Dee Fink's Integrated Course Design (Fink, 2003), which incorporates the backward design paradigm (Wiggins & McTighe, 1998): a three-stage design process that delays the planning of teaching and learning activities until clear and meaningful learning goals have been defined and feedback and assessment activities designed (Fig. 19.2).

Once course learning goals are established, identifying the feedback and assessment activities to know if students have mastered the goals is next. TBL is an assessment tool since it provides you and the students with immediate feedback along the way.

You should also use the backward design when developing a TBL module. Table 19.1 shows an example of a backward design table for a TBL module on 'the lower extremity'.

Fig. 19.3 shows the steps you need to follow to make TBL successful in your course, following the backward design process.

INSTRUCTOR'S PERSPECTIVE

TBL recurring steps

Step 1 – situational factors and learning goals

Identify important situational factors, e.g. students' prior knowledge. Write clear learning goals that answer the question "What do I want the students to be able

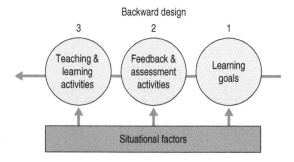

Fig. 19.2 Backward design.

Table 19.1 Backward design table for a TBL module on 'the lower extremity' **Situational factors:** Anatomy course, Year 1 students, little or no prior knowledge of the lower extremity

1. Learning goals	2. Feedback and assessment activities	3. Teaching and learning activities
• Identify and state the significance of all bony landmarks covered in the lab manual related to the lower extremity • Describe the pattern of cutaneous innervation in terms of dermatomes as well as areas supplied by specific nerves • Identify and describe the functions of structures associated with the joints of the lower extremity • Summarize the lymphatic drainage of the lower extremity • Identify and discuss the relevance of significant surface anatomy features of the lower extremity	• tAPP (graded) • iRAT, tRAT (graded)	Advance Assignment • A chapter in a recommended textbook • Online tutorials (lower extremity overview, neuromuscular, joints, imaging) • Dissection labs Instructor Clarification Review session

TBL Steps
Instructor's Perspective

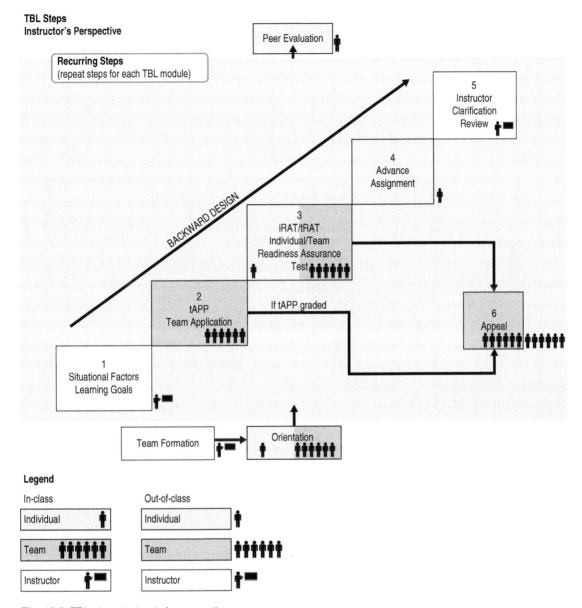

Fig. 19.3 TBL steps: instructor's perspective.

to DO?" Use action verbs such as describe, explain, calculate, differentiate, compare and analyze.

Step 2 – tAPP – team application

Create a Team Application exercise that:
- aligns with learning goals: assesses whether students can do what you want them to do
- is realistic and authentic
- challenges students: team power is required to solve problems
- encourages lifelong learning by having

teams utilize critical appraisal skills to resolve their uncertainty with the tAPP exercises.

Step 3 – iRAT/tRAT – individual readiness assurance test/team readiness assurance test

Create Readiness Assurance Test questions that:
- align with the tAPP: focused on the concepts needed to master for solving the tAPP
- avoid asking 'picky' questions just to see if they did the assignment

- are conducive to identifying knowledge gaps
- produce an individual's score that is tightly correlated with performance on any of the course's summative assessments.

 Write flawless multiple-choice questions (MCQs). If they are good questions and are foundational to the tAPP, then you don't have to worry about content coverage: the students will learn it and be able to use it.

Step 4 – advance assignment

Develop/select appropriate teaching/learning activities (readings, videos, labs, tutorials, lectures) for the Advance Assignment that:

- align with the iRAT/tRAT questions
- are effective and sufficient for content coverage
- encourage self-directed and lifelong learning and use of critical appraisal skills to evaluate resources.

Step 5 – instructor clarification review

Create an Instructor Clarification Review that:

- predicts/addresses gaps: focused on the concepts students are usually struggling to understand
- supports the development of critical thinking skills.

Step 6 – appeal

Consider a team's Appeal for an alternate answer to the one you have designated as 'best'. Each team must provide either:

- a clear and usable re-write of the question if they think it was poorly worded, or
- a rationale with references as to why their choice was as good as the 'best' chosen by the instructor.

TBL nonrecurring steps
Team formation

Assign students to teams: never let them self-select. Do so by distributing what you consider to be 'wealth factors' across teams, i.e. previous work experience in healthcare, completion of other graduate degrees in science, diversity backgrounds. Make your team selection process transparent so no student is wondering, "How was I put on this team?" Keep teams working together for the duration of the course or semester.

Orientation

Provide an orientation to TBL, using a sample TBL session that explains to students:

- why you are using TBL
- how it is different from previous group learning experiences

Peer evaluation

Create a peer evaluation instrument that:

- allows students to evaluate each of his or her teammates on their contributions to the team's success and their own learning
- has both a quantitative and qualitative component
- is accompanied by guidelines on how to provide helpful feedback.

Why does TBL work?

The following sections describe some key characteristics of TBL that make it work.

ACCOUNTABILITY

Students are accountable for being prepared for class. Most have gone even deeper in their exploration of the material. Although, at first, they feel accountable because part of their grade depends on the depth of out-of-class mastery of course content, they come to feel accountable to their teammates because they want to contribute all they can to their team's productivity.

IMMEDIATE FEEDBACK

A main driver for learning with TBL is the frequent and immediate feedback on both individual and team decisions.

SOLVING AUTHENTIC PROBLEMS

Once students have mastered course content and key concepts through the Readiness Assurance, they tackle complex problems that are similar to the ones they will encounter in their professional activities.

ENGAGEMENT WITH COURSE CONTENT

Students become fully engaged with course content both outside of class, with the Advance Assignment as a starting place, and in the classroom, with the set of activities that involve and embroil them in discussions on the course content. The tighter the fit of the instructor's components for the TBL module with the course learning goals and the greater the authenticity of the Team Application questions, the greater the student engagement.

LEARNING TO WORK COLLABORATIVELY

Teams stay together for as long as possible, and since there are clear incentives to collaborate for the good of the team, students learn how to communicate effectively with peers, resolve conflicts and stay focused on the tasks at hand.

What can go wrong with TBL?

Although they are clearly the exception rather than the rule, the most common stories of TBL going awry are the following.

1. **'The students hated it because they do not like to prepare for class.'**

   Solution: Prepare students for TBL.

   You must prepare your students for the shift to TBL in which they learn the content outside of class and apply it in the classroom. One of the quickest ways is to provide an orientation session for your students as a sample TBL session. You can create the sample session by using TBL content (based on a brief TBL article) or using the course syllabus as the first Advance Assignment (imagine students reading what the course is about before the first class!). The TBL Collaborative website (www.nbme.org) has a link called *Orienting Students* with more tips on how to introduce TBL to your students.

2. **'The students hated the RAT questions and argued so much with me that we had no time for the Team Application.'**

   Solution: Write good questions and use the Appeal process.

   A great source for writing effective MCQs is the National Board of Medical Examiners (NBME) Item Writing Manual, downloadable at their website (www.nbme.org).

   Use an Appeal process that enables students to challenge either the wording or content of a question.

3. **'The students hated it because they did so poorly on the RAT as individuals, and the team scores weren't so good either; the mood was grim and angry before we got to the Team Application.'**

   Solution: Adjust questions' level of difficulty.

   The mean iRAT score for the class should be close to their performance on any of the course's summative assessments; the tRAT mean score should be in the high 80s–90s. If the mean iRAT score is low, then your questions were poorly written and/or there is not a good fit between the questions and what they should have learned before class. Craft your Advanced Assignment so they know clearly what level of mastery is needed to 'pass' the iRAT. Sample questions with the Assignment are helpful.

4. **'Everything went well until it was clear we would not get through the Team Application because of time; then everyone was frustrated.'**

   Solution: Use fewer questions.

   Ensuring that there is enough time for the Team Application is essential, and the most common mistake is to include too many questions. It is far better to have just two to four really probing, thought- and debate-provoking questions that

   explore the 'why' and 'how' of the problem than trying to cover more content. Sometimes, it is best to separate the RAT from the tAPP by a few hours or even a day or two; consider having two sessions for the tAPP, the second one more challenging than the first.

5. **'It was chaos because the lecture hall has fixed seating, the acoustics were terrible and there was no room for any team clustering.'**

   Solution: Use efficient strategies to better organize the TBL session.

   Few institutions will have ideal space for TBL since either they have a lecture-based curriculum that uses the sage-on-the-stage design, or PBL is well-established and there are many small-group rooms and few larger ones. We have several suggestions about how to better organize your TBL classroom experience:

   - **Divide the TBL session into two groups:** There needs to be space in the classroom for clustering, so if the classroom is completely full with little room to spare, consider doing the TBL session twice after dividing the class in half.

   - **Require students to stand up when asking/answering questions:** Require that a student stand up when he or she speaks and face the class as much as possible. Almost always, when this happens the others will be quiet. If they are allowed to remain sitting when they speak, few can hear, and few will really pay attention. Re-state what is asked and what is said so that you are sure everyone in the class has heard.

   - **Develop systems for identifying teams and for simultaneous reporting:** Find some marker system so that you and everyone in the class knows where the teams are (e.g. poles or tents displaying team number), and when it is time for simultaneous reporting, have a way to display the choices. Methods used for posting answers include large colour-coded laminated cards with the options A, B, C, etc., and Audience Response System 'clickers'.

   - **Package materials in advance:** Keep the chaos factor down by having all TBL materials carefully prepared, packaged and ready to use at the team site, including IF-AT forms and clear instructions on how to record individual and team answers for grading. Ideally, you will keep all materials secure, meaning none of the materials leave the classroom.

6. **'The students got a lot out the Readiness Assurance but seemed unengaged in the Team**

Application because they felt the questions were too much like the Readiness Assurance ones.'

Solution: Design an effective Team Application.

Your case or problem for the tAPP must be authentic and closely resemble what students will be encountering soon in their careers, and it must require them to apply the content and concepts to solve. Be creative: use a video clip of a patient describing his or her symptoms; post laboratory or diagnostic information that is real but appears contradictory to the rest of the patient's presentation.

Is TBL worth the effort?

Designing an effective and successful TBL module can be labour intensive; however, there are many reasons that make it worthwhile, depending upon your context, how much time you have to plan ahead and your commitment to using classroom time for solving problems. Is it more work than putting together lectures? Yes, it is. But do you ever really know that your students are engaged with the course material in a lecture? At the end of your lectures, do you ever know if they could apply what you presented? When composing a lecture, do you ever consider *how* your students think?

Transforming your course or instructional unit to TBL will require that you shift from an emphasis on covering content to determining how students can apply content to answer meaningful questions. It also requires students to give up the expectation that 'spoon-feeding' lectures will provide them with what they need to know to pass the exams or be successful in their careers.

Some additional points to consider are the following.

ONE INSTRUCTOR; SAME MESSAGE

Only one instructor is needed without losing any of the benefits of 'small-group' learning, and the instructor need not be trained or talented in group process: he or she need only be a content expert and adhere to the structure and principles of the process. This provides the additional dividend of all students getting the same message, which is hard to achieve with multiple small-group instructors.

 Make your 'teaching moments' brief and in direct response to where you see gaps in student knowledge. The TBL process will provide you with continuous information about what your students know and don't know.

ONE CLASSROOM; NO SPREADING AROUND OR FINDING MORE FACULTY

An entire session is done in one classroom; no need for the small groups to be divided up and spread around the building or set of buildings. The classroom may become noisy, but the students are sharing, learning and very actively engaged in the process. There is no need to beg colleagues to leave their labs/clinics to come teach a small group or worry about how much they lecture in those small groups that were meant for discussion!

IN-CLASS MEETINGS; ALL HAPPENS IN THE CLASSROOM

Students do not have to meet outside of class to either prepare or complete any project. Except for the individual study as part of the Advanced Assignment, everything happens in the classroom.

INDIVIDUAL ACCOUNTABILITY; NO SOCIAL LOAFING

Social loafing is extinguished by the accountability components: 1) the iRAT counts as part of the course grade; 2) the tRAT counts as part of the course grade (and tAPP may also count); 3) peer evaluation.

SIMULTANEOUS REPORTING; NO PRESENTATIONS

Simultaneous reporting on specific choices and decisions eliminates having students take turns presenting findings, which students uniformly find boring and a waste of time.

INSTRUCTOR CLARIFICATION; IMMEDIATE FEEDBACK

There is a content expert, the instructor, who, at the appropriate times, does share his or her expertise to elucidate, clarify and amplify when the class gets stumped or needs new direction. Students master the course content (facts) and concepts because they have to apply both to solve the problems in the Team Application. Therefore, they complete a module feeling confident in what they know and how to apply it and are clear about what they don't know so that they might learn it before any next assessment.

NATURALLY FUNCTIONAL TEAMS; NO TEAMWORK INSTRUCTION

There is no need to instruct students in teamwork. They learn by doing, and the immediate feedback on their thinking both as individuals and as team members shapes collaborative behaviours. They become committed to the team's performance and make behavioural changes that lead to improved performance. It is extremely rare for there to be a dysfunctional team.

SELF-DIRECTED AND LIFELONG LEARNING

TBL helps promote self-directed and lifelong learning. Students realize their knowledge gaps and deficiencies vis-à-vis the Readiness Assurance process and in resolving their uncertainties during the Team Application exercises. Additionally, they develop critical appraisal skills of articulating specific questions, searching for answers, appraising the quality of their search results, and applying the results to the problem/case/question at hand in the Team Application exercise to make a specific choice. These same critical appraisal skills can be enhanced if an advance organizer is used that provides the students with the higher-order learning objectives associated with the tAPP problems or provides the cases for the tAPP problems, and then as part of the advance assignment asks them to generate their own self-directed learning goals that would help them achieve the higher-order learning objectives and/or help answer the case. This advance organizer can have students list which resources they utilized for their self-study and this list can be evaluated by the faculty after the in-class components for their quality and strength of evidence.

Summary

TBL can be an exhilarating learner-centred instructional strategy for both the instructor and students, providing students with regular opportunities to learn how to collaborate with peers. For an individual module or a whole course using TBL to be successful, one must adhere to the steps and principles emphasized in this chapter. Based on our many years of experience with TBL, we are convinced that it is ideal for medical education because of its emphasis on accountability, decision making, critical appraisal, and collaboration with peers: all essential competencies for healthcare professionals.

References

Fink, L.D., 2003. Creating Significant Learning Experiences: An Integrated Approach to Designing College Courses. Jossey-Bass Higher and Adult Education.

Haidet, P., McCormack, W.T., Kubitz, K., 2014. Analysis of the team-based learning literature: TBL comes of age. J. Excell. Coll. Teach. 25 (3&4), 303–333.

Huggins, C.M., Stamatel, J., 2015. An Exploratory Study Comparing the Effectiveness of Lecturing versus Team-based Learning. Teach. Sociol. 43 (3), 227–235.

Lubeck, P., Tschetter, L., Mennenga, H., 2013. Team-based learning: an innovative approach to teaching maternal-newborn nursing care. J. Nurs. Educ. 52 (2), 112–115.

McCormack, W.T., Garvan, C.W., 2014. Team-Based Learning Instruction for Responsible Conduct of Research Positively Impacts Ethical Decision-Making. Account. Res. 21 (1), 34–49.

Mennenga, H.A., 2013. Student engagement and examination performance in a team-based learning course. J. Nurs. Educ. 52 (8), 475–479.

Michaelsen, L.K., Parmelee, D.X., McMahon, K.K., Levine, R.E., 2008a. Team-Based Learning for Health Professions Education: A Guide to Using Small Groups for Improving Learning. Stylus.

Michaelsen, L.K., Sweet, M., Parmelee, D.X., 2008b. Team-Based Learning: Small Group Learning's Next Big Step. New Directions for Teaching and Learning. Jossey Bass.

Thomas, P.A., Bowen, C.W., 2011. A controlled trial of team-based learning in an ambulatory medicine clerkship for medical students. Teach. Learn. Med. 23 (1), 31–36.

Wiggins, G., McTighe, J., 1998. Understanding by Design. Merrill Education/ASCD College Textbook Series.

Online resources

Epstein Educational Enterprises, Immediate Feedback Assessment Technique (IF-AT) form: http://www.epsteineducation.com.

National Board of Medical Examiners (NBME) Item Writing Manual: http://www.nbme.org/publications/item-writing-manual-download.html.

Team-Based Learning Collaborative website: http://www.teambasedlearning.org.

20

Using digital technologies

R. H. Ellaway

Trends

- Digital technologies are now omnipresent in medical education.
- Medical teachers need to be proficient in selecting and using technologies in their teaching.
- Mobile technologies have become a critical medium for medical education.

Introduction

Education involves the systemization of teaching and learning. A key component in this is the use of a variety of technologies in support of teaching and learning. Medical education has long made use of educational technologies of many kinds and at different scales and levels. Books, buildings, photography and models have all played a critical role in shaping the direction and possibilities of medical education, and they continue to do so. Although there are many technologies employed in contemporary medical education, when we think about technology we tend to focus on digital technologies; the interconnected and interdependent computing devices, software, services, and network infrastructures that pervade our modern lives. There are many reasons for this, including the relative novelty of digital technologies (although that is fading), their pervasiveness, and their transformative power. Indeed, there is very little in medical education today that does not either involve the use of digital technologies or happen in the presence of digital technologies in some way or other.

There are two essential challenges facing medical teachers that will be explored in this chapter: how to use digital technologies in medical education, and how to be a medical teacher in a digital age. Medical teachers need to be literate in when and how to use (and not to use) digital technology in their teaching, not least because technologies are not just a means to an end, they change us and they change the ends

we are seeking to achieve. To that end, the modern medical teacher needs to be aware of the directing and disruptive nature of using digital technologies in medical education as well as their many affordances. This is particularly important in the contemporary sphere as we are currently training the last generation of doctors who can remember a time before the Internet, the first who will learn in an environment dominated by digital technologies and the first who will practice in a predominantly e-health environment. Medical teachers need to be attentive, reflective and considered in how they both use and respond to digital technologies.

 "We are training the last generation of doctors who can remember a time before the Internet."

The digital technology repertoire

Before exploring the use of digital technology in medical education, we need to set out the repertoire of tools and systems available to contemporary medical teachers.

- First and perhaps foremost is *content*; the data, information, and knowledge available through digital channels in different formats such as text, images, audio, and video. This includes generic materials and collections such as Wikipedia and YouTube, as well as medical–education-specific materials and study materials such as e-textbooks, reference materials such as pharmacopeia, along with patient or physician websites, study guides, virtual patients, games, and data sets.
- *Devices* are the digital technologies that provide the physical means by which humans can interact with digital media. This category includes generic devices that can serve many different purposes (such as computers, smartphones, and tablets) and education-specific devices (such as data projectors, simulators, cameras, digital stethoscopes, and laparoscopic simulators).
- The next layer of technology is made up of *tools* (the software, apps, and other services that run

on devices) that allow humans to access and manipulate digital content and to interact with other individuals and groups. This includes web browsers, calendars, writing tools, databases and spreadsheets.

- Tools may function as part of larger *systems* that may be generic (web, email, social media) or education-specific (learning management systems, quiz banks, assessment tools). These systems allow individuals to collaborate and to interact with shared resources.

- All of the above depend on *infrastructure*. While this is not usually a concern of the medical teacher, its weaknesses or failures can be a significant impediment to the use of technology or an incentive to use it less or not at all. Medical teachers should at least be aware of infrastructure issues in their teaching environments including Wi-Fi and cellular networks, security, electrical sockets and authentication.

These different technologies do not exist in isolation, using one often requires the use of others. Content needs tools in order to be accessed, tools need devices to run on and systems to interact with, and they all depend on infrastructure. Although the rest of this chapter will focus on the uses and impacts of digital technology in medical education, medical teachers should have a basic understanding of these dependencies so as to be able to make best use of the technologies available to them.

Using technology in medical education

Technologies have little value until they are actually used. Our primary focus as medical teachers should therefore be on how digital technologies can be best used to support and enable medical education. It is important to note that most technologies do not get used exactly as they were intended to; indeed, some of the most valuable applications involve various degrees of adaptation and improvisation. We should therefore be prepared to make use of the many affordances of digital technologies and not be limited by its intended uses.

Resources such as multimedia learning packages, podcasts and videos can be used in support of instruction, both in the classroom and for independent study. Online simulation resources such as virtual patients can be used to practise and hone skills such as clinical decision-making. Teachers and learners can communicate and collaborate with each other on educational projects and activities using a wide range of media (social media, webinars, wikis etc.) and they can publish the outputs of their work through blogs, websites, and media sites such as YouTube. Reference materials such as drug databases, clinical handbooks, and the research literature can be readily used in classroom, bedside, and independent learning activities, and the

results of their activities and the reflections on those activities recorded in clinical encounter logging systems and portfolios. Technologies are widely used in both formative and summative assessment in the form of online quizzes and formal computer-based proctored exams, and the results of those assessments can be tracked and analyzed in assessment and learning management systems. Curriculum maps can be used to facilitate curriculum planning, development and audit and can help teachers and learners to situate their work within the broader programme of study. Teachers and course organizers can use the tracking and analytics features in the tools they use to monitor their learners' progress and to identify individuals who need more support and observation. Clearly, almost every aspect of contemporary medical education practice does or can involve digital technologies.

These examples illustrate the many ways in which technologies can act as mediating artefacts; they are the medium for undertaking particular kinds of activities. Indeed, it is this mediating role that makes them both essential and peripheral to the focus or the outcomes of the activities they support. Thus, while medical teachers need to understand and have some facility in using technology, using technology is not their primary concern. The use of technology also depends to a great extent on the role the user is playing. The way a teacher uses PowerPoint or a learning management system is very different from the way their learners use these tools. Some technologies, such as tracking and analytics, are almost exclusively used by teachers or course leaders, while others, such as educational apps and virtual patients, are almost exclusively used by learners. Moreover, the uses of technology are not symmetrical; not everyone uses technology in the same way or to the same extent. In every class there will be students who are not interested in using digital technologies as well as those who actively embrace them. The contemporary medical teacher clearly has to encompass variation in technology use in many dimensions.

Why use digital technology?

Although there are a great many ways in which digital technologies can be used, we should ask; why use technology at all? Are there any aspects of medical education where using educational technologies is the best way to teach or learn? The gold standard for education typically involves face-to-face individual tutoring with little or no technology mediation, and there are few if any learning theories that are predicated on the use of technologies. So, again we can ask: why use technology at all? One answer can be found in the transforming nature of the Internet and the digital technologies that connect to it. We can encapsulate the strengths and weaknesses of Internet technologies as follows.

EXPONENTIAL CONNECTIVITY AND INTEGRATION

The Internet can be used to integrate a variety of services and information, reflected, for instance, in the proliferation of learning management systems such as Blackboard and Moodle. However, integration also means more interdependence, which can in turn make systems more and more vulnerable to errors and failures from one component in the system.

ACCELERATING SPEED OF ACTION AND RESPONSE

The Internet can make communication, processing, and access much faster. Although this means that tasks can be undertaken more quickly, there is less and less time to reflect on the consequences of one's actions and a lower tolerance for delays or things that take time to develop.

DEFEATING GEOGRAPHY AND TEMPORALITY

The Internet can significantly extend the reach of one's actions. For instance, geographically remote learners can study together and patients and physicians at different locations can be connected via telehealth networks. One reaction to this extended reach has been a tendency for students to value face-to-face encounters more than online ones.

OBSERVATION

Systems and tools can track and record almost any action their users make. While this provides the ability to provide rich feedback and modelling of learner behaviours, it can also reduce learners' autonomy to explore and their freedom to express themselves.

These affordances let us change the rules about how we work and how we interact with information and with each other. They can help teachers and learners to save time and effort in remembering, repeating, finding, recording and structuring information and knowledge. They can expand the reach of teaching and learning beyond physical limitations (potentially engaging more learners distributed across multiple locations). They can expand interaction beyond temporal limitations (teaching can be asynchronous – happening whenever is convenient rather than setting a single time for everyone). They can help to organize and connect learners and teachers in support of a multitude of learning activities, and they can help us to scrutinize, record, and track teacher and learner actions. If you need some or all of these advantages then technology can be an enabler in mediating your activities. However, you should also be aware of the less desirable implications that can accompany the benefits of using these technologies.

One key consequence of using digital technologies is that teachers and learners no longer have to be intimately connected to create learning opportunities. Indeed, designing and using digital technology in medical education creates many variations on teacher presence. Table 20.1 sets out a continuum between presence and absence and the different kinds of activities and tools that apply to these different settings.

Technology and instructional design

Using technology in medical education may happen relatively spontaneously but it is far more common (and advisable) for medical teachers to design and plan their use of technologies and to blend them into their

Table 20.1 A continuum of teacher presence and associated technology enhanced learning methods

	Face-to-face teacher presence	**Synchronous teacher telepresence**	**Asynchronous teacher telepresence**	**Teacher represented in software**
Location	Teacher and learners are in the same place at the same time using technology in a 'blended learning' mode	Teacher is online at the same time as their learners	Teacher interacts episodically and at different times to their learners	Software is designed to take on the role of the teacher
Activity	Learning activities are constructed between participants with little activity encoded in the artefacts and resources they use	Learning activities are constructed between the participants. Activities partly depend on the capabilities and functionality of the medium being used	Learning activities are very much defined by the capabilities and functionality of the medium being used	Learning activities and the range of variability within them is largely predefined and encoded in the software
Examples	Learning makes use of digital resources as part of a classroom activity or lecture	Learning is undertaken through webconferencing, videoconferencing or virtual worlds	Learning is undertaken through discussion boards, wikis or blogs	Learning is undertaken using self-study multimedia teaching packages and virtual patients

teaching practice. This is encapsulated in the practices of instructional design: "creating detailed specifications for the development, evaluation, and maintenance of situations which facilitate learning and performance" (Richey et al., 2011). There are two key areas of design involving technology: designing things to use (tools, materials) and designing things to do (activities). Both areas involve consideration of the following instructional design questions (expanding on Richey et al., 2011).

WHO ARE YOUR LEARNERS AND WHAT LEARNING PROCESSES WORK BEST FOR THEM?

As with all teaching and learning, it pays to understand what your learners' preferences and abilities are with respect to digital technologies. For instance, counter to popular opinion, not all young people are keen on using digital technologies. In any given class or cohort, there are likely to be some learners who are very interested in using technology and others who are not. Rather than assuming learner preferences and capacities it is better to discuss and negotiate what technology use works best for them.

WHAT ARE THE LEARNING AND PERFORMANCE CONTEXTS YOU ARE WORKING WITH?

The efficacy of using digital technologies can depend to a great extent on context, and it pays for medical educators to know about and, to an extent, be able to organize the contexts for medical education to support the use of digital technologies. This can involve making sure there is adequate Wi-Fi and electrical power for their learners' devices, setting clear expectations as to what constitutes appropriate and inappropriate uses of technology, and how to be a digital professional (see later section in this chapter).

WHAT CONTENT WILL BE INVOLVED, HOW SHOULD IT BE STRUCTURED AND SEQUENCED?

Although there are uses of technology that do not involve the provision of 'content' (such as discussion), many others do involve content, such as slide presentations, hand-outs, textbooks, reference materials, video and audio, and props and resources for practical exercises. Designing things to be used should draw on learning theories (such as those pertaining to sequencing and cognitive load) and empirical evidence, such as the work of Richard Mayer (2009). Mayer has synthesized a set of 'multimedia principles', heuristics to guide the design of media for instruction (Box 20.1). Other considerations include testing and ensuring the usability of learning resources (making sure that their design and presentation is clear, unambiguous and accessible), and making sure that copyright and other

> **Box 20.1 Multimedia principles – after Mayer (2009)**
>
> 1. Coherence: remove any material not relevant to the task in hand.
> 2. Signalling: add cues regarding the organization of the material.
> 3. Redundancy: images and narration are better than images, narration and text.
> 4. Spatial: corresponding words and images should be adjacent to each other.
> 5. Temporal: corresponding words and images should be presented at the same time.
> 6. Segmenting: user-paced segments are better than a single presentation.
> 7. Pre-training: learn key concepts before applying them.
> 8. Modality: image and narration is better than image and text.
> 9. Multimedia: words and images are better than words alone.
> 10. Personalization: using a conversational narrative style is better than using a formal one.
> 11. Voice: a real human voice is better than a machine-generated one.
> 12. Image: seeing the speaker's image, such as a 'talking head', does not improve learning.

licensing issues are addressed. The latter can be particularly daunting, and help from your library or other institutional supports may be advisable or even required.

WHAT INSTRUCTIONAL AND NON-INSTRUCTIONAL STRATEGIES SHOULD YOU USE?

Once you have a clear understanding of your learners, the learning context(s), and the content to be articulated, the next step is to select and design objectives for the learning activity, and the ways in which your learners will develop their knowledge, skills and attitudes. 'Activity design' is central to this step, as the medical teacher needs to decide what learners and teachers will be asked to do. Activities are typically based on an existing repertoire of approaches the teacher is familiar with and that are likely to afford the desired learning outcomes for the specific learners and learning circumstances they are working with. For instance, using an online discussion board can support peer mentoring and reflection while recorded didactic materials can be used in support of knowledge acquisition or revision for exams. It is beyond the scope of this chapter to describe the multitude of ways activities can be built around or using digital technologies.

However, as other chapters in this volume explore the many dimensions of contemporary medical education, the use of technologies is present, both explicitly and implicitly, throughout. One particular advantage to using technology is that it can help to break out of the traditional repertoire of medical education activities to create new and hybrid activities. For instance, a lecture is 'flipped' when the didactic materials are pre-recorded and put online for learners to study before class and the face-to-face time used for discussion and problem solving. Medical teachers are encouraged to think of activities and the uses of technologies as patterns can that can be combined and recombined to create innovative and effective responses to novel learning situations (Ellaway & Bates, 2015).

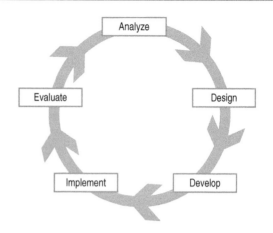

Fig. 20.1 ADDIE model for instructional design.

WHAT MEDIA AND DELIVERY SYSTEMS WILL YOU USE?

This step involves selecting the tools and devices that will be used. Selecting the digital technologies to be used in different educational activities often involves a compromise between the ideal and the practical. For instance, the cost of developing bespoke software to meet a specific teaching need means that this is rarely the path medical teachers take (although it is not unheard of). It is much more common for medical teachers to limit the choice of technologies they might use to those that are immediately available to them. Most schools have some kind of online learning management system (LMS – aka virtual learning environment or VLE) that provides basic course functions such as a file store, discussion, scheduling and announcements. There are many other generic educational tools and systems (Horton, 2006; Clark & Mayer, 2008), for instance many medical schools have online tools for portfolios, evaluation, clinical encounter logging, and assessment. More generic tools can also be used, such as wikis for collaborative writing, blogs for reflective writing, and webinar tools for distributed lecturing and small-group work. There are also tools and systems that are specific to medical education (Ellaway, 2007), including virtual patients, bedside reference materials (particularly for mobile devices), and procedural skills videos. Medical teachers can also use publicly accessible systems (particularly those that are free) such as YouTube for publishing videos, SoundCloud for publishing audio clips, SlideShare for presentations, and Skype for videoconferencing.

HOW WILL YOU ACTUALLY CONDUCT THE DESIGN PROCESSES?

This is about constructing, configuring, and/or deploying educational activities and the resources they employ. The ADDIE model has coalesced within the instructional design community as a way of guiding and structuring this process. First you analyze the situation and learner needs, and then you select (design) the kinds of things (activities, resources) that will be used. The next step is to build (develop) and implement the design, and finally the resulting learning is evaluated, which feeds back in to any changes that will be made to improve the learning situation the next time it is invoked (Fig. 20.1). Even if medical teachers don't create their own technologies, the ADDIE model can help to structure any kind of intentional use of digital technology in medical education.

Having set out strategies for using technology in medical education we can move on to look at more specific and emerging issues around the use of digital technology in medical education.

Mobile technologies

Within the last 10 years cell phones have been developed into smartphones with substantial computing power, while the design principles of smartphones and laptops have been merged to create tablet computers. Smart watches and other 'wearables' have also expanded the ways in which we can think about and interact with digital technologies. Mobile technologies are generally smaller and lighter than desktop and laptop computers, they are designed to be used in the hand (rather than on a lap or on a table) meaning they can be used at the bedside or any other location that larger devices cannot, and they have a wider range of network capabilities, again meaning they can be used in many locations. Another significant departure is that their tools are organized in the form of 'apps' (short for applications), which are available through the device on 'app stores' often for free, or for a small fee. The rise and rise of the use of mobile technologies has had a significant impact on medical education, not least because most (but not all) medical learners now have the power of these devices at their fingertips wherever they go, they have the convenience of their portability, and they have the autonomy of selecting their devices and tools with little or no oversight of their school or their teachers.

There are many applications of mobile technology in medical education including: logistics and personal information management; accessing content and reference materials (such as drug guides or procedural skills videos) at the bedside; collaboration with peers, using social media or polling in lectures; 'always-on' communication through texts, email and other tools; and practice, using a mobile device in consults and accessing electronic medical records. However, the value of using mobile technologies depends on the circumstances of use. We can consider a hierarchy of needs (adapted from Maslow's work) that puts the value of using mobile technologies in medical education in context (Fig. 20.2) (Masters et al., 2016).

Preparing for e-health

Physicians increasingly use digital technologies as a part of their practice. Indeed, e-health and telemedicine have become central to the provision of contemporary healthcare. As digital technologies have become part of professional practice, medical education has had to respond. In this case, technology use is both the medium and the objective of training activities. Key e-health technologies and systems include electronic health records (EHRs) and electronic medical records (EMRs), systems for imaging (such as picture archiving and communication systems [PACS]), laboratories, order entry and prescribing, point-of-care information resources, decision support systems and guidelines, logistic systems (for instance scheduling and tracking), tools for communicating with patients and colleagues, and information and support resources for the general population (such as public health websites, hotlines

and personal health records). All of these forms can be taught by using them for educational as well as practice purposes. For instance, an EMR can be populated with the cases learners will encounter in their PBL or clinical skills sessions. Clerking and managing patients using an EMR therefore becomes a part of the broader course experience. E-health competencies can frame the educational use of technologies in medical education. Box 20.2 sets out core e-health competencies for postgraduate medical education organized around CanMEDS roles (Ho et al., 2014) and these can be used to integrate the professional use of digital technologies in to medical education curricula.

Hidden curriculum and digital technologies

It is rare for the use of digital technologies to be undertaken and accepted without reservation. We should therefore consider the barriers, mixed messages, absences, and other socially constructed influences on the use of digital technology in medical education. We can do this in terms of the hidden curriculum, the informal curriculum, and the null curriculum of technology use in medical education (Ellaway et al., 2013):

- The hidden curriculum of digital technologies reflects the institutional expectations, policies, and cultural norms that influence their use. This can include situations where technology use is expected or even required (such as making the LMS the only way that course materials can be accessed), as well as where technology use is circumscribed (such as forbidding the recording of lectures or banning the use of digital devices in exams).

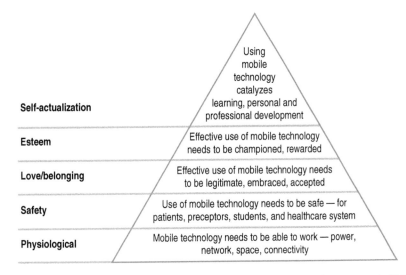

Fig. 20.2 A hierarchy of needs for using mobile technologies in medical education (Masters et al., 2016).

Box 20.2 Selected CanMEDS e-health competencies for postgraduate medical education (after Ho et al., 2014)

Medical expert:

- Use information and communication technologies to deliver patient-centred care and provide expert consultation to diverse populations in a variety of settings.
- Employ clinical decision support tools as an adjunct to clinical judgement in providing timely, evidence-based, safe interventions.
- Monitor and audit individual practice through the capture and analysis of health, quality and patient safety data.

Communicator:

- Document patient outcomes and safety considerations in an accurate, complete, timely, and retrievable manner, in compliance with legal, privacy, and regulatory requirements and in the interest of effective and efficient clinical decision making.
- Recognize how the capture, organization, tabulation and display of health information affect the care of patients, facilitate or impede information exchange, and influence the efficiency of the healthcare system.

Collaborator:

- Collaborate in the development, advancement, utilization and evaluation of electronic information and management systems, processes, and resources to facilitate best practice and the provision of safe, high-quality, and productive care.
- Share electronic information with other healthcare professionals collaboratively for the purpose of integrating and optimizing care and improving outcomes for individuals and populations.

Leader:

- Contrast the benefits and limitations of health information systems and apply this knowledge to patient management, patient safety, practice management, and continuous quality improvement in one's own practice and in all clinical and professional environments where one works.

- Acknowledge that human–computer interface issues, organizational culture, technological restrictions, and device and infrastructure malfunction may generate errors or distortion of data that negatively affect patient safety. Advocate for and implement harm reduction strategies in the workplace.

Health advocate:

- Employ health informatics to enhance quality of care and service delivery in the context of acute and chronic disease management in community settings.
- Advocate for balance between an individual's right to privacy and the needs of the healthcare system when using aggregated health information in decision making.
- Speak out against harmful medical misinformation portrayed in social media.

Scholar:

- Use information technologies to enhance knowledge, skill and judgement in the provision of evidence-informed patient care.
- Organize, maintain, appraise and continuously improve scholarly resource and health information management skills both for oneself and for others using information technologies throughout one's professional career.

Professional:

- Act to ensure technology preserves and strengthens the doctor–patient relationship, is of benefit to patients individually and collectively, and is used in a way that maintains public trust in the profession.
- Uphold professional obligations, comply with legislation, and maintain appropriate personal boundaries when engaging in the use of social media platforms and digital technologies to record, convey and respond to information.
- Adhere to organizational, professional, regulatory and legal tenets pertaining to privacy, confidentiality and security of data in health information systems.

- The informal curriculum of digital technology use reflects the individual interactions between learners and teachers that shape and direct their use. This can include situations where a teacher or preceptor is particularly keen on using technology (such as where a preceptor trades tips on apps and mobile devices with their students) or is against using technology (such as where a preceptor bans all use of mobile devices when around their patients).

- The null curriculum of digital technologies reflects the absences and omissions of technology use from the formal curriculum. For instance, the absence of e-health teaching, digital professionalism (see next section), or how to use digital tools for study and practice would each constitute a null curriculum.

These factors can interfere with providing a meaningful and deliberate technology presence in the medical education curriculum as well as redirecting or confounding objectives around technology use. This means that the potential benefits of using digital technologies may be reduced or they may not be realised at all.

Digital professionalism

The use of tools and systems such as social media has allowed learners (and sometimes faculty) to say or do things in public forums that impact their own reputations as well as those of their institution and profession. Of course, there have always been indiscretions; the difference with social media is that it makes an indiscretion far more public far more rapidly. While some institutions have responded by punishing or proscribing the use of social media around medicine or medical education, others have tried to take a more positive approach. We have previously defined the principles of digital professionalism as follows:

"Digital media are not an intrinsic threat to medical professionalism. Professionals should use digital media for positive purposes in ways that support principles of patient care, compassion, altruism, and trustworthiness. Professionals should be aware of the shaping nature of their relationships with digital media and they should maintain the capacity for deliberate, ethical, and accountable practice."

Ellaway et al., 2015

There are three dimensions to digital professionalism:

- *Proficiency:* digital professionals should be able to function effectively and safely, without making inappropriate use of time and resources, while avoiding unnecessary risks and distractions. This involves selecting and using technologies safely and efficiently, and making appropriate use of educational and support resources.
- *Reputation:* digital professionals should maintain their reputations as the basis for the trust that society places in them. Not only should professionals behave appropriately and respectfully in all venues with all media at all times, they should refrain from disclosing anything in any medium that they would not be comfortable defending as appropriate in a court of law or in front of a disciplinary panel.
- *Responsibility:* digital professionals are responsible for their actions; they should seek to develop and maintain positive and effective behaviours associated with using digital media. They should model positive behaviours in using digital media

to others including their students, peers, and patients.

Medical teachers should incorporate digital professionalism within broader professionalism training and assessment activities in the curriculum, they should clearly connect the day-to-day use of technology with the principles of professionalism, and they should model good digital professionalism to their students and colleagues.

The role of the medical e-teacher

The use of digital technologies for education has been popularly dubbed 'e-learning' even though it is usually defined and led by teachers rather than learners. It therefore helps to separate out two distinct kinds of practice: e-teaching (what the teacher does) and e-learning (what the learner does). Medical e-teachers select (and to an extent troubleshoot) the technologies used, they facilitate their learners' activities through and around digital media, and they evaluate and appraise how well they perform.

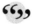

"There are two distinct kinds of practice: e-teaching (what the teacher does) and e-learning (what the learner does)."

Medical e-teachers also need to decide where their educational technology efforts are going to be targeted. The more efficient an educational artefact is the more it catalyses or otherwise supports learning for the greatest number of learners. However, it is an ongoing challenge for all educators that the best learners tend to make use of every opportunity afforded them and the problem learners do not. If the goal is to help less able learners then the resource needs to align with their needs and they ways that they approach their learning; simply making a resource available may increase the gap between the most and least able rather than closing it. Quizzes with targeted feedback can often help less able learners or those struggling with certain core concepts much more than multimedia-rich resources can.

It is also important for medical teachers to ensure that their technology-enabled activities are integrated into the curriculum; if they are not then they are unlikely to be used, particularly by those who need them most. Managing the alignment between e-teaching and programme objectives and outcomes is critical. Biggs (1999) stated that: "in aligned teaching there is maximum consistency throughout the system". This alignment should extend to the online as well as the offline aspects. If e-teaching is not in alignment with the rest of the curriculum then it introduces dissonance and confusion for the learner as well as hidden curriculum issues around what is and is not important. Furthermore, e-teaching does not sit in isolation from other methods and techniques; it interacts with, borrows from and ultimately better prepares teachers for more traditional face-to-face practise. The idea of blended learning (combining the best of traditional and new media and techniques) is now well established but the parallel concept of blended e-teaching is less so, although much blended e-learning clearly involves teaching. Negotiating alignment and the blend between e-teaching and other methods are skills that are best learnt from practical experience.

It is highly recommended that those wishing to take on an e-teaching role seek out opportunities to learn first-hand what it is like to be at the receiving end, perhaps as faculty development or continuing medical education activities. There are also opportunities to learn and develop through connecting with the many online e-teaching communities. One last issue, and one that experience as an e-learner will help to highlight, is that all technologies change. Some change quite rapidly while others change more slowly. Either way, focusing on operator skills alone will not suffice, developing an understanding of the broader issues of e-teaching is no longer an esoteric specialty but a core part of being a medical teacher.

Medical e-teachers also need to appreciate the roles and identities of their e-learners. There has been a tendency over the last decade, particularly in the media, to equate youth with greater computing skills and abilities than their seniors. Labels such as 'digital natives' or 'net generation' have become a powerful meme that has persuaded many learners and faculty (Ellaway and Tworek, 2012). This is problematic for a number of reasons. While some learners have certainly embraced a digital lifestyle, others have not. Every class will typically have a few students with strong IT skills while there will be others with relatively little practical ability. This can be exacerbated by learners' generally poor assessment of their ability to use digital technologies, typically they have greater confidence than competence. Faculty on the other hand often have less confidence than competence, perceive greater risks in using technologies and may as a result cede control of the digital to their learners on the belief that they are more able (Beetham, McGill and Littlejohn, 2009).

Despite the ability of educational technologies to track learners' activities, much of what learners do remains invisible to their teachers. For example, in the last few years the use of online social networking sites has become a staple online social activity for students worldwide, largely displacing such activity from university systems. Similarly, instant messaging allows discrete groups of learners to interact without the scrutiny or knowledge of their teachers. This includes interactions between learners at different institutions. Teaching materials from one school may be being used (and valued) by learners at another with no faculty involvement. Between learners seeking venues where they will not be observed and assessed by their faculty, and their participation in professional networks, many

of today's learners have become digital nomads even if they are not 'digital natives'.

Summary

This chapter is not intended to be a generic text on using digital technologies for educational purposes, not least because there are many excellent texts on this area already. The goal has instead been to provide a briefing on the wider themes and issues that accompany the use of digital technologies in medical education. Today's medical teacher has access to an unprecedented range of educational technologies to support their teaching.

From a practical point of view medical teachers need to be able to function in a range of different digitally enhanced environments, both as learners and as teachers. They need to be able to appreciate the dynamics of such environments; critiquing the options and selecting those tools and processes that best meet their needs. They also need to appreciate how e-health and other profession-focused digital developments intersect with the educational. Although there is likely to be an on-going role for educational technology specialists to cover the more strategic and involved aspects of digital medical education, all medical teachers are now to some extent medical e-teachers.

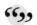 *"All medical teachers are now medical e-teachers."*

This chapter has set out a series of concepts around educational activities that allow both learners and their teachers to make much better use of their time both together and apart. The greatest promise of using digital technologies in medical education therefore may, and probably should be, to enhance and improve traditional models rather than to simply sweep them away. Future editions of this book will have the benefit of hindsight to validate or challenge this perspective.

References

Beetham, H., McGill, L., Littlejohn, A., 2009. Thriving in the 21st century: Learning Literacies for the Digital Age. Glasgow Caledonian University/JISC, Glasgow.

Biggs, J., 1999. Teaching for Quality Learning. OU Press, UK.

Clark, C.R., Mayer, R.E., 2008. e-Learning and the Science of Instruction. Pfeiffer, San Francisco.

Ellaway, R., 2007. Discipline Based Designs for Learning: The Example of Professional and Vocational Education. In: Beetham, H., Sharpe, R. (Eds.), Design for Learning: rethinking pedagogy for the digital age. Routledge, pp. 153–165.

Ellaway, R., Tworek, J., 2012. The Net Generation Illusion: challenging conformance to social expectations. In: Ferris, S.P. (Ed.), Teaching and Learning with the Net Generation: Concepts and Tools for Reaching Digital Learners.

Ellaway, R.H., Bates, J., 2015. Exploring patterns and pattern languages of medical education. Med. Educ. 49 (12), 1189–1196.

Ellaway, R.H., Coral, J., Topps, D., Topps, M.H., 2015. Exploring digital professionalism. Med. Teach. 37 (9), 844–849.

Ellaway, R.H., Fink, P., Campbell, A., Graves, L., 2013. Left to their own devices: medical learners' use of mobile technologies. Med. Teach. 36 (2), 130–138.

Ho, K., Ellaway, R., Littleford, J., et al. 2014. eHealth competencies for postgraduate medical education: CanMEDS 2015 eHealth Expert Working Group Report. Royal College of Physicians and Surgeons of Canada, Ottawa, ON.

Horton, W., 2006. E-Learning by Design. Pfeiffer, San Francisco.

Masters, K., Ellaway, R.H., Topps, D., et al., 2016. AMEE Guide 105: Mobile technologies in medical education. Med. Teach. 38 (6), 537–549.

Mayer, R., 2009. Multimedia Learning, second ed. Cambridge University Press, New York, NY.

Richey, R.C., Klein, J.D., Tracey, M.W., 2011. The instructional design knowledgebase: theory, research, and practice. Routledge, New York, NY.

Further reading

Ellaway, R., Masters, K., 2008. AMEE Guide 32: e-Learning in medical education Part 1: Learning, teaching and assessment. Med. Teach. 30 (5), 455–473.

Masters, K., Ellaway, R., 2008. AMEE Guide 32: e-Learning in medical education Part 2: Technology, management and design. Med. Teach. 30 (5), 474–489.

Instructional design

J. J. G. van Merriënboer

Trends

- Use of integrative objectives and whole-task approaches
- Diversification of delivery strategies and increased use of multimedia
- Teaching for transfer of learning to the workplace

Introduction

People learn in many different ways. They learn by studying examples, by doing and practising, by being told, by reading books, by exploring, by making and testing predictions, by being questioned, by teaching others, by making notes, by solving problems, by finding analogies, by rehearsing information and by many, many other activities. Learning is basic to all goal-directed human activity; people cannot deliberately do something without learning from it. This is not to say that learning is always optimal: there are many factors that may either hamper or facilitate learning. Instructional design is that branch of knowledge concerned with, on the one hand, research and theory about instructional strategies that help people learn and, on the other hand, the process of developing and implementing those strategies. Sometimes, the term instructional design (ID) is reserved for the *science* of doing research and developing theories on instructional strategies, and the term instructional systems design (ISD) is reserved for the *practical field* of developing, implementing and evaluating those strategies. The main aim of this chapter is to briefly introduce the reader to the field of ISD and ID.

 Instructional design is both a science and a practical field.

The ADDIE model

ISD models typically divide the instructional design process into five phases: (1) analysis, (2) design, (3) development, (4) implementation and (5) evaluation. In this so-called ADDIE model (Fig. 21.1), the evaluation phase is mainly summative, while formative evaluation may be conducted during all phases. Though the model appears to be linear, it does not have to be followed rigidly. Often, the model is repeatedly used to develop related units of instruction (iteration), phases are skipped because particular information is already available (layers of necessity) or later phases provide inputs that make it necessary to reconsider earlier phases (zigzag design). It is thus best seen as a project management tool that helps designers think about the different steps that must be taken. Moreover, the ADDIE model does not suggest or follow specific learning theories: it can be used for all instructional design projects irrespective of the preferred learning paradigm.

In the first phase of the ADDIE model (Fig. 21.1), the focus is on the analysis of the desired learning outcomes and on the analysis of fixed conditions. With regard to fixed conditions, analyses pertain to the analysis of the *context* (availability of equipment, time and money, culture, setting such as school, military or work organization etc.), the analysis of the *target group* (prior knowledge, general schooling, age, learning styles, handicaps etc.), and the analysis of *tasks and subject matter* (tools and objects required, conditions for performance, risks etc.).

 Optimal instructional strategies are determined by both desired outcomes and fixed conditions.

In the second phase of the ADDIE model, instructional strategies are selected that best help to reach the desired outcomes given the fixed conditions. A distinction may be made among organizational strategies (How is the instruction organized?), delivery strategies (Which media are used to deliver the instruction?) and management strategies (How and by whom is the instruction managed?). The basic idea is that both desired outcomes and fixed conditions determine the optimal strategies to select. For example, if the desired outcome is memorizing the names of skeleton bones, rehearsal with the use of mnemonics is a suitable organizational strategy, but if the desired outcome is

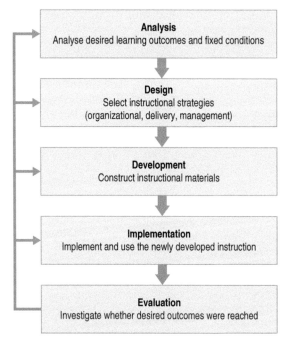

Analysis
Analyse desired learning outcomes and fixed conditions

Design
Select instructional strategies
(organizational, delivery, management)

Development
Construct instructional materials

Implementation
Implement and use the newly developed instruction

Evaluation
Investigate whether desired outcomes were reached

Fig. 21.1 The ADDIE model.

performing a complex surgical skill, guided practise with feedback on a wide variety of scenarios is a more suitable organizational strategy. In addition, if there is sufficient equipment or money available, the use of high-fidelity simulation might be a suitable delivery strategy for teaching a complex surgical skill, but if there is no equipment or money available, guided on-the-job learning is more suitable.

The remaining phases of the ADDIE model provide guidelines for the development, implementation and evaluation of selected strategies. Development refers to the actual construction of instructional materials, such as learning tasks and assignments, instructional texts, multimedia materials, slides for lectures, guides for teachers and so forth. Implementation refers to the introduction of the newly developed instruction in the setting in which it will be used and to the actual use of the instructional materials. Evaluation investigates whether the desired outcomes were actually reached and answers questions such as: Did the students achieve the expected outcomes? What did they learn? How can the instruction be improved? Each of these phases represents a whole field of research and development in itself. The remainder of this chapter will focus on ID models rather than ISD models, thus on the former two phases.

The universe of ID models

Close to 100 ID models have been described in the literature and on the Internet (see, e.g. www.instructional

design.org, http://thingsorganic.tripod.com/ Instructional_Design_Models.htm). ID models differ from each other in several dimensions. One dimension pertains to the learning paradigm they adhere to, which may reflect, for example, a behaviourist, cognitive or social-constructivist perspective. A second dimension, discussed in the next section, is between models directed at the level of message design, lesson design and course and curriculum design. A third dimension pertains to outcomes-based models and whole-task models.

 ID-models may take a behaviourist, cognitive or social-constructivist perspective.

OUTCOMES-BASED MODELS

Outcomes-based models typically focus on one particular domain of learning, such as the cognitive domain, psychomotor domain or affective domain (Anderson & Krathwohl, 2001), which roughly corresponds with the triplet knowledge, skills and attitudes. In one particular domain of learning, desired outcomes are analysed in terms of distinct objectives or learning goals, after which instructional strategies are selected for reaching each of the separate objectives. Gagné (1985) introduced a widely used taxonomy in the cognitive domain. His taxonomy makes a distinction between verbal information, intellectual skills, cognitive strategies, attitudes and psychomotor skills. The intellectual skills are at the heart of the taxonomy and include five subcategories:

1. Discriminations
2. Concrete concepts
3. Defined concepts
4. Rules
5. Higher-order rules.

This taxonomy reflects the fact that some intellectual skills enable the performance of other, higher-level skills. For instance, the ability to apply rules or procedures is prerequisite to the use of higher-order rules (i.e. problem solving). If you teach an intellectual skill, it is important to identify, in a so-called *learning hierarchy*, the lower-level skills that enable this skill. In teaching, one starts with the objectives for the skills lower in the hierarchy and successively works towards the objectives for the skills higher in the hierarchy.

Many researchers introduced alternative classifications of objectives. But a common premise of all outcomes-based models is that different objectives can best be reached by the application of particular instructional strategies (the *conditions of learning*; Gagné, 1985). The optimal strategy is chosen for each objective; the objectives are usually taught one by one and the overall educational goal is believed to be met after all separate objectives have been taught. For instance, if complex skills or professional competences are taught, each objective corresponds with one enabling or constituent skill, and sequencing the objectives naturally results in a part-task sequence. Thus, the learner is taught only one or a very limited number of constituent skills at the same time. New constituent skills are gradually added to practice, and it is not until the end of the instruction – if at all – that the learner has the opportunity to practise the whole complex skill.

Outcomes-based instructional design models are very effective for teaching objectives that have little to do with each other, that is, require little coordination. But in the early 1990s, authors in the field of instructional design started to question the value of outcomes-based models for reaching 'integrative' goals or objectives (e.g. Gagné & Merrill, 1990). For complex skills or professional competencies, which are dominant in the medical domain, there are many interactions between the different aspects of task performance and their related objectives: with high demands on coordination. Then, an outcomes-based approach yields instruction that is fragmented and piecemeal and thus does not work. Whole-task models provide an alternative because they pay explicit attention to the coordination of all task aspects.

 Outcomes-based instructional models are very effective for teaching isolated objectives.

WHOLE-TASK MODELS

Whole-task models explicitly aim at integrative goals, or *complex learning*. They take a holistic rather than atomistic perspective on instructional design (van Merriënboer, 1997). First, complex contents and tasks are not split over different domains of learning (e.g. knowledge is taught in lectures, skills are taught in a skills lab and attitudes are taught in role plays), but knowledge, skills and attitudes are developed simultaneously by having the learners work on whole, integrative tasks. Second, complex contents and tasks are not reduced into simpler elements up to a level where the single elements (i.e. isolated objectives) can be transferred to learners through presentation and/or practise, but they are taught from simple-to-complex *wholes* in such a way that relationships between the elements are retained. Thus, whole-task models basically try to deal with complexity without losing sight of the relationships between elements.

Rather than starting from a specification of objectives, instructional design starts with the identification of a representative set of real-life tasks and an analysis of the cognitive schemas that people need in order to perform those tasks (also called *cognitive task analysis* or CTA; Clark et al., 2012). Cognitive schemas can be seen as the building blocks of cognition and integrate knowledge, skills and attitudes. The process of competence development can be described as the

construction and automation of increasingly more complex cognitive schemas. Sub processes of schema construction are inductive learning and elaboration. Learners *induce* new cognitive schemas and modify existing ones as a result of their concrete experiences with a varied set of tasks. They *elaborate* their cognitive schemas by connecting newly presented information to the things they already know.

 Whole-task models start with the identification and analysis of a set of representative real-life tasks.

Sub processes of schema automation are knowledge compilation and strengthening. Learners *compile* new knowledge when they construct cognitive rules that always yield the same reaction under particular conditions. Repetition helps learners to *strengthen* these rules; each time the rule is used and yields desired effects, the chance it will be used again under similar conditions is increasing. Whereas schema construction helps learners to develop non-routine behaviours (problem solving, reasoning, decision making), schema automation helps them to develop routine behaviours. Typically, a mix of non-routine and routine behaviours is necessary to efficiently perform real-life tasks. From a design point of view, the specification of increasingly more complex schemas helps to define a series of simple to complex learning tasks. It also helps to identify the non-routine and routine aspects of performance, so that learners can be provided with the necessary information, feedback and assessments on all the different aspects of whole-task performance.

 Complex learning is driven by rich, meaningful learning tasks such as problems, projects or cases.

Whole-task models thus assume that complex learning takes place in situations where student learning is driven by rich, meaningful tasks that are based on real-life or professional tasks. Such tasks are called *problems* (in problem-based learning), *cases* (in the case method), *projects* (in project-based learning), and so forth. Van Merriënboer and Kirschner (2013) use the generic term 'learning tasks' to refer to all whole tasks that help learners reach integrative goals. Merrill (2013) compared a large set of whole-task models and found that they all shared five 'first principles of instruction', stating that meaningful learning is promoted when:

1. Learners are engaged in solving real-world problems
2. Existing knowledge is activated as a foundation for new knowledge
3. New knowledge is demonstrated to the learner
4. New knowledge needs to be applied by the learner
5. New knowledge is integrated into the learner's world.

Examples of ID models

This section will discuss three examples of ID models, at the level of instructional message design, lesson design, and curriculum and course design. All three models can be seen as whole-task models.

COGNITIVE LOAD THEORY

Nowadays, the most popular theories for instructional message design are Sweller's cognitive load theory (CLT) (van Merriënboer & Sweller, 2010) and Mayer's cognitive theory of multimedia learning (Mayer, 2010). Both theories have much in common; we will focus our discussion on CLT. The central notion of CLT is that human cognitive architecture should be a major consideration when designing instructional messages. This cognitive architecture consists of a severely limited working memory with partly independent processing units for visual/spatial and auditory/verbal information, which interacts with a comparatively unlimited long-term memory. The theory distinguishes between three types of cognitive load, dependent on the type of processing causing it, namely:

- *Intrinsic load.* This is a direct function of performing the task, in particular, of the number of elements that must be simultaneously processed in working memory. For instance, a task with many constituent skills that must be coordinated (e.g. dealing with an emergency) yields a higher intrinsic load than a task with less constituent skills that need to be coordinated (e.g. stitching a wound).
- *Extraneous load.* This is the extra load beyond the intrinsic cognitive load mainly resulting from poorly designed instruction. For instance, if learners must search in their instructional materials for information needed to perform a learning task (e.g. searching for the checklist of how to operate a piece of machinery), this search process itself does not directly contribute to learning and thus causes extraneous cognitive load.
- *Germane load.* This is related to processes that directly contribute to learning, in particular, to schema construction and schema automation. For instance, consciously connecting new information with what is already known and self-explaining new information are processes yielding germane cognitive load.

Intrinsic, extraneous and germane cognitive load are additive in that, if learning is to occur, the total load of the three together cannot exceed the available working memory capacity. Consequently, well-designed instructional messages should decrease extraneous cognitive load and optimize germane cognitive load in such a way that available cognitive capacity is not exceeded, otherwise cognitive overload with negative effects on learning will occur. A first set of principles generated by CLT aims to decrease extraneous cognitive load. The *goal-free principle* suggests replacing conventional learning tasks with goal-free tasks that provide learners with a nonspecific goal (e.g. ask students: "Please come up with as many illnesses as possible that could be related to the observed symptoms," rather than asking them "Which illness is indicated by the symptoms of this patient?"). Whereas conventional tasks force learners to identify the means to reach a specific goal, which causes a high cognitive load, goal-free tasks allow learners to reason from the givens to the goal, which causes a much lower cognitive load. Similar principles are the *worked example principle*, which suggests replacing conventional tasks with worked examples that provide a full solution learners must carefully study (e.g. let students criticize a ready-made treatment plan, rather than having them independently generate such a plan), and the *completion principle*, which suggests replacing conventional tasks with completion tasks that provide a partial solution learners must finish (e.g. let medical interns closely observe a surgical operation and only perform part of it, rather than having them perform the whole operation independently).

 Within the limits of available cognitive capacity, well-designed instructional messages should decrease *extraneous* cognitive load and increase *germane* cognitive load.

Other principles to decrease extraneous cognitive load are particularly important for the design of multimedia materials. The *split attention principle* suggests replacing multiple sources of information, distributed either in space (spatial split attention) or in time (temporal split attention), with one integrated source of information (e.g. provide students instructions for operating a piece of medical equipment just in time, precisely when they need it, rather than providing them the information beforehand). The *modality principle* suggests replacing a written explanatory text and another source of visual information (unimodal) with a spoken explanatory text and the visual source of information (multimodal, e.g. give students spoken explanations when they study a computer animation of the workings of the digestive tract, rather than giving them written explanations on screen). The *redundancy principle* suggests replacing multiple sources of information that are self-contained (i.e. they can be understood on their own) with one source of information (e.g. when providing learners with a diagram of the flow of blood in the heart, lungs and body, eliminate a description verbally describing the flow).

Another set of principles aims to optimize germane cognitive load. The *variability principle* suggests replacing a series of tasks with similar features with a series of tasks that differ from each other on all dimensions on which tasks differ in the real world (e.g. when describing a particular clinical symptom, illustrate it using patients with different sex, ages, physiques, medical histories etc.). The *contextual interference principle* suggests replacing a series of task variants with low contextual interference with a series with high contextual interference (e.g. if students practise different variants of a particular surgical task, order these variants in a random rather than a blocked order). The *self-explanation principle* suggests replacing separate worked examples or completion tasks with enriched ones containing prompts, asking learners to self-explain the given information (e.g. for students learning to diagnose malfunctions in the human cardiovascular system, present an animation of how the heart works and provide prompts that ask them to self-explain the underlying mechanisms).

NINE EVENTS OF INSTRUCTION

At the level of lesson design, Gagné's nine events of instruction (1985) provide general guidelines for the organization of lessons, which can be applied to a wide range of objectives or integrative objectives in the case of complex learning. Table 21.1 summarizes the nine events and illustrative remarks made by a teacher; they are roughly sequenced in the order in which they will typically occur in a lesson.

The first three events prepare the students for learning. First, their attention should be gained by presenting an interesting problem or a topical subject or asking them questions on a topic of their interest. This will help to ground the lesson and motivate the learners. Second, the goals of the instruction should be made explicit, so that learners know what they will be able to accomplish after the lesson. A demonstration might be given so that the students can see how they can apply the new knowledge. Third, the relevant prior

knowledge of the learners needs to be activated, by making explicit how the new knowledge is connected to the things they already know, providing them with a framework that helps learning and remembering or having them brainstorm on the topic of the lesson.

The next four events steer the actual learning process. First, the new knowledge is presented and examples or demonstrations are provided. Texts, graphics, simulations, figures, pictures and verbal explanations may all help to present the new knowledge. Second, the learners need to practise with the newly presented knowledge. Performance is elicited so that the learners do something with the newly acquired knowledge; for example, they apply new knowledge or practise new skills. Third, learners should receive guidance that helps them to be successful in the application of the new knowledge and skills. Guidance is different from the presentation of content because it primarily helps students to learn (e.g. help them to process new information). Fourth, the learners receive informative feedback, which helps them to identify weaknesses in their behaviour and provides hints for improvement.

 The presentation of new information should *always* be accompanied by guided practise and feedback.

The final two events mark the end of a lesson. First, learners' performance should be assessed to check whether the lesson has been successful and the learners have acquired the new knowledge and/or skills. Often, it is worthwhile to give the learners information on their progress over lessons. Second, explicit attention should be paid to enhancing retention and transfer of what has been learned. One might inform the learners about more or less similar problem situations in which the acquired knowledge and skills can be applied, let them review the lesson and come up with new situations in which the acquired knowledge and/or skills can be applied or actually let them perform in such transfer situations.

FOUR-COMPONENT INSTRUCTIONAL DESIGN (4C/ID)

At the level of course and curriculum design, four-component instructional design (van Merriënboer & Kirschner, 2013) is a popular whole-task model aimed at the training of complex skills and professional competencies. It provides guidelines for the analysis of real-life tasks and the transition into a blueprint for an educational programme. It is typically used for designing and developing substantial educational programmes ranging in length from several weeks to several years.

The basic assumption of 4C/ID is that blueprints for complex learning can always be described by four basic components, namely: (1) learning tasks, (2) supportive information, (3) procedural information

Table 21.1 Gagné's nine events of instruction

Event	Illustration
Gain attention	Did you hear about …?
Inform learner of objectives	Today we are going to …
Stimulate recall of prior information	Two days ago we learned how to …
Present information	This is a demonstration of how to …
Provide guidance	Now this is a guide for performing …
Elicit performance	Now you try it yourself
Provide feedback	Alright, but you need to …
Assess performance	We will now have a performance test
Enhance retention and transfer	Alright, now suppose you have to do it on the job

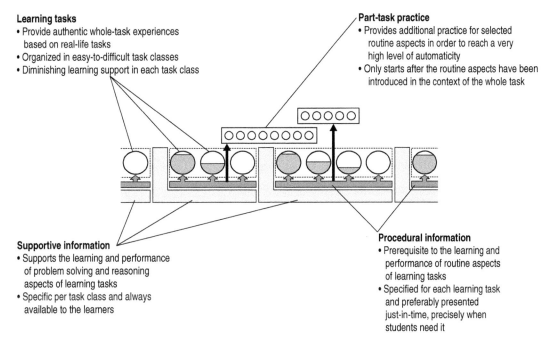

Learning tasks
- Provide authentic whole-task experiences based on real-life tasks
- Organized in easy-to-difficult task classes
- Diminishing learning support in each task class

Part-task practice
- Provides additional practice for selected routine aspects in order to reach a very high level of automaticity
- Only starts after the routine aspects have been introduced in the context of the whole task

Supportive information
- Supports the learning and performance of problem solving and reasoning aspects of learning tasks
- Specific per task class and always available to the learners

Procedural information
- Prerequisite to the learning and performance of routine aspects of learning tasks
- Specified for each learning task and preferably presented just-in-time, precisely when students need it

Fig. 21.2 Schematic overview of the four components in 4C/ID.

and (4) part-task practice. The four components are based on the four learning processes discussed previously: inductive learning, elaboration, compilation of rules, and strengthening. Learning tasks provide the backbone of the training programme; they provide learning from varied experiences and explicitly aim at transfer of learning. The three other components are connected to this backbone (Fig. 21.2).

Learning tasks include problems, case studies, projects, scenarios and so forth (indicated by the large circles in the figure). They are authentic whole-task experiences based on real-life tasks and aim at the integration of skills, knowledge and attitudes. The whole set of learning tasks exhibits a high variability of practice because learning from varied experiences facilitates transfer of learning (Maggio et al., 2015). The learning tasks are organized in easy-to-difficult task classes (indicated by dotted boxes around sets of circles) and have diminishing learner support and guidance within each task class (indicated by diminishing filling of the circles). The basic underlying process for learning from learning tasks is induction, that is, learning from concrete experiences.

Supportive information helps students learn to perform non-routine aspects of learning tasks, which often involve problem solving, diagnostic reasoning and decision making (indicated by L-shaped forms connected to equally difficult learning tasks or task classes). It explains how a domain is organized (e.g. knowledge of the human body) and how problems in that domain

are best approached (e.g. a systematic approach to differential diagnosis). It is specified per task class and is always available to learners. It provides a bridge between what learners already know and what they need to know to work on the learning tasks. The basic underlying process for learning from supportive information is elaboration, that is, learning by connecting the new information to what is already known.

 Supportive information is what teachers typically call 'the theory'.

Procedural information allows students to perform routine aspects of learning tasks that are always performed in the same way (indicated by the dark beam with upward pointing arrows to the learning tasks). It specifies exactly how to perform the routine aspects of the task (i.e. *how-to* information) and is best presented just in time, precisely when learners need it. This can be done by an instructor, but also by a quick reference guide, job aid or mobile application. It is quickly faded as learners gain more expertize. The basic underlying process for learning from procedural information is knowledge compilation, that is, learning by transforming new information into cognitive rules.

Finally, part-task practice pertains to additional practice of routine aspects so that learners can develop a very high level of automaticity for selected aspects for which this is necessary (indicated by the series of small circles). It is mostly used for critical task aspects

Table 21.2 Ten steps to complex learning

Blueprint components	Ten steps to complex learning
Learning tasks	1. Design learning tasks 2. Sequence task classes 3. Set performance objectives
Supportive information	4. Design supportive information 5. Analyze cognitive strategies 6. Analyze mental models
Procedural information	7. Design procedural information 8. Analyze cognitive rules 9. Analyze prerequisite knowledge
Part-task practice	10. Design part-task practice

(e.g. CPR, auscultation, stitching). Part-task practice typically provides huge amounts of repetition and only starts after the routine aspect has been introduced in the context of a whole, meaningful learning task. The basic underlying process for learning from part-task practice is strengthening, that is, automating routine skills through repetitive practice.

Van Merriënboer and Kirschner (2013) describe 10 steps that specify the whole design process typically employed by a designer to produce effective, efficient and appealing programmes for complex learning (Table 21.2). The four blueprint components directly correspond with four design steps: the design of learning tasks (step 1), the design of supportive information (step 4), the design of procedural information (step 7), and the design of part-task practice (step 10). The other six steps are auxiliary and are only performed when necessary. Step 2, in which task classes are sequenced: organizes learning tasks in simple to complex categories. They ensure that students work on tasks that begin simply and smoothly increase in complexity. Step 3, where objectives for the different task aspects are set: specifies the standards for acceptable performance. They are needed to assess student performance and to provide learners with useful feedback on all different aspects of whole-task performance. Steps 5, 6, 8 and 9, finally, pertain to in-depth cognitive task analysis. It should be noted that real-life design projects are never a straightforward progression from step 1 to step 10. As in the ADDIE model, new findings and decisions will often require the designer to reconsider previous steps, yielding zigzag design approaches.

Summary

Instructional design pertains, on the one hand, to the science of doing research and developing theories on instructional strategies, and, on the other hand, to the practical field of developing, implementing and evaluating those strategies. The latter is also called instructional

systems design and is characterized by the ADDIE model, which describes the process as a progression through the phases of analysis, design, development, implementation and evaluation.

Close to 100 instructional design models have been described in the literature. Outcomes-based models describe desired learning outcomes in instructional objectives and then select the best instructional strategy for each objective. Whole-task models aim at the development of complex skills or professional competencies; they describe desired learning outcomes as one integrative objective and then select instructional strategies that help students develop professional competencies in a process of complex learning by working on whole, meaningful learning tasks. Three representative examples of ID models on the level of instructional message design, lesson design, and course and curriculum design are, in order, Sweller's cognitive load theory, Gagné's nine events of instruction, and van Merriënboer's 4C/ID model.

In the field of medical education, we see an increased interest in integrative objectives and the development of competence-based curricula in order to facilitate transition from the school to the clinic. In addition, there is a diversification of delivery strategies with increased use of media such as medical simulation, animation and other e-learning applications. As a result, instructional design models are becoming more and more important to the field of medical education.

 ID models are becoming increasingly important in medical education because of the popularity of complex learning approaches and e-learning.

References

Anderson, L.W., Krathwohl, D.R. (Eds.), 2001. A Taxonomy for Learning, Teaching, and Assessing: A Revision of Bloom's Taxonomy of Educational Objectives. Longman, New York.

Clark, R.E., Pugh, C.M., Yates, K.A., et al., 2012. The use of cognitive task analysis to improve instructional descriptions of procedures. J. Surg. Res. 173 (1), e37–e42.

Gagné, R.M., 1985. The Conditions of Learning, fourth ed. Holt, Rinehart & Winston, New York.

Gagné, R.M., Merrill, M.D., 1990. Integrative goals for instructional design. Educ. Tech. Res. 38 (1), 23–30.

Maggio, L.A., ten Cate, O., Irby, D.M., et al., 2015. Designing evidence-based medicine training to optimize the transfer of skills from the classroom to clinical practice: applying the four component instructional design model. Acad. Med. 90 (11), 1457–1461.

Mayer, R.E., 2010. Applying the science of learning to medical education. Med. Educ. 44 (6), 543–549.

Merrill, M.D., 2013. First Principles of Instruction. Pfeiffer, San Francisco, CA.

van Merriënboer, J.J.G., 1997. Training Complex Cognitive Skills. Educational Technology Publications, Englewood Cliffs, NJ.

van Merriënboer, J.J.G., Kirschner, P.A., 2013. Ten Steps to Complex Learning, second ed. Routledge, New York.

van Merriënboer, J.J.G., Sweller, J., 2010. Cognitive load theory in health professions education: design principles and strategies. Med. Educ. 44 (1), 85–93.

Section 4

Curriculum themes

22

Basic sciences and curriculum outcomes

W. Pawlina, N. Lachman

Trends

- Frame classroom and laboratory activities in the basic science curriculum around "real-life" clinical contexts to promote authentic learning.
- Basic sciences should be presented as a dynamic tool inclusive of non-technical skills within team-based environment for solving real-life clinical problems.
- Students should maintain ownership of their own learning while maintaining partnership with a diverse teaching faculty to guide learning towards successful outcomes.

Introduction

The role of the basic sciences and, consequently, the role of the basic science educator in the medical curriculum have undergone significant change in the context of even more dramatic changes in both healthcare delivery systems and medical education. Over the last two decades, a debate has ensued challenging the very existence of basic science departments in medical schools. From this argument, it has been shown that a traditional delivery of the basic sciences no longer has a place within the medical curriculum. As medical curricula evolve, conventional courses need to adopt a new system of basic science instruction. As our understanding of the science of learning progresses, new knowledge transforms educational strategies in basic science. As clinical competencies adjust to the changing paradigm of health care delivery, integration and assessment of non-technical skill becomes an essential element of early courses in the medical curriuculm.

 Three tips for faculty teaching basic sciences in medical school:
- You are NOT teaching basic sciences to future basic scientists (… but to future physicians)
- When teaching basic sciences, you are NOT only teaching basic science content (… but other discipline-independent subjects)

- Teaching basic sciences should NOT be for 'breakfast' only (… but distributed as a regular 'meal' throughout the entire length of medical curriculum).

The changing medical curriculum

With the dissolution of input-based curricula that nurtured the traditional format of basic science teaching, the challenge now lies in teaching an 'old subject in a new world'. Regarding undergraduate programmes, a multiplicity of forces have changed the roles and responsibilities of medical educators. These forces include:

- Revision of medical curricula that progressively decreases the time allotted for basic sciences
- Adoption of student-centred, flexible curriculum design that promotes the well-being of students
- Move towards outcome-based education where the emphases are on the expecting learning outcomes and competencies
- Increased presence of innovations and electronic technologies
- Attention to the science of healthcare delivery systems with an emphasis on systems engineering
- Emphasis on clinical translational (bench-to-bedside) research
- Emphasis on value, safety, quality and other measurable outcomes in patient care
- Emphasis on interprofessional education (IPE) in basic sciences in which students of two or more professions learn with, from and about each other to improve collaboration and quality of care
- Inclusion of discipline-independent subjects such as professionalism, ethics, leadership and teamwork.

These concepts that once required a shift in paradigm, today form basic elements of a well-structured healthcare service driven curriculum.

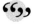

Therefore, educators must now produce scientifically competent graduates able to function as professionals in the climate change of healthcare reform. This means that they must practice evidence-based medicine, adhere to outcomes-based standards of care, translate scientific discoveries into clinical applications, work in interprofessional teams, utilize electronic information technology, comply with safety and quality measures and provide accessible, affordable, accountable and affable medical care (Srinivasan et al., 2006).

"Understanding the scientific foundation of medical practice and using this knowledge to inform decisions for patient care is an essential competency of a physician."

Fincher et al., 2009

The overarching objective of a basic medical science course is to provide fundamental scientific theories and concepts for clinical application. Traditionally, basic science subjects have included anatomy, histology, physiology, biochemistry, microbiology and pathology. The current teaching model includes genetics, cell and molecular biology, epidemiology, nutrition and energy metabolism and the science of healthcare delivery and bioinformatics. The medical curriculum has shifted from the Flexner model to an integrated model in which basic science courses are either paired with related clinical disciplines (e.g. anatomy/radiology, immunology/pathology, neuroscience/psychiatry) or taught in blocks by organ systems. Blocks are coordinated by faculty from both basic science and clinical departments, ensuring that students are given early exposure to patients in a clinical setting (Gregory et al., 2009).

Elements of an effective basic science course with distribution of faculty efforts:
* Specific course objectives (10%)
* Didactic component designed on the active learning platform supported by modern instructional technologies with critical thinking activities (60%)
* Formative feedback on students' performance (5%)
* Discipline-independent subjects (10%)
* Assessment of knowledge and skills (5%)
* Summative feedback on course performance and directions for professional development (10%).

Basic science courses that used to focus on content knowledge are morphing to incorporate the longitudinal objectives of the medical arts. Often termed 'holistic education', this movement encourages intellectual, social, creative and emotional development alongside knowledge acquisition. Technology offers new platforms upon which to build integrative innovations, but its use comes with many challenges. In e-learning, entire curricula are accessible via electronic content management systems on websites. This non-classroom didactic setting creates a challenge for the teacher when presented with the imperative to incorporate basic science into lessons in clinical medicine and professionalism through holistic learning. Teachers and learners alike must be flexible and adapt to this rapidly changing educational environment.

Authentic learning in basic science courses

In educational terms 'authentic learning' referes to a wide variety of pedagogical instructions and learning materials that connect what students are learning *in the classroom* to what is occurring *in 'real life'* scenerios, problems and applications that mirrors the real world of the active medical professional navigating their field (Lombardi, 2007; Herrington et al., 2014). Early exposure in basic sciences to 'authentic learning' provides an opportunity for specific knowledge acquisition in a setting that requires a student to become familiar with the realities of clinical reasoning, clinical problem solving, and use of other modalities such as clinical imaging in gross anatomy, laboratory test results in biochemistry and physiology, or interviews with affected patients in genetic courses (Pawlina & Drake, 2016). This approch also places emphasis on students' identity formation and team-forward behaviours in which development occurs alongside knowledge acquisition (Yardley et al., 2013).

Basic science material used for 'authentic learning' should have:
* *high intrinsic value*: thus the presented material needs be relavent to the medical field. In the last decade because of a reduction of teaching hours in basic sciences, educators have been forced to become selective in the material they present, and adopt educational strategies that focus on the most clinically relevant information.
* *high instrumental value*: thus the basic science content should be immediately useful. Recently, many anatomy courses are providing ultrasonography experience for medical students (Pawlina & Drake, 2015), which could be viewed as a practical extension of skills-based education with high instrumental value (Pawlina & Drake, 2016).

- *occupational realism*: thus simulating the clinical environment. For instance, histology material should be taught on the virtual system if such is utilized in the pathology sevices. Every effort should be placed to utilize available simulation centres in exploring cardiovascular or respiratory action of variouse pharmacological agents and simulated situations. This would allow students to practise the skills of building a differential diagnosis and defending their position using clinical evidence.
- *transportability*: thus internalizing concepts and skills associated with multiple curricular competencies (including nontraditional discipline-independent skills) with the ability to use them within settings that differ in many aspects from the familiar learning environment. Basic science knowledge should be regarded not as a collection of stored facts, but as a dynamic tool for real-life problem solving.

The active learning environment

Another didactic shift in this movement is the transition away from passive learning towards a more active learning environment. In active learning, students learn to restructure the new information and their prior knowledge into new knowledge (McManus, 2001). Among the most utilized formats for active learning are discussions in small groups (problem-based learning [PBL]), learning through clinical scenarios (case-based learning [CBL]), team-based learning (TBL) and learning through reflection (Lachman & Pawlina, 2006).

 "The basic science lesson can, through the implementation of creative exercises, present an ideal opportunity for initiating independent, self-directed learning that allows for integration and validation of key learning areas, both theoretically and practically."

Lachman & Pawlina, 2006

One of these approaches has become a commonly applied strategy in basic sciences: PBL (Bowman & Hughes, 2005). PBL shifts the emphasis from didactic instruction to self-directed learning. So for teachers with more experience in traditional education, the implementation of PBL requires not only a change in mindset, but also major adjustments in preparation to teach in this programme. The PBL approach is labour intensive, demanding more time for preliminary work to integrate appropriate skills and knowledge within the programme.

To facilitate student-centred learning, the TBL approach supports small-group activities where students teach one another. TBL was designed for use in large classrooms, and so TBL is often used in undergraduate courses such as anatomy, histology and microbiology during medical training. There is evidence that TBL has the ability to balance cognitive skills through group interaction of factual assimilation and application (Michaelsen et al., 2008). Since this type of strategy requires a small-group set-up and is highly collaborative in nature, teachers must master group facilitator skills while serving as content experts. Rather than lecturing, teachers debrief on the problems presented during TBL sessions (Michaelsen et al., 2008). While this level of interaction usually requires more in-depth understanding of the subject material by the facilitator, it also promotes more critical thinking and reflection.

 "As medical schools are creating integrated and interdisciplinary courses during the preclinical years, TBL is particularly useful because of its emphasis on teamwork, mastery of content, and problem solving for clinical application."

Vasan et al., 2009

CBL is learning stimulated by active discussion on clinical cases specifically constructed to emphasize basic science principles. Cases should portray authentic, often complex, problems resolved by applying basic science knowledge and critical analysis. Independently or in extracurricular study groups, students review the case ahead of the CBL session to identify and research the critical concept. During the CBL session, a facilitator advances learning objectives by asking a sequence of trigger questions that stimulate students to articulate their perspective: proposing problem-solving strategies, actively listening to group discussion and promoting reflection (Bowe et al., 2009). The multidisciplinary basic and clinical science faculty collaboration may enhance the outcomes of CBL sessions.

As coaches and facilitators instead of lecturers, teachers still manage the overall instructional process in which students have the opportunity to master course objectives and solve problems. As teachers continue to learn alongside their students, they serve as role models of lifelong learning. Additionally, mentorship may develop among teachers and students that self-select to serve as teaching assistants. In these apprenticeships, students find themselves on the way to becoming colleagues of their teachers, capable of working in effective, self-managed interprofessional teams and moving education forward.

Use of reflective practice, critical thinking and clinical reasoning

The use of reflection as a practical tool has become an important component of curriculum design for basic science. Reflective exercises support the practice of critical thinking for problem solving and the development of humanistic qualities desired in healthcare practitioners.

Within the learning environment, students may reflect individually through writing, or they may engage a team to explore or share experiences that lead to better comprehension and understanding. Reflection involves the synthesis of fragmented lessons, integration into one's personal experience, and application to the larger narrative in which students find themselves in the world. In this process, students cease to be educational automatons and develop personal epistemological initiative based on their values, which usually champion knowledge as a form of progress. From a theoretical standpoint, a student reflects by making an association with the learning objective, integrating the new concept with prior knowledge, validating the knowledge and, finally, applying the material (Lachman & Pawlina, 2006).

In designing a curriculum to include critical thinking through reflective exercises, it is important to leave the course methods open to challenge and review. Explicit training in clinical reasoning naturally begins with the basic science courses, as it is important for the development of a systematic and efficient approach to clinical cases. This foundation serves medical trainees well in all subsequent educational endeavors to come (Elizondo-Omaña et al., 2010). It entails bridging the gap between theory and practice, a chasm that can be crossed through reflection.

The implementation of reflective exercises may be achieved through the application of various techniques and learning activities. An effective way of teaching critical thinking and reflection in basic sciences is to encourage self-directed learning. Again, in this setting, the educator takes on the role of a facilitator rather than a director of knowledge. When assigned tasks that require investigation outside of the classroom, the student must reflect on the information given and decide upon a relevant interpretation of core objectives for the subject to be mastered. Critical thinking skills are further enhanced through collaboration and team interaction. The use of teamwork to facilitate conceptual understanding has proved to be effective in stimulating collective thinking. In many cases, this can be accomplished by utilizing e-learning technologies.

Reflection and clinical reasoning should also be incorporated into assessment strategies. Questions may be designed for critical thinking by including clinical cases that demonstrate core basic science concepts. Providing formative assessment allows students to monitor their own learning process. In many institutions, audience response systems (ARSs) are used to provide immediate feedback on individual student performance in relation to overall performance within the group. The use of a combination of questioning styles such as multiple-choice questions (MCQs) and short answer questions (SAQs) promotes both discernment and

writing skills. Additionally, peer and self-evaluation are effective assessments of critical analysis of teamwork dynamics.

 Conceptual knowledge:
- Understanding the process and concept rather than memorizing details
- Providing knowledge of resources for obtaining detailed information (e.g. finding gene structure and location on variety of genetic databases).

Applied knowledge:
- Applying content to situations that are clinically relevant
- Teaching reasoning skills through virtual patients/clinical cases
- Bridging the gap between basic science and clinical thinking.

Innovations in teaching basic sciences

Dramatic changes in basic science teaching are paralleled with advances in electronic media. The development of more powerful computers (tablet and notebook computers), 3D gaming and simulation, 3D printing, smartphones and mobile technologies, and high-speed wireless Internet connections has allowed medical educators to incorporate high-quality imaging, animations, virtual reality interactive training modules and learning management systems into the classroom. What were once considered advanced and sophisticated teaching methods and technologies are now commonplace or outdated (Pawlina & Lachman, 2004). The benefit of computer-assisted learning (CAL) is that it has great potential for enhancing knowledge acquisition as it appeals to the twenty-first-century learner (McNulty et al., 2009). However, educators must be aware that CAL has different characteristics when compared with conventional scenarios, especially as it impacts social communication, message exchange, cognitive load and participation of the learner.

However daunting, basic science teachers should take advantage of innovative technology. For example, the ARS serves as an interactive solution for teachers trying to engage their students in active learning. Employing ARS in the classroom allows students to continuously monitor their progress in the class (Alexander et al., 2009). Simulation laboratories are increasingly utilized in teaching basic sciences. Animal physiology laboratories have been replaced by simulation centres that utilize high-fidelity manikins that can demonstrate the basic physiological concepts, respond to pharmacological compounds, and encourage diagnostic reasoning skills in medical students (Rosen et al., 2009).

In addition to high-fidelity simulators, educators often use simple techniques and low-fidelity physical models in teaching the basic sciences. For instance, body painting in gross anatomy improves student knowledge of surface anatomy needed for palpation and auscultation in clinical practice (McMenamin, 2008). The active and kinesthetic nature of body painting, coupled with the strong and highly memorable visual images of underlying anatomy, contribute to the success of body painting as a learning tool. The use of simple physical models to demonstrate the spatial relationship of the represented structures within the human body aids understanding of its more complex function. These simple techniques and models serve as memory aids, reduce cognitive overload, facilitate problem solving, and arouse students' enthusiasm and participation (Chan & Cheng, 2011).

The use of new techniques and tools in basic science education is essential for the training of a medical student. Innovations must bear relevance to clinical practice and incorporate principles of functional science within integrated and practically digitized environments.

Basic science integration throughout the curriculum

In addition to preserving prior knowledge, undergraduate students must also incorporate recent advances that occur in clinical practice and correlate their understanding through the interpretation and integration of basic science concepts. Frequently, areas well known to the basic scientist but rarely explored by the clinical specialist become crucial to the success of new clinical procedures. For example, the use of surgical robots and interventional procedures with minimal access surgery, as in radiofrequency ablation of cardiac arrhythmias, necessitates a solid understanding not only of detailed anatomical relationships within the heart but also of the heart's electrophysiology. Detail once considered extraneous has renewed significance and is often critical to the success of a clinical procedure. Therefore, integration of basic sciences into the later years of the medical curriculum and, more so, in postgraduate specialization is growing in popularity. A return to the basic sciences during the latter years of medical curriculum, when students' clinical reasoning and analytical skills are more refined, enables learners to better integrate basic science concepts into their clinical experience (Spencer et al., 2008).

However, this also means that while modern medical education may not favour the retention of the classical basic scientist, the success of modern medical education is thoroughly dependent on the classical details of foundational medical sciences. Basic scientists can no longer exist in isolation from clinical disciplines and need to contribute to clinical outcomes. Whereas in the past their expertize was limited to the first few years of medical training, the new era of medicine requires the basic scientist to be engaged throughout the medical curriculum.

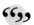
"The most effective leaders are those who can communicate effectively, generate trust, and motivate others to work together."

Jensen et al., 2008

Nontraditional discipline-independent skills

Moving forward, with the understanding that basic science will more likely extend throughout the curriculum (Spencer et al., 2008), basic science courses must therefore incorporate longitudinal objectives that will be revisited in clinical courses. These may include discipline-independent subjects such as leadership, teamwork, professionalism, effective communication (Evans & Pawlina, 2015) and promotion of students' well-being:

LEADERSHIP

- Skills fostered through team-based activities
- Demonstrated by the success with which a group is able to achieve set objectives under the direction of the designated team leader (Pawlina et al., 2006)

TEAMWORK

- Essential part of successful patient care
- Fosters collaboration in obtaining, sharing and presenting knowledge
- Involves learning teams as an instructional strategy (Michaelsen et al., 2008)

PROFESSIONALISM

- Entails acts of dutifulness and showing respect for others
- Based on traditional duties and responsibilities of the profession
- Anchored in clinical practice of medicine; also should apply to basic sciences (Lachman & Pawlina, 2006, 2015)

COMMUNICATION SKILLS

- Early emphasis equips students with the ability to effectively transfer information between the members of the team and later in the patient setting (Evans & Pawlina, 2015)
- Early introduction of peer and self-evaluations to enhance assessment skills (Lachman & Pawlina, 2015)

STUDENT WELL-BEING

- Protection of nonscheduled curricular time for self-learning, reflection and activities that promote well-being of learners

- Didactic review sessions and practise practical examinations utilizing format of final examinations
- Incorporation of flexible 'consolidation days' into the course curriculum with students' self-directed activities.

Early integration of nontraditional discipline-independent skills into basic science curricula positively impacts student awareness and their ability to apply these skills later in clinical training (Heidenreich et al., 2016). Establishing good practice in discipline-independent skill development involves formal assessment of these skills within a designed learning environment that provides students with opportunities to demonstrate these skills. Team-based learning environments that centre around consistent peer-to-peer interaction, rotational leadership roles and formal peer and self-evaluation are ideal. Providing clear objectives and expectations to students with regular feedback and teaching moments during laboratory sessions throughout the course encourages student awareness and subsequent development of nontraditional discipline-independent skills.

ASSESSMENT OF DISCIPLINE-INDEPENDENT SKILLS

Objective assessment of nontraditional discipline-independent skills is challenging since assessment is largely based on subjective evaluation. With this in mind, as students are evaluated faculty may want to consider categorizing assessment to include (1) cognitive skills: relating to a student's capacity to think (clinical reasoning), and (2) interpersonal skills: relating to how a student interacts with other individuals to contribute to overall team learning. In order to provide meaningful feedback to students in the form of quantitative assessment, faculty may consider the following:

- Faculty interaction with students during laboratory sessions should be maximized. Physically visiting work stations, posing critically thoughtful questions during tasks and guiding students through activities that are more technically challenging allow for better understanding of students ability.
- Regular and clear communication with students during the course is key for gathering information relating to student demonstration of targeted skills. Providing on-the-job and one-on-one feedback sessions allow faculty to assess student improvement and highlight areas for improvement.
- Increased cognizance of student disposition during class allows faculty to assess academic maturity (attentiveness, focus, punctuality, interaction with team members, contribution to discussions).

- Monitoring of student progress allows faculty to identify students at risk, and provide early intervention to promote student success.
- Maintaining paper trails and records of student interaction as well as student observation of good practice and insufficiencies provides data for feedback sessions.

As the current literature referenced in this section highlights the importance of nontraditional discipline-independent skills in healthcare, it must be reinforced that improvements in demonstration of these skills requires practise and repetition. Opportunities for integration of these skills within basic science curricula should be identified and developed so they may not only be meaningfully assessed but also interpreted and applied by students in a clinically meaningful way.

Learning basic science outside curricular structure

Advances in healthcare delivery are taking place at a staggering pace. There are many examples of lessons once strictly within the domain of basic science that are now a part of everyday clinical practice. Starting early in medical school, teaching faculty should advocate for, mentor and provide opportunities for students to be engaged in research projects that enrich their appreciation for translational research. Many schools have protected research time within the curriculum for medical students, usually dispersed among clinical clerkships. Others offer summer programmes for students who are interested in further research. In curricula without designated time for research activities, the basic science faculty should provide opportunities for students to participate in research activities during unstructured time in the medical curriculum. Under the guidance and direction of their mentors, students may elect to conduct research within a spectrum of possible projects including basic science bench research, medical education research and clinical research. Extracurricular research fosters closer relationships between students and their faculty mentors, gives students the opportunity to meet distinguished visiting physicians and scientists and allows them to gain experience in diverse laboratory and patient care settings.

These opportunities are likely to create a culture of scientific research as the students come to be clinicians (Fincher et al., 2009). If this approach generates an abundance of clinician-scientists, it will likely increase the translation of knowledge from the bench to the bedside and improve patient outcomes.

Summary

Basic sciences should no longer be taught in the traditional manner in the medical curriculum. The design of the contemporary medical curriculum incorporates clinical and translational research, an increased presence of electronic technology, the implementation of student-centred learning, and the increased emphasis on professionalism, ethics and interprofessional teamwork. Teachers should assume the roles of coaches and facilitators rather than directors within an authentic curriculum. They need to mentor students into becoming lifelong learners – apprentices on their way to becoming colleagues – capable of working within interprofessional communities. Students also need concrete knowledge of fundamental basic science alongside its application to clinical practice, and they must appreciate the process of scientific inquiry and translation (Fincher et al., 2009) within the digitized environment of electronic medical records and resources. Furthermore, basic scientists cannot exist in isolation from the clinical disciplines and must contribute to clinical outcomes. For the basic scientist, in framing a more modern concept of medical education, it will be necessary to shift the paradigm of tradition passed down over the centuries and integrate the foundations into clinical practice. Basic scientists must remain learners in this new age of medical education, and must strive to ensure that all efforts benefit their students: the future generation of healthcare providers.

References

Alexander, C.J., Crescini, W.M., Juskewitch, J.E., et al., 2009. Assessing the integration of audience response system technology in teaching of anatomical sciences. Anat. Sci. Educ. 2 (4), 160–166.

Bowe, C.M., Voss, J., Aretz, T.H., 2009. Case method teaching: an effective approach to integrate the basic and clinical sciences in the preclinical medical curriculum. Med. Teach. 31 (9), 834–841.

Bowman, D., Hughes, P., 2005. Emotional responses of tutors and students in problem-based learning: lessons for staff development. Med. Educ. 39 (2), 145–153.

Chan, L.K., Cheng, M.M., 2011. An analysis of the educational value of low-fidelity anatomy models as external representations. Anat. Sci. Educ. 4 (5), 256–263.

Elizondo-Omaña, R.E., Morales-Gómez, J.A., Morquecho-Espinoza, O., et al., 2010. Teaching skills to promote clinical reasoning in early basic science courses. Anat. Sci. Educ. 3 (5), 267–271.

Evans, D.J.R., Pawlina, W., 2015. The role of anatomists in teaching of nontraditional discipline-independent skills. In: Chan, L.K., Pawlina, W. (Eds.), Teaching Anatomy: A Practical Guide, first ed. Springer International Publishing, New York, pp. 319–329.

Fincher, R.M., Wallach, P.M., Richardson, W.S., 2009. Basic science right, not basic science lite: medical education at a crossroad. J. Gen. Intern. Med. 24 (11), 1255–1258.

Gregory, J.K., Lachman, N., Camp, C.L., et al., 2009. Restructuring a basic science course for core competencies: an example from anatomy teaching. Med. Teach. 31 (9), 855–861.

Harden, R.M., 2015. Interprofessional education: the magical mystery tour now less of a mystery. Anat. Sci. Educ. 8 (4), 291–295.

Heidenreich, M.J., Musonza, T., Pawlina, W., et al., 2016. Can a teaching assistant experience in a surgical anatomy course influence the learning curve for nontechnical skill development for surgical residents? Anat. Sci. Educ. 9 (1), 97–100.

Herrington, J., Reeves, T.C., Oliver, R., 2014. Authentic learning environments. In: Spector, M.J., Merrill, M.D., Elen, J., Bishop, M.J. (Eds.), Handbook of Research on Educational Communications and Technology, fourth ed. Springer Science+Business Media, New York, pp. 401–412.

Jensen, A.R., Wright, A.S., Lance, A.R., et al., 2008. The emotional intelligence of surgical residents: a descriptive study. Am. J. Surg. 195 (1), 5–10.

Lachman, N., Pawlina, W., 2006. Integrating professionalism in early medical education: the theory and application of reflective practice in the anatomy curriculum. Clin. Anat. 19 (5), 456–460.

Lachman, N., Pawlina, W., 2015. Peer and faculty assessment of nontraditional discipline-independent skills in gross anatomy. In: Chan, L.K., Pawlina, W. (Eds.), Teaching Anatomy: A Practical Guide, first ed. Springer International Publishing, New York, pp. 299–309.

Lombardi, M.M., 2007. Authentic Learning for the 21st Century: an Overview. EDUCAUSE Learning Initiative, Boulder, CO.

McManus, D.A., 2001. The two paradigms of education and the peer review of teaching. J. Geosci. Educ. 49 (5), 423–434.

McMenamin, P.G., 2008. Body painting as a tool in clinical anatomy teaching. Anat. Sci. Educ. 1 (4), 139–144.

McNulty, J.A., Sonntag, B., Sinacore, J.M., 2009. Evaluation of computer-aided instruction in a gross anatomy course: a six-year study. Anat. Sci. Educ. 2 (1), 2–8.

Michaelsen, L.K., Parmelee, D.X., McMahon, K.K., Levine, R.E., 2008. Team-Based Learning for Health Professions Education: A Guide to Using Small Groups for Improving Learning, 229. Stylus Publishing LLC, Sterling, VA.

Pawlina, W., Drake, R.L., 2015. New (or not-so-new) tricks for old dogs: ultrasound imaging in anatomy laboratories. Anat. Sci. Educ. 8 (3), 195–196.

Pawlina, W., Drake, R.L., 2016. Authentic learning in anatomy: a primer on pragmatism. Anat. Sci. Educ. 9 (1), 5–7.

Pawlina, W., Hromanik, M.J., Milanese, T.R., et al., 2006. Leadership and professionalism curriculum in the gross anatomy course. Ann. Acad. Med. Singapore 35 (9), 609–614.

Pawlina, W., Lachman, N., 2004. Dissection in learning and teaching gross anatomy: rebuttal to McLachlan. Anat. Rec. B New Anat. 281 (1), 9–11.

Rosen, K.R., McBride, J.M., Drake, R.L., 2009. The use of simulation in medical education to enhance students' understanding of basic sciences. Med. Teach. 31 (9), 842–846.

Spencer, A.L., Brosenitsch, T., Levine, A.S., Kanter, S.L., 2008. Back to the basic sciences: an innovative approach to teaching senior medical students how best to integrate basic science and clinical medicine. Acad. Med. 83 (7), 662–669.

Srinivasan, M., Keenan, C.R., Yager, J., 2006. Visualizing the future: technology competency development in clinical medicine and implication for medical education. Acad. Psychiatry 30 (6), 480–490.

Vasan, N.S., DeFouw, D.O., Compton, S., 2009. A survey of student perceptions of team-based learning in anatomy curriculum: favorable views unrelated to grades. Anat. Sci. Educ. 2 (4), 150–155.

Yardley, S., Brosnan, C., Richardson, J., 2013. The consequences of authentic early experience for medical students: creation of mētis. Med. Educ. 47 (1), 109–119. Anat. Sci. Educ. 8(3):195–196, 2015.

23 Social and behavioural sciences in medical school curricula

J. Harden, J. E. Carr

Trends

- Social and behavioural sciences (SBS) are core subjects in medical education.
- Integrated curricula offer opportunities to include SBS.
- Revising curricula to include SBS may require faculty development to ensure the required expertize to design, deliver and assess SBS.

Introduction

Medicine faces significant challenges from an array of non-communicable diseases, contributed to by increasing societal problems including addiction, poor nutrition, obesity, violence, chronic disease, and healthcare issues of aging populations. Medical educators must ensure that graduates are provided with the knowledge and skills required to successfully address these challenges. The majority of these problems are readily addressed by treatment and prevention strategies derived from social and behavioural sciences (SBS) research. This chapter highlights key issues and offers practical guidance to those who may already include SBS in the curriculum, or are considering how best to do this. It addresses the following key questions:

- **Why** are SBS important in medicine?
- **What** should be considered core SBS content for medical education?
- **Where and when** should SBS be included in the medical curriculum?
- **Who** should be involved in developing and delivering SBS in the medical curriculum?
- **How** can SBS be taught and assessed to enhance students' learning?

Why are the social and behavioural sciences important in medicine?

 "There are a number of compelling reasons for all physicians to possess knowledge and skill in the behavioral and social sciences".

Institute of Medicine, 2004

The importance of social and behavioural factors in the aetiology of medical disorders is well established. Research worldwide consistently shows that illnesses subject to social and behavioural influence cover the entire medical spectrum and include communicable diseases as well as non-communicable diseases such as cancer, heart disease, poor pregnancy outcomes, type II diabetes, immune system disorders, accidental injuries, indeed, diseases and disorders associated with every organ system. A significant challenge is the array of non-communicable diseases (NCDs) that are the leading causes of mortality worldwide, causing more deaths than all other causes combined, striking hardest at the world's low- and middle-income populations. These diseases are especially challenging and of epidemic proportions in some countries, yet they could be significantly reduced, saving millions of lives, through reductions of their social and behavioural risk factors, early detection, and timely prevention (WHO, 2010).

This mounting body of research on social and behavioural determinants of health has prompted reports in the United States (AAMC, 2011) and United Kingdom (Frenk et al., 2010) calling for reforms in medical education to properly equip graduates with the skills to address these new health challenges, to identify societal and behavioural factors that caused them or impeded their treatment, and develop strategies

Table 23.1 World Federation for Medical Education: global standards for quality improvement
Medical School Accreditation: social and behavioural sciences World Federation for Medical Education: global standards for quality improvement

2.4 Behavioral and social sciences, medical ethics and jurisprudence

Basic standards:

The medical school must
- in the curriculum identify and incorporate the contributions of the:
  - behavioural sciences. (B 2.4.1)
  - social sciences. (B 2.4.2)
  - medical ethics. (B 2.4.3)
  - medical jurisprudence. (B 2.4.4)

Quality development standards:

The medical school should
- in the curriculum adjust and modify the contributions of the behavioural and social sciences as well as medical ethics and medical jurisprudence to
  - scientific, technological and clinical developments. (Q 2.4.1)
  - current and anticipated needs of the society and the healthcare system. (Q 2.4.2)
  - changing demographic and cultural contexts. (Q 2.4.3)

http://wfme.org/standards/bme/78-new-version-2012-quality-improvement-in-basic-medical-education-english/file

for successful intervention or prevention. Thus, medical education requires the inclusion of the social and behavioural sciences as well as the physical and biological sciences in medical school curricula, providing a foundation for more efficacious, comprehensive and integrated biopsychosocial clinical care. The relevance of SBS is also increasingly reflected in regulatory frameworks. Within the United Kingdom, the General Medical Council's statement of outcomes for graduates includes SBS as a requirement for medical schools, while in the United States, SBS are required portions of the Medical College Admission Test (MCAT) and the accreditation standards for the Licensing Committee on Medical Education (LCME), the accreditation body for MD degree programmes in the United States. As countries adopt accreditation standards comparable to the World Federation for Medical Education (WFME) (Table 23.1) or the LCME, instruction in SBS will be an accreditation requirement.

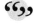 *"The behavioural and social sciences, medical ethics and medical jurisprudence would provide the knowledge, concepts, methods, skills and attitudes necessary for understanding socio-economic, demographic and cultural determinants of causes, distribution and consequences of health problems as well as knowledge about the national health care system*

and patients' rights. This would enable analysis of health needs of the community and society, effective communication, clinical decision making and ethical practices."

World Federation for Medical Education, 2012

The challenge for medical educators has been to move from a curriculum focused on the traditional *biomedical model*, which, as the name implies, focused solely on biological determinants, to one that also incorporates SBS. The *biopsychosocial model* (Engel, 1977) has called attention to the importance of social and behavioural factors, conceptualized as a hierarchy of multiple biological and psychosocial determinants of disease and resultant illness processes. However, as originally conceived, it did not address the mechanisms by which biological and SBS processes interacted. Subsequent advances in multidisciplinary research clearly established bidirectional interdependencies between biological and social-behavioural processes, leading to a more advanced biopsychosocial model, which emphasizes the importance of integrating the biological and the social and behavioural sciences, and the necessity for clearly illuminating the complex mechanisms by which these aetiological processes interact and affect health and disease (Carr, 1998).

What topics should be included in the curriculum?

Key institutions in the United States, (including the Institute of Medicine, National Institute of Heath, American Association of Medical Colleges) and the United Kingdom (General Medical Council, Behavioural and Social Science Teaching in Medicine, Public Health Educators in Medical Schools), have identified core SBS curricular content and learning outcomes (Institute of Medicine 2004; BeSST, 2010, 2015), which include the following major topics.

BIOLOGICAL MEDIATORS OF SBS FACTORS AND HEALTH

The optimal curricula will familiarize students with the physiological mechanisms by which environmental, psychological, behavioural, developmental and socio-cultural stressor conditions alter physiology. Essential to understanding the mediators of SBS influence is appreciating the role homeostatic systems play in the survival of the organism, their interconnections and central neuroendocrine regulation, and how the stressor conditions that challenge homeostasis contribute to failed homeostatic adaptation and resultant disease or dysfunction. Curricula should familiarize students with the mechanisms by which epi-genetic factors such as environmental, social, behavioural and cognitive stressor events impact gene expression, how such factors interact with and affect developmental processes, and how they contribute to chronic medical problems, like chronic pain, and somatization. It is essential that students understand that SBS factors such as beliefs, attitudes, familial perceptions and sociocultural sanctions can influence biological functioning as well as influence perception of illness, and receptivity to treatment.

SOCIAL AND CULTURAL DETERMINANTS OF HEALTH, ILLNESS AND DISEASE

In order to provide appropriate care to patients from differing social, ethnic, cultural and economic backgrounds, and at different stages in their lifespan, prospective physicians need to understand the way health and illness is shaped by these factors. It is well established that morbidity, mortality, and disability rates are linked to social factors such as gender, ethnicity, race, cultural identity, education, income, occupation and workplace. Students should be aware of the profound influence that these factors have on patients' health-related behaviours, choices, and outcomes. The ability to understand and effectively treat individuals from diverse populations and backgrounds requires cultural competence, i.e. recognition of and sensitivity to the sociocultural context of a patient's illness, as well as cultural humility, i.e. recognition of one's limited knowledge of the patient's beliefs and experience, awareness of one's biases and assumptions, and a willingness to learn and redress the imbalance of power inherent in the doctor–patient relationship.

PATIENT BEHAVIOUR

Primary care physicians can potentially be effective in changing patients' unhealthy behaviours (e.g. smoking, alcohol abuse, diet, stressful lifestyle, treatment adherence etc.) but many lack the training in principles of behaviour change to develop and apply effective techniques for behaviour change counselling. Training in important basic principles from psychology and sociology such as classical conditioning, cognitive/social learning theory, positive/negative reinforcement, stages of change model, social action theory etc. are essential for effective behavioural change counselling. Essential to medical training is instruction and experience with techniques such as Motivational Interviewing (Miller & Rose, 2009). This approach enables the physician to assist the patient in assessing the patient's barriers to change. The Stages of Change Model (Prochaska & Prochaska, 2011) outlines progressive step-wise strategies for addressing barriers to change in order to more effectively enable patients to adhere to diets, seek preventive healthcare such as breast cancer screening, reduce alcohol consumption, and adhere to medication regimens.

 Training in applying the Stages of Change Model and Motivational Interviewing skills should emphasize that these methods focus on both sociocultural as well as individual barriers to change. (For further information on training in Stages of Change and Motivational Interviewing see https://www.bcm.edu/education/programs/sbirt/index.cfm?pmid=25042.)

THE EXPERIENCE OF ILLNESS

Students should be aware of the potential disruption that illness can cause for all aspects of life (including work, family and relationships) and to the patient's sense of self or identity. Teaching students how to access and understand patients' illness narratives (the way patients make sense of illness onset and its impact) is essential both to the moral exercise of medicine, in ensuring that patients are listened to, but also has direct clinical relevance in developing accurate diagnoses and developing optimal treatment plans.

 "It is clinically useful to learn how to interpret the patient's and family's perspective on illness. Indeed the interpretation of narratives of illness experience … is a core task in the work of doctoring, although the skill has atrophied in biomedical training."

Kleinman, 1988

PHYSICIAN–PATIENT INTERACTIONS

The quality and quantity of information required to correctly diagnosis and appropriately treat the patient is dependent upon the physician's social and communication skills. Students must learn to not only inquire comfortably about patients' biomedical aetiology but also about their personal and social concerns, emotions and behaviours. Students must develop skills that promote respectful and compassionate communication, and demonstrate an appreciation for patients' understanding of, and expertize in living with their condition, and their expectations regarding medical care. Productive physician–patient interactions are based on the ability to establish rapport and build trust through empathic listening, elicit adequate information while at the same time understanding and addressing patient concerns, and facilitating patient involvement in a mutual exchange of information and shared decision making.

PHYSICIAN ROLE AND BEHAVIOUR

SBS curricula can encourage students to reflect on the meanings of professionalism and the ethical guidelines that have been the foundation of medical care since Hippocrates first defined them. Students must develop an awareness of how their personal values, attitudes, biases, and their own health and well-being can influence their care of the patient. Students should learn that physicians' social accountability and responsibility extends beyond the individual patient. They must have experience and training in working in integrated interdisciplinary healthcare teams in clinics and hospitals, and develop the interpersonal and administrative skills required to work effectively within organizations and the community at large.

 SBS facilitates students' awareness of their wider roles and addresses the potential impact of their own values and beliefs on practice.

HEALTH POLICY AND ECONOMICS

Prospective physicians must be well informed about the influence of political and economic factors on patients' health and healthcare. Those aspects of living conditions, environments, occupations, income, adequacy of diet, and access to healthcare resources that are determined by public policy and economic conditions significantly influence individual choices regarding health behaviours and healthcare decisions. Accessibility to healthcare depends upon financial resources of the patient, public resources made available by national healthcare systems and policies, insurance carriers, or combinations thereof. Therefore, appropriate treatment planning must involve an appreciation of the financial and political constraints, as well as the social and cultural limitations, imposed upon the patient and the physician. In addition, the physician must be knowledgeable about the complexities of both the formal and informal indigenous healthcare system and how they influence the accessibility of healthcare for the patient.

Where and when should SBS be presented in the curriculum?

Where and when SBS should be presented depends upon the current structure of the school's curriculum and may relate to the disciplinary organization of courses within the curriculum. Three models are discussed below, which relate to a wider discussion of curriculum integration discussed elsewhere in this book.

DISCIPLINE-SPECIFIC CURRICULA

If the curriculum is organized along discipline-specific biomedical lines, then SBS content may be more readily presented initially as a stand-alone course in the first year, in concert with other basic science courses (e.g. microbiology, anatomy/physiology, etc.). However, a disciplinary approach may reflect the 'isolation' (Harden, 2000) of SBS from other disciplines with minimal reference to what is being taught in other parts of the curriculum, making it appear to be less relevant.

 The efficacy of discipline-specific courses in the curriculum depends upon the application of these same principles/techniques in subsequent clinical courses.

If the curriculum and faculty fail to reinforce the SBS clinical applications in other subsequent courses and clinics, students will conclude that SBS is of limited relevance to medicine, and SBS training will have little lasting impact.

MULTIDISCIPLINARY

It is also possible to adopt a multidisciplinary curricular design, where SBS has allotted time within a course to address its particular take on the theme or topic being discussed. This may be likened to the 'sharing' model of integration (Harden, 2000). SBS content can be presented within the context of clinical case studies, standardized patient experiences, team-based learning, or clinical rounds. Problem-based learning courses can also offer opportunities for a multidisciplinary integration of SBS and basic science content. This approach familiarizes the student with the comparative contribution of SBS and biomedical approaches, although it may not necessarily explain the mechanisms of their interaction. Also, since there is competition for curricular time within the multidisciplinary model, instructors must ensure that SBS content is adequately presented.

INTERDISCIPLINARY

A development on the above method is the *interdisciplinary* approach, where SBS is integrated as part of a holistic curriculum design in which disciplinary labels disappear. Often utilizing case-based learning, cases are discussed within the context of the interdependency of the various aetiological factors, the mechanisms of their interaction, and the application of this knowledge to the selection of appropriate combined bio-behavioural interventions in their treatment. Again, the efficacy of any inclusion of SBS in the curriculum requires continuous subsequent review of SBS aetiologies, biopsychosocial interactions, and derivative behavioural medicine interventions throughout the curriculum. Interdisciplinary integration may present challenges for curriculum development in relation to identifying where and when SBS content is being included. For example, the interdisciplinary approach may offer limited opportunities for students to develop understanding of core SBS conceptual tools that would be offered in stand-alone courses. Therefore, medical educators must ensure that foundational tools are taught early in the curriculum sequence.

As implied above, comprehensive integration of SBS into a medical school curriculum may ultimately require a comprehensive restructuring of the curriculum to ensure that biological, social, and behavioural science integration is inherent and continuous throughout all years of training. Such initiatives are challenging, and it may be useful for schools considering this to review the experiences of US medical schools that were awarded grants by the National Institutes of Health to integrate behavioural and social sciences education in undergraduate medical school or graduate medical education curricula (Office of Behavioral and Social Sciences Research).

 In evaluating the outcomes for different models of integration, it is important to identify what impact the varying degrees of integration have on the outcomes, as opposed to changes in content, delivery format or faculty development.

Who should do the teaching design and delivery?

While all medical school faculty members should optimally possess training and clinical experience in biopsychosocial medicine, and should be familiar with the current conceptual and empirical research on SBS factors in medicine, including health related aspects of psychology, sociology, anthropology and economics, such expectations may not be realistic (Russell et al., 2004). The potential for conflict between clinicians and SBS specialists arising from the different world views can present challenges for them to work together (Satterfield et al., 2004). However, combining SBS specialists who possess experience and/or research backgrounds in selected medical areas, with clinicians in those same areas (a 'dynamic duo'" teaching team) has been shown to be effective, especially as they work together and integrate their knowledge in the course of teaching students (Carr, 1998).

Integrating SBS into the curriculum requires a clear and detailed plan for

1. bringing together a carefully selected group of appropriately trained and experienced faculty, committed to developing an innovative integrated curriculum

2. educating other faculty through continuing education programs

3. recruiting new faculty with a demonstrated biopsychosocial orientation, experience and expertize

4. developing and implementing the curriculum

5. mentoring students who will themselves become experienced biopsychosocial clinicians and teachers.

How can SBS be learnt, taught and assessed?

Developments in medical education present opportunities for innovative approaches to students' learning,

Box 23.1 Top tips for teaching SBS

- Encourage active learning
- Ensure learning opportunities provide added value
- Connect to the real world
- Be realistic about time
- Provide clear learning guidance

including problem-based learning; case-based learning; team-based learning; blended learning; flipped classrooms and community-based learning. Such approaches are discussed in detail elsewhere, including the relevant chapters of this book, and so will not be described here. This section presents 'top tips' that address pertinent issues to consider together with practice advice and examples for teaching SBS within a medical school curriculum (Box 23.1).

- *Encourage active learning*: Like all subjects in the curriculum, SBS subjects are best learnt through students' involvement in discussing, reading, thinking about, researching, and applying knowledge.

Example: Students can be asked to identify a clinical concern based on the topic area being addressed. Working in small groups, they develop a 'problem tree'(Snowdon et al., 2008) to establish the SBS causes of the problem (roots) and its effects (branches). Based on this, the students can then identify potential solutions relating to specific aspects of the causes (roots). This is a useful exercise in encouraging students to not only identify SBS influences on clinical problems but also to discuss the challenges of developing interventions to bring about change.

- *Ensure learning opportunities provide added value.* Consider how best to use the contact time with students and whether 'being there' is worth it for the student. In classes where the material from a textbook is simply reproduced, students may choose not to attend because they could read the book in their own time without having the inflexibility and additional time commitment of the lecture.

Example: If a one-hour lecture is allocated to addressing the topic of health inequalities between socioeconomic groups, it is important to ask whether some of the 'knowledge' you want to impart can be acquired· in other ways. While important statistical evidence of health inequalities can be presented in the lecture, it may be more useful to provide a brief summary (in note form or as a short video) of this evidence for students prior to the lecture. This approach, drawing on the idea of the flipped classroom, where some instruction is transferred from the class into individual learning time, allows the lecture time to be used differently. Rather than using class contact time to provide basic, albeit core information, which could be provided in other ways, the time can be used more constructively to provide learning experience that could not be achieved without being present in class, for example using the lecture time for a question and answer session with a panel of experts in the field of health inequalities.

- *Connect to the real world*: In presenting SBS concepts to medical students, it is important to focus upon the medical relevance and clinical application of concepts. This can be achieved through the use of examples including case presentations, research findings, patients' or clinicians' experiences.

Example: Community-based learning can be appropriate for connecting students' learning to reallife contexts, for example in schools, charitable organizations, and nursing homes, enhancing the application and meaningfulness of the students' learning. It is also important to ground class-based work in real examples. For example, discussing young people's experiences of illness, present short video interviews with teenage patients (for example those provided by the online resource www.healthtalk.org) and ask students to consider the challenges illness may present at this stage in life and the implications for medication adherence.

- *Be realistic about time*: Medical students must constantly balance the conflicting demands of studying with socializing, part-time work, and family commitments. Thus, in planning training experiences, it is important to work with the students, keeping their learning stage, level of experience, and demands on their time in mind. This requires an accurate assessment of the time required to complete the assigned SBS work (contact time, independent study, and assessment) for a module/unit/course.

Example: Students are allocated 3 hours of study preparation for a case tutorial discussing Anna, a 28-year-old woman, whose mother has recently been diagnosed with Huntington's disease. There are a number of different perspectives to be explored, including biomedical, ethical, and SBS, that require more than 3 hours of work. Hence, it is important to be clear about the objectives you want the students to achieve in their preparation for and participation in the tutorial, and to collaborate with the session organizer to ensure these objectives can be realistically achieved in the time given. If an objective is "to be aware of relatives' reactions when a family member is diagnosed with Huntington's," it may be possible to direct students to resources that present relevant patient stories. If

an objective is "to identify factors that shape genetic testing decision making in families with Huntington's," an appropriate (at the right level and length) academic paper may be a useful source.

- *Provide clear learning guidance*: Some medical students may be new to studying independently and new to studying SBS. This presents students with challenges (particularly in year 1) in identifying what they 'need to know' and how best to learn. While this may be a broader concern it is particularly an issue for SBS topics because many students may have little or no experience studying these subject areas.

Example: Provide a clear indication of what is required of students with focused learning objectives. Structure students' learning (until more experienced as independent learners and with SBS subject areas), for example by offering guidance on how to read academic SBS papers and how to use sources to address the learning objectives. Also, consider ways to provide formative guidance to students. Individual feedback on written work is valued by students and can provide significant help in understanding SBS concepts and acquiring core academic skills. If adequate time and resources are not available to support independent feedback, feedback to the whole class following assessments can be used effectively. It is also important to consider ways to support students who may be interested in pursuing the subjects further. For example, students can be given an annotated list of further resources (book chapters, journal articles, websites, audio/visual clips) to facilitate their investigation of the topics in more depth.

Assessment

 "The choice of assessment method(s) should be appropriate to the content and purpose of that element of the curriculum."

General Medical Council, 2010

Discussion relating to assessment methods highlights the challenges of balancing different requirements relating to validity, reliability and feasibility. Increasingly, undergraduate medical assessment is assessed via extended matching questions (EMQs), single best answer (SBA) and objective structured clinical examination (OSCE). While well written EMQs and SBAs can be developed to assess some SBS learning objectives, it is important to consider *what* is being assessed, in order to develop appropriate modes of assessment. If students are being assessed on their reflective skills, or ability to discuss issues, free-text response questions (either in exam or in course assessments such as essays, reports or reflective writing) may be more appropriate.

The level of integration reflected in the curriculum structures described above (disciplinary, multidisciplinary and interdisciplinary) will influence the modes of assessment. When delivery is integrated it is important to ensure that SBS content is included in assessment (Litva & Peters, 2008). Consideration should be given as to how best to address SBS objectives in assessment, and the extent to which SBS concepts and information should be assessed separately or integrated with other clinical material. For example, OSCEs may offer the opportunity to integrate SBS information into clinical assessments.

How do we implement an SBS curriculum?

None of the above will occur without the full support of the officers and administration of the medical school (i.e. Dean, Executive Committee, Chairs of key departments etc.) who must be informed as to the importance of the SBS in healthcare, and their inclusion in medical school curricula. Any curricular change must therefore involve an array of complementary strategies that must be initiated simultaneously with, if not in advance of, the steps below.

1. Identify faculty members who support SBS in the curricula. Encourage them to seek assignments to key curriculum planning committees. Encourage faculty to participate and promote interdisciplinary teaching in collaboration with other departments and disciplines.

2. Circulate to medical school administrators and officers research reports and proposals from governmental agencies and NGOs calling for SBS integration in medical school curricula, and calls for social and behavioural medicine clinical services in the state, region, country.

3. Organize conferences, continuing medical education workshops, and invite speakers on the topic of SBS factors in clinical care, medical education and public health.

4. Enhance research-teaching links by encouraging faculty with SBS expertize to develop clinical outcome studies on the efficacy of social and behavioural medicine approaches to clinical disorders of particular interest to governmental bodies, and other departments/ disciplines. Encourage applications for grants in research on the influence of SBS factors in health care.

5. Establish a social and behavioural medicine clinic or consultation service (where appropriate), and offer services to all other departments and clinical services. As part of that service, offer teaching consultation to the students/residents of the requesting department/clinic as an additional perk.

6. Provide the Dean and key administrators with periodic reports, publishable articles, and press releases on the services being provided, cases being seen, and public problems being addressed by the medical school, underscoring the school's service to the community and nation.

Summary

Social and behavioural sciences should have a core place within medical curricula in order to ensure that medical students acquire all the relevant skills enabling them to become effective practitioners. SBS curricular content should address: biological mediators of SBS factors and health; social and cultural determinants of health, illness and disease; patient behaviour; the experience of illness; physician–patient interactions; physician role and behaviour; health policy and economics. SBS should be integrated into the curriculum in a way that ensures adequate consideration is given to the relevance of SBS content throughout all stages of students' learning. Effective integration requires collaboration between clinical and SBS faculty, drawing on the expertize of both to ensure that SBS content design, delivery and assessment is appropriate, timely and relevant. Whether at the early stage of introducing SBS to the medical curriculum or further developing its integration, implementing an SBS curriculum requires the support of the medical school administration. Institutions whose faculty and administration have both the vision and commitment will succeed in developing and implementing a comprehensive, integrated, biopsychosocial curriculum.

References

AAMC. Behavioral and Social Science Foundations for Future Physicians. Report of the Behavioral and Social Science Expert Panel, 2011, Association of American Medical Colleges.

BeSST. A Core Curriculum for Psychology in Medical Education: a Report of the BeSST Steering Group for Psychology. 2010. Available at: https://www.heacademy.ac.uk/resource/core-curriculum-psychology-undergraduate-medical-education. (Accessed December 2015). Behavioural and Social Science Teaching in Medicine.

BeSST. A Core Curriculum for Sociology in Medical Education: A Report of the BeSST Steering Group for Sociology. 2015, Behavioural and Social Science Teaching in Medicine.

Carr, J.E., 1998. The need for an Integrated Science Curriculum in medical education. Teach. Learn. Med. 10 (1), 3–7.

Engel, G., 1977. The need for a new medical model: a challenge for biomedicine. Science 196, 129–136.

Frenk, J., Chen, L., Bhutta, Z.A., et al., 2010. Health professionals for a new century: transforming education to strengthen health systems in an interdependent world. Lancet. 376 (9756), 1923–1958.

General Medical Council. Standards for Curricula and Assessment Systems. 2010. Manchester, UK.

Harden, R., 2000. The integration ladder: a tool for curriculum planning and evaluation. Med. Educ. 34, 551–557.

Institute of Medicine, 2004. Cuff, P.A., Vanselow, N.A. (Eds.), Improving Medical Education: Enhancing the Behavioral and Social Science Content of Medical School Curricula. National Academies Press, Washington, D.C.

Kleinman, A., 1988. Illness Narratives: Suffering Healing and the Human Condition. Basic Books.

Litva, A., Peters, S., 2008. Exploring barriers to teaching behavioural and social sciences in medical education. Med. Educ. 42 (3), 309–314.

Miller, W., Rose, G., 2009. Toward a theory of motivational interviewing. Am. Psychol. 64 (6), 527–537.

NIH, Office of Behavioral and Social Sciences Research. Enhancing behavioral and social sciences in undergraduate medical education. Available at: https://obssr.od.nih.gov/scientific-initiatives/bss-consortium/. (Accessed 9 January 2017).

Prochaska, J.O., Prochaska, J.M., 2011. Behavior change. In: Haverling, A., Reilly T. (Eds.), Population health creating a culture of wellness. Jones and Bartlett Learning, LLC.

Russell, A., van Teijlingen, E., Lambert, H., Stacy, R., 2004. Social and behavioural science education in UK medical schools: current practice and future directions. Med. Educ. 38 (4), 409–417.

Satterfield, J., Mitteness, L., Tervalon, M., Adler, N., 2004. Integrating the social and behavioural sciences in an undergraduate medical curriculum: the UCSF essential core. Acad. Med. 79 (1), 6–15.

Snowdon, W., Schultz, J., Swinburn, B., 2008. Problem and solution trees: a practical approach for identifying potential interventions to improve population nutrition. Health Promot. Int. 23 (4), 345–353.

WHO. Global Status Report on Noncommunicable Diseases, 2010, World Health Organization.

World Federation for Medical Education. Global Standards for Quality Improvement, 2012.

Further reading

Alder, B., Abraham, C., van Teijlingen, E., Porter, M., 2009. Psychology and Sociology Applied to Medicine. Churchill-Livingston, London.

Fadem, B., 2014. Behavioral Science, sixth ed. Walters Kluwer, Philadelphia, PA.

Feldman, M.D., Christensen, J.F. (Eds.), 2014. Behavioral Medicine: A Guide to Clinical Practice, fourth ed. McGraw-Hill, New York, NY.

Sahler, O.J., Carr, J.E. (Eds.), 2012. The Behavioral Sciences and Health Care, third ed. Hogrefe, Cambridge, MA.

Wedding, D., Stuber, M.L., 2010. Behavior and Medicine, fifth ed. Hogrefe, Cambridge, MA.

24

Clinical communication

J. R. Skelton

Trends

- Everyone knows that communication matters
- The educator's job is to sensitize people to it, and to give them a vocabulary to discuss it with
- But it's increasingly integrated within other areas, often as part of 'professional development'
- Communication in many different contexts increasingly foregrounded – both spoken and written
- No consensus at present about what to teach, or where, under the banner of clinical communication

Introduction

The importance of clinical communication is now taken for granted. It is routinely taught and tested at undergraduate and postgraduate level in many countries, often with a set of 'communication skills' in mind, which are perceived as the conduit for patient-centred medicine. The most fully developed list of skills derives from Silverman et al. (2005) and is available online, and Maguire and Pitceathly (2002) give a brief summary of what they term 'key communication skills'. As regards other approaches, Makoul (2001) reports on the approach of the Kalamazoo Statement, which began by synthesizing some of the key "models" put forward for doctor–patient communication, and produced "seven sets" of communication "tasks", such as "build[ing] the doctor–patient relationship", "open[ing] the discussion" and so on. As these are at a greater level of abstraction, they have the advantage of seeming less prescriptive.

There have been a number of recent developments, however. First, as regards 'skills', it is self-evident that any skill is ineffective taken to the extreme. What counts as 'appropriate' eye-contact, for example, is dependent on an indefinitely large set of variables (gender, age, culture etc.). What matters, therefore, is being able to communicate flexibly. This may be termed a type of "creativity" (Salmon & Young, 2011).

"Making choices" rather than "performing skills" is at the heart of good communication (Skelton, 2008), and the teaching of communication is therefore, at heart, about sensitizing people to choice.

Secondly, the relationship between communication and broader concepts of "professional development" has changed (Stern and Papadakis, 2006), to the extent that communication teaching is often seen as part of a professional development strand. This context has been around for some time, and one difficulty at present is how to keep distinct the different strands of professional development, while acknowledging the need to integrate them. The United States Medical Licensing Examination (USMLE), for example, distinguishes between "communication and interpersonal skills," on the one hand, and "professional and ethical/legal" "interactions", on the other (Box 24.1). More recently, in United Kingdom the Francis Report into the problems at one English Hospital Trust has brought the word 'culture' to the fore (as in a phrase like: "the culture of medicine"). The recent initiative from the GMC, *Promoting Excellence*, also picks up this term, and puts together "communication, partnership and teamwork".

Thirdly, there is growing awareness of the many types of communication doctors need to undertake: the quasi-counselling model of communication with patients is no longer enough on its own.

The centrepiece of most clinical communication teaching remains doctor–patient interaction, however. And the central methodology continues to be role play.

Using role play

RATIONALE

'Role play' is an unfortunate label: even in the United Kingdom, it has overtones of amateur dramatics, and in the United States it has perhaps even less credibility. But alternative labels for similar activities (e.g. 'simulated patients') are unfortunately used in different ways, so the term 'role play' has been retained to mean a serious, challenging educational activity.

Box 24.1 USMLE on 'communication', 'professionalism' and 'interaction'

Communication and Interpersonal Skills
Fostering the relationship
Gathering information
Providing information
Making decisions
Supporting emotions
Enabling patient behaviours
Using a translator.
Professionalism, including legal and ethical issues
Professionalism/legal/ethical issues in interaction with patients and families
Professionalism/legal/ethical issues in interactions with patients and families related to death and dying
Professionalism/legal/ethical issues in interactions with other health professionals
(http://www.usmle.org/pdfs/tcom.pdf on *USLME Physician tasks/competencies*).

The fundamental rationale for role play is that it provides a safe environment for mistakes and experimentation and can offer the same educationally useful performance repeatedly.

Behind this rationale are other important characteristics. Education through role play is essentially inductive in nature; it moves from a focus on a particular case to a discussion that seeks to induce general principles. For example, "Mr Smith responded in this way – is this typical of how people might respond in these circumstances?" It therefore fits well with contemporary educational practice in starting with individual cases rather than lecture-based generalities. It also fits neatly into the common pattern of clinical life: contact with patients, one by one.

FORMATS FOR ROLE PLAY

There are unlimited variations of the role play formats outlined below, which are indicative rather than prescriptive.

- *Forum theatre*: One role player, one or two facilitators. Audience of any size up to several hundred, e.g. in lecture theatre. One hour in length.

  Role player and facilitator act out a scenario in a less-than-perfect way. Facilitator subsequently invites comments from audience (or second facilitator does, with roving microphone). Repeat scenario, building in changes suggested. Draw conclusions.

- *Large group*: Role player and facilitator, audience of 8–20. This can be done as a version of forum theatre, but the smaller group size makes it more flexible. Two hours in length. 'Time outs' can be introduced, so that everyone (including role player and facilitator) can stop, review, ask questions or make suggestions.

With a group of this size, it becomes reasonable to ask participants to play the part of the doctor. Depending on levels of confidence, other participants can offer detailed advice beforehand (this shares the burden of responsibility if things go badly) or none at all.

With a group of up to 20, it isn't usually realistic to offer everyone a chance to role play. Notoriously, those most in need are least likely to volunteer, but it may be reasonable to allow some to take a back seat, participating in targeted observation. This means asking individuals to look for certain key elements – "How is the doctor achieving empathy?" or, at a lower level, "How many open questions is the doctor asking?" (A variant of this, particularly with students on attachment, is to make explicit use of the clinical tutor as a model, with students looking at the tutor's clinical communication in practice.) This kind of activity can form part of the feedback offered. Discussion often lasts at least as long as the role play itself, and is at least as interesting. The best role players are essentially educators, and contribute detailed feedback.

- *Small group*: Role player and facilitator, or facilitator only, group of up to eight. With this number of participants it becomes realistic to offer everyone a chance to role play, either seeing a consultation through from beginning to end or undertaking part and then handing over to someone else during a time out.

Educators often suggest asking health professionals to take the part of patients. Where the budget doesn't run to a professional role player, this is inevitable. Most people can at least play a version of themselves tolerably well ("Just imagine that you personally are in this situation.").

A standard (but costly) variant is to subdivide a larger group into smaller groups of four to six, each with a facilitator, and with a number of role players rotating round the groups.

- *Single participant role play*: Role player–facilitator, or role player plus facilitator, one participant.

It's clear that this is an expensive resource but, particularly in cases where the aim is remedial support, the intensity of the contact and the possibility of very detailed discussion make it cost effective. A 2-hour session can make a real difference. And it is very likely to reveal a great deal about other areas such as attitude.

CONDUCTING A ROLE PLAY SESSION

Of central importance is that the atmosphere is right. If participants have never undertaken role play before, they may be nervous and, often for this reason, sceptical. It's therefore vital that the facilitator and role players are confident, matter-of-fact and serious.

This brings us to the question of feedback. At an elementary level (for example, with junior undergraduates or for remedial support), there is a need for feedback centred on the basic skills: questioning styles, body language, checking of understanding and so on. This is vital, partly because it may be done poorly, but mostly so that participants are made aware of these skills and have a vocabulary with which to discuss them.

This is, however, basic stuff: a course in 'advanced eye contact' is hardly plausible. One of the real values of role play is the opportunity it gives for discussion at a higher level, for reflection about oneself and others and about the profession. In fact, there is a basic hierarchy of questions (Box 24.2), which perhaps most

people employ, but is seldom made explicit. Again: good communication is not the mechanical application of skills but insightful choices about when to deploy them.

Level 1, clearly, deals with behavioural skills. The facilitator's role here is to ensure that the participant and observers can describe accurately what they have seen, and evidence it. Thus, not "You were very empathic," but "When you leaned forward and murmured, 'Take your time' that made you appear very empathic." And – moving as quickly as possible on to the next level in the hierarchy – to ensure that they can justify what was done. The third level in the hierarchy represents the classic movement of inductive teaching: it compares the particular instance against general patterns. A common way of linking the two is through the facilitator or one of the participants, saying, "This happens a lot – I had a patient once …"

The higher-order questions are invitations to reflect. "What do you make of this patient?", "What kind of person are they?" or, "What does this role play tell you about being a doctor?"

Move as quickly as you can up the 'hierarchy of questions': the higher the level of the questions, the more interesting the session.

The wider context

OTHER ASPECTS OF SPOKEN COMMUNICATION

This section begins with non-verbal behaviour, since it is often misunderstood. As Henry et al. (2012) point out, studies have tended to focus on controlled rather than naturally occurring language. This makes findings dubious – indeed, the wild claims that are sometimes still made for non-verbal communication (e.g. that it accounts for 90% or more of communication) are almost all based on a misunderstanding of experiments in a controlled environment from the late 1960s. The idea is evident nonsense (if you disagree, explain why, without using words: see Max Atkinson's blog for details [http://maxatkinson.blogspot.co.uk/]). Nevertheless, Henry et al. unsurprisingly argue that findings identify a link between apparent "listening" and "warmth" of non-verbal communication, and patient satisfaction. Having said that, "creating an impression of warmth" is a matter of changing behaviour to a limited extent only, and perhaps rather more a conceptual issue (What kind of person do you want your patient to think you are?). As so often, the performance of behaviours seems only to scratch the surface. In general, the identification of 'good' and 'bad' non-verbal behaviour in one-to-one interaction, beyond the blindingly obvious (don't look out of the window and yawn) is likely to be situation-specific. Again, what matters is sensitization: for 'tone of voice', e.g. every actor has tried out exercises such as those suggested.

Box 24.2 Hierarchy of question types after role play

1. *Describing skills*: Did you maintain eye contact? The right amount? How do you know?
2. *Justifying skills*: Why did you do it that way? What if you'd done it differently?
3. *Generalizing skills*: Are there general principles here, e.g. about how to defuse aggression? ("I had a patient who …")

Higher-order questions

4. *Assessing people*: What was the patient like? Is this typical or unusual for patients of this type, or with this problem?
5. *Assessing self*: What kind of person are you? What did the experience tell you about, e.g. your response to stress, breaking bad news … how did it make you feel?
6. *Assessing the profession*: In the light of this scenario, what does it mean to be a doctor? What kind of things do doctors do?

Exercises for learners: Sensitization to tone of voice
Practise dialogues like this, thinking of as many contexts as possible – a fan and a film star, a gangster and someone who owes him money … think of more dialogues!
A: Who are you?
B: Don't you know?
A: You're not …?
B: Yes I am

Nevertheless, there has been some success in identifying what one might call broad brushstroke body language in other areas: in presenting to audiences, for example. Thus, alongside routine verbal markers of shifts of theme ("now …", "let's turn to …" etc.) good presenters will not only change tone of voice but will more or less subconsciously make a small postural change – it might be no more than shifting one's weight from one foot to the other. The key way to teach this is to video participants, make them aware of what they do, and build on their strengths.

Exercises for learners: Reflecting on body language
Video yourself.
Don't worry – no-one looks quite as silly as they think they do when they first see themselves.
Monitor what you do with your hands, your arms (how big an area do you cover with your gestures?), your gaze, your smile.
What do you do physically to interrupt someone (lean forward? Put your hand out?)

Exercises for learners: Making oral presentations
As above – video! (And don't worry).
Observe how you change the subject: Do you say "OK", "Well then …"
How do you introduce a topic: Do you say "Next I want to discuss …" "Let me turn now to …"
Work out what works.
Have a look at online videos – e.g. Ted Talks. What styles work, and what styles can you imagine using yourself?

The other side of the coin is the need for awareness of what is lost when interviews are not face to face (e.g. on the telephone). The picture here is confused by the different goals of many such interactions. Telephone consultations are, for example, often used to triage patients into those who do and those who do not need an urgent visit. This may account at least in part for the suggestion that telephone interaction demonstrates less evidence of the traditional attributes associated with "patient-centredness" (Innes et al., 2006).

MEDICAL RECORDS

There are demands made on doctors in this area as never before. There is a general view, supported by research (e.g. Shachak & Reis, 2009) that electronic medical records (EMRs) have "a positive impact on information exchange" (they help ensure the doctor asks appropriate clinical questions) but "a negative influence on patient centredness" (their attention is on the record, not the person). Possible approaches, where a doctor is having problems in this area, are to advise separating out the consultation and the EMR more or less completely, or to build the EMR into the meeting – "Right, let me just put that into the record – I'll forget if I don't do it now." Or to simply increase computer literacy.

COMMUNICATION AND HI-FIDELITY SIMULATION

Clinical communication happens in a context and setting: a busy ward, a meeting room and so on. Often it is a matter of seconds rather than minutes, which makes the counselling model less relevant. Yet the doctor who spends 10 seconds with a patient is creating a foundation of trust, which might be of considerable importance.

The most detailed form of clinical communication teaching is what happens on simulated wards, and is often associated with the teaching of human factors (Leonard et al., 2004). This kind of work deals head-on with the relationship between communication and aspects of professionalism. This suggests that the agenda – the list of topics – for clinical communication teaching will need substantial recasting in the near future (Box 24.3).

COMMUNICATION BETWEEN COLLEAGUES

A key aspect of this is handover skills, often taught using 'SBAR' (NHS Institute, 2011): situation, background, assessment, recommendation. (SBAR was first developed in an aviation context). The idea is that, at any stage of the patient's journey, the template can be used to 'shape' communication between colleagues. It is for this reason that SBAR teaching is particularly useful – it forms a good general template, relevant for many kinds of reporting. As regards teaching, it lends itself to a wide variety of different approaches. A paper case can be offered to a group, for example, and they can be invited to agree what elements matter, that is, how to fill the SBAR template. This is obviously a good prioritization task in itself. One of the participants can then actually report the case, perhaps under psychological pressure (it's the middle of the night, you're on the phone, the consultant is horrible …). Some people have great difficulty disentangling information that matters from the background noise. As a real exercise, or as a thought experiment, they can be given

Box 24.3 Topics for clinical communication

Contexts of communication

Speaking/listening:
Doctor–patient interaction
Oral presentations
SBAR handovers
Telephone communication
Colleague-to-colleague communication
Rich contexts, multiple people (e.g. human factors)
Effective listening (e.g. to lectures: includes note-taking)

Writing/reading:
Referral letters
Medical records
Letters to patients
Writing for publication
Reading research papers
Writing reports

an impossible instruction: "Here is a case. Present it in SBAR format using a maximum of 30 words." (Stress beforehand that the task is deliberately impossible, and for the purpose of raising awareness!)

Other common issues centre on aspects of teamwork, leadership, negotiation and the like. Here, there are issues of what is known as *register*, i.e. how to express the correct level of formality and, by extension, appear appropriately polite without being obsequious (with seniors) or patronizing (with juniors). This evidently also lends itself to role play, but there are simple consciousness-raising activities that are possible as well. Most TV dramas with a hospital setting represent atrocious professional interaction: usually people shouting at each other for dramatic purposes, and reworking a brief piece of dialogue is useful (copyright permitting).

READING AND WRITING

'Critical reading' is a well-established concept. Generally, critical reading courses (see also Greenhalgh, 2006) incorporate some aspects of 'reading skills', as the phrase is normally used. What is often missing is the kind of standard reading exercise done in other disciplines: exercises in skimming, reading for gist and so on. This type of exercise is often undertaken against the clock; for example, "Here's a *JAMA* article without its abstract. In 20 seconds, tell me what the authors acknowledge as the main shortcomings of their paper." This confirms for participants that 'good reading' can consist of things other than reading a piece intensively

from beginning to end: professional life involves quick, sensible choices about what to read and at what level of detail. It also requires readers to know where they are likely to find shortcomings stated (by convention, usually early in the discussion section), and this in turn gives them an understanding of the structure of academic papers (see also Chapter 50, *Medical Education Research*).

The core of successful teaching of academic writing is an understanding of how its very highly conventionalised structure is put together. A personal favourite activity to sensitize participants to aspects of structure is to invite them, in a group of up to six, to write up an imaginary randomized controlled trial (RCT) to test the hypothesis contained in a well-known proverb such as 'a stitch in time saves nine'.

Shorter pieces of writing are best handled not in the 'writing class' but in the context of professionalism. The doctor who doesn't fill in handover notes, or makes poor records on the ward of tasks to do and tasks done is a risk to patient safety. Of the tasks which are slightly longer, a key one is reading and writing referral letters. Rewriting tasks work well in these areas, for example improving a letter too vague or discourteous to be effective (see Exercises for Learners for an example).

LANGUAGE, CULTURE AND THE INTERNATIONAL MEDICAL GRADUATE (IMG)

IMGs, and for that matter international medical students, are likely to encounter substantial difficulties (Whelan, 2005), even when they are fluent speakers of the main local language. There are many doctors who speak vigorous, confident South Asian, West African or other well-established (and equally good) varieties of English or French, say, but do not practice in their local cultures. Often, these doctors struggle with 'communicative competence', that is, they *know* the language, but cannot *use* it: they know the phrase: "That's wrong" and the phrase: "I wonder if I could possibly disagree?", but are at risk of using them with the wrong people. Such issues become serious everyday hurdles: "Who should I be on first-name terms with?" "How should I talk to a junior nurse?"

The best advice for the IMG is usually exposure to the target culture (e.g. through local friends, TV and radio). In addition, they should listen for, make a note of and practise the words and phrases they hear others using to make requests, offer a suggestion, ask a difficult question, etc. (Note that the Medical Council of Canada have recently launched a new initiative to support IMGs with communication and cultural competence.)

Of course, the multicultural nature of many parts of the modern world is such that many doctors encounter dozens of different cultural groups in the course of a year. Learning the rules of communicative competence for all these groups would be impossible.

Professionalism

'Communication' is a term that, exasperatingly, can mean more or less anything. The clothes we wear 'communicate', as does our accent, or the architectural style of the local town hall, which perhaps 'communicates' the bourgeois values if its builders. It's impossible to set precise boundaries. For example, the relationship between written communication and the intellectual ability to construct an academic argument has been hinted at above, as has the relationship between communicating well and taking due professional care.

The boundaries set on 'clinical communication' will vary in place and time. This seems to be particularly well-illustrated in the area of remedial support. 'Poor communication' is often given as a frequent cause of patient or colleague complaint, but it is often the symptom rather than the disease. Common sense suggests that the doctor who communicates bad news in a manner perceived as uncaring may actually *be* uncaring rather than merely poorly skilled.

'Communication' is a label that gets slapped on many of the nonclinical, professional problems that doctors encounter and is often the entry point for remediation. Thus particular doctors may be perceived as bullying (with the 'poor communication' being that they shout at people, for example), and this may in turn be because they are anxious, or set impossible standards and so on. Or perhaps they 'lack leadership qualities', meaning that they don't talk much: which in turn may mean that they need to find a leadership style that allows them to be their true, quiet selves, yet carry authority and so on.

Assessment

Assessment of clinical communication, at least for doctor–patient interaction, is well accepted. Typically, summative assessment happens through OSCEs with role players. The only major difficulty here is instructive. The more one tries to break down the 'good consultation' into its constituent skills, the more it turns communication into a mechanistic exercise, but the more holistic one is, the more subjective the judgement. This is an area where the discipline of assessment is finally making a firm case. See, for example, the central point of van der Vleuten et al. (2010) that "objectivity does not equal reliability". As they say, this insight has "far-reaching practical consequences. Most importantly, it justifies reliance on (expert) human judgement." This gives the assessor freedom from the pitfalls of reductionism.

Other types of assessment include simple observation and feedback, 360-degree appraisal and the like. It is difficult to be sure, however, what the level of expertize is of the raters under these circumstances, or whether they all understand 'communication' the same way. This perhaps makes them more appropriate for formative assessment.

Conclusion

Doctor–patient communication as a concept, and an important clinical competence, is well-established. What the discipline is now engaging with, however, is the need to integrate with the wider issue of professional development, while retaining its identity. The fundamental educational background of the discipline, however, and particularly the fact that role-play and simulations generally are superbly flexible methodologies, mean that the discipline continues to be well placed to have its voice heard.

References

Greenhalgh, T., 2006. How to Read a Paper, third ed. Blackwell, Oxford.

Henry, S.G., Fuhrel-Forbis, A., Rogers, M.A.M., Eggly, S., 2012. Association between non-verbal communication during clinical encounters and outcomes: a systematic review and meta-analysis. Patient Educ Couns. 86 (3), 297–315.

Innes, M., Skelton, J., Greenfield, S., 2006. A profile of communication in primary care physician telephone consultations: application of the Roter Interaction Analysis System. Br. J. Gen. Pract. 56 (526), 363–368.

Leonard, M., Graham, S., Bonacum, D., 2004. The human factor: the critical importance of effective teamwork and communication in providing safe care. Qual. Saf. Health. Care. 13 (Suppl. 1), i85–i90.

Maguire, P., Pitceathly, C., 2002. Key communication skills and how to acquire them. Br. Med. J. 325 (7366), 697–700.

Makoul, G., 2001. Essential elements of communication in medical encounters: the Kalamazoo consensus statement. Acad. Med. 76 (4), 390–393.

Salmon, P., Young, B., 2011. Creativity in clinical communication: from communication skills to skilled communication. Med. Educ. 45 (3), 217–226.

Shachak, A., Reis, S., 2009. The impact of electronic medical records on patient–doctor communication during consultation: a narrative literature review. Version of Record online: 10 JUN 2009 | doi:10.1111/j.1365-2753.2008.01065.x. (Accessed 28 January 2017).

Silverman, J., Kurtz, S.M., Draper, J., 2005. Skills for Communicating with Patients, second ed. Radcliffe.

Skelton, J., 2008. Language and Clinical Communication: This Bright Babylon. Radcliffe, Oxford.

Stern, D.T., Papadakis, M., 2006. The developing physician – becoming a professional. NEJM 355 (17), 1794–1799.

van der Vleuten, C.P.M., Schuwirth, L.W.T., Scheele, F., et al., 2010. The assessment of professional competence: building blocks for theory development. Best Pract. Res. Clin. Obstet. Gynaecol. 24 (6), 703–719.

Whelan, G., 2005. Commentary: Coming to America: the integration of international medical graduates into the American medical culture. Acad. Med. 81 (2), 176–178.

Relevant websites

1. For the Francis Report, see: http://webarchive.nationalarchives.gov.uk/20150407084003/http://www.midstaffspublicinquiry.com/report

2. For USMLE (United States Medical Licencing Examination), see: http://www.usmle.org/pdfs/tcom.pdf

3. For Medical Council of Canada support for IMGs, see: http://physiciansapply.ca/orientation/about-the-communication-and-cultural-competence-program/

4. For the recent General Medical Council document on standards, see: http://www.gmc-uk.org/Promoting_excellence_standards_for_medical_education_and_training_0715.pdf_61939165.pdf

5. For Max Atkinson's always witty and profound insights into (amongst other things) the exaggerated claims made for non-verbal communication, see his blog at: http://maxatkinson.blogspot.co.uk/

Teaching resources available online

The amount of interesting, easily accessible material for use with students or doctors learning about – or simply reflecting on – clinical communication is considerable. This is a sample only.

1. Examples of role play in a clinical setting are available on the following website, which emanates from St. George's: www.virtualpatients.eu/resources/other-resources-2/communication-skills-online

2. Tokyo Medical University has an extensive website (in English) to support medical students and doctors. It is designed to support non-native speakers of English, but is of considerable value for anyone, and includes both reading support and videos of consultations: www.emp-tmu.net This website (also of value for many educational areas) looks in detail at the approach associated with Silverman, Kurtz and Draper: www.skillscascade.com/models.htm#Calgary-Cambridge. (Accessed 27 January 2017).

3. The Picker Institute, which promotes patient-centred care, has interesting information on clinical communication: www.pickereurope.org

4. Although this is more properly 'patient narrative' rather than communication in itself, there is a great deal of potential value for teaching and learning communication in this extensive website: www.healthtalkonline.org

5. EACH (European Association for Communication in Healthcare) has extensive resources that are worth looking at. Medilectures in partnership with the UK Council of Clinical Communication in Undergraduate Medical Education offers a series of simulated consultations for medical students: www.ukccc.org.uk/consultations-e-learning
NHS Institute for Innovation and Improvement: Situation, background, assessment, recommendation: SBAR. http://www.institute.nhs.uk/safer_care/safer_care/Situation_Background_Assessment_Recommendation.html, 2011. (Accessed 27 January 2017).

Support for the international doctor

1. By far the best-known language textbook for those at an intermediate level of English is the following. Glendinning has worked in this area for many years: Glendinning EH, Holmström BAS: *English in Medicine*, Cambridge, 2005, Cambridge University Press.

2. There is a huge tradition in applied linguistics of support for reading and (especially) writing skills. In fact, most of what is known and taught is of value to doctors in their first language as well. A key text is: Swales JM, Feak CB: *Academic Writing for Graduate Students: Essential Tasks and Skills*, ed 2, Ann Arbor, MI, 2004, University of Michigan Press.

3. The concept of 'communicative competence' dates back to the following (quite technical) paper: Hymes D: On communicative competence. In Pride JB, Holmes J, editors: *Sociolinguistics: Selected Readings*, Harmondsworth, 1972, Penguin Books, pp. 269–293.
There is a strong tradition in the United States of support for IMGs based on collaborations between language teachers and medical educationalists. See, for example, English Language and the Medical Profession: Instructing and Assessing the Communication Skills of International Physicians. Emerald Group. Barbara J. Hoekje, Sara M. Tipton - 2011

Ethics and attitudes

T. C. Voo, C. H. Braddock III, J. Chin, A. Ho

Trends

- Medical ethics education should be integrated into the medical curriculum so that students can engage with ethics as a core aspect of good clinical care.
- Ethics teaching should include three dimensions: knowledge, habituation and action.
- Contemporary professional qualities as well as time-honoured virtues in medicine should both be fostered.
- Teaching and assessment should take into account stage of student development and type of learners.
- Challenges include countering the hidden curriculum, and demonstrating the effectiveness of ethics education in developing clinical ethical competence and its impact in improving patient care or outcomes.

Introduction

 Current accepted standards of medical ethics education:
Multidisciplinary and multi-professional
Academically rigorous and related to research
Fully integrated horizontally and vertically
Focused on clearly defined outcomes
Sound teaching methods and valid assessment.

Medical ethics has seen a remarkable development in the last three decades across the globe. There is international consensus that it should be an important part of any medical curriculum (WHO, 1995; WMA, 2005).

As the field 'comes of age' (Goldie et al., 2000; Miles et al., 1989), there is now wide acceptance that medical ethics education has to be multidisciplinary and multi-professional; academically rigorous and related to current research and debates in its field; and fully integrated into the medical curriculum, both horizontally (i.e. with the basic science and clinical teaching) and vertically (i.e. through all stages of a doctor's education from medical school, residency and continuing education), so that there is seamlessness between what is being taught at any given time and pertinent ethical issues, along with continuous reinforcement for professional growth.

Although the vast majority of medical schools teach medical ethics to some extent, there is considerable variation in terms of how it is taught, who teaches it and how frequently. These findings were reported by Mattick and Bligh (2006) in a survey of medical schools in the United Kingdom where, in spite of having a well-accepted core curriculum in medical ethics, there is wide diversity in teaching, assessment methods and staffing levels (GMC, 1993; Consensus Statement, 1998 [updated in Stirrat et al., 2010]). There is no clear and consistent picture in the current literature of the efficacy of existing forms of ethics education (Campbell et al., 2007).

This chapter illustrates the practical implementation of the current standards of medical ethics teaching, using the undergraduate curricula taught by the authors of this chapter as case studies. It also highlights the ethical values, skills and attitudes that the future practitioner must acquire, through a discussion of the critical challenges facing the medical profession. To nurture the ethical doctor, ethics education must be based on clearly defined outcomes and matching assessment methods in the key areas of students' ethical development, that is, knowledge, habituation and action. Theoretical and practical issues with the assessment of ethics and professional attitudes will be discussed.

Critical challenges

 Challenges for medical ethics education:
Profound social change and the meaning of professionalism
Global standards and cultural diversity
Countering the hidden curriculum.

CHALLENGE 1: THE CHANGING DOCTOR–PATIENT RELATIONSHIP

In the last 20 years, international trends to privatize medicine have nurtured a 'healthcare industry' aimed primarily at profit. This has created role conflicts for medical practitioners, who are caught between their responsibilities to patients and the notion of 'entrepreneurship' that encourages personal business acumen combined with loyalty to corporate employers (Breen, 2001).

Thus, the search for new standards by the medical profession has to focus on those values that distinguish medicine from business, that define fiduciary responsibilities to the vulnerable sick and that bind doctors together as a committed body of persons with judgement and stewardship of knowledge and skill (Pellegrino, 2002; Working Party of the Royal College of Physicians, 2005). To meet this challenge, medical ethics education must emphasize qualities that all patients look for in a practitioner: they seek a trustworthy advocate, committed first and foremost to patient welfare, empathetic, reflective and able to face up to the complexity of the rapidly changing world of medical practice. But today's doctors also have to be stewards of scarce resources: they should seek just uses of finite healthcare budgets that provide the best available healthcare for patients, balancing fee-for-service care to meet growing (and at times unrealistic) consumer demands with publicly provided healthcare (Michels, 1999). To do this, they have to create effective relationships with corporate administrators that preserve rather than absolve or diminish professional responsibility (Breen, 2001). This stewardship will also involve assessing the effectiveness of new healthcare delivery channels, including 'disruptive' technologies such as telemedicine and Internet medicine.

The changing doctor–patient relationship
"Until recently, physicians generally considered themselves accountable only to themselves, to their colleagues in the medical profession and, for religious believers, to God. Nowadays they have additional accountabilities – to their patients, to third parties such as hospitals and managed healthcare organizations, to medical licensing and regulatory authorities, and often to courts of law."

WMA, 2005

The growth of the pharmaceutical and biomedical research industries has exerted additional pressures on doctors' professionalism. As they are increasingly encouraged to help recruit patients for clinical trials and to occupy the often uneasy role of 'clinician researchers', a whole new range of ethical skills must be learned, such as medically responsible participant enrolment in approved randomized controlled trials, and research integrity.

CHALLENGE 2: CULTURAL PLURALISM

Globalized societies must deal with bewildering questions about the translation of standards and ethical paradigms across diverse cultural contexts. No wholesale application of global standards, including in medicine, is possible.

Multiculturalism
"The process of bridging the cultural divide does not imply uncritical acceptance of all cultural norms as being intrinsically equal, as there may not always be room for compromise. It does imply, however, that discussion about values should be open and transparent and that questions of cultural conflict arising from the inevitable collision of different paradigms of health, illness, society, law and morality should be debated in a critical and reflective manner."

Irvine et al., 2002

One implication of this for medical ethics is that patients will differ in their beliefs concerning matters such as human suffering and illness, obligations to others in decision making or the extent of interventions upon nature. Today's doctors must be prepared to test their own ethical beliefs and cultural assumptions against other cultural frameworks. But how will 'ethical contours' be discerned in a world that is increasingly flattened by late capitalist imperatives of individualism, universalism, commodification and unrelenting conquest of, and dissociation from, the natural world? Some emerging considerations include greater attention to deep and longstanding cultural values that place ethically and ecologically important limits on medical interventions; the relationships of family and community in the lives of individuals and their impact on decisions; the avoidance of cultural stereotypes and genuine embrace of an ethics of virtue that commands trust and values patient autonomy (through, for example, shared decision making), as contrasted with a mere ethics of obligation that emphasizes only procedural requirements in dealing with disagreement or outright conflict of values (Irvine et al., 2002).

CHALLENGE 3: THE POWER OF THE HIDDEN CURRICULUM

It has long been established that the 'hidden curriculum' can have harmful effects on the ethical development of medical students and junior doctors (Hafferty & Franks, 1994). While medical education professes explicit commitment to traditional values such as altruism, the milieu in which medicine is practiced may engender tacit, non-reflective acceptance of detachment and professional self-interest instead (Coulehan & Williams, 2001). This easily leads to a narrowing of professional identity to that of the competent technician, devaluing relational approaches to medicine. It is commonplace that medical graduates' spirits can be broken by the tough discipline of hospital managers and senior clinicians, and fair to say that the educational model of most hospital internship programmes may be likened to a hierarchical 'militaristic' command structure (Leeder, 2007). The 'soft' influence of pharmaceutical companies in undergraduate medical education is also an area of concern, particularly its effects on the practice of evidence-based medicine. Students' interaction with industry is found to be associated with positive attitudes towards industry marketing, including the reception of gifts, and scepticism about possible negative influence on their prescribing patterns (Austad et al., 2011).

Hidden curriculum – teaching teachers
"Character formation cannot be evaded by medical educators. Students enter medical school with their characters partly formed. Yet, they are still malleable as they assume roles and models on the way to their formation as physicians."

Pellegrino, 2002

How can this 'hidden curriculum' be countered? Part of the answer lies in the teacher–student relationship, which prefigures the student–patient relationship (Reiser, 2000). As Reiser puts it, "Students first learn about the use of authority in medicine from the faculty: how those with power and knowledge treat those who lack it." But beyond this, as he points out, there is enormous educational potential for good or ill in the policies and pronouncements of the medical school, its traditions and ceremonies, and the atmosphere of scientific, technical and ethical commitment that its entire staff in unison with administrative personnel creates. Formal ethics training can contribute to cultural reformation by encouraging critical and independent thinking and rejecting the false idea that seniority alone is a guarantee of ethical perceptiveness and considered judgement. That is why 'teaching the teachers' must be an integral part of medical ethics education.

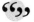

"As we expect greater professionalism from our students, we need to expect the same from teachers and organizational leaders. Anything else is disingenuous. For example, students have every right to expect that mistreatment by residents and faculty is taken just as seriously as unprofessional behaviour on the part of students."

Stern & Papadakis, 2006

Undergraduate education

ORGANIZING UNDERGRADUATE ETHICS EDUCATION

The nuts and bolts of setting up an ethics curriculum are best explained with reference to specific examples, and we focus here on the undergraduate medical school programme at the National University of Singapore's Yong Loo Lin School of Medicine (taught by Ho, Voo, Chin and Campbell); and the MD programme at the David Geffen School of Medicine at the UCLA (University of California, Los Angeles) (taught by Braddock).

National University of Singapore Yong Loo Lin School of Medicine (NUS YLLSoM)

NUS YLLSoM is an undergraduate medical school where students enter directly from high school (with the exception of male Singaporean citizens or residents, who are required to serve a compulsory 2-year National Service after high school unless they successfully applied for disruption to complete medical school). Recognizing that medical ethics is essential to achieving professionalism and excellence in patient care, YLLSoM established the Centre for Biomedical Ethics in 2007, whose main responsibility is to implement an integrated longitudinal track in Health Ethics, Law and Professionalism (HeLP) for the 5-year MBBS programme (Fig. 25.1). From setting course objectives and content to assessing student learning, a core collaborative group of bioethicists and clinicians (trained in medical ethics and law) designs and implements the curriculum. To emphasize the clinical relevance of HeLP, clinical educators from hospitals and private practices are also involved as lecturers and tutors throughout the longitudinal programme.

HeLP aims to develop students' sensitivity to the humanistic aspects of medicine; an understanding of the doctor–patient relationship and its ethics; knowledge of professional codes, ethical guidelines, laws and regulations that frame clinical decision making; the ability to apply ethical reasoning tools and approaches, taking into account relevant facts and competing or conflicting values of a given case; and professional attributes.

While it is accepted that medical ethics teaching is ultimately aimed at improving the quality of patient care, there is debate on whether the best way to achieve this aim is through character development or ensuring behavioural competencies (Carrese et al., 2015). HeLP blends the two schools of thought by specifying the attributes or 'virtues' (honesty and integrity; responsibility and participation; respect and sensitivity; compassion and empathy) deemed essential to medical professionalism, and entrustable professional activities (EPAs) for each attribute to form a basis of tracking and assessing curriculum outcomes and student competencies. EPAs define specific activities that students are expected to be able to perform, taking into account the amount of guidance needed at the end of each phase or year of their training. For example, as an EPA under the professional attribute of compassion and empathy, students should, with ample guidance, strive to understand patients' and families' physical and emotional needs

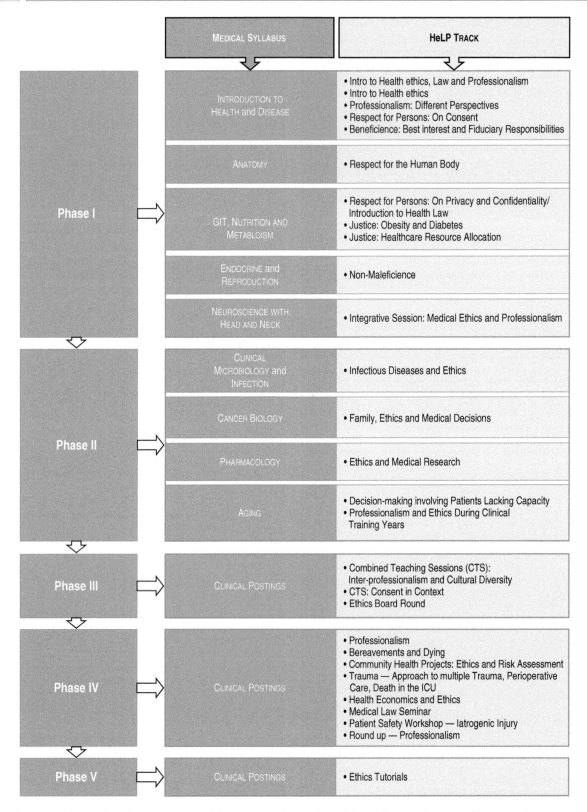

Fig. 25.1 Integration of ethics education into the medical curriculum at the National University of Singapore Yong Lin School of Medicine (Academic Year 2016-2017)

Table 25.1 EPA for compassion and empathy (professional attribute)

Compassion and empathy			
Strives to understand fellow students' needs and respond appropriately	4	4	4
Strives to understand patients' and families' physical and emotional needs	2	3	4
Strives to meet patients' and families' physical and emotional needs when appropriate	2	2	3
Reflects on observed caring attitudes toward patients in PBP* (as evidenced by contributions to discussion groups and reflection log)	3	-	-
Demonstrates a caring attitude toward patients (directly or as evidenced by feedback from staff and peers)	-	3	4

Standard: 1 = unable to achieve outcome; 2 = requires a lot of guidance to achieve outcome; 3 = requires little to moderate amount of guidance to achieve outcome; 4 = able to achieve outcome with no guidance (entrustment); 5 = has the ability to guide/teach others.
*PBP (patient-based program): A program that introduces early and meaningful patient contact to students through clinic/hospitals visits, patient narratives and case-based learning, and simulated/skills-lab training sessions.

at the end of both Phase I and Phase II, and they are entrusted (i.e. expected to achieve this outcome on their own) in Phase IV (Table 25.1).

In the pre-clinical years of Phases I and II, emphases are placed on facilitating identity formation as students begin their journey to become medical professionals, and promoting an understanding of pertinent bioethical principles as they apply to the broad ethical, legal and professional responsibilities of the medical student and doctor. Topics such as respect for the human body and persons, confidentiality and patient rights, the best interest of the patient, and justice in healthcare, are introduced in lectures and then strengthened in interactive and case-based tutorials.

Utilizing spiral learning that increases complexity and reinforces previous learning, our HeLP curriculum in the clinical years of Phases III to V provides more in-depth analysis of various ethical, legal and professional considerations as they arise in students' domestic and international clinical postings. Integrating conceptual understanding with practical guidance, students learn about professional and ethical issues and considerations as regards conscientious objections, international postings and mission trips, end-of-life care and allocation of life-sustaining interventions, patient safety and error disclosure etc.

David Geffen School of Medicine at UCLA (DGSOM)

Like most US medical schools, students matriculate after 4 years of undergraduate education, typically at a university. Hence, the typical medical student in the United States is in their early 20s, and many have life experiences beyond their schooling. These differences create a fundamentally different set of opportunities and challenges for medical education in ethics and professionalism. For example, even more than younger learners, these students are more clearly adult learners, and as such need even more explicit connections made between learning and recent or future real-world experiences. This and other observations about the adult learner have greatly informed the approach of medical education and ethics education in the United States.

At DGSOM, the medical curriculum incorporates principles of adult learning. Basic science teaching is organized not in discipline-based courses, such as physiology and biochemistry, but rather into integrated organ-based 'blocks', each of which provides instruction in complementary disciplines aligned around specific normal states of health and common disease states. Furthermore, the application of these scientific concepts is reinforced from the earliest weeks of medical school. One classic adult-learning-oriented approach that DGSOM uses is problem-based learning (PBL). Developed in the 1960s, PBL is a teaching method in which students working in groups are presented with clinical cases. As they move through interpretation of the clinical data, the group formulates 'learning issues', specific learner-originated topics for research and reading, the goal of which is to acquire new knowledge specifically to aid them in discernment of the appropriate differential diagnosis, evaluation, and management of a hypothetical patient. Furthermore, PBL begins to cultivate a mode of thinking that mirrors that of clinicians in practice – students are learning to 'think like doctors'.

It is in this context that we approach education in ethics and professional attitudes within DGSOM. Our curriculum has thematic 'threads' that have continuity across the first three years of medical school, and within which small-group exercises can take place. For example, a PBL case in which the teenager with a sexually transmitted illness who does not want their parents to know, can prompt learners to explore the ethics and legal dimensions of confidentiality, public health responsibilities for communicable disease reporting, and more. These conversations build on lectures and readings earlier in the curriculum that provide the foundation regarding ethical principles and professional values upon which rest subsequent learning.

In our 'Doctoring' thread, these small-group, learner-centred discussions continue, triggered by critical readings, cases, videos, standardized patient interview, and other prompts, facilitated by faculty trained to elicit reflection and learning that deepens conceptual understanding. In the third year of Doctoring, these groups become interprofessional, including nursing students, so that the focus can expand to include interprofessional interactions and teamwork. Finally, as fourth-year students, numerous team-based simulation activities are used, which stretch students to think as physicians and interact as a team, in high-fidelity simulation scenarios.

By embracing concepts of adult learning, we gain the advantage of learning guided by the learner's own sense of what they need to apply to a problem they are facing, and help prepare them to think on their feet. It also gives them valuable practice in small groups, learning how to interact professionally and respectfully with colleagues, a key value of professionalism.

Assessment of ethical and professional attitudes

FITTING OUTCOMES AND INNOVATIVE METHODS

Ethics education in a medical school should aim to create a valid programme for educating and certifying graduates who are knowledgeable, ethically sensitive and reflective and able to act with clinical ethical competence. These are key areas of a medical ethics education, the development of which can be illustrated with an ascending pyramid with specific learning outcomes and matching methods of assessment (Fig. 25.2). For example, at the YLLSoM, student assessments include selected short-answer and multiple-choice questions to test content knowledge for selected HeLP

topics in the overall final exams as well as case-based group presentations and objective structured clinical examinations (OSCE) to evaluate students' understanding and application of HeLP to clinical scenarios.

ASSESSMENT: SOME DIFFICULTIES

Much research is now focused on measuring medical professionalism and ethical attitudes, after a sustained period of scepticism about the possibility of making such assessments. Efforts in this area have led to better understanding of the limits of measurement (Parker, 2006), and a growing realization of the conceptual and practical issues involved in assessment (Self et al., 1992).

First, an interesting study by Hodges (2006) identified four models of competence found in competency assessments around the world: competence as knowledge, competence as performance, competence as reliable test score and competence as reflection. It discovered that overemphasis on an aspect of competency may lead to 'hidden incompetence', such as poor integration of knowledge with performance. For example, a student who had acquired knowledge competency but clearly displayed a kind of incompetence asked a patient, "Madam, do you have higher conjugated or unconjugated bilirubin?" Other types of hidden incompetence include a performance 'checklist' mentality and lack of appropriate interpersonal behaviour, merely producing portfolios without appropriate self-awareness and remedial self-learning. Critics of the reflection model have noted that self-assessment often correlates poorly with peer assessments, as well as performance (Hodges, 2006; Kaslow et al., 2007).

Secondly, there are also problems in assessment design. For example, clinical vignettes are often used to assess ethical sensitivity and reasoning, but there are unanswered questions about how these attributes can be properly measured, and whether ability to

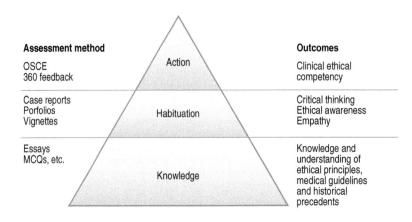

Fig. 25.2 Outcomes and assessment methods

(adapted from Miller GE: The assessment of clinical skills/competence/performance, Academic Medicine 65(9 Suppl):S63–S67, 1990).

analyze cases correlates to it (Herbert et al., 1992). No obvious connection has been shown between helping students to reason things out and defend their point of view and acting in an ethically acceptable manner in the future. Indeed, increase in reasoning ability seems a minimal criterion for measuring success in ethics education: necessary, no doubt, but is it sufficient? Goldie attempted to assess the effect of ethics teaching using an instrument he calls "consensus professional judgement". This was a set of vignettes in which there was a consensus on the best way of resolving a given dilemma, both from the literature and from experts who were consulted about the issues in the vignette. They were administered to measure how far ethics teaching improved the students' ability to make judgements that were consistent with what would be the judgement of the experts (Goldie et al., 2000).

Part of the solution in addressing these difficulties is helping students to integrate knowledge, skills, dispositions, self-perceptions, motives and belief-attitudes, and fostering the capacity for reflective lifelong learning (Kaslow et al., 2007).

The special nature of attitudes

While the possibility of objective measurement of competence is highly defensible so that no excuse can be made for failure to implement such assessments (Cruess & Cruess, 2006; Stern & Papadakis, 2006), it is important to note the special nature of attitudes and their evaluation. Parker points out that we can reasonably assume that students have basic attitudinal competence upon entry to medical school, but a requirement of positive demonstration of such competence across a slew of 'summative hurdles' assumes precisely the opposite! Assessment of attitudes, he argues, is rather like evaluating a person's decisional capacity, where it is up to the doctor to rebut the presumption of decision-making competence. It is easier to come to a consensus that a person lacks (falls below a certain threshold of) a capacity than to agree that he or she has it, and at what precise level. In practice, this type of assessment can be done by setting clear expectations of behaviour, training teachers to deal with issues of misconduct and providing a remedial mentoring program (Field, 2008). Repeated misdemeanours such as absenteeism, dishonesty, unreliability, disrespect or recalcitrance should trigger a need to decide whether a student fails the ethics and professionalism course. Consensus is usually not difficult at this point, as Parker observes (Parker, 2006).

Consistent expectations

The medical school's programme of certifying students professionally competent should be consistent with expectations of professionalism later in their careers (Carrese et al., 2015). Standards should therefore be congruent with those of licensing boards, but levels of competency must be adjusted suitably in line with student experience.

Summary: effecting culture shift

Medical ethics education is in a progressive phase, and ideas about implementation are burgeoning. Success in medical ethics education is measured in terms of producing ethically reflective, self-regulating doctors. To this end, a culture shift towards concerted teaching and assessment of professional attitudes and ethical behaviour must be affected.

References

Austad, K.E., Avorn, J., Kesselheim, A.S., 2011. Medical students' exposure to and attitudes about the pharmaceutical industry: a systematic review. PLoS Med. 8 (5), e1001037.

Breen, K.J., 2001. The patient–doctor relationship in the new millennium: adjusting positively to commercialism and consumerism. Clin. Dermatol. 19 (1), 19–22.

Campbell, A.V., Chin, J., Voo, T.C., 2007. How can we know that ethics education produces ethical doctors? Med. Teach. 29 (5), 431–436.

Carrese, J.A., Malek, J., Watson, K., et al., 2015. The essential role of medical ethics education in achieving professionalism: the Romanell Report. Acad. Med. 90 (6), 744–752.

Consensus Statement by Teachers of Medical Ethics and Law in UK Medical Education, 1998. Teaching medical ethics and law within medical schools: a model for the UK core curriculum. J. Med. Ethics 24 (3), 188–192.

Coulehan, J., Williams, P.C., 2001. Vanquishing virtue: the impact of medical education. Acad. Med. 76 (6), 598–605.

Cruess, R.L., Cruess, S.R., 2006. Teaching professionalism: general principles. Med. Teach. 28 (3), 205–208.

Field, L., 2008. Deciding when students are not fit to practice. Student BMJ. 16, 64–65.

General Medical Council, 1993. Tomorrow's Doctors: Recommendations on Undergraduate Medical Education. GMC, London.

Goldie, J., Schwartz, L., Morrison, J., 2000. A process evaluation of medical ethics education in the first year of a new curriculum. Med. Educ. 34 (6), 468–473.

Hafferty, F.W., Franks, R., 1994. The hidden curriculum, ethics teaching, and the structure of medical education. Acad. Med. 69 (11), 861–871.

Herbert, P.C., Meslin, E.M., Dunn, E.V., 1992. Measuring the ethical sensitivity of medical students:

a study at the university of Toronto. J. Med. Ethics 18 (3), 142–147.

Hodges, B., 2006. Medical education and the maintenance of incompetence. Med. Teach. 28 (8), 690–696.

Irvine, R., McPhee, J., Kerridge, I.H., 2002. The challenge of cultural and ethical pluralism to medical practice. Med. J. Aust. 176 (4), 175–176.

Kaslow, N.J., Rubin, N.J., Bebeau, M.J., et al., 2007. Guiding principles and recommendations for the assessment of competence. Prof. Psychol. Res. Pr. 38 (5), 441–451.

Leeder, S.R., 2007. Preparing interns for practice in the 21st century. Med. J. Aust. 186 (7).

Mattick, K., Bligh, J., 2006. Teaching and assessing medical ethics: Where are we now? J. Med. Ethics 32 (3), 181–185.

Michels, R., 1999. Medical education and managed care. NEJM 340 (12), 959–961.

Miles, S.H., Lane, L.W., Bickel, J., et al., 1989. Medical ethics education: coming of age. Acad. Med. 64 (12), 705–714.

Miller, G.E., 1990. The assessment of clinical skills/competence/performance. Acad. Med. 65 (9 Suppl.), S63–S67.

Parker, M., 2006. Assessing professionalism: theory and practice. Med. Teach. 28 (5), 399–403.

Pellegrino, E.D., 2002. Professionalism, profession and the virtues of the good physician. Mt. Sinai J. Med. 69 (6), 378–384.

Reiser, S.J., 2000. Wear, D., Bickel, J. (Eds.), Educating for Professionalism: Creating a Culture of Humanism in Medical Education. University of Iowa Press, Iowa.

Self, D.J., Baldwin, D.C. Jr., Wolinsky, F.D., 1992. Evaluation of teaching medical ethics by an assessment of moral reasoning. Med. Educ. 26 (3), 178–184.

Stern, D.T., Papadakis, M., 2006. The developing physician health ethics, law and professionalism becoming a professional. NEJM 355, 1794—1799.

Stirrat, G.M., et al., 2010. Medical ethics and law for doctors of tomorrow: the 1998 Consensus Statement updated. J. Med. Ethics 36 (1), 55–60.

WHO, 1995. The Teaching of Medical Ethics: Fourth Consultation with Leading Medical Practitioners. World Health Organization, Geneva.

WMA, World Medical Association: Medical Ethics Manual. Ferney, Voltaire, France/Online. Available at: http://www.wma.net, 2005.

Working Party of the Royal College of Physicians: Doctors in Society: Medical Professionalism in a Changing World, London, 2005.

Professionalism

H. M. O'Sullivan

Trends

- Interest in students' and junior doctors' professionalism online, especially on social media sites
- Increasing awareness of the cultural dimensions of professionalism
- Focus on developing and assessing emotional competence as part of professionalism

Introduction

Medical professionalism is now widely accepted as a key part of medical education and often features directly or indirectly in the educational standards of national medical bodies. As far back as Ancient Greece, the Hippocratic Oath symbolized the regard that is paid by the medical professional to the standards that it expects of its members. However, although its importance is well understood, finding ways to integrate the development of professionalism into the curriculum and then measuring its achievement remains a challenge. It is arguably easier to identify students who exhibit unprofessional behaviour and the importance of identifying students who are not fit to practise has been in focus in recent years.

 "Professional status is not an inherent right, but is granted by society."

Cruess & Cruess, 1997

This gained even more importance when Maxine Papadakis (Papadakis et al., 2004) presented evidence of a link between unprofessional behaviour in medical school and subsequent poor performance or unethical behaviour in practice. There is a risk that professionalism is defined negatively and that the opportunity for students to develop and be assessed on positive behaviours is lost. This chapter will outline some of the ways that educators can integrate the development

and assessment of professionalism into their curricula.

Defining professionalism

The first task when integrating professionalism into the curriculum is to agree on a definition acceptable to the institution that you are working in. A quick search of the literature will make it clear that professionalism has been defined in many different ways. There is still a lack of complete consensus. Within your institution, setting the values intrinsic to professionalism in the context of the changing societal pressures on medicine and healthcare in your country, culture and institution is essential. This section gives a brief roundup of the different approaches to defining professionalism but for a more complete account see van Mook et al., 2009c or Birden, et al., 2014.

 "In simple words, professionalism means the skill, good judgement and polite behavior expected from a trained person in order to do the job well, namely good conduct."

Mahmood et al., 2015

Public perceptions of the role of the doctor have changed. This has been reflected in an increasing focus in the media on the behaviour and role of healthcare practitioners (van Mook et al., 2009c). The rapid expansion of medical knowledge and skills, the revolution in information technology, the desire for more equal engagement between patients and healthcare practitioners, multidisciplinary teamwork and the diversity of healthcare providers in different parts of the world, all challenge the power originally held by doctors. At the same time, profound changes have taken place within the workforce itself with reduction in working hours and changes in doctors' attitudes to their vocation as more emphasis is placed on the quality of life outside work; all these impact on the original understanding of medicine as a vocation (van Mook et al., 2009c; Cruess et al., 2015).

In the 1980s the American Board of Internal Medicine (ABIM) started to focus on the humanitarian aspects of a doctor's work. This resulted in *Project Professionalism* a decade later. The ABIM attempted to spell out what professionalism means to contemporary society. They identified key elements: altruism, accountability, duty, excellence, honour, integrity and respect for others (Project Professionalism, 2002). The move was influential. Medical schools became increasingly aware that professionalism should have an explicit place in the curriculum, and by 2006 most UK medical schools were reporting that professionalism was part of the curriculum (Stephenson et al., 2006).

> *"Unprofessional behaviours are known to be associated with impediment of communication, collaboration, information transfer, and workplace relationships, poor adherence to guidelines, low staff morale and turnover, medical errors, adverse outcomes and with malpractice suits."*
>
> *van Mook et al., 2015, p 559.*

In 2005, the Royal College of Physicians produced a report that described the nature and role of medical professionalism at a time when the UK healthcare system was undergoing enormous change. Six major themes emerged in the report: leadership, teamworking, education, career pathways, appraisal and research. The report set the tone for UK definition and frameworks with the statement that "Medical professionalism signifies a set of values, behaviours and relationships that underpin the trust the public has in doctors." (Royal College of Physicians, 2005). Other useful frameworks from around this time were provided by Hilton and Slotnick (2005) and Arnold and Stern (2006).

> *"Our current understanding of professionalism is further complicated by the fact that the literature largely reflects a Western (Anglo-Saxon) notion of professionalism."*
>
> *Jha et al., 2015*

Yet, to date there is no common understanding of what the term *professionalism* actually means. The North American approach views professionalism as a mainly theoretical construct, described in abstract idealistic terms, mirroring character traits rather than observable behaviours. Common elements are altruism, respect for others, honour, integrity, ethical and moral standards, accountability, excellence and duty. These terms are easily identifiable and difficult to challenge but are not very concrete or specific. They do not translate into tangible measurable learning outcomes. In contrast, a move to frame professionalism as observable behaviours from which norms and values can be visualized stems from the Netherlands. This offers advantages for assessment (van Mook et al., 2009a).

However, the complexity of the relationship between external professional behaviour and internal attitudinal values remains poorly understood. There has been some recent interest in the role that psychological models such as emotional intelligence might play in developing professionalism (Cherry et al., 2012, 2014).

Setting expectation: agreeing a framework for professionalism

Once the definition of 'professionalism' for the context of your environment has been agreed, the next step is to ensure faculty, students and other key stakeholders understand the definition and agree with it. Areas where there are differences of opinion should be highlighted at an early stage and resolved so that there is a common consensus and understanding of the values that are articulated. The exercise itself develops a sense of ownership for the integration of professionalism into the curriculum. Holding a workshop where faculty, students and junior doctors develop a shared code of conduct for everyone to abide by can help with student engagement and can also be used to call attention to faculty or clinical colleagues whose own behaviour occasionally falls short of expected standards.

Role model the positive behaviours that you wish to observe in your students.

It is important to pay particular attention to the professional guidelines in operation in your country, if in existence. For institutions where there is an existing framework, it is useful to have a refresher session every few years to ensure that the understanding of the professional values is still shared and agreed. At the end of this process you will almost certainly have a number of areas or domains of professionalism in which you would like your students to demonstrate a threshold standard. It is then important to set standards and generate outcomes in these domains. Some of these will be developed across the whole of the programme (such as communication or ethics) whilst others (such as adherence to code of practice, rules of confidentiality) might require competency at the programme threshold standard to be demonstrated by the end of year one.

> *"Despite radically different cultural and healing traditions, physicians around the globe subscribe to professional values."*
>
> *Arnold & Stern, 2006*

Setting out these outcomes as clearly stated observable behaviours in a framework is essential. The institution's expectations can be made very clear to students at the beginning of the programme and provide the stimulus for students to contribute to the planning of their professional development. It enables students to understand from the beginning of their studies that the standards of behaviour expected are different to those of non-vocational students. In countries where students enrol for medical school straight from school, this expectation of high demonstrable standards of professional behaviour at all times presents a rather stark contrast to their peers on other courses. Graduates who have already had the more liberal freedom of university and hold greater life experience may well be at an advantage but there is no firm evidence to suggest this is the case. Activities at the beginning of a programme such as lectures from senior faculty and students taking a public, professional oath of ethical conduct can help bring home the message about the behaviour that is expected.

Once definitions and standards are agreed, it is possible to review the existing learning opportunities in the curriculum and map these onto the professionalism framework. Opportunities for developing professionalism should be clearly identified and be appropriate for the stage of development of the student. There are lots of innovative ways to develop professionalism; for a review see van Mook et al., 2009b.

Developing a culture of professionalism: role modelling and the hidden curriculum

However professionalism is defined, the state of being a professionals is conceived as a set of behaviours, values and attributes that are developed over time. Students don't simple pass a professionalism test and become a professional. Hilton and Slotnick coined the term 'proto-professionalism' to describe the lengthy state in which the learner develops the skills and experiences that they need in order to be a professional. They suggest that a key component of being a professional is the acquisition of *phronesis*; a practical type of wisdom that can only be gained through experience. So, while it is possible for a student to behave in a professional way, at this stage, they are proto-professionals (Hilton & Slotnick, 2005).

 "To remain trustworthy, professionals must meet the obligations expected by society."

Cruess & Cruess, 1997

In discussing the development of professionalism Hilton and Slotnik developed a model (Fig. 26.1).

In this model there are two types of forces that influence the development of the proto-professional. *Attainment* is the acquisition of positive professional values and behaviours that result from observing positive role models and reflecting on experiences in a positive environment. *Attrition* is the development of negative behaviours and values or the seeping away of positive values through proximity to negative role models and a damaging culture. If the balance of influences is towards attainment then students and developing doctors finally reach the stage of phronesis and professionalism. If the prevailing influences are negative then the students' natural idealism on entering training can be turned into cynicism, self-interest and even self-preservation.

Educators therefore need to pay attention to values and behaviours that students see in the educational or training setting and (importantly) in clinical practice.

 Provide a safe space for medical students and junior doctors to debrief and reflect when they have witnessed unprofessional behaviour.

The unwritten and unintended lessons that medical students learn from their interactions with educators, peers, clinical supervisors and other clinical staff is known as the hidden curriculum as these lessons are often unacknowledged. It can be problematic because the values and behaviours on display can be contradictory to the values and behaviours being espoused in the formal curriculum causing students to be confused and in conflict about which code of behaviour to follow. The problems of the hidden curriculum and the necessity of identifying the impact that it has on the education and training of junior doctors has been well established (Hafferty, 1998), but it has been questioned recently whether this is now such a problem, given that so much scrutiny has ensured these issues are now far from hidden (MacLeod, 2014). Regardless of this debate, educators need to acknowledge and identify factors that might be contributing to attrition in Hilton and Slotnick's model and ensure students have the opportunity to reflect on these and discuss their impact. There are many ways to achieve this but reflective logs, critical incidence reporting and small-group discussions can all help.

 Use a workshop format to agree a code of conduct for students and faculty.

The faculty and clinical staff that we trust with educating our students and trainees need to demonstrate professional behaviour themselves and provide positive role models. It can be difficult to address this issue directly, but through staff development sessions that discuss teaching and assessment of professionalism, the values and behaviours that we expect to see demonstrated to our students can be emphasised and addressed.

 Using clips from medical dramas such as *ER* and *House* can stimulate group discussions about professionalism.

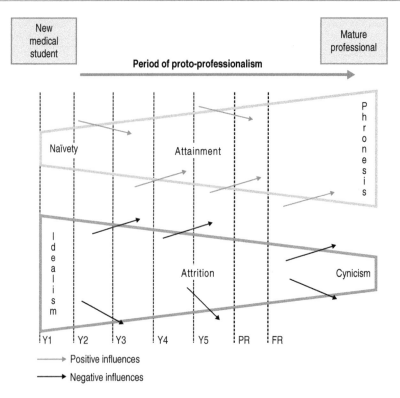

Fig. 26.1 Proto-professionalism.

(From Hilton, S. R. and Slotnick H. B: Proto-professionalism: how professionalization occurs across the continuum of medical education, Medical Education 39(1): 58–65, 2005.) Reproduced with permission.

The model of proto-professionalism also highlights the importance of developing and assessing professionalism in ways that are appropriate for the stage of education or training. Students' psychosocial and moral development as well as their judgement and reflective skills will proceed at different rates throughout their training. By creating teaching materials and assessments that acknowledge this staged approach, students can demonstrate that they have developed the incremental stages needed to become a full professional.

Digital professionalism

For the last 15 years or so, medical educators have been evolving ways to define and develop professionalism in students and trainees and during this time, the proliferation of social media has changed the way that we interact online. The fundamental principles and behaviours that we expect are the same but the way that these are expressed through social media can give rise to new problems in professionalism. These issues can be grouped into three main areas:

Reputational issues – bringing the school, university or healthcare institution into disrepute though online activity or comments that would be seen as inappropriate or offensive by members of the public.

Privacy – the same principles of confidentiality and privacy apply to online activity, but the ubiquity of cameras on mobile devices as well as the instantaneousness of platforms such as Twitter can turn inexperienced indiscretion into a national scandal.

Distraction – social media has a beneficial presence in a healthcare setting but it is also an opportunity for distraction, which can lead to loss of productivity and potentially, medical errors.

In addition, things that were reasonably straightforward in the past such as professional boundaries and professional identity can be blurred if patients or colleagues become part of your social network.

 Don't wait until there is an 'incident' on social media to educate students on digital professionalism.

Appropriate use of social media and other online activities should form a part of any professionalism framework and professionalism curriculum. Medical educators have a fantastic opportunity to help students and trainees to understand the value and pitfalls of being online, but this can be tricky if the educators feel that they know less about current trends in social media than the students! In addition, students and younger trainees appear to be tech savvy but have often grown up without questioning the amount of information that they are sharing or the appropriateness of it.

Educating faculty on social media

A good place to start is by holding a workshop to educate faculty on the most common forms of social media, how they are used and how privacy settings work. It can also be helpful to examine case material where there have been unintended consequences of online activity and look at some common pitfalls that students might get into. A useful activity is to challenge each other to find material online that pertains to you or your colleagues' social or family life. This can have a sobering effect on the participant and cause them to attend to their own privacy settings!

BUILDING IN GUIDANCE ON THE USE OF SOCIAL MEDIA

Many schools, universities and healthcare workplaces now have guidelines on the professional use of social media, but if yours doesn't you should develop guidance so that you can give your students and trainees clear expectations of the behaviour that you expect. Some international medical associations have published their guidance; the one below is from the British Medical Association but there are similar ones from the Canadian Medical Association (http://policybase.cma.ca/dbtw-wpd/Policypdf/PD12-03.pdf) the General Medical Council (http://www.gmc-uk.org/guidance/ethical_guidance/21186.asp) and the
American Medical Association (http://journalofethics.ama-assn.org/2015/05/nlit1-1505.html)

 Guidance for doctors on the use of social media from the British Medical Association (BMA)
- *Social media can blur the boundary between an individual's public and professional lives*
- *Doctors and medical students should consider adopting conservative privacy settings where these are available, but be aware that not all information can be protected on the web*
- *The ethical and legal duty to protect patient confidentiality applies equally on the Internet as to other media*
- *It would be inappropriate to post informal, personal or derogatory comments about patients or colleagues on public Internet forums*
- *Doctors and medical students who post online have an ethical obligation to declare any conflicts of interest*
- *The BMA recommends that doctors and medical students should not accept Facebook*

friend requests from current or former patients
- *Defamation law can apply to any comments posted on the web made in either a personal or professional capacity*
- *Doctors and medical students should be conscious of their online image and how it may impact on their professional standing.*

BMA, 2011

Assessing professionalism

Given that assessment is a powerful stimulant for learning, it is important to find ways to assess professionalism that are robust, defensible, reliable and valid.

 "Our failure to measure professionalism sends a conflicting message to both students and practicing physicians."
Arnold & Stern, 2006, p 5

A single, definitive tool for assessing professionalism has not been identified but there are several common approaches including peer assessment, direct observation by faculty, reflective portfolios, critical incident report and objective structured clinical examinations. A summary of the types of assessment methods and their uses can be found in the article on assessing professionalism by van Mook and colleagues (van Mook et al., 2009a). More important than choosing individual tools is to think about the assessment strategy for professionalism. Should you assess professionalism as an overall construct or build up a picture through assessments of individual components? Who should assess professionalism: faculty, clinical tutors, peers, patients? Individual assessment tools may measure different things or have lower validity than more traditional methods but through triangulation a robust summative assessment can be built up of an individual student.

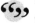 *"They don't respect what you expect, they respect what you inspect."*
p v Jordan Cohen (Arnold & Stern, 2006)

Lambert Schuwirth has written extensively on the subject of programmatic assessment (most recently, Heeneman et al., 2015), which is intended to maximize the benefits of learning to the student and enable schools to make more informed summative decisions about the students' demonstration of the programme outcomes. This approach can be used to assess professionalism even if there is not a full programmatic assessment strategy in the school. Students gain meaningful feedback from assessment activities to enable them to learn and develop and to gain ownership of their learning so that their performance can be better in the next assessment. As students become more mature and used to this approach they can direct their own learning and have some say in selecting the development activities that they need to undertake. This longitudinal flow of information about learners replaces a single high-stakes assessment. More practical advice on how to implement programmatic assessment can be found in van Der Vleuten et al., 2015.

Most people working in medical education will be familiar with 'Miller's Pyramid' (Miller, 1990) – a way of visualizing the stages that are needed in a competency-based education model. The stages of knows (knowledge), knows how (competency), shows how (performance) and does (action) has been enormously influential in shaping assessment strategies in medical education in general, and particularly important in assessing professionalism. Cruess et al. (2016) have recently suggested that Miller's Pyramid should have an additional layer on top of the pyramid, namely, *is (being)*. This layer represents professional identity and the complete integration of professional values and beliefs that are essential to professional behaviour. Wide acceptance of their suggestion would add a useful dimension to the way that professionalism might be assessed with the development of tools specifically designed to measure the acquisition of a defined professional identity.

Summary

Professionalism is now considered to be a routine part of the medical curriculum but there is no agreed definition, and the values and behaviours that educators want to develop in students and trainees can vary depending on the cultural context. Many national medical bodies have professionalism codes and requirements, and it is important to reach an agreed and widely shared understanding of professionalism for your students, faculty and clinical colleagues. Teaching and assessing professionalism is most effective when it is integrated into the curriculum and there should be a variety of learning opportunities and ways for students to learn from formative feedback before summative assessments are made. Specific guidance on digital professionalism with reflection on case studies can help students navigate social media without causing themselves or their profession any reputational damage. It is important to develop robust summative assessments that are respected by students and that test observable behaviours. It must be possible for students to 'fail' professionalism if attempts at remediation and support are to no avail as there is a link between unprofessional behaviour in medical school and practice. The key to establishing appropriate development opportunities is setting a culture of professionalism through positive role modelling and calling attention to unprofessional behaviour by students, faculty or clinical colleagues.

References

Arnold, L., Stern, D.T., 2006. What is medical professionalism? In: Stern, D.T. (Ed.), Measuring medical professionalism. Oxford University Press, New York, pp. 15–37.

Birden, H., Glass, N., Wilson, I., et al., 2014. Defining professionalism in medical education: a systematic review. Med. Teach. 36 (1), 47–61.

Cherry, M.G., Fletcher, I., O'Sullivan, H., Dornan, T., 2014. Emotional intelligence in medical education: a critical review. Med. Educ. 48 (5), 468–478.

Cherry, M.G., Fletcher, I., O'Sullivan, H., Shaw, N., 2012. What impact do structured educational sessions to increase emotional intelligence have on medical students? BEME Guide No. 17. Med. Teach. 34 (1), 11–19.

Cruess, R.L., Cruess, S.R., Steinert, Y., 2016. Amending Miller's pyramid to include professional identity formation. Acad. Med. 91 (2), 180–185.

Hafferty, F.W., 1998. Beyond curriculum reform: confronting medicine's hidden curriculum. Acad. Med. 73 (4), 403–407.

Heeneman, S., Oudkerk Pool, A., Schuwirth, L.W.T., et al., 2015. The impact of programmatic assessment on student learning: theory versus practice. Med. Educ. 49 (5), 487–498.

Hilton, S.R., Slotnick, H.B., 2005. Proto-professionalism: how professionalisation occurs across the continuum of medical education. Med. Educ. 39 (1), 58–65.

Jha, V., McLean, M., Gibbs, T., Sandars, J., 2015. Medical professionalism across cultures: A challenge for medicine and , medical educators. Med. Teach. 37, 1–7.

MacLeod, A., 2014. The hidden curriculum: is it time to re-consider the concept? Med. Teach. 36 (6), 539–540.

Miller, G.E., 1990. The assessment of clinical skills/competence/performance. Acad. Med. 65 (9 Suppl.), S63–S67.

Papadakis, M.A., Hodgson, C.S., Teherani, A., Kohatsu, N.D., 2004. Unprofessional behavior in medical school is associated with subsequent disciplinary action by a state medical board. Acad. Med. 79 (3), 244–249.

Project Professionalism, M. P., 2002. Medical professionalism in the new millennium: a physicians' charter. Lancet 359 (9305), 520–522.

Royal College of Physicians, 2005. Doctors In Society: Medical Professionalism in a Changing World. London, Royal College of Physicians, Report of a Working Party.

Stephenson, A.E., Adshead, L.E., Higgs, R.H., 2006. The teaching of professional attitudes within UK medical schools: reported difficulties and good practice. Med. Educ. 40 (11), 1072–1080.

van Der Vleuten, C., Schuwirth, L., Driessen, E., et al.,
2015. Twelve tips for programmatic assessment.
Med. Teach. 37 (7), 641–646.

van Mook, W.N., Gorter, S.L., O'Sullivan, H., et al.,
2009a. Approaches to professional behaviour
assessment: tools in the professionalism toolbox. Eur.
J. Intern. Med. 20 (8), e153–e157.

van Mook, W.N., van Luijk, S.J., de Grave, W., et al.,
2009b. Teaching and learning professional

behavior in practice. Eur. J. Intern. Med. 20 (5),
e105–e111.

van Mook, W.N., van Luijk, S.J., O'Sullivan, H.,
et al., 2009c. The concepts of professionalism and
professional behaviour: conflicts in both definition
and learning outcomes. Eur. J. Intern. Med. 20 (4),
e85–e89.

Evidence-based medicine

L. A. Maggio

Trends

- Evidence-based medicine (EBM) instruction is a fixture in medical student training.
- EBM instructors are encouraged to be flexible in selecting teaching modalities that best fit the needs of their learners and institutions.
- The optimal teaching of EBM may require development of faculty EBM skills and teaching approaches.

Introduction

Because of the continually expanding availability of biomedical information, it is not possible for physicians to rely on the information they learned in their medical training to deliver optimal patient care. Instead, physicians must act as lifelong learners continually seeking and integrating new evidence into their practice. In the early 1990s, evidence-based medicine (EBM) was proposed to help physicians bridge this gap between their current knowledge and the increasingly available biomedical evidence. Now associated with physicians' lifelong learning skills and improved patient care, EBM has become an expectation of clinical practice and a fixture in medical education training (Tilson et al., 2011).

 EBM is *"the conscientious, explicit and judicious use of the best current evidence in making decisions about the care of individual patients".*

Sackett et al., 1996

The practice of EBM and EBM training initiatives are often characterized by the following steps of EBM:

- Asking a clinical question related to a knowledge gap
- Acquiring information to fill the gap
- Appraising the found information
- Applying the found evidence in conjunction with clinical expertise, and the patient's values

- Assessing practice.
  Dawes et al., 2005

These steps have commonly been referred to as the 5As. However, educators have suggested a sixth A or precursor step be added, which recognizes the importance of practitioners and learners acknowledging knowledge gaps in their practice. Dubbed 'Step Zero' this recognition of knowledge gaps further aligns EBM with learner and practitioner needs to act as self-regulated learners.

Currently there is no gold standard approach for teaching EBM to medical students and the recognized steps of EBM are taught to varying degrees (Maggio et al., 2013). For example, one institution might require students to attend multiple EBM lectures that focus on critical appraisal, another might feature hands-on sessions in computer labs that tackle all the steps of EBM, and yet another may introduce EBM by challenging students to identify and answer clinical questions derived from their clerkship experiences. This lack of standardization has resulted in calls for centralized EBM teaching guidelines (Blanco et al., 2014). However, recent systematic reviews of the EBM teaching methods have concluded that based on current evidence there is no clear superior approach to teaching EBM, therefore making it difficult to promote such standards (Ilic & Maloney, 2014; Ahmadi et al., 2015). Yet, on the flip side this allows EBM instructors great flexibility in selecting and implementing teaching modalities that best fit their institutions' and learners' needs.

 Consider the unique needs of your institution and learners when selecting an approach to EBM teaching.

In this chapter we present a variety of approaches to teaching EBM, presenting evidence of efficacy when possible, to familiarize medical educators with common approaches and enable them to select those relevant to their needs. This chapter focuses on broad approaches to teaching EBM and does not zoom in on training approaches particular to EBM skills. See Table 27.1 for examples of step-focused learning exercises that could be integrated into the below broader approaches. We also address who is teaching EBM, the timing of

Table 27.1 Examples of EBM step-focused learning exercises

EBM step	Learning exercise
Acknowledge	During a clerkship rotation, students are required to identify a knowledge gap for each patient that they manage.
Ask	Using a video of a patient encounter, students are asked to develop a clinical question that includes the patient, intervention, comparison, if appropriate, and the patient's hoped-for outcome.
Acquire	Students are given three clinical questions and challenged to retrieve relevant evidence from three different information resources.
Appraise	Students are provided a randomized controlled clinical trial and challenged to critically appraise its clinical value.
Apply	Prior to a standardized patient encounter, students are provided evidence, asked to appraise it, and then engage in making a shared decision with the patient based on the evidence.
Assess	Following a clerkship, students are asked to write or record a short reflection on how the integration of particular evidence impacted the recent rotation and how they think it may impact their future practice.

EBM training, resources for teaching EBM, the assessment of EBM skills, and potential future directions for EBM training.

Approaches to teaching EBM

BUILDING-BLOCK APPROACH

EBM is often taught in relation to its steps, with some educationalists advocating for an atomistic or building-block approach. Using a building-block approach, instructors present each EBM step discretely and then after practising these steps independently expect that leaners will be able to assemble the steps to execute the complete process of EBM. For example, an instructor might present their medical students with a series of EBM sessions such that the students are presented a session on formulating clinical questions in their first term, followed the next term with a session on literature searching, and then several sessions on critical appraisal and application of evidence later in their curriculum. After these step-focused practise opportunities, students are challenged to piece together the discrete steps in a capstone session or assignment.

Building-block approaches provide learners opportunities to master each step of the process over time and buffer them from being overwhelmed when being introduced to new skills. However, building-block approaches have been associated with fragmentation of knowledge and difficulties in transferring knowledge from different contexts (van Merriënboer & Kirschner, 2013) suggesting that EBM educators may want to consider the use of this approach in conjunction with other strategies.

WHOLE-TASK APPROACH

In contrast to the building-block approach, EBM educators also utilize using whole-task approaches, which have been associated with increased transfer of knowledge (van Merriënboer & Kirschner, 2013). Whole-task approaches challenge learners to undertake all the component steps of a task in a cohesive manner. In the context of EBM, a learner might be provided a clinical case and be asked in a single session to formulate a clinical question, locate and appraise relevant evidence, consider how the evidence might integrate into their care of the patient, and evaluate this experience in light of their current and future practice. In this ways, whole-task approaches provide learners a holistic model of how EBM is practiced, which can more easily transfer from one situation to another as is needed in clinical care.

 For further information on designing and implementing whole-task approaches consult Dolman's "twelve tips" article (Dolmans et al., 2013), and the related AMEE Guide (Vandewaetere et al., 2015).

INTEGRATION WITH OTHER COURSES AND CONTENT

EBM is generally integrated with other courses and content. For example, some institutions introduce and teach EBM within the context of their problem-based learning curriculum, which is felt to promote overlapping skills sets such as the ability to effectively recognize knowledge gaps and search the biomedical literature. Additionally, some institutions teach EBM alongside other curricular topics such as shared decision making, ethics, biostatistics and clinical exam skills. This integration provides learners multiple opportunities to practise EBM, allows learners to observe synergies between EBM and other topics, and in some cases does not require the addition of extra sessions to already packed curricula. The integration of EBM with other content has been linked to improving learners' attitudes towards EBM, satisfaction with EBM training, and attainment of EBM knowledge (Ilic & Maloney, 2014).

CLINICAL INTEGRATION

EBM training is frequently integrated with clinical experiences, which has been demonstrated to have a slight positive effect on students' EBM skills (Ahmadi et al., 2015). Clinical integration is commonly achieved by integrating EBM into clerkship experiences, including daily patient care tasks, but has also been described in early clinical preceptorship experiences (Maggio et al., 2013). For example, a student in their paediatrics clerkship may be required to complete an assignment that requires that they identify a gap in their knowledge based on a patient encounter and carryout the steps of EBM, including sharing their findings with their patient care team. To support clerkship integration, some institutions have reported incorporating EBM training into their transition to clerkship curriculum courses to refresh learners' EBM skills (Maggio et al., 2016). Clinical integration has also been achieved by inviting clerkship students to actively participate in student-run or departmental journal clubs that incorporate and emphasize the elements of EBM, such as locating biomedical information and its critical appraisal. In some cases, medical students are tasked with particular responsibilities within the structure of the journal club, such as the search and retrieval of the relevant evidence.

COMPUTER ASSISTED AND ONLINE LEARNING APPROACH

Computer assisted and online learning approaches for teaching EBM have been found to be as efficacious as delivering EBM training using in-person approaches (Ahmadi et al., 2015) and provide instructors increased flexibility in their content delivery. Examples of computer assisted and online EBM training include online tutorials, recorded videos, podcasts, web-based worksheets, clinical question banks, and EBM subject guides. In some cases, online training stands alone; however, EBM is more generally taught using a model that blends both in-person and online approaches. For example, following the trend of the flipped classroom model, online materials are increasingly being used to prepare students for in-class sessions in which the learners will be challenged to apply the content delivered in the online materials. In many cases, instructors using this approach are utilizing videos that introduce foundational EBM skills and/or feature EBM practitioners describing their clinical use of EBM. The use of these materials enables instructors to decompress in-class time, provide flexibility for students to choose when to complete training, alleviate scheduling difficulties for faculty, and reach learners at clinical sites that may be at a distance.

 Ask students about technologies they use to keep track of knowledge gaps. Consider adopting them in your instruction.

Timing of EBM

There is no consensus on the ideal timing of EBM training for medical students. Some institutions offer EBM early in the pre-clerkship phases of their curriculum, while others wait until students are immersed in clinical activities in their clerkship rotations. In some rare instances, institutions take a longitudinal approach to providing EBM instruction, which includes multiple sessions taught throughout a student's medical school tenure.

Early EBM exposure has been viewed as an opportunity to provide trainees multiple opportunities to learn about and practise EBM with the hopes of increasing learner readiness for applying EBM skills upon entering clerkships. However, concerns have been raised that trainees early in their medical school career may lack the clinical context to appreciate the importance of EBM and find it irrelevant at that point in their studies (Maggio et al., 2016). To address this issue and provide context, institutions have increasingly incorporated authentic clinical cases into their EBM teaching and recruited physicians to share their experiences of EBM through in-class presentations and recorded interviews.

The timing of EBM sessions impacts the number of training sessions that an institution might offer. For example, the late introduction of EBM may diminish the number of potential EBM sessions. Researchers have identified that multiple EBM interventions versus single interventions are more efficacious in improving student EBM knowledge and skills (Young et al., 2015). This suggests that when designing EBM training, instructors should consider carefully the optimal number of EBM sessions for their institution. Although lack of curricular time has been identified as a barrier to implementing EBM education (Blanco et al., 2014), educators should consider some of the above approaches, such as integration with other courses and content, to expand EBM training without having to add curricular hours.

EBM instructors

Physicians most commonly teach EBM trainings (Maggio et al., 2013). However, clinicians often co-teach with other professionals, including information scientists/librarians, biostatisticians, and other allied health professionals, such as nurses and social workers. In some cases, a subject matter expert might take the lead in covering a component of EBM related to their area of expertise. For example, librarians frequently lead training on the formulation of clinical questions and literature searching and biostatisticians often provide training on critical appraisal.

 Reach across professions to recruit EBM instructors.

In addition to formal training, trainees learn EBM by observing clinician role models engage or in some cases not engage in EBM while caring for patients.

Researchers have raised concerns about the suboptimal nature of EBM role modelling, worrying that faculty may demonstrate subpar EBM skills, disparage the practice of EBM, or fail to make explicit their EBM processes (Maggio et al., 2016). In the context of EBM, this is especially concerning as students have reported that faculty role models play a major role in whether or not they will engage in EBM in the future (Ilic, 2009). The identification of suboptimal role models has led to calls for faculty development (Blanco et al., 2014). Specifically, educators have noted the need for training that improves faculty EBM skills but also encourages and teaches faculty to explicitly make visible their cognitive EBM processes, such as when a faculty member recognizes a gap in their knowledge. The routine recognition and demonstration of these steps will help to normalize and encourage the practice of EBM.

Learning resources for EBM

There are a variety of learning resources to support EBM instruction, including online tutorials, interactive tools such as EBM search engines, instructive journal articles and textbooks. While some of these resources cover EBM broadly, many focus on supporting particular steps of EBM. For example, the Oxford Centre for Evidence-Based Medicine makes available their CAT-Maker tool (http://www.cebm.net/catmaker-ebm-calculators/), to assist in the critical appraisal of studies. As these resources are constantly evolving, several medical libraries and EBM centres have curated online guides to facilitate identifying and accessing these resources (Table 27.2).

Information resources for finding evidence also act as learning resources for EBM. Traditionally, instructors have taught students to acquire evidence by using biomedical databases, such as PubMed. However, the biomedical information landscape has evolved to include a variety of point-of-care (POC) information resources

Table 27.2 EBM resource guides

Resource	URL
Cornell EBM Guide	http://med.cornell.libguides.com/ebm
McMaster Resources for Evidence-Based Practice	http://hsl.mcmaster.libguides.com/ebm
Oxford Centre for Evidence-Based Medicine	http://www.cebm.net/category/ebm-resources/
Government of Southern Australia EBM Resources	http://salus.sa.gov.au/ebm
Centre for Evidence-Based Medicine – Toronto	http://ktclearinghouse.ca/cebm/
University of Illinois at Chicago EBM Guide	http://researchguides.uic.edu/ebm

that synthesize available evidence for quick use at the patient bedside. These tools are now frequently used in patient care and students observe physician role models incorporating them in their practice. While many POC tools are user friendly and may not require training for their operation, it remains important for instructors to introduce them in the context of EBM and to provide instruction on how to critically consume this type of information. Failure to acknowledge POC tools may send students a mixed message indicating that EBM teaching is out of sync with practice.

There are also a host of learning resources to support instructors in designing EBM curriculum. For example, the online repository MedEdPORTAL (www.mededportal.org) features course materials, cases and guides for teaching EBM that are freely available. Additionally, there are several training opportunities, offered both online and in-person, focused on equipping instructors with specific skills to design and teach EBM instruction. For example, Duke's Teaching and Leading EBM programme (http://sites.duke.edu/ebmworkshop), McMaster's Evidence-Based Clinical Practice workshop (http://ebm.mcmaster.ca) and Oxford's Teaching Evidence-Based Medicine provide hands-on opportunities for honing EBM teaching skills and approaches.

EBM assessment

Educators have approached the assessment of students EBM skills and training using a variety of methods. To assess students' EBM skills, educators have developed and utilized multiple-choice exams, case-based exercises, critical appraisal challenges, and objective structured clinical examinations (OSCEs). Educators have also used the more formal Berlin Questionnaire (Fritsche et al., 2002) and Fresno Test (Ramos et al., 2003), both of which are psychometrically robust, but can be lengthy to administer. More recently, the ACE (Assessing Competency in EBM) Tool, which incorporates elements of the Berlin Questionnaire and Fresno Test, has been proposed specifically for assessing medical students' EBM competence (Ilic & Maloney, 2014). The ACE Tool is based on a patient scenario, features 15 yes/no items, and has been found to have moderate validity and internal reliability. As the number of available EBM assessment tools grows, EBM instructors may find the Classification Rubric for EBP Assessment Tools in Education (CREATE) (Tilson et al., 2011) useful for classifying the purpose of EBM trainee assessment tools and selecting the approach most relevant to their users and needs.

Future directions for EBM teaching

As the nature of medicine and biomedical information continues to evolve, EBM educators will be challenged to adapt their training to take into consideration new developments and practice directions. For example, as the use of electronic medical record (EMR) systems becomes ubiquitous, EBM instructors might consider training that empowers students to integrate resources built into EMRs, such as info buttons, links to information resources and embedded decision tools, into their EBM workflow. Additionally, as patients increasingly have access to and bring information to their appointments, EBM educators should consider training approaches that prepare students to discuss this information with patients and if appropriate integrate it into the decision-making process.

 Keep evolving your EBM training to keep pace with changes in practices.

Summary

The practice of EBM can help physicians bridge the gap between their current knowledge and the increasingly available biomedical evidence. Currently there is no standard or best approach to teaching EBM for medical students, which affords instructors flexibility in adopting learning approaches appropriate for their learners. This chapter presented several learning approaches and addressed EBM instructors, the timing of EBM training, resources for teaching EBM, the assessment of EBM skills, and potential future directions for EBM training.

References

Ahmadi, S.F., Baradaran, H.R., Ahmadi, E., 2015. Effectiveness of teaching evidence-based medicine to undergraduate medical students: a BEME systematic review. Med. Teach. 37 (1), 21–30.

Blanco, M.A., Capello, C.F., Dorsch, J.L., et al., 2014. A survey study of evidence-based medicine training in US and Canadian medical schools. J. Med. Libr. Assoc. 102 (3), 160–168.

Dawes, M., Summerskill, W., Glasziou, P., et al., 2005. Sicily statement on evidence-based practice. BMC Med. Educ. 5 (1), 1.

Dolmans, D., Wolfhagen, I., van Merriënboer, J.J.G., 2013. Twelve tips for implementing whole-task curricula: how to make it work. Med. Teach. 35 (10), 801–805.

Fritsche, L., Greenhalgh, T., Falck-Ytter, Y., et al., 2002. Do short courses in evidence based medicine improve knowledge and skills? Validation of Berlin questionnaire and before and after study of courses in evidence based medicine. BMJ 325 (7376), 1338–1341.

Ilic, D., 2009. Teaching evidence-based practice: perspectives from the undergraduate and post-graduate viewpoint. Ann. Acad. Med. Singap. 38 (6), 559–565.

Ilic, D., Maloney, S., 2014. Methods of teaching medical trainees evidence-based medicine: a systematic review. Med. Educ. 48 (2), 124–135.

Maggio, L.A., Tannery, N.H., Chen, H.C., et al., 2013. Evidence-based medicine training in undergraduate medical education: a review and critique of the literature published 2006-2011. Acad. Med. 88 (7), 1022–1028.

Maggio, L.A., Ten Cate, O., Chen, H.C., et al., 2016. Challenges to Learning Evidence-Based Medicine and Educational Approaches to Meet These Challenges: A Qualitative Study of Selected EBM Curricula in U.S. and Canadian Medical Schools. Acad. Med. 91 (1), 101–106.

Ramos, K.D., Schafer, S., Tracz, S.M., 2003. Validation of the Fresno test of competence in evidence based medicine. BMJ 326 (7384), 319–321.

Sackett, D.L., Rosenberg, W.M., Gray, J.A., et al., 1996. Evidence based medicine: what it is and what it isn't. BMJ 312 (7023), 71–72.

Tilson, J.K., Kaplan, S.L., Harris, J.L., et al., 2011. Sicily statement on classification and development of evidence-based practice learning assessment tools. BMC Med. Educ. 11, 78.

van Merriënboer, J.G., Kirschner, P.A., 2013. Ten Steps to Complex Learning: A Systematic Approach to Four-Component Instructional Design. Routledge, London.

Vandewaetere, M., Manhaeve, D., Aertgeerts, B., et al., 2015. 4C/ID in medical education: How to design an educational program based on whole-task learning: AMEE Guide No. 93. Med. Teach. 37 (1), 4–20.

Young, T., Rohwer, A., van Schalkwyk, S., et al., 2015. Patience, persistence and pragmatism: experiences and lessons learnt from the implementation of clinically integrated teaching and learning of evidence-based health care - a qualitative study. PLoS ONE 10 (6), e0131121.

Patient safety and quality of care

28

L. A. Headrick, D. E. Paull, K. B. Weiss

Trends

- Training in healthcare quality and patient safety must be based on an understanding of developing and maintaining complex systems of patient care, and the role of the healthcare professionals in providing care within those systems.

- A healthy healthcare organization is not dependent on the heroic actions of individuals to maintain safety but rather the systems they have built to capture errors before they reach the patient.

- The just culture accepts that healthcare professionals are fallible and that errors will occur but acknowledges the underlying latent, organizational, environmental and device factors that made the error more likely to occur in the first place.

- Team training, based on Crew Resource Management (CRM) principles, is associated with better patient outcomes, improved staff morale, and an enhanced patient safety culture.

- Education in patient safety sciences and quality improvement needs to be continual throughout training, thereby modelling this as a part of normal professional expectations rather than as a task to be conducted to complete training.

- Since healthcare is a team effort, interprofessional learning experiences in healthcare quality and patient safety will be required, increasing the complexity.

- Healthcare educators need to work closely with healthcare system leaders to design and implement healthcare quality and patient safety education programmes.

Introduction

Each year from 3% to 16% of hospitalized patients suffer patient safety events (Jha et al., 2010), and an untold number of events related to ambulatory care. Regardless of where in the world healthcare quality is being measured, the findings suggest there are

substantial opportunities for improving basic aspects of acute and chronic patient care.

Patient safety and healthcare quality sciences, methods and skill development are recognized as important to medical education internationally (Walton et al., 2010). Medical education leaders emphasize that patient safety and healthcare quality are essential topics in a successful medical education curriculum (Irby et al., 2010). In the United States, recent education and training in healthcare quality and patient safety is rapidly entering the mainstream of medical education (USMLE, 2015; Wagner et al., 2016).

Creating and deploying a successful curriculum in the sciences of healthcare quality and patient safety is challenging. As with other aspects of medical education, the educational objectives need to focus on knowledge acquisition, skill development, clear milestones that define progression, and tools for assessment of educational outcomes. This evolution in the medical curriculum requires faculty development in both the practice of and teaching of patient safety and quality improvement. However, unlike some of the areas in medical education, which primarily centre on the dyad of the physician and his or her patient (and family), patient safety and healthcare quality requires the engagement of the physician and patient dyad along with a commitment from the leadership of their clinical learning environment as well as collaboration with other members of the healthcare team.

This chapter focuses on three objectives; (1) to provide an brief introduction to healthcare quality and patient safety to those educators who are new to these sciences; (2) to provide an introduction on how to construct an educational experience in these fields for medical students, residents and fellows; and (3) to identify some resources to help the reader organize and implement successful learning experiences in patient safety and healthcare quality.

 Education in healthcare quality and patient safety must be based on understanding of developing and maintaining complex systems of patient care, and the role of the healthcare professionals in providing care within those systems.

Introduction to patient safety, the tragedy of preventable harm

Why is it important for students to learn about patient safety? Let's examine this question through the lens of a story about Lewis, a teenage patient (Gibson & Singh, 2003). Lewis was scheduled for a surgical procedure to correct a congenital deformity (pectus excavatum) at a prestigious academic medical centre. Postoperatively, Lewis was maintained on both an epidural catheter and regular injections of a medicine (labelled with warnings of possible bleeding or perforated ulcer).

On Sunday, two days postoperatively, Lewis developed abdominal pain described as the "worst pain imaginable". Over the course of the day, at the insistence of Lewis' mother, several residents saw Lewis, each concurring with a working diagnosis of an ileus; an ulcer or its complications were not considered. Clinical efforts were directed towards increased ambulation. A blood test was not ordered nor was an attending physician consulted. By Monday morning, Lewis' condition deteriorated further. He developed tachycardia, hypotension and cardiac arrest. Autopsy disclosed a perforated, bleeding ulcer with litres of blood within the peritoneal cavity.

Lewis' death was preventable. It was not primarily the lack of 'technical skills' among the staff that led to this tragic outcome. 'Non-technical' leadership, teamwork, communication skills and knowledge of human factors would promote questioning a diagnosis amidst contradictory findings and facilitate calling for help earlier. These skills transcend professional and specialty boundaries. Unfortunately, stories such as that of Lewis are not uncommon.

New competencies and patient safety

Patient safety is defined as the prevention of inadvertent harm or injury to patients. The goal is the prevention of harm **not** the elimination of errors. Humans are not perfect. Medical teachers must foster the belief among their learners that the "most dangerous person in the room" is the person who does not believe their own patients are at risk (Bagian, 2005). A healthy organization is not dependent on the heroic actions of individuals to maintain safety but rather the systems they have built to capture errors before they reach the patient.

 A healthy organization is not dependent on the heroic actions of individuals to maintain safety but rather the systems they have built to capture errors before they reach the patient.

Reporting and learning from adverse events and close calls

An 'adverse event' has been defined as "an injury related to medical management, in contrast to complications of disease. Medical management includes all aspects of care, including diagnosis and treatment, failure to diagnose or treat, and the systems and equipment used to deliver care" (World Health Organization, 2005). The patient safety system is dependent on the reporting of adverse events: "You cannot fix what you do not know about." (Bagian, 2005). Trainees must learn what to report and how to report. Successful healthcare organizations will overcome the barriers to reporting by providing staff and learners with a confidential, easy to use reporting mechanism replete with feedback as to what actions were taken to correct the unsafe condition reported.

The reporting of adverse events is insufficient for patient safety. After all, a patient had to be injured. 'Close call' reporting represents a proactive approach to patient safety. A close call is a serious error that has the potential to cause an adverse event but fails to do so because of chance or because it is intercepted (World Health Organization, 2005). Not only are close calls hundreds of times more abundant than adverse events but they are often easier for providers to discuss since no patients were harmed. Case-based learning, where learners determine whether an event was an adverse event or close call, represents an effective adjunct to lecture.

Patient safety education requires that we learn from adverse events and close calls in order to prevent recurrence of these same events. One patient safety sense-making tool is Root Cause Analysis (RCA). RCAs are performed on those adverse events or close call reports prioritized because of their association with either real or potential catastrophic harm. An interprofessional team reviews the medical record, interviews staff involved in the incident, reviews literature and guidelines, and determines the underlying systems-based factor(s) contributing to the event. Actions to address the root cause(s) are developed and implemented, along with a plan to monitor whether such actions were successful in preventing a recurrence.

Medical teachers can provide learners the necessary tools to succeed as a member or leader of a RCA team including the ability to create flow, cause and effect, and fishbone diagrams to analyze patient safety incidents, learning delivered through observed structured clinical examinations (Gupta & Varkey, 2009).

Establishing the just culture

James Reason states that human errors in healthcare can be viewed in one of two ways: a "person approach" or a "systems approach" (Reason, 2000). The person approach views adverse events as due to an individual

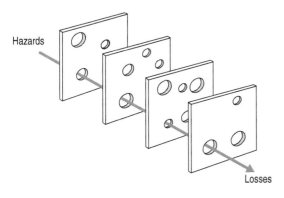

Hazards

Losses

Fig. 28.1 Swiss Cheese Model.

Redrawn from Reason, J. Human error: Models and management. BMJ, 320, 768-770, 2000.

provider's carelessness. In this model, the involved provider is "shamed, blamed and retrained." However, this approach does not often prevent a recurrence of a similar adverse event. The systems approach accepts that physicians are fallible and that errors will occur but acknowledges the underlying latent, organizational, environmental and device factors that made the error more likely to occur in the first place. The "Swiss cheese" diagram (Reason, 2000) illustrates the systems approach to error (Fig. 28.1). In this model the patient safety system consists of multiple slices of Swiss cheese. One slice might represent automation, another teamwork, and yet another policy. Automation like barcoding helps prevent medication errors, and team training improves communication. But these barriers intended to prevent errors from reaching the patient are not perfect. They have holes, and under a particular set of circumstances the holes in the barriers line up so that the error reaches the patient. Holes or vulnerabilities include ineffective or ambiguous policy, automation failure or its unintended consequences, and lack of recurrent team training. The Swiss cheese model allows us to identify and address specific risks that led to a given adverse event or close call.

The reporting of adverse events and close calls are dependent on the establishment of a 'just culture'. A just culture is an atmosphere of trust in which people are encouraged to speak up with safety-related information (Leonard & Frankel, 2010). Individuals trust they will not be held accountable for system failures, and are also clear about where the line must be drawn between acceptable and unacceptable behaviour. In a just culture, humans involved in an error would be consoled not disciplined. Actions include redesigning the system to make it less likely for the adverse event to recur. The just culture also administers disciplinary action when individuals commit a deliberately unsafe act (e.g. disruptive behaviour). Again, case studies where learners decide whether a particular course of action represented non-blameworthy human error, at risk

behaviour, or a blameworthy deliberately unsafe act have proven useful educational instruments.

 The just culture accepts that healthcare professionals are fallible and that errors will occur but acknowledges the underlying latent, organizational, environmental and device factors that made the error more likely to occur in the first place.

Teamwork skills and a deeper understanding of human factors

The root cause for most serious adverse events in healthcare relates to a failure in communication. The Institute of Medicine recognized this in *To Err is Human*, recommending aviation-based Crew Resource Management (CRM) team training as a possible remedy. CRM has been defined as using all available resources including information, personnel and equipment to ensure safe care. CRM-based team training encourages everyone to speak up with concerns, even when faced with an authority gradient (Haerkens et al., 2015). Another CRM concept is situational awareness (SA). During CRM training, students learn to recognize red flags indicating low SA: two pieces of clinical information that contradict one another; confusion; team members taking short-cuts for standard safety policies and procedures (so-called 'normalization of deviance'); and a patient's condition failing to respond to a treatment plan. Learners are taught to 'step back', re-assess the patient, and make use of additional resources (information, personnel, equipment).

Other CRM principles and behaviours include briefings and debriefings, checklists, closed loop communication (e.g. repeat backs), and safe handoffs. Team training has been associated with better patient outcomes, improved staff morale, and an enhanced patient safety culture (Haerkens et al., 2015; Sculli & Paull, 2015). Team training is more effective when incorporated into the healthcare system as a recurring phenomenon as opposed to a one-time workshop. These CRM teamwork and communication tools and techniques can be practised with simulation ranging from simple role plays to more sophisticated high-fidelity simulations.

 Team training, based on Crew Resource Management (CRM) principles, is associated with better patient outcomes, improved staff morale, and an enhanced safety culture.

Human factors represent "the study of the inter-relationship between humans, the tools and equipment they use in the workplace, and the environment in which they work" (World Health Organization, 2005). Patient safety is concerned with threats to patients and providers from environmental, equipment, biological and chemical sources. Providing learners with experiences in medical device usability testing will begin to address the deficiencies in product design for safety that afflict healthcare. Including Human Factors Engineering (HFE) experts on medical school faculty and RCA teams will lead to more sustained solutions to the causes of adverse events.

Introduction to health care quality

The end goal for any patient safety issue is quality improvement. Calls for physician involvement in quality improvement have been long standing; dating back as far back as Sir Thomas Percival – most known for his code of medical ethics – who in the 1800s called for physicians to maintain registries of the work they do for the purposes of quality audit. Similarly, in the 1800s Florence Nightingale called for the need to document the quality of care through the emerging field of epidemiology. In the mid-1800s a Viennese physician, Ignaz Semmelweis, identified through observations that hygienic practices (washing hands) was associated with patient outcomes; a quality concern that continues to vex healthcare to this day. In the 1900s Earnest Codman, a Boston surgeon, called for the maintaining of patient registries and that payment should be linked to the quality of patient outcomes.

The major impetus for what is currently viewed as contemporary (early twenty-first century) efforts in quality improvement emerged from an early twentieth-century industrial model of quality improvement as developed in the United States by Walter Shewhart. His focus was on studying the variability in processes and outcomes (special and common cause variation), and using data on variability to drive continual process improvement process—the Plan, Do, Study, Act (PDSA) cycle of improvement. In the 1970s Wennberg and Gittelsohn used large database analysis to bring variability in healthcare process and outcomes to the field of medical care (Wennberg & Gittelsohn, 1973). The actual introduction of the Shewhart (PDSA) improvement cycles did not occur until the early 1990s through the collaborative efforts of the National Demonstration Project and subsequently Berwick, 1991. While there are many theories and methods for quality improvement that are currently being used around the world, it seems that the most accessible and easiest to initiate for early learners such as medical students, residents and faculty, is the Model for Improvement (Langley et al., 2009) with its set of simple questions and use of the Shewhart's (PDSA) cycles (Fig. 28.2).

The Institute of Medicine of the National Academy of Sciences in the United States dramatically heightened the focus on the issues of healthcare quality and patient safety both in the United States and internationally, through two seminal publications that declared, at least in the United States, that patients were being unnecessarily harmed and healthcare was in urgent

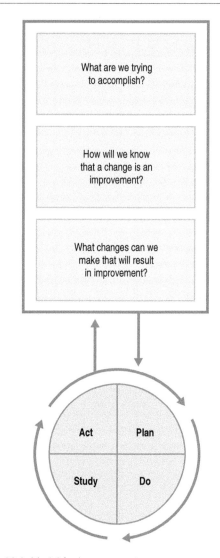

Fig. 28.2 Model for Improvement.

Redrawn from Langley GJ, et al.: The improvement guide: a practical approach to enhancing organizational performance. 2nd ed. San Francisco, CA: Jossey-Bass, 2009.

need of improvement (Institute of Medicine, 2000, 2001). By 2004 the movement for both healthcare quality improvement and patient safety became global (Donaldson & Philip, 2004).

Teaching healthcare quality and patient safety

A CONTINUUM OF PHYSICIAN PROFESSIONAL DEVELOPMENT IN QUALITY AND SAFETY

Creating and sustaining the high quality, safe care that our patients need and deserve requires physicians and other health professionals to improve healthcare and patient safety as a core part of professional practice. Like other professional competencies, excellence in quality and safety demands a continuum of professional development, from the beginning medical student (novice) to the graduating resident (competent) to the accomplished practising clinician (proficient) to scholars who advance the field (masters) (AAMC, 2013).

By medical school graduation, physicians should be able to (1) critically evaluate the knowledge base supporting good patient care, (2) determine the gap between prevailing practices and best practices, and (3) participate in closing the gap between prevailing and best practices (AAMC, 2001). The resident about to enter practice must "demonstrate the ability to investigate and evaluate their care of patients, to appraise and assimilate scientific evidence, and to continuously improve patient care based on constant self-evaluation and life-long learning" (ACGME, 2013). The proficient practising clinician incorporates feedback into practice, works effectively in interprofessional teams, and views improving systems of care as an integral component of professional identity (AAMC, 2013).

Strategies for teaching quality and safety

The following five principles are helpful in the design of learning experiences related to quality and safety across multiple levels of physician development (Wong et al., 2010; Armstrong et al., 2012):

1. *Employ a combination of didactic and experiential learning strategies.* Even novice health professional learners repeatedly remind the faculty that improving healthcare quality and safety, like other professional activities, requires skills that must be practised, with opportunities for feedback and reflection.

2. *Find ways to include interprofessional learning, since interprofessional collaboration is key to quality improvement and patient safety.* The World Health Organization (WHO) defines interprofessional education to be "when students from two or more professions learn about, from and with each other to enable effective collaboration and improve health outcomes" (WHO, 2010). It is a truism in quality improvement that one cannot effectively improve someone else's process. While some aspects of quality improvement and patient safety might be learned in discipline-specific activities, successful changes in practice require the ability to engage the perspective, knowledge and collaboration of everyone involved.

3. *Remember that clinically based learning is usually more powerful than classroom-based learning.* In their landmark report, *Calls for Reform of Medical Education by the Carnegie Foundation for the Advancement of Teaching: 1910 and 2010,* Irby and colleagues call for the integration of formal learning with clinical experience, citing the advantages of medical education processes that closely represent the nature of physicians' learning and work (Irby et al., 2010). Their argument is validated by generations of medical students who report the remarkable sustainability of lessons acquired in the context of meaningful patient care.

4. *Take advantage of the power that comes when one aligns with clinical quality improvement efforts.* The Accreditation Council for Graduate Medical Education's *Clinical Learning Environment Review (CLER) Report of Findings* from its first round of site visits to US academic teaching centres highlighted the value of shared goals and strategies between education and clinical leadership (Bagian & Weiss, 2016). Learners in clinical settings are front-line personnel whose insights may be essential to improvement. Learner-generated improvement efforts may be exciting, but are difficult to sustain if they are not sufficiently in sync with organizational priorities to attract partners and other resources. Coalescing education and clinical improvement efforts around shared goals can generate important learning experiences in the context of demonstrable benefit to patients.

5. *Role model improvement as an education leader.* Educators demonstrate the importance of measurement, feedback and improvement by incorporating these into their own work in a way that is visible to learners. It is essential that faculty be developed as role models in patient safety and healthcare quality.

Innovative faculty have created learning experiences in quality improvement and patient safety in the classroom, the simulation centre and in clinical settings (Headrick et al., 2012). Examples include learners using a paper case to work through the steps of a quality improvement effort, practising safe handoffs in the clinical simulation centre, and taking on a specific aspect of a larger improvement effort that can be accomplished in a limited time period. Many argue for a series of learning experiences over time, perhaps starting in the classroom but progressing rapidly to clinically based activities.

 In patient safety, sciences and quality improvement needs to be continual throughout training, thereby modelling this as a part of normal professional expectations rather than as a task to be conducted to complete training.

Table 28.1 Typology of educational outcomes for learner assessment and programme evaluation

Outcome	Example
1. Learner Reaction	Written feedback
2a. Modification of attitudes/ perceptions	Pre/post-learner assessment
2b. Acquisition of knowledge/skills	Pre/post-learner assessment
3. Behavioural change	Checklist-driven faculty ratings of student performance in the clinical setting
4a. Change in organizational practice	Improvements in clinical processes
4b. Benefits to patients/clients	Clinical outcomes

Adapted from Barr H, et al.: Effective Interprofessional Education: Argument, Assumption and Evidence. Oxford, UK: Blackwell Publishing, 2005, p 43.

Assessment and evaluation

Strategic measurement can provide feedback to both learners ("How have I progressed?") and educators ("How well did these strategies meet our goals?"). As modified by Barr and colleagues, the Kirkpatrick typology of educational outcomes provides a comprehensive approach that addresses learner, organizational and patient outcomes (Barr et al., 2005). Table 28.1 provides details and examples. Peer-reviewed resources include the *Readiness for Interprofessional Learning Survey* (RIPLS) (Parsell & Bligh, 1999) and the Quality Improvement Knowledge-Acquisition Tool (QIKAT-R) Singh et al., 2014).

 Since healthcare is a team effort, interprofessional learning experiences in healthcare quality and patient safety will be required.

Challenges that are somewhat unique to establishing a patient safety and healthcare quality educational programme

With the introduction of any new content to the medical education curriculum there will be challenges. Listed below are a few that should be addressed early in the design of curricula in this area.

1. Meaningful clinical improvement experiences for all learners probably requires the integration of quality improvement (QI) and patient safety (PS) into core clinical practice (the way we do our work every day).

2. For education about QI/PS to occur in the context of routine professional work, faculty members must practise and teach QI/PS in their roles as clinicians, educators and researchers.

3. Patient safety and healthcare quality take place in the complex learning environment that we call clinical care. Aligning education and clinical improvement efforts increases the chance that learners will experience successful change as it is designed, implemented and sustained.

 Healthcare educators need to work closely with healthcare system leaders to design and implement healthcare quality and patient safety education programmes.

Summary

The fields of patient safety and healthcare quality improvement have emerged as essential to the practice of clinical medicine. Over the past decade, there has been international recognition of the need to include these subjects in medical school curricula as well as in all clinical training and practice thereafter. Training in these fields is challenging in that it requires close collaboration between the learner and their faculty, along with the other practitioners and administrators who are part of the healthcare environment (clinical learning environment) in which education takes place. There are excellent resources available to assist faculty in developing curricula on these subjects. Robust educational curricula and outcomes on these subjects will create benefits to both learners and patients.

References

Accreditation Council for Graduate Medical Education (ACGME), (2013). Common Program Requirements. Chicago, IL, http://www.acgme.org/acgmeweb/Portals/0/PFAssets/ProgramRequirements/CPRs2013.pdf. (Accessed March 2016).

Armstrong, G., Headrick, L., Madigosky, W., Ogrinc, G., 2012. Designing education to improve care. Jt. Comm. J. Qual. Patient Saf. 38 (1), 5–14.

Association of American Medical Colleges (AAMC), (2001). Medical School Objectives Project. Report V Contemporary Issues in Medicine: Quality of Care. Washington, DC.

Association of American Medical Colleges (AAMC), Teaching for Quality: Integrating Quality Improvement and Patient Safety Across the Continuum of Medical Education. Washington, DC, 2013. https://members.aamc.org/eweb/upload/Teaching%20for%20Quality%20Report.pdf. (Accessed March 2016).

Bagian, J.P., 2005. Patient safety: what is really at issue? Front. Health Serv. Manage. 22, 3–16.

Bagian, J.P., Weiss, K.B., 2016. The overarching themes from the CLER National Report of Findings 2016. J. Grad. Med. Educ. 8 (2 Suppl. 1), 21–23.

Barr, H., et al., 2005. Effective Interprofessional Education: Argument, Assumption and Evidence. Blackwell Publishing, Oxford, UK.

Berwick, D.M., 1991. Controlling variation in health care: a consultation from Walter Shewhart. Med. Care 29, 1212–1225.

Donaldson, L., Philip, P., 2004. Patient Safety, a global priority. Bull. World Health Organ. 82, 12.

Gibson, R., Singh, J.P., 2003. Wall of silence. LifeLine Press, Washington DC.

Gupta, P., Varkey, P., 2009. Developing a tool for assessing competency in root cause analysis. Jt. Comm. J. Qual. Patient Saf. 35, 36–42.

Haerkens, M.H., Kox, M., Lemson, J., et al., 2015. Crew Resource Management in the Intensive Care Unit: a prospective 3-year cohort study. Acta. Anaesthesiol. Scand. 59, 1319–1329.

Headrick, L.A., Barton, A.J., Ogrinc, G., et al., 2012. Results of an effort to integrate quality and safety into medical and nursing school curricula and foster joint learning. Health Aff. (Millwood) 31, 2669–2680.

Institute of Medicine (IOM), 2000. Kohn, L.T., Corrigan, J.M., Donaldson, M.S. (Eds.), To Err Is Human: Building a Safer Health System. National Academy Press, Washington, D.C.

Institute of Medicine (IOM), 2001. Crossing the Quality Chasm. Crossing the Quality Chasm: A New Health System for the 21st Century. National Academy Press, Washington, D.C.

Irby, D.M., Cooke, M., O'Brien, B.C., 2010. Calls for reform of medical education by the Carnegie Foundation for the Advancement of Teaching: 1910 and 2010. Acad. Med. 85, 220–227.

Jha, A.K., Prasopa-Plaizier, N., Larizgoitia, I., Bates, D.W., 2010. Patient safety research: an overview of the global evidence. Qual. Saf. Health Care 19, 42–47.

Langley, G.J., Moen, R.D., Nolan, K.M., et al., 2009. The Improvement Guide: A Practical Approach to Enhancing Organizational Performance, second ed. Jossey-Bass, San Francisco, CA.

Leonard, M.W., Frankel, A., 2010. The path to safe and reliable healthcare. Patient Educ. Couns. 80, 288–292.

Parsell, G., Bligh, J., 1999. The development of a questionnaire to assess the readiness of health care students for interprofessional learning (RIPLS). Med. Educ. 33, 95–100.

Reason, J., 2000. Human error: models and management. BMJ 320, 768–770.

Singh, M.K., Ogrinc, G., Cox, K., et al., 2014. The Quality Improvement Knowledge Application Tool Revised (QIKAT-R). Acad. Med. 89 (10), 1386–1391.

Sculli, G., Paull, D.E., 2015. Building a High-Reliability Ogranization: A Toolkit for Success. HCPro, Brentwood, TN.

USLME, Changes to the USLME 2015-2016. www.usmle.org/pdfs/Changes_to_USMLE_handout.pdf. (Accessed March 2016).

Wagner, R., Koh, N., Patow, C., et al.; for the CLER program, 2016. Detailed findings of the Clinical Learning Environment Review Program, 2016. JGME (in press).

Walton, M., Woodward, H., Van Staalduinen, S., et al.; for and on behalf of the Expert Group convened by the World Alliance of Patient Safety, as Expert Lead for the Sub-Programme, 2010. The WHO patient safety curriculum guide for medical schools. Qual. Saf. Health Care 19, 542–546.

Wennberg, J., Gittelsohn, A., 1973. Small Area Variations in Health Care Delivery: a population-based health information system can guide planning and regulatory decision-making. Science 182, 1102–1108.

Wong, B.M., Etchells, E.E., Kuper, A., et al., 2010. Teaching quality improvement and patient safety to trainees: a systematic review. Acad. Med. 85, 1425–1439.

World Health Organization, 2005. WHO Draft Guidelines for Adverse Event Reporting and Learning Systems. Retrieved from: http://osp.od.nih.gov/office-clinical-research-and-bioethics-policy/clinical-research-policy-adverse-event-reporting/world-health-organization-who-draft-guidance-adverse-event-reporting-and-learning-systems. (Accessed 25 January 2016).

World Health Organization, (2010) Framework for Action on Interprofessional Education & Collaborative Practice. Geneva, Switzerland. http://apps.who.int/iris/handle/10665/70185. (Accessed March 2016).

29 Medical humanities

J. Y. Chen, H. Y-J. Wu

Trends

- Medical humanities taking root in undergraduate education with particular interest in Asian medical schools
- Blended learning as an approach for curriculum delivery
- Sub-disciplines such as public health humanities

Introduction

 "Knowing the tools of evidence-based practice is necessary but not sufficient for delivering the highest quality patient care. In addition to clinical expertise, the clinician requires compassion, sensitive listening skills, and broad perspectives from the humanities and social sciences. These attributes allow understanding of patients' illnesses in the context of their experience, personalities, and cultures."

Guyatt et al., 2000

The fundamental remit of medical schools around the world is to nurture the development of future doctors who will provide safe, competent care. This includes proficiency in the biomedical realm together with the requisite clinical skills, but most tellingly from the experts in evidence-based medicine, must also comprise the attributes, attitudes and broad perspective drawn from humanistic fields of study to understand illness in patients' own personal contexts. Understanding the patient as a person and the individuality of illness and suffering is the first step towards relieving suffering, arguably the primary goal of medicine (Cassell, 1999). Whatever illness a patient has, the issues concerning the human condition – suffering, death, love and friendship, for example – are the real concerns that grip the person, and which the doctor must address. The medical humanities (MH) have been recognized and adopted in myriad ways in undergraduate medical education as a means to emphasize, celebrate and critically explore the human aspect of medicine. This chapter will describe what the medical humanities are

and the rationale for their inclusion in the medical curriculum, provide an overview of key educational approaches using the experience at The University of Hong Kong (HKU) as a case study, and discuss some of the practical considerations and challenges of developing a medical humanities curriculum.

What are the medical humanities?

As of yet, there is no universally agreed definition of the medical humanities, or the more inclusively termed 'health humanities.' Scholars in the field have suggested conceptualizations of medical humanities, which encompass a list of disciplines whose subject matter spans ethics to art to philosophy to cultural studies, as a set of goals or roles in medical education leading to greater insight into the human experience in general, and health and illness in particular, as a programme of moral development for acquiring the values of good doctoring, and as a supportive friend to whom we turn for enjoyment and wisdom (Brody, 2011; Gordon & Evans, 2013). A comprehensive and nuanced discussion of the origins, evolution and definitions of the medical humanities grounds a treatise on how a refocused critical medical humanities in medical education can help shape medical students (Bleakley, 2015), and is well worth reading. Equally useful, is a practical and pragmatic definitionthat emphasizes the interdisciplinary nature of medical humanities and the centrality of their application to healthcare proposed by the Division of Medical Humanities at the New York University School of Medicine.

 "We define the term 'medical humanities' broadly to include an interdisciplinary field of humanities (literature, philosophy, ethics, history and religion), social science (anthropology, cultural studies, psychology, sociology), and the arts (literature, theater, film, multimedia and visual arts) and their application to healthcare education and practice. The humanities and arts provide insight into the human condition, suffering, personhood, and our responsibility to each other. They also offer a historical perspective on healthcare. Attention to literature and the arts help to develop and

nurture skills of observation, analysis, empathy, and self-reflection – skills that are essential for humane healthcare. The social sciences help us to understand how bioscience and medicine take place within cultural and social contexts and how culture interacts with the individual experience of illness and the way healthcare is practiced."

New York University School of Medicine

Considering medicine from these diverse perspectives can illuminate more fully what is meant about the human condition, the nature of suffering and the greater context in which the doctor and patient engage together in seeking meaning from illness and healing (Hurwitz, 2003). It also enables training the process of critical thinking with the expectation that students "be capable of rigorous and independent thought, to account for their decisions, to be creative, imaginative and tolerant of ambiguity"(Gordon & Evans, 2013). Facilitating this understanding and nurturing such skills lead to the promise of more insightful patient care, professional development and personal wellbeing.

How do the medical humanities contribute to medical education?

In addition to bringing balance to the biomedical focus of the medical curriculum, medical humanities are useful for their "instrumental role" in preparing students for clinical practice and also for their intrinsic value in broadening perspective and in personal development (Macnaughton, 2000).

PREPARATION FOR MEDICAL PRACTICE

 "You never really understand another person until you consider things from his point of view … until you climb inside of his skin and walk around in it."

Harper Lee

Particularly for undergraduate medical students in Europe, Australia and Asia, where admission to medical school is predominantly gained directly from secondary school, medical humanities provide vicarious life experience through stories told through literature, poetry, film, art and narratives. They allow students to inhabit the character whose story is being told. Encountering the loss of a parent, the darkness of depression, or the feelings about dissecting a cadaver through stories, and reflecting on personal responses in a safe environment can help reveal hidden fears and internal biases and 'prepare' students before they encounter these situations in a real-life clinical setting. Through drama or visual arts students can learn to interpret emotions and reflect on the communication between individuals, including what not to say or do.

This can offer opportunities to practise verbal communication skills and appropriate body language by re-imagining and role-playing a scene in an alternate, more patient-centred way.

Perhaps most importantly, the medical humanities address the neglected curriculum in medicine: "What makes us human?"; "What gives our lives meaning?"; "What is the nature of suffering?"; "What can we do when there appears to be no cure or hope for improvement?"; "How does one face uncertainties, mistakes and develop appropriate responses?" In tackling these questions, students generate new inquiries and reflections, which build awareness to equip them better to face the analogous complexities and ambiguities of issues involved in medical care and practice. They also learn to appreciate the wider context of the nature and meaning of suffering of their patients and their aim to live a life of meaning because of and despite their illness.

PERSPECTIVE AND PERSONAL DEVELOPMENT

The medical humanities provide a wider lens with which to view the world, beyond the narrow focus of medical training. The learning about man himself is an education that shapes the kind of person one will become, which is of particular importance in good doctoring, which is built on a foundation of trust. Through the medical humanities, students can observe and uncover knowledge about patients, themselves and their own values and challenge preconceived beliefs (Macnaughton, 2000), thereby developing an increasing sense of self-awareness.

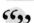 *WANTED: The 21ˢᵗ Century Physician Altruistic, compassionate, courageous, intellectually curious, frugal scholar, gifted in history, philosophy, politics, economics, sociology, and psychology. Must have working knowledge of biology, chemistry, physics, and medicine … Physical endurance, emotional maturity, and technical-manual skills sufficient to take apart and reassemble the human body and mind at levels ranging from the micromolecular to the gross are required; must have flexibility to master all knowledge, sift and discard that no longer applicable, while discovering new data at the bench, in clinical practice, in both general and subspecialty medicine. Should be able to prevent and cure disease, including the depredations of advancing age; physical disarray; and spiritual, mental, emotional, and economic illnesses. Will need to function effectively and efficiently in both intensive care units and urban slums … This is a 24 hour per day commitment. Should make house calls.*

Fitzgerald, 1996

In the prevailing climate of medical education and medical practice of unremitting professional demands, punishing schedules and resultant burnout and psychological distress among medical students and healthcare professionals, self-awareness as a first step towards self-care is crucial. Through self-awareness and the exercise of judicious and ethical decisions, students can learn to be humane to themselves and to their colleagues, to take care in the face of punishing work schedules, to recognise the limits of one's expertise and to avoid as much as possible (or face up to) making mistakes. Medical humanities as personal development can also provide guidance for medical students to look after their physical and mental health better, given the demanding nature of medical training and the realities of a profession that they will one day join. It is one tied up with dealing with human suffering and death, making difficult and sometimes complex decisions, and above all, recognizing stress and guilt arising from the fallibility of human beings when medical errors are made despite the best attempts at prevention. Aside from this, literature, film, music and drama quite simply bring pleasure and joy to people, providing a welcome escape into an imaginary world.

BRING BALANCE TO THE MEDICAL CURRICULUM

 "I am in a profession that has succeeded because of its ability to fix. If your problem is fixable, we know just what to do. But if it's not? The fact that we have had no adequate answers to this question is troubling and has caused callousness, inhumanity, and extraordinary suffering."

Gawande, 2014

The training of medical students and the practice of medicine have undergone a paradigm shift in that success in medical care is perceived to be based on an understanding of our genes, in advances made through biomedical sciences, in the availability of cutting edge medical technology and in the development of personalized medicine and stem cell–based therapies. In the pursuit of such goals underpinned by the promise from science and technology, the medical profession appears to be in danger of forgetting that the practice of medicine is based on the basic tenets of 'cure sometimes, care often and most importantly comfort always' for the patient entrusted to his or her care. Understanding and alleviating the suffering of patients with chronic illnesses and incurable diseases is often seen as a lower priority in terms of modern day medicine compared to the quest of goals such as to cure cancer, delay ageing and reverse neurodegenerative disorders. We need very much to remind ourselves that the human and humane aspects of medical practice go hand in hand with the benefits reaped through science and

technology beginning with a more balanced medical curriculum that addresses disease but also suffering (fear, loss, isolation, stigmatisation, despair) and cure but also healing (love, respect, trust, hope, compassion). Medical humanities help students to appreciate and recognize the diverse ways and different contexts in which we can explore suffering as human experience and as part of the human condition; to understand the social, societal and cultural factors that influence illness and healing; and to create new avenues for the doctor and patient to engage together in seeking meaning of illness and therapy.

What educational approaches are useful in medical humanities?

Many medical schools around the world have already been incorporating medical humanities in undergraduate medical curricula with a special issue in *Academic Medicine* dedicated to providing a sampling of these (Dittrich, 2003), and in more recent times, Asian medical schools in Taiwan, Singapore, Hong Kong and China have also come on board. There is a wide variety of educational approaches described and also summarized in more recent overviews on medical humanities in medical education (Bleakley, 2015; Gordon & Evans, 2013). These address the structural aspects of a medical humanities curriculum or learning activity, the content and delivery of such learning, and the assessment of outcomes. In medical humanities, as with medical education in general, the most appropriate kind of learning is dependent on the setting of the individual medical school that makes good practice highly contextual.

Curriculum structure

FRAMEWORK

The details on developing a medical humanities curriculum can be demonstrated using a case example from HKU that captures some of the considerations when embarking on such an initiative, including how to conceptualize, structure, teach, integrate and assess. This MH programme is underpinned by a conceptual framework that begins with knowledge and self-exploration, then progresses to skill development, and finally to embodiment of attitudes and behaviours nurtured through medical humanities in clinical practice (Fig. 29.1). It a 6-year, compulsory longitudinal curriculum taught by medical and non-medical teachers often concurrently, which is built around five designated themes (patient and doctor stories; culture, spirituality and healing; history of medicine; death, dying and bereavement; and humanitarianism and social justice), which are explored via five genres (narrative and literature, film, performance, visual art and experiential learning [mindful practice, historical immersion and service]).

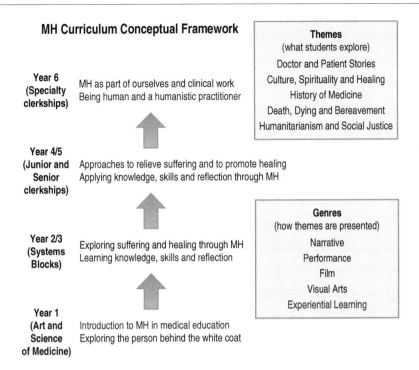

MH Curriculum Conceptual Framework

Year 6 (Specialty clerkships) — MH as part of ourselves and clinical work / Being human and a humanistic practitioner

Year 4/5 (Junior and Senior clerkships) — Approaches to relieve suffering and to promote healing / Applying knowledge, skills and reflection through MH

Year 2/3 (Systems Blocks) — Exploring suffering and healing through MH / Learning knowledge, skills and reflection

Year 1 (Art and Science of Medicine) — Introduction to MH in medical education / Exploring the person behind the white coat

Themes (what students explore)
Doctor and Patient Stories
Culture, Spirituality and Healing
History of Medicine
Death, Dying and Bereavement
Humanitarianism and Social Justice

Genres (how themes are presented)
Narrative
Performance
Film
Visual Arts
Experiential Learning

Fig. 29.1 MH Conceptual Framework.

OUTCOMES-BASED APPROACH TO STUDENT LEARNING (OBASL)

A medical humanities activity or curriculum, like other teaching and learning in medical education, can be designed and structured in a pedagogically rigorous way. The outcomes-based approach to student learning (OBASL) is based on sound educational principles and also reflects the competency-based curriculum design already familiar to many medical schools in which the attainment of specific outcomes or competencies is the goal. In OBASL, the curriculum design is centred on stated learning outcomes that make it clear to the student exactly what they need to know. The expected outcomes govern what kind of teaching and learning activities are constructed to achieve the learning outcomes, and the assessment task is then designed to assure that the outcomes are met. It makes the planning of the activity, course or programme much more explicit, focused and accountable. The inter-reliance of outcomes, learning activities and assessment is shown in (Fig. 29.2), which uses one of the learning outcomes for the Year 1 MH curriculum at HKU to illustrate the curriculum alignment.

ASSESSMENT

The learning outcome desired for a particular medical humanities initiative will determine the form of assessment. The skills-based outcomes such as being able to reflect or to critically appraise can be assessed using more conventional means such as essays, reflective logbooks or presentations based on desired rubrics. On the other hand, attitudinal and behavioural outcomes, such as being empathic or compassionate, are harder to measure though portfolios, and reflective writing can be useful. There are instruments that have been validated for this purpose. The bigger question is whether assessing the 'immediate' outcomes after an activity or a course are meaningful given that the ultimate outcome of better patient care, which medical humanities are striving for, is years removed from medical school and subject to many confounding factors that make it difficult to evaluate.

INTEGRATION

Integration into the core medical curriculum helps to underline the relevance of the MH to medical study and practice. In pre-clinical years, a respect ceremony and reflection on one's first clinical teacher, the cadaver, and MH-themed issues within a case study or problem-based learning case trigger are well-received. In clinical years, MH can be embedded in the clinical teaching and learned experientially. For instance, encounters with suffering during a clinical clerkship (whether it be an unexpected diagnosis or an elderly woman's depression) can be debriefed and discussed with reference to Eric Cassell's article on the nature of suffering.

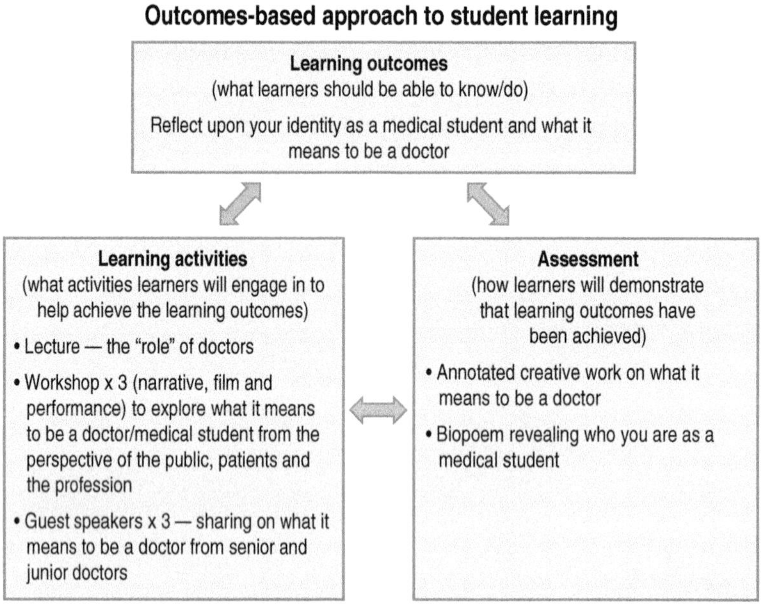

Outcomes-based approach to student learning

Learning outcomes
(what learners should be able to know/do)

Reflect upon your identity as a medical student and what it means to be a doctor

Learning activities
(what activities learners will engage in to help achieve the learning outcomes)

- Lecture — the "role" of doctors

- Workshop x 3 (narrative, film and performance) to explore what it means to be a doctor/medical student from the perspective of the public, patients and the profession

- Guest speakers x 3 — sharing on what it means to be a doctor from senior and junior doctors

Assessment
(how learners will demonstrate that learning outcomes have been achieved)

- Annotated creative work on what it means to be a doctor

- Biopoem revealing who you are as a medical student

Fig. 29.2 Example of OBASL in MH.

Among clerkship preparatory readings at the University of Washington is a poem about a patient who appeals to his doctors to be seen as a person (*When you come into my room* by Stephen A Schmidt) and a story about the most uninteresting patient on the ward who turns out to be not so uninteresting (*Curiosity* by Faith T Fitzgerald), and in residency programmes, shared stories are incorporated into hospital rounds (http://www.nytimes.com/2008/10/24/health/chen10-23.html?_r=0), all of which bring the medical humanities explicitly to the clinical realm.

COMPULSORY OR ELECTIVE

How the medical humanities are positioned in the curriculum is variable, and dependent on the educational philosophy of the institution but also on practical considerations like curriculum time and resourcing. More often, programmes in undergraduate medical education have the medical humanities as electives or special study modules (SSMs) in which students take structured courses or self-initiate a learning experience in the humanities. These allow self-selected students to pursue an area of interest or to try an unfamiliar area of inquiry. In contrast, medical humanities can also be a compulsory area of study just like anatomy or clinical skills or paediatrics, which is subject to some form of summative assessment. This makes explicit the importance MH have in the curriculum and exposes all students to MH principles as part of their core medical education.

Content and delivery

NARRATIVE BASED

Narrative medicine is about developing the textual, creative and affective skills through close reading of text to be able to recognize, absorb, interpret and be moved by the stories of illness (Charon, 2004) in a therapeutic alliance with patients to make meaning of illness and move towards healing. The study of narratives exposes students to different explanatory models of suffering and healing from different perspectives and can be revealed through various written narrative forms as short stories, novels, poetry, or visual forms like painting, photographs or film. Students are compelled to see and experience life from different angles by writing, sharing, reading or actively listening to stories, either factual or fictional.

In addition to guided close reading and analysis of text and responding verbally or in writing, students can experiment creating alternative forms to examine their response to the narrative. Students can, for instance, make four-box comic strips or a micro movie to explore the significance of "perspectivism" (Kleinman, 1988) triggered by watching a video in which various perspectives of disease causations or treatment contest each other. The scene between the doctor and patient about his diagnosis in the film *Angels in America*, is a powerful juxtaposition of explanatory models of illness from the perspectives of healthcare provider, public health planner, patient, family and activists of marginalized community. By exploring the inter-subjectivity of these narratives, students use their moral imagination ("What would I do if I were in the same situation?"), examine their affective reactions ("How does this interaction make me feel?") and realize the complexity and challenges in their clinical and social roles.

ARTS BASED

Aesthetic education is a learning method concerned with the process of perceptually engaging with something new, of being introduced to media that are originally unfamiliar to learners and nurtures an intensified awareness for various aspects of humanity (Beardsley, 1982). With regard to medical training, it helps students to sharpen their perception and gaze into body structure and the image of disease/disability. It also helps discover new ways of looking at, listening to, moving in and speaking of illness or healing experiences. Since aesthetic quality is inherent in art, various arts-based approaches, music, dance and movement, drama and the visual arts can all be useful media to develop aesthetic awareness. Visual analysis of portraits can help students observe and reflect on the state of mind and emotional state of a person. Under the guidance of a drama educator, students play out a scene and discover the powerful messages that can be delivered through body language and tone and how in the clinical setting this can affect healthcare professionals and the therapeutic relationship with patients.

E-LEARNING

In the digital era, e-learning (web-based learning or online learning) is a promising approach to learn medical humanities, especially for large classes or for periods when students are in distant attachments. For example, the exploration of illness narratives through written and multimedia applications supplemented with interactive online discussion forums could be an intriguing approach. However, the opportunities created for face-to-face debates and the conflicting values generated through the dynamics of real-time free-style discussion in conventional humanities classes are difficult to replicate in the e-learning environment making a blended learning approach useful, incorporating the best of both worlds.

EXPERIENTIAL LEARNING

Mindful practice

The themes of self-care, spirituality and healing are common in medical humanities curricula and may take the form of mindful practice. Mindfulness is the quality of having moment-to-moment non-judgemental awareness. Through guided workshops and immersing themselves in the practice, medical students can acquire this skill that helps develop self-awareness, which in turn can reduce psychological distress and improve clinical interpersonal skills such as attention, awareness, compassion and the capacity to deal with the witnessing of human suffering.

Historical visits

When learning about the history of medicine, students gain a sense of why contemporary medicine is practised the way it is, which contributes to the development of their collective professional identity. Reading, hearing about and discussing significant historical events such as the plague outbreak in Hong Kong in 1894 help students see parallels in how crises are handled in comparison with the SARS outbreak in 2003, how cultural beliefs and racial discrimination affected medical care and the public health changes that came about as a result. But, experiencing actual places where events took place add a new dimension. Places make connections across time, giving them a unique ability to create an empathetic understanding of what happened and why.

Service learning

Service learning is a widespread educational approach to prepare students to serve and to encourage the desire to serve while actually contributing something concrete to a community. As part of MH curricula, service learning provides pragmatic opportunities to explore social justice and humanitarianism in settings where narratives of illness and pressing concerns in disease management are real and confronted face to face. Such 'experiential narrative' not only helps students to further refine the reflective skills they learn in protected settings it also helps them.

What are some practical considerations and challenges?

TEACHERS

Traditionally, medical teachers are content experts in their field when the field is defined by a discipline. In the medical humanities curricula, where the discipline is multi- and cross-disciplinary, and teachers are academic experts in medicine or humanities or the arts or expert practitioners in any of those fields, it is difficult to define an expert medical humanities teacher and who should teach medical humanities (Box 29.1). Teachers in medical humanities programmes therefore bring expertise from their respective backgrounds and often join because of personal interest, and, with the contribution of many teachers, collectively enrich the medical humanities as a whole. However, faculty development to standardize understanding of the intent and goals of a particular medical humanities activity or programme is important. In addition, teachers who are trained as scientists or clinicians may benefit from the revisiting the concepts of health and diseases from a humanities and social sciences viewpoint looking at

> **Box 29.1   Tips for developing medical humanities in the curriculum.**
>
> - Draw on the expertise of the medical humanities and medical education communities, and the many resources available online and in print.
> - Develop a solid conceptual framework and structure based on sound educational principles such as OBASL.
> - Base content on the needs, goals and desired outcomes of the medical curriculum in the given context of the medical school.
> - Integrate with existing teaching and try to have co-teaching by medical/clinical and non-medical/clinical teachers to visibly reinforce the relevance of the MH as core learning.
> - Make it count so that there is explicit and tangible acknowledgement of the value of the MH learning.
> - Engage students in the planning process and encourage peer-to-peer teaching to develop a sense of ownership of the programme and sustainability.
> - Take a concurrent bottom-up and top-down approach as it is essential to have the Dean's support as well as that of front-line teachers who can commit to supporting the activity/programme.
> - Invest in professional development for skill-development among interested teachers, and to promote medical humanities among those who may not know they are interested, which will help broaden the base of teachers, sustain interest and build a community of practice.
> - Most importantly, have a passionate champion who will drive the initiative as the process will be time and energy intensive and will undoubtedly face as many deterrents as rewards.

basic historiographies of medicine, narrative representation of illness, social and cultural factors on health and diseases. Similarly, humanities-trained teachers can be familiarized with medical education principles to help frame their expertise for their learners.

SUSTAINABILITY

Students often do not realize how useful the core agenda of medical humanities is until they engage with patients in their senior years or even until after many years of practice. Sustainability of the curriculum is related to buy-in from the students and faculty members as well as perceived relevance to clinical practice, which is often challenging for medical humanities curricula.

Integrating medical humanities in the core medical curriculum and clinical teaching normalizes it as part of the curriculum that isn't 'finished' once an activity or course is completed. Student participation in planning groups and in peer teaching can help develop a sense of ownership in the programme. Innovative research approaches and longitudinal follow-up to investigate the impact of medical humanities on student and patient outcomes beyond the pre/post course evaluations can provide evidence of the value of MH and support its continuation. Moreover, creating and maintaining a critical mass of manpower to support teaching is important and can be achieved through faculty development and partnerships with non-medical faculties, museums and art galleries, as well as alumni and retired doctors.

CHANGING ROLE OF DOCTORS

Patient expectations and the scope of issues that impact practice have grown and are reflected in the evolving objectives of undergraduate medical education. These now address global health issues and a wider range of social and cultural determinants of health and disease, such as the increasing costs on healthcare, the widening gap between the rich and the poor, and improving health literacy among the general population, and reflect a medical learner's role as a world citizen and responsibilities as a future doctor. In response to such change, the teaching and learning of medical humanities is also evolving with the emergence of sub-disciplines of medical humanities such as public health humanities, which helps medical learners to understand, in a more nuanced way, the influence of social, cultural and financial contexts on health behaviours and to empathize with people in difficult circumstances (Saffran, 2014).

CROSS-CULTURAL AND LINGUISTIC ISSUES

All medical schools are set in communities with their own sociocultural norms and disease patterns, and the medical humanities curriculum, like the medical curriculum, needs to reflect the community in which their graduates will practise. Care must be taken in selecting medical humanities learning materials that best suit the cultural context. In Hong Kong, the general population speaks Cantonese, the local Chinese dialect, but the medium of instruction in the medical school is English. Most students' native language is Cantonese and conversation among students within and outside the classroom is almost always in Cantonese. While students respond insightfully to the Western-based texts discussed in the medical humanities curriculum, many prefer Chinese-language books, blogs and movies. Making use of works created by local authors, artists and filmmakers and presented in the local language may resonate more strongly with students and consequently stimulate more interest and enthusiasm.

In addition, while medical educators have been highlighting the importance of cultural competency, there is a call to shift the focus to cultural competency that is more rigorous in explaining intricate health and disease problems. Structural competency focuses on the forces that influence health outcomes at levels beyond individual clinical interactions to issues of poverty and inequality that might be shielded by presumed cultural representations. With such an approach, students gain critical awareness of the complexity regarding realistic goals of medical treatment and care (Metzl & Hansen, 2014). For example, Anne Fadiman's *The Spirit Catches You and You Fall Down*, has been widely used in medical schools to teach students about cultural barriers and non-compliance to therapy. However, in this complex story, it is the politics and international relations beyond the discussion of culture that are as critical in determining the family's resistance to modern medicine not only their superstitious help-seeking behaviour.

REALITIES OF PRACTICE

There is clear evidence for the benefits of mindfulness meditation, expressive art practice, and narrative-based medical practice in the wellbeing of medical learners themselves and in potentially improving the quality of their future careers. But sadly, students face a grim external reality when they emerge from the relatively protected confines of medical school into clinical work with its demanding work and schedule, consumerism-oriented pressures and potential lawsuits. Medical humanities may help equip students to better cope with these realities but hopefully will also begin a shift in mindset and medical culture to address the structural problems of higher training and practise.

Summary

Medical humanities are primarily critical endeavours that explore the human condition and the greater context through which the patient and doctor make meaning of health and illness through the broader perspective of the humanities, arts and social sciences but also contribute to wellbeing and personal development.

A large number of medical schools around the world have adopted the medical humanities in some form into their curricula, and there is great diversity in the way they are conceptualized, structured, taught and assessed.

Robust educational principles should underpin the teaching and learning, which should also be tailored to suit the context, and a variety of educational approaches can be used including narrative, arts based, experiential and e-learning.

Conceptual and practical issues include the definition of medical humanities, who should teach them, sustainability, evaluation of impact or effectiveness of medical humanities teaching, and sensitivity to cultural, linguistic and realities of practice.

Acknowledgement

With immense gratitude to Professor LC Chan (1951–2015), a passionate medical educator and tireless champion of the medical humanities in the medical school curriculum at HKU and beyond.

References

Beardsley, M., 1982. The Aesthetic Point of View. Cornell University Press.

Bleakley, A., 2015. Medical Humanities and Medical Education: How the medical humanities can shape better doctors. Routledge, Milton Park.

Brody, H., 2011. Defining the medical humanities: three conceptions and three narratives. J. Med. Humanit. 32 (1), 1–7. doi:10.1007/s10912-009-9094-4.

Cassell, E.J., 1999. Diagnosing suffering: a perspective. Ann. Intern. Med. 131 (7), 531–534.

Charon, R., 2004. Narrative and Medicine. NEJM 350 (9), 862–864.

Dittrich, L., 2003. The humanities and medicine: reports of 41 US, Canadian and international programs (preface). Acad. Med. 78 (10), 951–952.

Fitzgerald, F.T., 1996. Wanted: 21st century physician. Ann. Int. Med. 124 (1 pt 1), 71.

Gawande, A., 2014. Being mortal: illness, medicine and what matters in the end. Metropolitan Books, New York.

Gordon, J., Evans, M., 2013. Learning medicine from the humanities. In: Swanwick, T. (Ed.), Understanding Medical Education: evidence, theory and practice, second ed. John Wiley and Sons, pp. 213–226.

Guyatt, G.H., Haynes, R.B., Jaeschke, R.Z., et al., 2000. User's guides to the medical literature: XXV. Evidence-based medicine: principles for applying the user's guides to patient care. Evidence-based Medicine Working Group. JAMA 284 (10), 1290–1296.

Hurwitz, B., 2003. Medicine, the arts and humanities. Clin. Med. (Lond) 3 (6), 497–498.

Kleinman, A., 1988. The Illness Narratives: Suffering, Healing and the Human Condition. Basic Books, New York.

Macnaughton, J., 2000. The humanities in medical education: context, outcomes and structures. Med. Humanit. 26 (1), 23–30. doi:10.1136/mh.26.1.23.

Metzl, J.M., Hansen, H., 2014. Structural competency: theorizing a new medical engagement with stigma and inequality. Soc. Sci. Med. 103, 126–133.

NYU School of Medicine, n.d. Humanities, social sciences and the arts in relation to medicine and medical training. http://medhum.med.nyu.edu/about. (Accessed February 2016).

Saffran, L., 2014. 'Only connect': the case for public health humanities. Med. Humanit. 40 (2), 105–110. doi: 10.1136/medhum-2014-010502.

30 Integrative medicine in the training of physicians

A. Haramati, S. R. Adler, B. Kligler

Trends

- Graduating physicians need to be knowledgeable about complementary and integrative medical practices so they can advise their patients about the judicious use of these therapies to improve health and healing.

- Most medical schools include aspects of complementary and integrative medicine in the curriculum to achieve learning outcomes in knowledge acquisition and clinical skills building about complementary and alternative medicine (CAM), and innovative institutions are including experiential mind-body medicine sessions to foster self-awareness and self-care of the students and faculty.

- The incorporation of integrative medicine in clinical training can be synergized with other elements such as interprofessional education and cultural competency to create robust clinical skills examinations.

- Integrative medicine is becoming an important component of the curriculum in residency training programmes focusing on primary care, and fellowship training is evolving the field into a sub-specialty designation.

Introduction

In virtually all developed countries that practice conventional medicine, a significant percentage of the public seeks complementary and alternative medicine (CAM) to enhance health and healing. These include mind-body therapies such as meditation, imagery and spirituality; body-based therapies such as chiropractic and osteopathic manipulation and massage; nutritional supplements, herbs and botanicals; energy healing interventions such as Reiki and acupuncture; and systemic approaches such as Traditional Chinese Medicine (TCM), Ayurvedic medicine and many other traditional and indigenous healing rituals.

The past 30 years has seen the emergence of integrative medicine in which the physician, working usually with a team of practitioners, seeks to combine the best approaches from both conventional and complementary therapies to treat illness and foster wellbeing. Integrative medicine, as defined by the Academic Consortium for Integrative Medicine and Health, reaffirms the importance of the relationship between practitioner and patient, focuses on the whole person, is informed by evidence, and makes use of all appropriate therapeutic and lifestyle approaches, healthcare professionals and disciplines to achieve optimal health and healing (Academic Consortium for Integrative Medicine and Health, 2015). In this chapter, we will explore the rationale for teaching physicians about integrative medicine in medical school, and the strategies that have been employed to incorporate integrative medicine into undergraduate and graduate medical education.

 "Integrative medicine reaffirms the importance of the relationship between practitioner and patient, focuses on the whole person, is informed by evidence, and makes use of all appropriate therapeutic and lifestyle approaches, healthcare professionals and disciplines to achieve optimal health and healing."

Academic Consortium for Integrative Medicine and Health, 2004

Integrative medicine in undergraduate medical education

The rationale for incorporating integrative medicine into the medical school curriculum is that graduating physicians should be able to understand advances in the field and provide guidance to their patients on what works, what is dangerous and what seems to be of no use. Thus, in most academic institutions around the world, there is at least a mention of CAM and integrative medicine within the curriculum, although the amount of time and degree of depth these elements are taught varies widely. In 1999, the National Center for Complementary and Alternative Medicine (now called the National Center for Complementary and Integrative Health) at the National Institutes of Health in the United States provided significant funding to 14 conventional medical and nursing schools to develop curricula and exemplars of how best to incorporate

CAM and integrative medicine into the training of health professionals. The lessons learned were summarized in a series of articles published in *Academic Medicine* in 2007 and disseminated at international conferences, especially those focusing on medical education. The significance of that initiative, along with others publishing in a number of countries, is that many more institutions were willing to bring CAM and integrative medicine into their classrooms and clinics.

PRE-CLINICAL YEARS

Kligler et al. published a recommended set of competencies in integrative medicine for medical school curricula, and delineated knowledge, skills, attitudes and values that educators from 23 academic health centres felt were fundamental to the field (Kligler, 2004). Most schools focus on teaching students *about* CAM and integrative medicine, rather than *how to practice*. In the pre-clinical years, this manifests as seamless integration of content into the required course structure. Thus, lectures on acupuncture and other non-pharmacologic approaches to management of pain appear in neuroscience and in physiology, manipulation and massage might be added to an anatomy course, and mindfulness meditation becomes part of the discussion on the physiology of stress—with the focus on how to reduce stress. Virtually all pharmacology courses now include material on herbs and botanicals. This information serves not only to educate students on the most common non-vitamin, non-mineral supplements that their patients may be taking but also to caution on potentially serious herb–drug interactions that might ensue, especially if the patients are not inclined to inform their healthcare provider of what they are taking.

Adding CAM and integrative medicine can also help achieve curricular goals regarding understanding patient preferences and cultural competence. In this regard, many schools have included CAM in their 'doctoring' courses on the practice of medicine, and in courses that address patient, physician and society. Some have gone on to include CAM in their clinical skills training and add awareness of these dimensions and considerations to the assessment component as part of an objective structured clinical exam.

EXPERIENTIAL LEARNING

Perhaps the most effective instructional strategy is to provide opportunities to experience CAM first-hand: either by offering integrative clinics as part of the student's ambulatory rotation in the community or by creating immersion experiences as electives. In both cases, students get to experience some of the therapies first-hand, and also observe the practice of integrative medicine and relationship-centred principles in action. For many students, this experience also provides an important opportunity to research the state of the

evidence for many modalities and to engage in directed self-learning.

Another way in which CAM and integrative medicine has been incorporated into the pre-clinical curriculum has been through elective courses that emphasize mind-body skills to foster self-awareness and self-care. Teaching students meditation, imagery and tools for self-reflection as a way to reduce stress and build resilience, has become increasingly prevalent, with prominent schools such as Monash University in Australia, Charite University in Germany and Georgetown University in Washington, DC, leading the way. Outcomes from these initiatives suggest that the programmes are effective in achieving multiple competencies ranging from knowledge and skills to attitudes (Lee et al., 2007).

 "...graduating physicians should be able to understand advances in the field of complementary and integrative medicine and provide guidance to their patients on what works, what is dangerous and what seems to be of no use."

CLINICAL YEARS

In addition to ensuring that all students achieve core competencies through required foundational content, the goal of teaching integrative medicine in the pre-clinical years is to provide skills training in clerkships, as well as advanced electives for students interested in pursuing a higher level of proficiency. One challenge of teaching integrative medicine, however, persists in the form of the disproportionate need to justify the inclusion of content, particularly where there is a pervasive sense that existing curricula are overly full.

Thus, it is important to take a strategic and context-aware approach to the selection of material and teaching methods in the clinical years. Designing curricula for the third and fourth years of medical school requires the same systematic, evidenced-based approach to content selection (e.g. reviewing and mapping a school's existing integrative medicine content, designing an 'ideal' curriculum, and then developing strategies to address the gaps between the existing and ideal forms). Over the last two decades of designing curricula, most medical schools have developed a set of strategies for maximizing the quality, integration, and impact of integrative medicine content.

Clerkships

CLINICAL PEARLS TOOLKIT

Increasingly, medical educators are acknowledging the imperative for tomorrow's physicians to be educated regarding CAM issues. This growing awareness is often expressed as the need for students to be able to interact appropriately with patients and advise them in a manner that contributes to high-quality, comprehensive care. As medical students transition from the classroom to clerkships, however, they face the challenge of applying integrative medicine knowledge and skills (often learned out of context) to real patient encounters.

One tool that has been developed at the University of California San Francisco (UCSF) to help students distil the key elements to review and reinforce on the wards is a collection of 'clinical pearls', that is, an annotated collection of small bits of free-standing, clinically relevant information (Saba et al., 2010). As part of a larger effort to design a social and behavioural sciences curriculum, faculty at UCSF worked with clerkship directors and medical students to review the pre-clinical integrative medicine content and identify key concepts that students would find most useful throughout all clerkships. These 'pearls' take the form of summaries (1–2 pages) to remind students of what to focus on in clinical encounters. (They also help further efforts at curriculum integration by informing clerkship directors, faculty preceptors, and house staff of the integrative medicine content students have been taught prior to the third year.) For example, one pearl is *Communicating with Patients about Integrative Medicine: Suggestions for Talking with Patients about CAM.* The one-page summary includes definitions of key terms, questions and prompts for discussions with patients, and key references. This curricular resource has proven extremely effective in aiding students' recall of important integrative medicine information and guiding their application of the content during their clerkship experience.

INTERPROFESSIONAL STANDARDIZED PATIENT EXAM

An increasingly recognized challenge for health professions students is moving from education in silos to adapting to a team environment. With the evolution from the solo clinician to team-based care, it is important to include integrative medicine in the systematic interprofessional education that is necessary for true collaboration: the curriculum must reflect the real-life experience of clinical teams in order to prepare students for the diverse scenarios and dynamic environments they will encounter in practice.

 "The synergy between integrative medicine and interprofessional education was inherent in designing the Interprofessional Standardized Patient Exam (ISPE), which assesses the common goals of team-based, community-focused, and patient-centered care, and is required of all health professions students at University of California San Francisco."

The fields of integrative medicine and interprofessional education share many values, including effective communication between practitioners, shared problem solving and decision making, and integration of different knowledge structures into comprehensive action plans. The synergy between the two fields was inherent in designing an assessment to promote the common goals of team-based, community-focused, and patient-centred care. Effective interprofessional education engages participants in authentic tasks, settings and roles. Using these guiding principles, faculty at UCSF developed an interprofessional standardized patient exam (ISPE) that is required of all UCSF medical, dental, nurse practitioner, pharmacy and physical therapy students. In collaboration with a multidisciplinary team, including colleagues from geriatrics and palliative care, an integrative medicine case was developed in which the patient presents to establish care and discuss therapeutic options, including acupuncture and mindfulness meditation, for chronic low back pain and depressive symptoms. The learning objectives include effective communication regarding integrative medicine and respecting and negotiating the patient's preferences. This required ISPE not only assesses students' integrative medicine knowledge, skills, and attitudes, but, because of the 'capital' of the high-stakes exam, it provides an opportunity to validate the importance of integrative medicine and endorse its role in interprofessional education.

FOURTH-YEAR ADVANCED ELECTIVES

Despite the tremendous gains evident in some medical school curricula, the scope of required content in integrative medicine for many medical students remains limited. Students are frequently merely introduced to integrative medicine without the necessary depth of exposure. Given the structural limitations of many medical school curricula, including insufficient time, the best form of advanced experience may be the fourth-year elective.

Many medical schools have developed electives that permit a deeper exploration for students interested in advanced study. Typically, this two to four week block includes a contextualizing overview of the historical and sociocultural context of integrative medicine, followed by didactic sessions (e.g. patterns of CAM use in the United States, Traditional Chinese Medicine (TCM), Ayurveda, CAM for medically underserved populations), experiential sessions (tai chi, mindfulness meditation, guided imagery, acupuncture), joint sessions with interprofessional students (group discussions and activities with students from a local TCM college), and community preceptorships (shadowing local acupuncturists, naturopaths, chiropractors). This model of advanced exploration (Adler, 2013) has been used successfully in the design of other long-standing integrative medicine electives and has proven ideal for providing greater breadth and depth of instruction in the field; offering real-world experiences in integrative, team-based care; and proposing practical options for pursuing additional clinical or research study in integrative medicine.

Although some of the difficulties faced by educators in teaching integrative medicine are unique, such as historical scepticism on the part of the biomedical field, many of the curricular challenges have already been faced by other medical school faculty endeavouring to incorporate content outside of the existing canon (e.g. the social and behavioural sciences). As is the case with other previously non-traditional topics, it is important to find ways to institutionalize integrative medicine content. It is always helpful to have a high-level champion within a school to promote integrative medicine education, but a great deal can also be accomplished through a deliberate, strategic approach to curricular integration.

As curricular reform and renewal takes place in many medical schools, there is opportunity to engage and collaborate with students, who are widely recognized as particularly effective curricular change agents. Specifically, while keeping the goals of the broader medical school curriculum in mind, faculty and students can suggest integrative–medicine-themed solutions to existing curricular challenges. For example, there are opportunities to apply cultural competence concepts through communication with standardized patients about complementary and integrative medicine use. Another area is in the teaching of evidence-based medicine, where the rigors and limitations of trial designs can be examined by reviewing recent acupuncture studies and trying to understand the impact of the clinical encounter and the power of placebo.

Integrative medicine in graduate medical education

RESIDENCY

The first published set of curriculum goals and objectives for residency-level training in complementary and integrative medicine was developed by the Society of Teachers of Family Medicine in 2000 (Kligler et al., 2000). Because of its explicit commitment to the biopsychosocial philosophy and to a whole person model of care, family medicine as a specialty was a natural fit for integrative medicine training. Although these were recommended rather than required guidelines, they helped set the stage for a rapid spread of curriculum interventions in family medicine programmes around the United States. Most of these were offered as electives, but a number of programmes did begin at that point to require basic training in complementary/integrative medicine as part of core family medicine training.

These early curriculum experiments, and a sense that a more uniform approach to delivering knowledge

and skills in integrative medicine was needed, ultimately led to the development of the Integrative Medicine in Residency (IMR) programme in 2007 by the University of Arizona Center for Integrative Medicine (Lebensohn et al., 2012). The IMR programme is a 200-hour online curriculum designed to be imported into any primary care residency programme, supplemented with onsite activities led by a faculty mentor. The programme was originally piloted in eight family medicine programmes and is now being used in over 60 sites around the United States and Canada. The competencies outlined for the IMR project were deliberately keyed to existing ACGME competencies as a strategy to facilitate widespread integration and acceptance of this curriculum by residency programme directors. The curriculum is modular and can be distributed through the course of residency in a variety of different ways depending on the needs and structure of a given residency programme.

 "The Integrative Medicine in Residency (IMR) programme was originally piloted in eight family medicine programmes and is now being used in over 60 sites around the United States and Canada, and expanded to other primary care training programmes."

The IMR programme has now expanded beyond family medicine residency and is being offered in a number of specialty training programmes including paediatrics, internal medicine, and preventive medicine. A variation of the curriculum aimed specifically at paediatric programmes is currently in pilot testing at six residency sites around the United States. Of the over 60 sites currently offering the IMR, many do so as a track for residents specifically interested in integrative medicine, and others as a required curriculum element for the whole programme. Evaluation of the programme has shown it to be effective in increasing knowledge of integrative medicine content and residents' confidence in their ability to effectively counsel patients in this area. There is also an explicit self-care component in the IMR curriculum to address issues of physician burnout and resilience.

The development of integrative medicine education at the graduate medical education (GME) level has been significantly advanced with the recent entry of the federal Health Resources and Systems Administration (HRSA) into this arena. HRSA is an agency of the US Department of Health and Human Services, which over the past four years has funded several significant projects to expand the scope of GME training in integrative medicine. The first of these was the Integrative Medicine in Preventive Medicine Education (IMPriME) programme, which supported the development of competencies in integrative medicine for preventive medicine as a specialty, as well as the development of curricular innovations to transmit those competencies (Jani et al., 2015). Following on this initiative, HRSA is now funding a number of preventive medicine residency programmes that are explicitly committed to including integrative medicine as a focus of their required curriculum.

In a bold move to take integrative medicine training beyond the boundaries of medical education and into the interprofessional arena, HRSA is also funding the National Center for Integrative Primary Healthcare, a national initiative aimed at developing uniform competencies and curriculum across the spectrum of health professions involved in primary care. This project—a collaboration between HRSA, the University of Arizona Center for Integrative Medicine, and the Academic Consortium for Integrative Health and Medicine— includes in its scope not only the primary care medical specialties (family medicine, internal medicine, paediatrics, and preventive medicine) but also nursing, pharmacy, behavioural health, chiropractic, acupuncture, naturopathy, public health and dentistry. A consensus set of competencies for this project has been developed and published (Box 30.1).

Box 30.1 Competencies for integrative primary healthcare

1. Practise patient-centred and relationship-based care.
2. Obtain a comprehensive health history that includes mind-body-spirit, nutrition, and the use of conventional, complementary and integrative therapies and disciplines.
3. Collaborate with individuals and families to develop a personalized plan of care to promote health and wellbeing, which incorporates integrative approaches including lifestyle counselling and the use of mind-body strategies.
4. Demonstrate skills in utilizing the evidence as it pertains to integrative healthcare.
5. Demonstrate knowledge about the major conventional, complementary and integrative health professions.
6. Facilitate behaviour change in individuals, families and communities.
7. Work effectively as a member of an interprofessional team.
8. Engage in personal behaviours and self-care practices that promote optimal health and wellbeing.
9. Incorporate integrative healthcare into community settings and into the healthcare system at large.
10. Incorporate ethical standards of practice into all interactions with individuals, organizations and communities.

The 45-hour online core curriculum will enter a pilot phase in 2016. The ultimate goal of this project is to create, test and disseminate the set of educational resources needed to eventually support an experience in integrative healthcare as part of the required curriculum in every health profession participating in the primary care environment. As healthcare moves to a more team-based, interprofessional approach, these resources will enable the development of effective teams ready to deliver integrative medicine in the primary care setting.

The question of whether integrative medicine is primarily a subspecialty, requiring fellowship-level training programmes, or primarily an approach to the practice of medicine as a whole that should be incorporated into training at all levels and for all specialties, has been hotly debated for two decades. The de facto outcome of this debate has been a two-pronged approach to training including both the broad-based strategies described above and an evolving landscape of fellowship-level training programmes as well.

FELLOWSHIP

Fellowship-level training in integrative medicine dates to 1996 with the inception of the residential programme at University of Arizona. This was a two-year residential fellowship with an emphasis on clinical training and leadership. This programme was later converted into a two- year, 1000-hour distance-learning programme (which still includes three residential weeks over the two years), which over the past ten years has graduated over 1000 fellows, with almost every medical specialty represented. Meanwhile, residential fellowships, most of them one year in duration, have proliferated at academic settings around the Unites States, with roughly 20 programmes enrolling fellows as of late 2015. The growth in the number of fellowship spots has been somewhat constrained by the current status of integrative medicine as a non-accredited fellowship, which has led to a lack of access to the federal training dollars that support much of fellowship training in the United States. A set of core competencies for fellowship-level training, developed by the Academic Consortium for Integrative Medicine and Health, was published in 2014, and will most likely be used eventually as the framework for credentialing and accrediting fellowship programmes in this field (Ring et al., 2014).

Summary

The field of integrative medicine has emerged over the past 30 years as the public sought therapeutic options for chronic conditions that were not being addressed adequately with conventional medical approaches. Researchers and clinical investigators followed with a renewed focus on studying the efficacy of non-pharmacologic approaches to management of pain, symptoms from cancer treatment, stress and other conditions. Physicians need to be knowledgeable about complementary and integrative medical practices so they can advise their patients about the judicious use of these therapies to improve health and healing. Most medical schools and many residency programmes now include aspects of complementary and integrative medicine in the undergraduate and graduate curriculum, in ways that advance competencies in knowledge, skills and attitudes. Moreover, integrative medicine in clinical training can be synergized with other elements such as interprofessional education and cultural competency to create robust clinical skills examinations and competent skilled healthcare practitioners that can meet the public need.

References

Academic Consortium for Integrative Medicine and Health: Definition of Integrative Medicine. Available at: http://imconsortium.org/about/about-us.cfm. (Accessed 27 January 2017).

Adler, S., 2013. Benedict's Lens: Medical Students' Perspectives on Integrative Medicine Education. EXPLORE-NY 9 (5), 331.

Jani, A.A., Trask, J., Ali, A., 2015. Integrative medicine in preventive medicine education: competency and curriculum development for preventive medicine and other specialty residency programs. Am. J. Prev. Med. 49 (5 Suppl. 3), S222–S229. doi:10.1016/j.amepre.2015.08.019.

Kligler, B., Maizes, V., Schachter, S., et al., 2004. Core competencies in integrative medicine for medical school curricula: a proposal. Acad. Med. 79, 521–531.

Kligler, B., Gordon, A., Stuart, M., Sierpina, V., 2000. Suggested curriculum guidelines on complementary and alternative medicine: recommendations of the Society of Teachers of Family Medicine Group on Alternative Medicine. Fam. Med. 32 (1), 30–33.

Lebensohn, P., Kligler, B., Dodds, S., et al., 2012. Integrative medicine in residency education: developing competency through online curriculum training. J Grad Med Educ. 4 (1), 76–82. PMID: 23451312.

Lee, M.Y., Wimsatt, L., Hedgecock, J., et al., 2007. Integrating complementary and alternative medicine instruction into medical education: organizational and instructional strategies. Acad. Med. 82, 939–945.

Ring, M., Brodsky, M., Low Dog, T., et al., 2014. Developing and implementing core competencies for integrative medicine fellowships. Acad. Med. 89 (3), 421–428.

Saba, G., Satterfield, J., Salazar, R., et al. The SBS Toolbox: Clinical Pearls from the Social and Behavioral Sciences. MedEdPORTAL Publications; 2010. Available from: http://dx.doi.org/10.15766/mep_2374-8265.7980.

Global awareness

P. K. Drain, A. M. Wylie

Trends

- Global awareness is a fundamental element to practising modern medicine, and teaching and learning global health starts by understanding local health issues.

- The methods of integrating global awareness into medical education and teaching activities are evolving.

- The six major learning objectives are the following: Global Burden of Disease, Socio-Economic and Environmental Determinants of Health, Health Systems, Global Health Governance, Human Rights and Ethics, and Cultural Diversity and Health.

- Students and faculty should be encouraged to pursue global health field educational and elective experiences to promote good global health awareness practices.

Introduction

The world has become increasingly interconnected during the last century with more international travel and trade, integration of global economies and an increasingly mobile global work force. While this improves the dissemination of science, knowledge and technology, an interconnected world can lead to a more rapid spread of infectious diseases. This globalization has shifted the burden of disease in many resource-limited countries to include more chronic non-communicable diseases, such as cardiovascular disease, diabetes and cancer (Bhutta et al., 2010). The emerging field of global health is a combined medical and public health discipline that aims to improve the lives of all people by principally reducing health disparities and inequalities, and identifying and addressing modifiable social determinants of health. The principles of global health have grown from the previous disciplines of tropical medicine and international health to include a more comprehensive approach to achieving equity in health for all people worldwide(Koplan et al., 2009). While understanding the global health principles may

be critical to maintaining stable, healthy populations and reducing conflict, the teaching of those principles has been slowly incorporated into the curriculum of various health science programmes. The aim of this chapter is to describe the rationale for including global awareness in health science education, particularly medical and nursing curricula, and to provide some practical lessons for planning and integrating global health education into an existing curriculum.

The rationale for global awareness

The changing global landscape and advances in educational practices fostered a recent opportunity to re-examine the delivery of health science education. In 2010, the Commission on Education of Health Professions for the 21st Century was formed to advance health by recommending changes to develop a generation of health professionals who will be better equipped to address present and future health challenges (Bhutta et al., 2010; Frenk et al., 2010). The Commission, co-chaired by Dr Julio Frenk, then Dean of the Harvard School of Public Health, and Dr Lincoln Chen, President of the China Medical Board, was formed to coincide with the 100th anniversary of the Flexner report and to acknowledge the global health initiatives that have underscored the critical importance of the health workforce and health systems. These new educational approaches, which recognize changing patterns of health determinants, population movements, technological advances, and health systems innovations, can better address the pressing needs for global awareness and local sensitivity.

The Commission's report highlighted severe institutional shortages both between and within countries, as well as a distribution of expenditures for health professional education that was poorly aligned with population size or burden of disease (Bhutta et al., 2010). China, India, Brazil, and the United States have an abundance of medical schools (Fig. 31.1), while 36 countries had no medical school. Global accreditation systems were described as weak and unevenly practised, and there was an overall scarcity of information on research about health professional education. A major

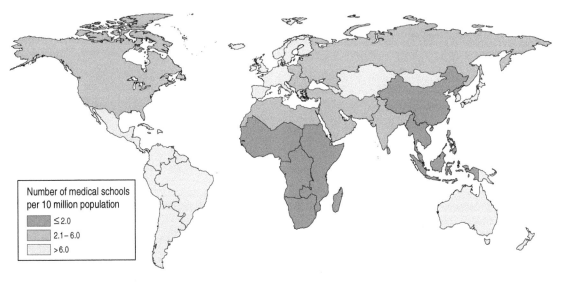

Fig. 31.1 Density of medical schools by region.

(From Frenk et al., Health professionals for a new century: transforming education to strengthen health systems in an interdependent world. The Lancet 376(9756): 1923–1958, 2010.)

recommendation from the report was to implement instructional reforms that "adopt competency-driven approaches to instructional design; and adapt these competencies to rapidly changing local conditions drawing on global resources." In addition, the Commission highlighted the benefits of medical schools in all countries forming twinning programmes that foster exchange, share resources, and undertake collaborative work for the goal of mutual advance.

The Commission's findings and recommendations were built upon both empirical research and expert opinion on the changing cause of morbidity and mortality. The World Health Organization (WHO) has detailed a global increase for mortality related to chronic non-communicable diseases, and a global decrease for mortality related to infectious diseases. Additional changes in human migration, conflict, medical tourism and mass travel have further reinforced the need to integrate global health principles into medical education.

Exploring and understanding a patient's social determinants of health, including racial and ethnic background, occupation, and use of alcohol and tobacco, constitutes an essential part of the medical examination (Behforouz et al., 2014). The expansion of the patient 'social history' is necessary to understand not only their determinants of disease but also their resources and abilities to achieve good health. The expanded patient history should include cultural healthcare beliefs, perception of healthcare, and ability to access and utilize healthcare services. Thus, taking a more comprehensive patient social history is one method to include global awareness in each medical encounter, which can lead

to individualized care plans that take into account a patient's personal and structural barriers to good health as well as a patient's abilities, opportunities and resources.

With enhanced global awareness, the next generation of clinicians should be well equipped to provide personalized, appropriate and sustainable care, within the parameters of their medical role. Clinicians who have a more comprehensive awareness of their patient's global environment and beliefs will be able to optimize clinical judgement and patient management (Wylie & Holt, 2010). Addressing the social determinants that either impede or promote good health can lead to providing optimal cost-effective medical care, which may also bring satisfaction to both patients and providers.

Understanding the global health agenda for medical education

In 2012, *The Lancet* published six proposed learning themes with 21 specific outcomes to teach global health in medical curricula (Box 31.1) (Johnson et al., 2012). These themes and outcomes provide some guidance, but a dissemination of innovation and good practices requires continued collaboration and dialogue. While Box 31.1 provides a blueprint for teaching global awareness to medical students, the changing nature of global health may require frequent refinements of these learning themes and objectives.

In 2015, the United Nations adopted 17 sustainable development goals (SDGs), which were agreed upon

1. Global burden of disease

- Discuss communicable and non-communicable disease at the global level.
- Discuss the impact of international travel and migration on the diseases at the local level.
- Discuss the causes and control of global epidemics.

2. Socio-economic and environmental determinants of health

- Demonstrate awareness of the non-clinical determinants of health, including social, political, economic, and environmental and gender disparities.
- Examine how health can be distributed unequally within and between populations in relation to socially-defined measures.
- Describe how the environment and health interact at the global level.

3. Health systems

- Discuss the essential components of a health system using the WHO model.
- Recognize that health systems are structured differently and function differently across the globe.
- Recognize the inequitable distribution of the international workforce, and explain the migration of health- care workers.
- Examine the causes and scale of inequalities in health workforce distribution.

4. Global health governance

- Demonstrate awareness of the complexity of global health governance, including the roles of international organizations, the commercial sector and civil society.

- Discuss the role of the WHO as the international representative body of national governments for health.
- Discuss how health-related research is conducted and governed globally.

5. Human rights and ethics

- Respect the rights and equal value of all people without discrimination and provide compassionate care for all.
- Examine how international legal frameworks impact on local healthcare delivery.
- Discuss and critique the concept of a right to health.
- Describe the particular health needs of vulnerable groups and migrants.
- Discuss the role of doctors as advocates for their patients, including the importance of prioritizing health needs over other concerns and adhering to codes of professional conduct.

6. Cultural diversity and health

- Demonstrate understanding that culture is important and may influence behaviour, while acknowledging the dangers of assuming that those from a particular social group will behave in a certain way.
- Communicate effectively with those from different ethnic, religious and social backgrounds, where necessary using external help.
- Work effectively with colleagues from different ethnic, religious and social backgrounds.

by United Nations member countries, to represent a framework for global development through to the year 2030. While all of the SDGs influence the approach to global health principles, only the third goal (SDG-3) relates directly to health and achieving equity in health for all people worldwide. SDG-3 has nine measureable targets for the global health community to achieve over the next fifteen years. These targets relate to maternal and child health, infectious diseases, chronic non-communicable diseases, as well as substance abuse, injuries, health systems and environmental health (United Nations, 2015). http://www.un.org/sustainable development/sustainable-development-goals/.

All students in undergraduate or graduate health science education should be aware of the sustainable development goals. Students should receive regular encouragement or recognition for actively pursuing the goals of the common global health agenda. One pathway

for students to participate in this agenda is to join or form a student interest group or organization, such as International Federation of Medical Students Association (IFMSA), the American Medical Student Association (AMSA) in the United States, or MEDSIN in the United Kingdom.

Integrating activities and resources for global awareness

At most medical schools curriculum planning and reviewing is an on-going process with frequent minor revisions and periodic major restructuring. The major changes are often influenced by regulatory bodies, changing healthcare priorities or resources, and advances in educational and pedagogical research. This chapter offers a general approach for medical curricula, with the caveat that specific details might need to be adapted to the local context.

Some global health curricula have adopted a 'vertical strand' or 'spiral curriculum' to allow students to build a systematic and advancing body of knowledge and skills. A vertical strand is a topic or subject that is integrated throughout the curriculum that maintains relevance to the core content and builds on existing knowledge and skills. A spiral curriculum applies several topics or subjects to the current context of core learning principles (Wylie & Holt, 2010). Both tools should be structured around a core set of principle knowledge or clinical competencies. By integrating the teaching and skills-based practice this approach avoids having an isolated module or lecture without relevant context. In this manner, global health education will become an integral part of the medical education (Wylie, 2011). For modular or specific global health sessions, a facilitator might explore open-ended questions about the cause of health and disease (Johnson et al., 2012).

Teaching global health principles should include informational topics, clinical encounters and practical experiences, and begin as early in the student's medical training as possible. Throughout the curriculum, faculty and students should be regularly encouraged to explore the most relevant global health topics. By periodically coming back to the same questions, students may progress in relation to their clinical learning, which would enable them to gain insight into some of the basic principles of global health. How this option is implemented and assessed will vary, but the process should be guided and accountable, based on evidence and informed by scholarly inquiry, practical experience and a respectful debate.

 Faculty and students should ask and explore the following questions:
- What causes health and what causes disease?
- Why and how do patterns of morbidity and mortality vary?
- What modifiable risk factors influence patterns of disease?
- How should the medical profession respond to global health inequalities?

Global health training starts by understanding local health issues

Students matriculate into medical school with wide varieties of background and experience. Some will have rather extensive experience conducting health-related work in a resource-limited setting, while others will have little or no understanding of the relevant issues or principles of global health. Not every medical student will be interested in travelling to far off destinations to treat patients with neglected tropical diseases, but almost every medical student will encounter patients who are facing socio-behavioural, cultural, economic challenges, and determinants of health that impede either access to or delivery of quality healthcare. Thus, every medical student and junior doctor will face global health issues within their local community.

Starting with local issues is a way to engage all students in global health issues. At the start of medical school, students could conduct mapping exercises to plot the salient features that impact health issues within their local neighbourhood. The exercise might include determining access to healthcare (by calculating the distance to a clinic or hospital or pharmacy) or evaluating the possibility of eating well (by determining the price of fresh fruit and vegetables). Students could assess the ethnic diversity of the local population, and ask neighbouring clinics if language translators or interpreters are available for the commonly spoken languages.

Early clinical encounters will almost certainly include patients from various ethnic backgrounds, recent immigrants, or visitors from foreign countries. Discussion of these patients' health needs should include various health issues and potential diagnoses within a global context. For example, a patient presenting with a fever after recently travelling to a malaria-endemic country in West Africa should be suspected of having malaria. Knowing about certain genetic and ethnic-related diseases is important. For example, sickle cell anaemia or thalassemia may have variable penetration within a local community, and a clinician lacking global health awareness and training would be unaware and unsuspecting. During student's clinical encounters, supervising physicians should review global health principles and diagnoses with medical students and junior physicians.

As medical students advance to the senior years, they will likely improve their medical interviews with a patient-centred approach. This approach focuses on the patient who has a symptom or disease, and not solely on the patient's symptom or disease. By focusing on the patient, a full history might uncover signs or symptoms, medical beliefs or health behaviours linked to a patient's social and ethnic context. As medical students learn various approaches to behaviour change and motivational interviewing, they should be informed of cultural sensitivities, local resources and possible social support.

At many medical schools, teaching about communications skills is integrated into the core medical curricula and periodically reinforced. Students should be taught how and when to use translation and interpreter services. Students should also be aware of the potential for misunderstanding, breach of confidentiality, coercion, and the vulnerability of patients. The description of symptoms, medical concerns and information received can often be complex and misunderstood (Wylie, 2011). There may also be unspoken concerns about the costs of medical diagnostics and/or treatments. Some patients may expect a paternalistic approach, rather than a patient-centred approach. Medical students will need to learn to ascertain a reliable medical history, and explain a clear diagnostic and treatment plan, whether or not they use a medical interpreter.

The more complex global health issues should be reinforced and strengthened for senior medical students. For example, while a junior student may not know the most relevant clinical questions to ask an immigrant patient who speaks another primary language, senior students should be training to work with language interpreters and cultural mediators so that they can ask the appropriate questions, including the spiritual, religious and cultural beliefs. In addition, senior students should be able to develop a treatment plan that will be suitable to meet the patient's needs and to explain a diagnosis and care plan with cultural sensitivity.

Senior students should have already begun to explore the larger context of global health. In this manner, senior students might be encouraged to take a broader perspective of population-level interventions. During these years, additional lectures and didactics could expand the teaching topics. Relevant topics for these students might include an understanding of different healthcare systems, issues related to the delivery of care in resource-limited settings, and health matters related to income inequality and poverty. As senior students gradually gain a more comprehensive under-standing of global health issues they will or should aspire to become articulate well-informed advocates for their patients.

Upon completion of medical training, students should appreciate the complexity of healthcare provisions, the concept of shared clinical decision making, and an understanding of various ethnic and cultural issues, including genetic predisposition and patient vulnerability. Most high-income countries have very diverse ethnic and multicultural populations, each one having different systems and goals for healthcare and a varied understanding of medicine. Patients place confidence in clinicians to address their medical needs in a safe and appropriate manner, and developing these skills amongst physicians relies on the integration of global awareness in medical training.

Assessment

The assessment of medical students drives their individual learning. Therefore, the learning objectives for a given curriculum should be assessable with an acceptable standard or format. Objective knowledge forms a significant part of medical curricula and is generally amenable to knowledge-based assessment formats such as multiple-choice questions. Conversely, many learning objectives in global health are more complex and are not easily reducible to multiple-choice questions. As such, assessment of understanding global

health should be carefully and thoughtfully planned. This is easier to accomplish at the time of the curricula development.

Consider the vertical strand and spiral curriculum approach to global health learning outcomes. In the early years of medical school this may relate to some facts and knowledge. For example, evaluating common global health statistics and trends could be assessed with single best answer questions. As students progress in their training they could be asked to write short essays about the identified global health issues. This process allows them to fully understand the issues, review the literature, and critique the authorized data sources. Students who participate in an international clinical rotation might be asked to submit a report, reflective essay or assessment presentation upon their return. These reflective-type assignments encourage the medical students to present their knowledge and experience in descriptive terms, which allows them to articulate the complexity of health inequalities, healthcare systems, and the role of resource allocation and governance.

 Assessment approaches need to be planned during the curriculum development process. They need to be appropriate to the learning outcomes, pragmatic, reliable and appropriately resourced.

Medical students must acquire and demonstrate competent skills when interviewing a patient and performing a medical examination in the clinic setting. The objective structured clinical examination (OSCE) is an established method to observe and assess a medical student performing a medical consultation on a stand-ardized patient (Wylie & Holt, 2010). The OSCE can also be used to teach and assess students' knowledge and ability to address global health issues. For example, a medical student might be asked to perform a consulta-tion while using the services of a medical interpreter. The goal of this encounter would be to assess how well a student is able to ascertain symptoms and present a diagnostic and treatment plan with patients who have a different primary language. This should be a common skill among physicians, and one that could be systemati-cally assessed with an OSCE.

Other possible OSCE scenarios could be a traveller who has returned with a geographically limited infec-tion, or a person from a particular ethnic group present-ing with a known high-risk disease. Senior medical students, who are expected to demonstrate an advanced understanding of global health issues, could also be evaluated by an OSCE. In this scenario, senior medical students should be able to identify different cultural beliefs and practices, barriers to healthcare access, and socio-behavioural impediments to good health.

Medical students and doctors will need to effectively communicate with a variety of patients who have different cultural, ethnic and religious backgrounds. Any approach will need to depend on several factors including the language skills of the patient and the medical student. However, all medical students should be required to demonstrate competency for using a medical interpreter, demonstrating cultural sensitivity and professionalism, and exercising sound judgement when treating patients with a different ethnic background or cultural beliefs.

Preparing students for international experiences and electives

International travel for clinical rotations, research, and volunteer opportunities can be a meaningful and even transformative experience for students. Travel abroad can also be challenging and entail risks that may be different from those to which healthcare trainees and providers are accustomed at home. Adequate preparation for any international clinical rotation is essential to stay safe and healthy while abroad so the student can make the most of the experience. Reliable resources are available to cover these aspects in great detail, along with listings of pre-travel vaccinations and medical evacuation options. In this section we address only the most salient topics.

All students should visit a travel clinic to obtain pre-travel vaccinations as well as medications for pre- and post-exposure prophylaxis if indicated. Most domestic health insurance plans do not cover expenses related to illness or injury sustained abroad or the costs of emergency evacuation. Therefore, students should check with their institution to understand the coverage, and purchase supplemental insurance if needed. Students going to resource-limited settings should consider obtaining medical evacuation insurance. While many options are available, a comprehensive travel insurance plan would include travel health insurance, medical evacuation, emergency medical expenses, and repatriation.

Before departure, students should familiarize themselves with the safety and security situation at their destination. Many governments, including the US State Department (http://travel.state.gov), publish up-to-date travel advisories and warnings by country. The United Kingdom's Foreign and Commonwealth Office (FCO) also issues current travel information. Country-specific health information is available online from the World Health Organization (http://www.who.int/countries/en/) and the Centers for Disease Control and Prevention (http://wwwn.cdc.gov/travel/destinationList.aspx). Upon arrival, students should seek local safety advice from in-country hosts. Finally, awareness, appreciation, and respect of the local culture are essential, and these preparations should be part of the trip planning.

 Global health is "an area for study, research, and practice that places a priority on improving health and achieving equity in health for all people worldwide"

(Koplan et al., 2009).

Faculty development for global awareness

 It is probable that many clinical practitioners, knowingly or not, incorporate some global health concepts into their clinical care and practice without having any global health expertise. We need to recognize and build on this.
In addition, faculty could look at SDG-3, and consider implications for the practice and teaching. http://www.un.org/sustainable development/sustainable-development-goals/.

Faculty development for global awareness is critical for students to receive proper global health education and training. Faculty physicians need to possess the knowledge and skills of competent and compassion clinicians, which requires some degree of global awareness. In order to fully understand the risk factors for certain diseases, a clinician needs at least a minimal understanding of their patients' demographic background and recent travel history. For example, a concentration of specific ethnic groups can result in localised health beliefs and practices that lead to certain diseases. A globally aware competent clinician will be able to obtain a more detailed clinical history, be aware of recent global health activities, and integrate that knowledge into their care and treatment plan. Some faculty may also take a more active role to raise awareness of local health problems and become involved in developing appropriate solutions.

Clinician educators should to be supported to improve their global awareness and to optimize their ability to provide patient care and medical teaching. Since some faculty may not have received prior global health training, these services should be provided to the entire faculty. In addition, all faculty should have access to appropriate learning and teaching resources. Enabling medical educators to play a significant role in the assessment of students and the medical curriculum should be an integral part of the process.

There are several methods of providing global awareness development to medical faculty. First, medical schools could offer continuing medical education programmes or conferences for medical faculty to learn about relevant global health issues and topics. Second, departments could offer seminars or workshops that are specific to a particular medical specialty. In this scenario, clinicians who have global health experiences can share their cases and lessons with other faculty members. Third, schools could offer innovative online teaching modules for those wanting to understand more in-depth global awareness issues such as the disease epidemiology of the local immigrant population.

To increase faculty participation, medical schools could provide incentives for attendance at development workshops. Perhaps the contribution to global health awareness within the medical community could be reimbursed or linked to promotion criteria. Clinician educators should be rewarded for exceeding expectations and improving their clinical knowledge and skills through global health awareness.

Ethical issues and international electives

Medical students and professionals engaged in international health electives are often eager to provide their energy and skills to make meaningful contributions to the medical needs at a host site. Occasionally, well-intentioned visitors mistake the lack of resources for a lack of knowledge or capability of the staff, which can cause confusion or unintended insult. In more severe cases, students who dismiss the capacity of the local healthcare system may result in causing significant harm to patients. In general, local staff have a wealth of knowledge of the diseases and medical practices within their healthcare setting. The visiting student or faculty member has much to gain by observing and learning about local practices, which are linked to local resources and the expertise of the healthcare providers.

Medical trainees who seek opportunities to work in regions lacking an adequate supply of well-trained healthcare professionals often face difficult ethical issues (Elit et al., 2011). Some trainees encounter situations or circumstances in which they are expected to perform duties beyond their competence level and without adequate supervision. Although the student may want to help, medical trainees should avoid actions and responsibilities for which they have not received adequate training or qualifications. The resulting impact may have severe consequences for patient outcomes and also impact negatively on the relations with the host clinicians. Both of these outcomes will erode global health partnerships. Qualified physicians-in-training should ensure that their medical insurance and malpractice coverage is active abroad, and may still consider purchasing an additional insurance plan.

Summary

Global health has become an integral aspect of clinical practices and public health intervention. Therefore global health should be a regular component to both undergraduate and postgraduate medical education. However, challenges remain to develop learning outcomes and assessments within integrated medical curricula. All medical educators from various specialties should bring global health awareness as a learning objective into their specific core curriculum. We have described methods and tools to help medical educators prepare students to become proficient in their evolving profession and provided guidance for more senior students embarking on an overseas medical elective.

Awareness of ethical issues and professional behaviour remain paramount regardless of where a clinician practices. Clinicians must work within the context of local need and be aware of their own limitations, competencies and skills. Healthcare needs and priorities will change over time within countries and regions; therefore, clinicians need to be able to access valid, reliable and trustworthy information from appropriate sources, know how to critique and interpret complex and contested data, be politically aware and prudent with resources. These goals are achievable by integrating global awareness into the core curriculum with appropriate methodologies to assess student learning. As medical educators, we are charged with the responsibility of making global health present and relevant in the standard medical curriculum. The evolution of our global healthcare systems will depend in part on how well we met our responsibility.

References

Behforouz, H.L., Drain, P.K., Rhatigan, J.J., 2014. Rethinking the social history. NEJM 371 (14), 1277–1279.

Bhutta, Z.A., Chen, L., Cohen, J., et al., 2010. Education of health professionals for the 21st century: a global independent Commission. Lancet 375 (9721), 1137–1138.

Elit, L., Hunt, M., Redwood-Campbell, L., et al., 2011. Ethical issues encountered by medical students during international health electives. Med. Educ. 45 (7), 704–711.

Frenk, J., Chen, L., Bhutta, Z.A., et al., 2010. Health professionals for a new century: transforming education to strengthen health systems in an interdependent world. Lancet 376 (9756), 1923–1958.

Johnson, O., Bailey, S.L., Willott, C., et al., 2012. Global health learning outcomes for medical students in the UK. Lancet 379 (9831), 2033–2035.

Koplan, J.P., Bond, T.C., Merson, M.H., et al., 2009. Towards a common definition of global health. Lancet 373 (9679), 1993–1995.

United Nations, 2015. Transforming out world: the 2030 Agenda for Sustainable Development United Nations.

Wylie, A., 2011. Health Promotion in General Practice. A Textbook of General Practice. A. Stephenson. London, HodderArnold.

Wylie, A., Holt, T., 2010. Health Promotion in Medical Education: From Rhetoric to Action. Radcliffe Publishing, Oxford.

Medical education in an era of ubiquitous information

J. Patton, C. P. Friedman

Trends

- Information is available more and more in digital form.
- Biomedical knowledge via the Internet is making point of care reference easier.
- Learning health systems are enabling healthcare to continuously improve, reducing quality improvement latency by years.
- Because new evidence is being generated in real time, clinicians need to be able to deal with uncertainty of evidence when making decisions.
- Comfort with clinical reasoning and decision aids must continue to increase.

Ubiquitous information

In the modern world, health information is everywhere. Increasingly, this information is in digital form, which makes it accessible not only to people but also to devices that can store it and add value to it through computation. Information is available to everyone who participates or has an interest in health and healthcare including health professionals and their patients, organizations that pay for healthcare, educators, as well as researchers and quality improvement specialists.

Perhaps the greatest change in recent years is the availability of health-related information to the general public, including both their personal health data and general medical knowledge. Patients as recipients of healthcare have access to data about them generated by healthcare, and, increasingly, they are capturing their own data through sensors and mobile devices.

Information is a resource that can lead to better health and healthcare, but this does not happen automatically. All participants in healthcare must learn to be careful generators, skilled navigators, and discriminating users of information. They must approach information with a healthy scepticism about its accuracy. They must know how to filter information to avoid what has been called drinking from a fire hose (Friedman et al., 2016).

Data, information, knowledge

Understanding the distinction between data, information and knowledge allows us to develop different strategies to teach learners to interact in the digital healthcare environment. 'Information' is typically used as an umbrella term for the continuum of data to knowledge, and we follow suit in this chapter. Anchoring the continuum on the data side are the strings of symbols that we are familiar with as raw data. Anchoring the continuum on the knowledge side are rules and hypotheses that help us analyze complex situations. In our current environment it has all become ubiquitous as it is increasingly stored in a digital format.

 "Perhaps more than any other recent advance, health information technology (HIT) is rapidly becoming a key foundation for all aspects of patient care. As the complexity of healthcare increases, so does the complexity of collaboration needed between different members of the healthcare team. To evaluate the effectiveness of new treatments and the quality of care in specific populations, individual providers or the team as a whole must be able to rapidly and efficiently collect, analyze, and select intervention and performance data. Regardless of their chosen field, all medical students will have to manage vastly increased amounts of biomedical and clinical data."

Triola et al., 2010

When knowledge is in a computable form it can also advise us as to what course of action to take. Knowledge has existed for decades in the form of journal articles and other tomes. While available, it is not easily accessed and its ability to give on-demand advice is non-existent. In the last decade we have seen digital knowledge being leveraged in the form of risk prediction calculators and computable clinical guidelines. The ability to access this knowledge in the moment is a competency that will increasingly be necessary for clinicians.

The ability to access the right information, about the right patient, at the right time to deliver quality and effective care is a benefit that electronic health records give to healthcare providers across the globe. The generation of data by the patients themselves, in addition to all of the data generated by the healthcare system, and the continued explosion of medical knowledge at exponential rates has created a dynamic, fluctuating information environment in healthcare. As clinicians, the ability to recognize what medical knowledge needs to be intrinsic to one's self, what knowledge can be obtained when needed and where to obtain that knowledge becomes another waypoint that must be navigated. The partnership between people and technology is continuing to develop and can fulfil this need. As educators, we must ensure that our learners are able to maximize the partnership between themselves and digital information resources.

Healthcare in the digital age (and biomedical knowledge in the cloud)

In the digital world, information can easily be moved from where it is to where it is needed. The current healthcare environment is evolving to supply data and information from electronic health records, emerging knowledge from the learning health system, and biomedical knowledge repositories in the cloud. As these technologies take a foothold, they have effects on medical education and we will explain the impact of each of these in turn. Increasingly, in this digital environment, and with the explosion of biomedical knowledge, information technology will be required in addition to the decision-making done in clinical practice. This will require a shift on the part of the profession to recognize that best practice will begin to increasingly rely on aids to clinical reasoning and decision making, such as clinical decision support systems.

ELECTRONIC HEALTH RECORDS

A multitude of global sources predict that the movement of healthcare documentation from analogue to digital will continue to evolve, and at a rapid pace. In the United States, expert opinion suggests that by 2019 80% of care will be documented in electronic health records rather than paper records. Electronic health records have been abundant in the United Kingdom since the 1990s, and the continued adoption of digital documentation for acute care continues. Northern European nations, such as Denmark and the Netherlands, have converted to nearly digital systems. A nationwide implementation of the open source VistA electronic health record occurred in Jordan in 2009. In developing nations, such as Malawi, that are still implementing critical infrastructure, efforts to implement electronic health records at the point of care have created networks of healthcare information that improve the quality of care for patients. This continued evolution from paper records to digital ones has several benefits, including increased access for authorized individuals and the ability to perform analyses with greater ease.

In addition to providers who benefit from increased access to their patients' digital information, there are two additional beneficiaries – other providers on a national or international infrastructure, and the health system itself. As the exchange of health information from one location to another becomes more seamless, having a fuller picture of a patient available to them, physicians on the other side of a country or on the other side of the world, are able to provide the best possible care to a patient with increased precision.

LEARNING HEALTH SYSTEMS

This same information is available to the health system at large, allowing it to study and improve itself. The concept of the 'learning health system' is continuing to grow in the United States and in Europe. This infrastructure affords simultaneous virtuous learning cycles on a variety of specific health problems. A learning cycle consists of three key phases: (1) the aggregation and analysis of data; (2) the creation of knowledge and its application to change clinical practice; and (3) recording the results of the application and continuous improvement thereafter. The learning health system has a large number of uses, from public health tracking and managing epidemics to the surveillance of drugs newly released to market, to the discovery of new best practices for the treatment of common diseases such as asthma.

 "A more efficient, effective, and safe health care system requires a more rapid progression of knowledge from the lab bench to the bedside."
Friedman et al., 2010

BIOMEDICAL KNOWLEDGE IN THE CLOUD

As this new knowledge is generated, it is often digitally available before it reaches print, if it ever reaches physical print at all. As both biomedical information (general information about the human body and health) and knowledge (in the form of checklists, best practices guidelines, models and algorithms) become available on the Internet, it can be represented in both human readable and computable forms. Both formats will give rise to the 'knowledge cloud', available anytime and anywhere with a connection to the Internet. Over the coming decade, the ability to pose biomedical questions to the knowledge cloud, or for the cloud to offer clinical decision support based on the best available evidence will emerge as the best clinical practice.

AIDS TO CLINICAL REASONING AND DECISION MAKING

Even in the present day, clinical decision support from local systems serves as an aid for the brain capacity of physicians. This, however, is not a new concept. Handbooks are a common item found in the lab coats of physicians across the world. The amount of information that one is required to remember in order to deliver immediate care versus what can be referenced has long since been recognized. The dilemma we face at the present day, and will continue to face in the future, is that the volume of information that we will have to store external to our own brains will continue to increase. The medical profession will need to be ever more comfortable with relying on external sources to provide it with the information needed to deliver effective and safe care to patients. As educators, it is equally important that we are comfortable with this mode of patient care. We must recognize our own biases and current practices. This will aid us in helping our learners develop their own practices based on their innate abilities – understanding what they need to know and what they need to know how to retrieve. This changes the lens with which we examine our learners' performance and the expectations we have for them and that they have for themselves.

 "It must be acknowledged, first, that the development of health information technology will require (or enable) cognitively-based physicians to delegate many tasks that they previously held closely."

Blumenthal, 2010

The digital native learner

Many educators will assume that because our younger learners have grown up with Google and smartphones that they will instantly have proficiency with the digital tools that we supply to them. This is far from true, and is a pitfall that many of our colleagues fall into when approaching the so-called digital native learner.

Research has yet to show that the generation that has grown up with digital tools is at large competent with those tools or that those competencies transfer to the academic environment (Gallardo-Echenique et al., 2015). Since these learners are not as competent as you may anticipate, it is important to at first ensure the baseline competencies necessary to engage with digital healthcare environment.

It is probably best to begin with understanding how comfortable your learners are with technology. From an experience of teaching a classroom of younger learners in the same age range, chapter author Patton found the learners' facility with the tools provided to them to be widely variable. While a few of the learners could easily access a virtual private network and log on to the simulated electronic health record, other learners had difficulty just logging in to the computer itself. This was Patton's first indication that a section on this topic would be necessary. Prior to this, he had been quite presumptuous in the learners' collective ability to successfully navigate commonplace technology.

We recommend that, as a baseline, learners will need to be competent in computer and mobile hardware; have facility with accessing the Internet and other digital resources; and be capable of rudimentary searches. Developing the basic information retrieval competencies of our learners may not be so easy. Thompson (2013) found that while learners are facile with rapid communication technologies like text messaging, their ability to perform deep, meaningful searches was lacking. The first step then would be to build up the learners' ability to create search terms that will be appropriate to yield valuable information. This will be covered later in the chapter.

The generational differences that we assume between the 'digital native' learners and the 'digital immigrant' faculty are an artificial boundary created by our assumptions of the environment that our learners born after 1980 have grown up in, and reinforced by, the popular media (Gallardo-Echenique et al., 2015). As educators, we should instead focus on 'digital learners', regardless of the generation they belong to. This allows us to engage with physician learners across the spectrum of their career, and focus on what a digital learner needs at baseline in order to be successful in acquiring the competencies we will outline in the second half of this chapter.

Three key competencies at a time of ubiquitous information and educational strategies to support the digital learner

A medical education curriculum at a time of ubiquitous information requires changes or additions to current educational goals and strategies. We introduce three key competencies for physician learners, along with the accompanying strategies for curriculum design, delivery and assessment. These are our suggestions to effectively prepare physicians for the information-based future of clinical practice in 2020 and beyond.

METACOGNITION AND SENSING GAPS IN ONE'S KNOWLEDGE

In the age of ubiquitous information, it may be more important for a physician to know whether their approach to and knowledge about a clinical situation are correct or incorrect rather than it actually be correct. If their assessment of the situation is flawed, and the physician is able to recognize that it is flawed, their ability to access and interpret knowledge from sources external to themselves proves invaluable and they are able to course correct. Physicians that believe that they are correct will not routinely consult available resources. Their unaided actions could presumably put patients' health and wellbeing at risk. The first competency that we are recommending is that the competent physician must be aware of what they do and do not know, and have some insight into how they process information – they must know when to ask for help when making clinical decisions in real time because they have reached the limit of their knowledge about the situation. Collectively, these skills and attitudes fall into the realm of metacognition.

METACOGNITION

Metacognitive skills are the hallmark of a learner that will be capable of lifelong learning. Mark Quirk (2006) describes the five key metacognitive skills of the physician learner to be (1) definition and prioritization of goals, (2) anticipation and assessment of their specific needs in relation to the goals, (3) organization of their experiences to meet their personal needs, (4) definition of their own and recognition of differences in others' perspectives, and (5) continuous monitoring of their knowledge and problem solving. The fifth skill, continuous monitoring of one's knowledge, plays a critical role in the day-to-day of clinical practice. Not discounting the other skills, which are necessary for professional development over one's lifetime, helping learners develop the ability to appraise their knowledge level in the moment could potentially prove to be life saving. By providing an environment that allows learners to acquire and utilize these skills, we allow these future physicians to develop the confidence that they will need in order to act decisively in difficult situations.

CONFIDENCE CALIBRATION

Described by Friedman et al. (2016), the Confidence Calibration Matrix (Fig. 32.1) displays what happens when a clinician is correct or incorrect when their appraisal about their knowledge is correct or incorrect. The physician is typically safe when they are properly calibrated and appropriately access information. There is the possibility, however, that sub-optimal use of information resources results in the clinical assessment switching from correct to incorrect. Using the strategies outlined below we can guard against this.

The first type of miscalibration occurs when a physician is correct but believes that they are incorrect. While typically safe, this form of miscalibration results in slower clinical decision making, which could be hazardous in some clinical situations. The second type of miscalibration occurs when the physician is incorrect but believes that they are correct. This is the most dangerous situation because the physician will not seek assistance from the appropriate information resources.

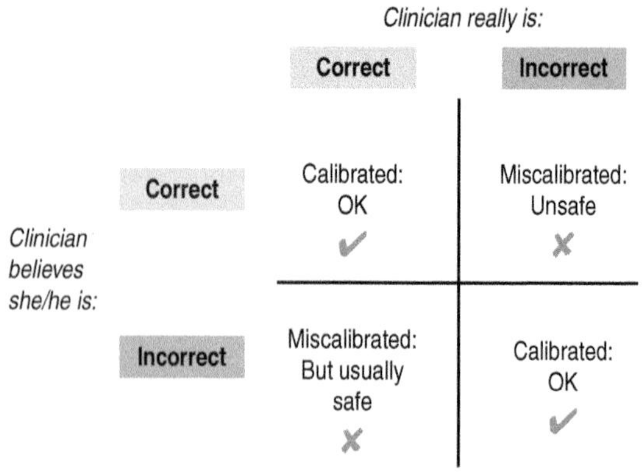

Fig. 32.1 The Confidence Calibration Matrix.

(Originally published in Friedman CP, Donaldson KM, Vantsevich AV: Educating medical students in the era of ubiquitous information. Medical Teacher, 38(5):504–509, 2016.)

Even when decision support tools sense a problem, this physician will likely ignore the advice.

It is difficult to guard against this second type of miscalibration. Individuals in this state will not seek help, and others will only recognize their deficiency once a medical error is made. Preventing learners and physicians from entering this state by reinforcing the following point is the best cure for this ailment.

The salient identification for medical teachers is the learner that is incorrect and recognizes that they are incorrect. This requires a change in culture where not knowing the answer but recognizing one's knowledge gap and knowing how to bridge the gap in one's own knowledge is equal to or greater than having the right answer. The learners that meet this competency will be able to understand their own thought process and knowledge; access and retrieve available resources; and utilize those resources to make corrections to their thoughts and actions.

Demonstration and assessment of metacognition

A strategy to have learners demonstrate this behaviour could be used during rounds when learners are presenting on patients, or similarly in small groups discussing scientific principles. Preceptors should routinely ask the learners about their level of confidence in the assessment they have made and what evidence brought them to that conclusion. This promotes the behaviour of consciously considering one's confidence level. With habituation this will be a routine inner dialogue for the learner – to evaluate their confidence about the assessment of a clinical situation.

To reinforce this approach, practising physicians should model these same types of behaviours. As medical educators we will need to become more introspective about, aware of, and willing to discuss our own confidence and levels of calibration.

 The value of reflection continues to be questioned by learners. Be certain to help them understand the value of such activities to create buy-in and allow them to do meaningful work.

Reflection of this type is a good way to assess this metacognition competency. Through carefully designed guided reflections, learners will be able to self-monitor and receive feedback from others (Sandars, 2009). Assessment of the reflection should include comments on the depth of reflection, examination of one's own perspective, and inclusion of the perspective of others.

Information retrieval and the ability to form an appropriate question

While the first competency addresses the ability to recognize gaps in one's knowledge, the second competency ensures that the skills are in place for the learner to frame a good question and access available resources to improve their incomplete knowledge. However, in order to know where to look, there must be some basic understanding of the subject at hand.

To illustrate the point, consider three potential states of being for the learner or physician before interacting with digital resources (Fig. 32.2). In the first state, the individual has insufficient knowledge about the problem of interest to frame an appropriate question. The learner in this state will not be able to obtain assistance from any resources and will be unable to address their current situation. In the second state, the learner has partial knowledge about the problem of interest and will be able to frame a good question. In the third state, the learner's personal knowledge is already complete. In this final state consultation with information resources is not needed; however, as the volume of biomedical knowledge continues to explode, learners are unlikely to reach this state by the end of their careers.

FOUNDATIONAL, ADVANCED AND SPECIALIZED MEDICAL KNOWLEDGE

Delivering this competency to learners requires a shift in focus from providing every possible piece of knowledge to learners before they exit our doors, to one of learning what they need to know in order to frame an appropriate question. This educational approach places an emphasis on the organization of knowledge in curricula to adequately describe what is truly foundational knowledge for learners, compared to what would be advanced knowledge or even specialized knowledge. This is a departure from teaching a large volume of

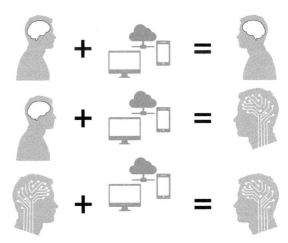

Fig. 32.2 Effects of ubiquitous information on different states of knowledge. *Top* With insufficient knowledge, the person cannot frame a question and does not increase their knowledge. *Middle* With partial knowledge, the person can pose questions to the available resources and increase their knowledge. *Bottom* With (nearly) perfect knowledge additional information is not needed.

(Image created from modifications of Brain by Wes Breazell from the Noun Project; Cloud Server by Creative Stall from the Noun Project; Computer Icon by Creative Stall from the Noun Project; Mobile Phone by Cengiz SARI from the Noun Project.)

knowledge and a shift to teaching foundational knowledge that serves as a scaffold to prepare learners for advanced, and subsequently specialized, medical knowledge.

 Curriculum inventory software, including several free to use packages, simplify the task of compiling curriculum data. Sharing, making visualizations, and deriving meaning from the data become easier.

Cataloguing the existing curriculum is the first step in reorganizing it to effectively deliver the right knowledge to the learner at the right time. Many schools are beginning to inventory what they teach and where, documenting learning objectives for each session that they give to their learners (Dexter et al., 2012). To fully realize the potential of what has been collected, tagging content according to its level of abstraction from facts to high-level principles will help filter what must be taught from what can be sought by the learner. Once this inventory is available it becomes relatively easier to restructure the curriculum to deliver foundational scaffolding knowledge to early students, advanced knowledge to your more senior medical students, and supply specialized knowledge to those who will need it in their practice.

FRAMING AN APPROPRIATE CLINICAL QUESTION

Informationists and librarians play a key role in educating physician learners about framing an appropriate clinical question. Once an appropriate search has been devised, assessing which sources of information can best answer that question can be guided by the librarian. Librarians use heuristics like reputation of source, methodology of creation and date of publication to help them make recommendations. Learners and medical teachers can also use these heuristics to evaluate sources of information.

Physician learners will require practise in formulating good questions to prepare them for the digital information supported practice of the future. In order to accomplish this, information retrieval sessions could employ currently available versions of cloud knowledge resources that are mature enough to provide valid advice – even if these tools are not yet mature enough to be deployed in clinical practice. In doing this, we can take advantage of the fact that simulated clinical problems posed in the classroom mirror future practice. Even though this technology is still being developed, it can be used in these situations to help learners develop skills they will need in a future when that technology is more mature and widely deployed. In general, the curriculum should challenge learners with problems that require use of the digital information resources, whatever the state of those resources might be at that point in time.

ASSESSMENT OF INFORMATION RETRIEVAL AND ANALYSIS

In order to assess the ability to frame an appropriate question and retrieve the appropriate information, examinations should allow learners to demonstrate this competency via 'open book' exams. This shift from 'closed book' exams aligns with the shift from learning a large fund of knowledge to knowing what you need to know in order to learn more. Given the ubiquitous nature of information in the digital age of healthcare, there is little justification to continue the custom of 'closed book' exams at the level we currently practice.

Enacting this assessment strategy can be accomplished using a modification of the triple jump exercise introduced at McMaster University (Smith, 1993) (Fig. 32.3). The first pass is a closed book exam based on the learner's personal knowledge only. This first pass provides a 'scaffold score', which assesses their foundational knowledge. In the second pass, the learner can access information resources to provide a refined answer to the problem at hand. This second exercise provides two scores: a 'process score' related to how well they were able to use the available information resources and an 'exam score' of how well the learner was able to perform assisted by the information in

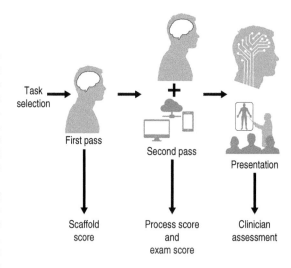

Fig. 32.3 The Triple Jump exercise in the era of ubiquitous information.

(Image created from modifications of Brain by Wes Breazell from the Noun Project; Cloud Server by Creative Stall from the Noun Project; Computer Icon by Creative Stall from the Noun Project; Mobile Phone by Cengiz SARI from the Noun Project.)

their environment. In the final jump of the assessment, the learner presents their findings from the second exercise to an assessor that can interrogate the learner's knowledge and process in the moment. The final jump verifies the learner's ability to access knowledge and understand their thought process in real time.

 Following the learner's digital trail, collection of experience data can be achieved via the Experience API (xAPI) and a Learner Record Store. http://experienceapi.com/overview.

Evaluating and weighing evidence to make decisions; recognizing patients and interprofessional colleagues as additional sources of information

A discriminating user of all the information resources and knowledge repositories of our digital healthcare environment must be able to deal with and handle uncertainty. The third competency ensures that learners will have the knowledge and skills to evaluate, include/exclude and weigh all available evidence. Some of the evidence will come from clinical guidelines and e-textbooks. Real-time evidence will be generated from the learning health system, and the responses that the system generates will be accompanied by confidence measures for the results. In many scenarios, clinicians will be faced with incomplete and/or conflicting information. Therefore, part of the knowledge scaffolding of the physician in the digital age must relate to decision making under uncertainty.

 Rather than teaching evidence-based medicine as a block early or late in a programme, consider threading it through every year.

In order to achieve the delivery of this competency to learners, increased curricular attention must be given to topics like formal decision modelling and analysis; evidence based decision making; critical evaluation of the literature; meta analysis; and data mining and signal detection. In recent years, medical schools have begun to introduce to the topic of evidence-based medicine to our learners, and it has become more prevalent in clinical practice. It has been a struggle to make this appear relevant to learners and practising physicians alike. The need for this competency across the continuum of learners will become increasingly apparent as we continue to move into the era of ubiquitous information.

ASSESSMENT OF UNCERTAINTY/SHARED DECISION MAKING

Objective structured clinical examinations (OSCEs) can be designed to assess for this competency. A complex clinical case, with a patient that has several social or cultural considerations involved as determinants of the decision, would serve as an excellent example. Learners would need to demonstrate their ability to gather the necessary information and incorporate statements about their confidence in the knowledge they have, or have obtained, into the explanation of their decision.

 How learners weigh evidence and handle uncertainty can be incorporated into Mini-CEX assessments.

Summary

It is an exciting time in healthcare as more of the information about patients and medical knowledge become available digitally. While there are baseline competencies that are required for practice in this new era of ubiquitous information, the three key competencies we have outlined will be critical to the success of physicians in clinical practice beyond the next decade.

The ability to sense the gaps in one's knowledge will serve to reduce medical errors by improving the confidence of physicians in their medical knowledge. The ability to quickly form appropriate clinical questions and access relevant, reliable sources of information will prevent physicians from becoming overwhelmed by the large volume of information at hand. Finally, the ability to evaluate and weigh the available information will help physicians handle the uncertainty that exists in their environment.

References

Blumenthal, D., 2010. Expecting the unexpected: health information technology and medical professionalism. In: Medical Professionalism in the New Information Age. Rutgers University Press, New Brunswick, NJ, pp. 8–22.

Dexter, J., Koshland, G., Waer, A., Anderson, D., 2012. Mapping a curriculum database to the USMLE Step 1 content outline. Med. Teach. 34 (10), e666–e675.

Friedman, C.P., Wong, A.K., Blumenthal, D., 2010. Achieving a nationwide learning health system. Sci. Transl. Med. 2 (57), 57cm29.

Friedman, C.P., Donaldson, K.M., Vantsevich, A.V., 2016. Educating medical students in the era of ubiquitous information. Med. Teach. 38 (5), 504–509.

Gallardo-Echenique, E.E., Marques-Molias, L., Bullen, M., Strijbos, J.W., 2015. Let's talk about digital learners in the digital era. Int. Rev. Res. Open Distrib. Learn. 16 (3), 156–187.

Quirk, M.E., 2006. An emerging paradigm for medical education. In: Intuition and Metacognition In Medical Education: Keys to Developing Expertise. Springer Pub. Co., New York, NY, pp. 1–10.

Sandars, J., 2009. The use of reflection in medical education: AMEE Guide No. 44. Med. Teach. 31 (8), 685–695.

Smith, R.M., 1993. The triple-jump examination as an assessment tool in the problem-based medical curriculum at the University of Hawaii. Acad. Med. 68 (3), 366–372.

Thompson, P., 2013. The digital natives as learners: technology use patterns and approaches to learning. Comput. Educ. 65, 12–33.

Triola, M.M., Friedman, E., Cimino, C., et al., 2010. Health information technology and the medical school curriculum. Am. J. Manag. Care 16 (12 Suppl. HIT), SP54–SP56.

Section 5

Assessment

33 Concepts in assessment including standard setting

J. Norcini, D. W. McKinley

Trends

- Validity is not obtained or achieved. Instead, evidence is collected to support the interpretation of assessment results. These interpretations, or validity arguments, are supported through information that is collected over time. A framework to view assessments through this validity lens is provided in the chapter.

- As attention shifts to competency-based, student-centred learning, more attention has been paid to formative assessment, with an emphasis on supporting and creating learning. Research has begun to identify the effectiveness of formative assessment that emphasizes feedback, particularly in workplace settings.

- While it is not unusual for institutions to use fixed scores in order to pass assessments, this practice can generate a number of problems. Fixed passing scores ignore differences in student ability and test difficulty. There are ways to address these issues, however. Information on score equivalence and standard setting are introduced in the chapter.

Even a cursory review of the assessment literature reveals a bewildering array of dichotomies and concepts. These are often overlapping, and authors sometimes use them with less precision than is desirable, especially for the clinical teacher attempting to make sense of assessment for the first time. The purpose of this chapter is to identify some of these concepts and provide background to their meaning, development and use.

Measurement theories

Test theories or psychometric models seek to explain what happens when an individual takes a test (Crocker & Algina, 1986). They provide guidance about how to select items, how long tests need to be, the inferences that can be drawn from scores, and the confidence that can be placed in the final results. Each model makes different assumptions and, based on those assumptions, different benefits accrue. There are many psychometric models, but three deserve attention here because they are used frequently in medical education.

CLASSICAL TEST THEORY (CTT)

CTT has been the dominant model in testing for decades, with roots in the late nineteenth and early twentieth centuries (Lord & Novick, 1968). It assumes that an individual's score on a test has two parts: true score (or what is intended to be measured) and error. To apply CTT to practical testing situations, a series of very restrictive assumptions need to be made. The bad news is that these assumptions are often violated in practice, but the good news is that even when this happens it seldom makes a practical difference (i.e. the model is robust with respect to violations of the assumptions).

A number of useful concepts and tools have been developed based on CTT (De Champlain, 2010). Among the most powerful is reliability, which indicates the amount of error in observed scores. Also very useful has been the development of item statistics, which help with the process of test development. CTT has contributed significantly to the development of a series of excellent assessments and it continues to be used and useful today.

GENERALIZABILITY THEORY (GT)

Although it has its roots in the middle of the twentieth century, GT rose to prominence with the publication of *The dependability of behavioral measurements*, by Cronbach, Gleser, Nanda, and Rajaratnam in 1972. Like CTT (which is a special case of GT), it assumes that an individual's score on a test has two parts: true score and error. However, compared to CTT, GT makes relatively weak assumptions. Consequently, it applies to a very broad range of assessments and, like CTT, even when these assumptions are violated it usually makes little practical difference.

GT offers a number of advantages over CTT (Brennan, 2001). For example, GT allows the error in a test to be divided among different sources. So in a rating situation, GT allows the error associated with the rater to be separated from the error associated with the rating form they are filling out. Likewise, GT supports a distinction between scores that are intended to rank individuals as opposed to scores that are intended to represent how much they know. Given these advantages, GT has special applicability to the types of assessment situations found in health professions education.

ITEM RESPONSE THEORY (IRT)

With considerable interest starting in the 1970s, the use of IRT has grown substantially, especially among national testing agencies (Hambleton et al., 1991). Unlike GT, IRT makes very strong assumptions about items, tests and individuals. These assumptions are difficult to meet, so there are a number of different IRT models, each with assumptions that are suitable for particular assessment situations.

When the assumptions are met, many practical benefits accrue (Downing, 2003). For example, individual scores are independent of exactly which set of items are taken and item statistics are independent of the individuals who take the test. So individuals can take completely different test questions but their scores will still be comparable. As another example, IRT supports the creation of tests that are targeted to a particular score, often the pass-fail point. This permits a shorter test than would otherwise be the case because IRT allows the test to be constructed with most precision (reliability) at the pass-fail point.

 Compared to CTT, GT and IRT provide different but powerful advantages. However, for most practical day-to-day work any of the test theories are sufficient.

Types of assessment

Assessments can be classified in a variety of different ways and many of them are reasonable. One useful classification of assessments is as formative, summative or diagnostic (Hanauer et al., 2009). Although some assessments are designed to simultaneously serve more than one purpose (e.g. be summative but also provide formative information), it is very difficult to do this well and one of the purposes usually dominates. In the end, it is better to develop a good *system* of assessment that incorporates different tests methods, each of which serves a single purpose well.

FORMATIVE ASSESSMENT

An assessment of trainees during an educational intervention is often referred to as formative. The purpose of these assessments is twofold. First, they provide feedback to students and their teachers that is intended to guide learning. Second, there is recent work indicating that the act of assessment itself creates learning, so formative assessment is integral to education.

 "Over the past 50 years, considerable energy has been devoted to the development of summative assessment. Although much work remains, good summative assessments of medical knowledge, clinical skills, and other competencies are now readily available. More recently, the focus has shifted to formative assessment and its focus on supporting and creating learning. We need to develop a much better understanding of how to build and use these types of assessments. Research has begun to identify the effectiveness of formative assessment that emphasizes feedback, particularly in workplace-settings."

Lefroy et al., 2015

There are many examples of these types of assessments, one class of which is workplace-based assessment (e.g., mini-CEX, direct observation of procedural skills). These often require some form of direct observation followed by assessment and then immediate feedback. Despite the fact that formative assessment is central to learning, insufficient attention has been paid to the development and refinement of these types of instruments. Of particular relevance recently has been research on the provision of feedback (e.g. DiVall et al., 2014).

SUMMATIVE ASSESSMENT

An assessment of trainees at the end of a period of time is generally referred to as summative. The purpose of these assessments is to determine whether the trainee has learned what has been taught. These are assessments that are associated with decisions of some type; consequently, these assessments are usually cumulative and indicate whether the trainee is competent to move on in training or practice.

Examples of summative assessments are the examinations that occur at the end of units, courses, semesters and years. Also summative are tests for graduation, licensure, certification and so on. These tests are so pervasive, especially in medical school, that when most students are asked about it they describe all assessment as summative.

DIAGNOSTIC ASSESSMENT

An assessment of trainees relevant to a particular educational intervention, and usually before exposure to it, is generally referred to as diagnostic. Analogous to medicine, the purpose of these assessments is to determine the trainees' educational needs with the goal of optimizing learning. Often they produce a profile that identifies areas of strength and weakness.

Examples of this type of test are most common in continuing medical education, where participants select, or are assigned to, a particular educational experience based on their performance. In some settings, diagnostic assessment takes place when physicians have been out of practice for a period of time (e.g. Varjavand et al., 2012). In general, they are underutilized in formal training where the focus remains largely on educational process. With the movement to competency-based education, these types of assessments should increase in importance.

Qualities of a good assessment

There are many ways to judge the quality of an assessment. Historically, there was emphasis on the measurement properties of the test alone (reliability and validity). More recently, van der Vleuten (1996) expanded the list of qualities, pushing beyond the traditional measurement characteristics to include issues related to the test's effect, acceptability and feasibility. These criteria were reaffirmed and added to in a consensus statement of the 2010 Ottawa Conference, which resulted in the following criteria for good assessment (Norcini et al., 2011).

- **Validity or coherence**. There should evidence that is coherent ('hangs together') and that supports the use of the results of an assessment for a particular purpose.
- **Reproducibility or consistency**. The results of the assessment would be the same if repeated under similar circumstances.
- **Equivalence**. The same assessment yields equivalent scores or decisions when administered across different institutions or cycles of testing.
- **Feasibility**. The assessment is practical, realistic and sensible, given the circumstances and context.
- **Educational effect**. The assessment motivates those who take it to prepare in a fashion that has educational benefit.
- **Catalytic effect**. The assessment provides results and feedback in a fashion that creates, enhances and supports education; it drives future learning forward.
- **Acceptability**. Stakeholders find the assessment process and results to be credible.

 "Over time, most of these criteria have been presented in detail by a variety of authors and their importance is clear. More recently, however, particular emphasis has been placed on the catalytic effect. This criterion refers to how well the assessment provides results and feedback in such a way that learning is created, enhanced and supported. It is central to the evolving view of assessment as means of generating learning

as well as deciding the degree to which it has occurred."

Norcini et al., 2011

VALIDITY THEORY

Determining the purpose of an assessment and then ensuring that test development, test construction, and scoring support that purpose is a particular concern in health professions education. Validity theory presents a useful framework for considering this concern, and there is a long history of its development (e.g. Cook & Beckman, 2006). For purposes of this chapter, a framework outlined by Kane (2013) provides a useful introduction. The framework has four components and Kane contends that validation is a matter of accruing evidence around each of them.

 "In determining validity, it is important to collect evidence that supports interpretations made based on test scoring, generalization, extrapolation, and interpretation/decisions."

Cook & Beckman, 2006

The scoring component is concerned with developing evidence that the assessment is administered fairly, that students are assessed appropriately, and that any criteria developed are applied consistently. When the assessment is given, evidence that conditions are the same for all students supports the argument that testing is fair and testing conditions are similar, regardless of location or who administers the test. This is also referred to as standardization. The level of difficulty of the task should be well matched to the group being tested. Scoring criteria should be applied equally to all students taking the test. No one group should have an advantage over others. The evidence collected to support the scoring argument includes meeting the criteria for reproducibility (reliability).

The generalization component requires evidence that the content of the test adequately represents the domain from which it is drawn and that enough of it is sampled to produce scores and/or decisions that are reasonably precise. Evidence of generalizability is often supported by reliability coefficients from classical test theory, or generalizability coefficients from generalizability theory.

The extrapolation component requires evidence that the scores are relevant to the construct of interest, and this includes demonstrating that they were not influenced by things that are unrelated to this construct. This evidence shows that the assessment is 'coherent', and scores relate in a manner that is expected. Additional information about this component is presented in the next section, Score interpretation.

The interpretation/decision component requires that evidence be collected that shows a link between test usage and assessment results. For example, if pass/fail decisions are being made, evidence should be gathered to support the process and usefulness of the classification of those being assessed. More information about this component of validity theory is provided in the section on standards.

Score interpretation

A score is a letter or number that reflects how well an individual performs on an assessment. When a test is being developed, one of the first decisions to be made is how the scores will be interpreted: norm-referenced or criterion-referenced (Glaser, 1963). This decision has implications for how the items or cases are chosen, what the scores mean when they are being used by students, teachers and institutions, and how the reliability or reproducibility of scores is conceived (Popham & Husek, 1969).

NORM-REFERENCED SCORE INTERPRETATION

When scores are interpreted from a norm-referenced perspective they are intended to provide information about how individuals perform against a group of test takers. For example, saying that a student's performance was one standard deviation above the mean indicates that he or she did better than 84% of those who took the test. It says nothing about how many questions the student answered correctly.

Norm-referenced score interpretation is especially useful in situations where there are a limited number of positions and there is a need to select the best (or most appropriate) of the test takers. For example, in admissions decisions, there are often a limited number of seats and the goal is to pick the best of the applicants. Norm-referenced score interpretation aids in these types of decisions. However, it is not useful when the goal is to identify how much each individual knows or can do.

CRITERION-REFERENCED SCORE INTERPRETATION

When scores are interpreted from a criterion-referenced perspective (sometimes called domain-referenced) they are intended to provide information about how much an individual knows or can do given the domain of the assessment. For example, saying that a student got 70% of the items right on a test means that he or she knows 70% of what is needed. It says nothing about how the student performed in comparison to others.

Criterion-referenced score interpretation is particularly useful in competency testing. For example, an assessment designed to provide feedback intended to improve performance should yield scores interpreted from a criterion-referenced perspective. Likewise, an end-of-course assessment should produce scores that indicate how much material students have learned. However, criterion-referenced score interpretation is not useful when the goal is to rank students. Scores from criterion-referenced assessments can be particularly useful in outcome- or competency-based education programmes.

One common variation on criterion-referenced score interpretation is called a *mastery* test. In a mastery test, a binary score (usually pass or fail) connotes whether the individual's performance demonstrates sufficient command of the material for a particular purpose.

Score equivalence

When an assessment is given, there are many instances when it is desirable to compare scores among trainees, against a common pass-fail point, and/or over time. Clearly, if all the trainees take exactly the same questions or encounter exactly the same patients, it is possible to compare scores and make equivalent pass-fail decisions. Some methods, like multiple-choice questions (MCQs) and standardized patients (SPs), were created in part to ensure that all trainees would face exactly the same challenge and their scores would mean exactly the same thing.

There are also a variety of important assessment situations when scores are not equivalent where adjustments can be made. For example, in an MCQ or SP examination, the test items or cases are often changed over time and, despite maintaining similar content, these versions or forms of the same assessment differ in difficulty. With these methods of assessment, the issue can be addressed through test *equating* (Kolen & Brennan, 1995; van der Linden & Hambleton, 1997). Equating is a set of procedures, designs and statistics that are used to adjust scores, so it is as if everyone took the same test. Although this provides a way to adjust scores, it is complicated, time intensive and labour intensive. Consequently, it is used often in national assessments and less frequently for locally developed tests.

There are also a variety of important assessment situations where scores are not equivalent and where good adjustment is not practical or possible. For example, virtually all methods of assessment based on observed trainees' encounters with real patients yield scores (or ratings) that are not equivalent because patients vary in the level of challenge they present and observers differ in how hard they grade. Attempts to minimize these unwanted sources of influence on scores usually take the form of wide sampling of patients and faculty (to hopefully balance out the easy and difficult patients), training of observers, and certain IRT-based methods that statistically minimize some of the differences among observers (Linacre, 1989). None of these is wholly satisfactory, however, and although these types of assessments are essential to the training and credentialing of doctors, the results must be interpreted with some caution when used for summative purposes. They are well suited to formative assessment.

Standards

Assessments can be given for many reasons. At times they are used by teachers to check what students have learned. In other cases, they are used to provide feedback or to decide who is admitted to a programme or awarded a licence or other qualification. While the goals of an assessment may differ, there may be decisions associated with the use of these instruments—decisions regarding the competency or proficiency of individuals. Sometimes, it may be important to categorize performance on a test, usually as pass or fail (although there may be times when more than two categories are needed). The score that separates passes from fails is called the standard or pass-fail point. It is an answer to the question, "How much is enough?" A standard is the score that separates success from failure on these assessments. Standard setting is the process of translating a description of the characteristics denoting the desired level of performance into a number that applies to a particular test. There are two types of standards: relative and absolute (Norcini, 2003).

 "Standard setting is the process of translating a description of the characteristics denoting the desired level of performance into a number that applies to a particular test. The credibility of standards depends to a large degree on the standard setters and the method they use. The standard setters must understand the purpose of the test and the reason for establishing the cut score, know the content, and be familiar with the examinees. The specific method chosen to set standards is not as important as whether it produces results that are fit for the purpose of the test, relies on informed expert judgement, demonstrates due diligence, is supported by a body of research, and is easy to explain and implement."

McKinley & Norcini, 2014

RELATIVE STANDARDS

For relative standards, the pass-fail point is chosen to separate individuals based on how well they performed compared to each other. For example, a cutting score might be selected to pass the top 80% of students (i.e. the 80% of students with the best scores). Relative standards are typically used in the same circumstances as norm-referenced tests, where the performance of the group taking the test is important.

Relative standards are most appropriate in settings where a group of a particular size needs to be selected.

For instance, in an admissions setting where the number of seats is limited and the purpose is to pick the best students, relative standards make the most sense. Relative standards are much less appropriate for assessments where the intention is to determine competence (i.e. whether a student knows enough for a particular purpose).

ABSOLUTE STANDARDS

For absolute standards, the pass-fail point is chosen to separate individuals based on how much they know or how well they perform. For example, a cutting score might be selected to pass the students who correctly answer 80% of the questions.

Absolute standards are most appropriate in settings where there is a need to determine competence. This type of standard is useful with criterion- (or domain-) based assessment. For instance, in an end-of-year assessment where the purpose is to decide which students learned enough to progress to the next year, absolute standards make the most sense. Absolute standards are much less appropriate for assessments where the intention is to select a certain number or percentage of students for a particular purpose.

The characteristics of the process of selecting the pass-fail point of an assessment contribute to the evidence of the credibility of the standard and its associated cut score (Norcini & Guille, 2002; Norcini & McKinley, 2009). The method selected should be easy to explain to those participating in the process and should be supported by research. The process should be designed to meet assessment goals. Those participating should be engaged in thoughtful effort (due diligence). Methods that are based on global judgements and done quickly are not as defensible, but the process should not take many days either. The process should show that considerable effort was made in conceptualization of the standard and determination of the score associated with that standard.

Blueprints

The content included in an assessment is essential to the quality of the results and to provide evidence of the validity and credibility of the scores and decisions emanating from it. A good assessment starts with a good blueprint (sometimes called a table of specifications), which specifies in appropriate detail what content needs to be covered (Downing & Haladyna, 2006). This blueprint should be shared with anyone being assessed, well in advance of the actual examination.

For example, the American Board of Internal Medicine publishes its blueprint for the certifying examination in internal medicine (www.abim.org). It specifies 'patient task', using patient demographics (e.g. Women's Health is 6%) to determine examination content (American Board of Internal Medicine, 2016). More than 50% of the questions must require synthesis or judgement to reach the correct conclusion. The blueprint specifies in detail the percentage of the items devoted to each of the medical content categories (e.g. cardiovascular disease is 14%, infectious disease is 9%, psychiatry is 4%) and there is a cross-cutting classification for areas like geriatric medicine (10%) and prevention (6%). Each test contributes to a primary content category and may contribute to a cross-cutting category as well (e.g. a prevention question in cardiovascular disease). Because this is a national assessment and there is so much at stake, the blueprint is very detailed. For local assessments and/or those based on fewer items or cases (e.g. an OSCE), this level of detail is unnecessary, but a blueprint is still essential to provide evidence of the validity of the results.

 "For a credentialing examination, such as certification, the content and blueprint should be based on the nature of practice, not the nature of training. Consequently, the blueprints for such examinations are often based on a job analysis. This supports the validity of the scores by creating an explicit link between the test content and what is done in practice."

Colton et al., 1991

The source of content for an assessment will depend on its purpose. For example, if it intended to determine what has been learned as part of a course then the content should be drawn from the syllabus. However, if it is intended to indicate readiness for practice then it should be based on the patient problems that constitute that practice. There are a variety of sophisticated designs and statistical methods for supporting the development of a blueprint that are suitable for assessments where the stakes are high (Downing & Haladyna, 2006).

Self-assessment

Self-assessment has occupied a central role in medical education for some time. In general, it is assumed that the individual chooses what he or she believes is important to assess, selects how the assessment will be done, and then uses the results of the assessment to confirm strengths and address weaknesses. Within this context, virtually all methods of assessments can be used for self-assessment.

 "Of the 20 comparisons between self- and external assessment, 13 demonstrated little, no, or an inverse relationship and 7 demonstrated positive associations. A number of studies found the worst accuracy in self-assessment among physicians who were the least skilled and those who were the most confident. These results are consistent with those found in other professions."

Davis et al., 2006

For society to grant doctors and other professionals the ability to self-regulate, it must assume that they are able to self-assess accurately. This ability has in turn been expected to drive day-to-day practice and lifelong learning. As important, accurate self-assessment is what allows doctors to limit their practices to areas of competence. Given this critical role, it is not surprising that medical education is expected to develop this ability in trainees and practitioners.

Despite its importance, there is good evidence that doctors and other professionals are not very good at self-assessment. A recent review of the literature by Davis and colleagues (2006) concluded that although the literature was flawed, doctors have a limited ability to self-assess accurately. Eva and Regehr (2005) added that self-assessment "is a complicated, multifaceted, multipurpose phenomenon that involves a number of interacting cognitive processes". Given its complexity, there is neither the research nor the educational strategies available at the moment to suggest that self-assessment in its purest form can be relied upon.

Three important suggestions have been offered to make self-assessment more effective by ensuring that it is guided (Galbraith et al., 2008). First, it is essential that the self-assessment be chosen to be relevant to the learning or practice experience of the student or doctor; it should not be completely self-selected. Second, the self-assessment should be directly linked to educational experiences that can remediate difficulties. Third, the results of self-assessment should be periodically validated by external assessments.

Objective versus subjective assessments

In the literature, it is not unusual for authors to refer to some forms of assessment as 'objective' and others as 'subjective'. Generally speaking, objective assessments have one or more clearly correct or incorrect responses or behaviours that can be readily observed. Examples of objective assessments include MCQs and checklists. In contrast, subjective assessments often require judgements about a response or set of behaviours. Examples of subjective assessments include essay questions and rating forms.

 "There is much research comparing checklists (seen as objective) and global ratings (seen as subjective). In fact, scores from checklists are slightly more reliable and global ratings are slightly more valid. But the differences are relatively small, so that using either methodology can produce good results."

Norcini & Boulet, 2003

In many ways, this is not a useful dichotomy. MCQs are arguably the most objective of the assessment methods. Nonetheless, judgements are made through the test construction, scoring and standard-setting process. Creation of the blueprint requires a number of judgements about importance and frequency. When individual items are written, the author makes judgements about the patient's age, the site of care, which diagnostic tests and treatments are included among the potential responses and so on. For scoring, judgements need to be made as to whether/how much to weight each response, how to aggregate those weights, what scale to report them on, and where the pass-fail point will be.

All assessment requires judgement

The only difference among the various methods is the way in which those judgements are gathered and the number of experts involved. MCQs have an advantage because many experts can contribute to test creation so that items can be eliminated, various different perspectives can be represented, and the product (i.e. the final test) can be endorsed by the group. In addition, many different clinical situations can be sampled efficiently. The exact same judgements are made in a bedside oral examination, but the method limits the number of experts and clinical situations that can be included. To the degree that the number of experts and patients can be increased, the 'objectivity' of the oral examination approaches that of MCQs.

Summary

The purpose of this chapter is to identify some of the concepts fundamental to assessment and to provide background to their meaning, development and use. The test theories underlying assessment have been briefly described as have the types of assessment to which they apply and the criteria against which to judge their success. The importance of test content, as highlighted by the blueprint, plays a central role in the quality of an assessment and more technical matters like score interpretation, equivalence and standards must be aligned with the purpose of assessments so they perform as intended. Finally, much is written about self-assessment and subjective versus objective measurement. The chapter has suggested some potential concerns and clarifications around these popular topics.

References

American Board of Internal Medicine. Internal Medicine Certification Examination Blueprint. Available at: http://www.abim.org/~/media/ABIM%20 Public/Files/pdf/exam-blueprints/certification/ internal-medicine.pdf. (Accessed 2016).

Brennan, R.L., 2001. Generalizability theory. Springer-Verlag., New York.

Colton, A., Kane, M.T., Kingsbury, C., Estes, C.A., 1991. Strategies for examining the validity of job analysis data. J. Educ. Meas. 28 (4), 283–294.

Cook, D.A., Beckman, T.J., 2006. Current Concepts in Validity and Reliability for Psychometric Instruments: theory and Application. Am. J. Med. 119 (2), 166.e7–166.e16.

Crocker, L., Algina, J., 1986. Introduction to classical and modern test theory. Harcourt, Brace, & Jovanovich, Fort Worth TX.

Cronbach, L.J., Gleser, C.G., Nanda, H., Rajaratnam, N., 1972. The dependability of behavioral measurements. Wiley, New York.

Davis, D.A., Mazmanian, P.E., Fordis, M., et al., 2006. Accuracy of Physician Self-assessment Compared With Observed Measures of Competence: a Systematic Review. JAMA 296 (9), 1094–1102.

De Champlain, A.F., 2010. A primer on classical test theory and item response theory for assessments in medical education. Med. Educ. 44 (1), 109–117.

DiVall, M.V., Alston, G.L., Bird, E., et al., 2014. A Faculty Toolkit for Formative Assessment in Pharmacy Education. Am. J. Pharm. Educ. 78 (9), 160–169.

Downing, S.M., 2003. Item response theory: applications of modern test theory in medical education. Med. Educ. 37 (8), 739–745.

Downing, S.M., Haladyna, T.M. (Eds.), 2006. Handbook of test development. Erlbaum, Mahwah, NJ.

Eva, K.W., Regehr, G., 2005. Self-Assessment in the Health Professions: a Reformulation and Research Agenda. Acad. Med. 80 (10Suppl), S46–S54.

Galbraith, R.M., Hawkins, R.E., Holmboe, E.S., 2008. Making self-assessment more effective. J. Contin. Educ. Health Prof. 28 (1), 20–24.

Glaser, R., 1963. Instructional technology and the measurement of learning outcomes: some questions. Am. Psychol. 18 (8), 519–521.

Hambleton, R.K., Swaminathan, H., Rogers, H.J., 1991. Fundamentals of Item Response Theory. Sage Press, Newbury Park, CA.

Hanauer, D.I., Hatfull, G.F., Jacobs-Sera, D., 2009. Active Assessment: Assessing Scientific Inquiry. Springer.

Kane, M.T., 2013. Validating the Interpretations and Uses of Test Scores. J. Educ. Meas. 50 (1), 1–73.

Kolen, M.J., Brennan, R.L., 1995. Test equating: Methods and practices. Springer-Verlag, New York.

Lefroy, J., Watling, C., Teunissen, P.W., Brand, P., 2015. Guidelines: the do's, don'ts and don't knows of feedback for clinical education. Perspect. Med. Educ. 4 (6), 284–299.

Linacre, J.M., 1989. Many-facet Rasch measurement. MESA Press, Chicago.

Lord, F.M., Novick, M.R., 1968. Statistical theories of mental test scores. Addison-Welsley Publish Company, Reading MA.

McKinley, D.W., Norcini, J.J., 2014. How to set standards on performance-based examinations: AMEE Guide No. 85. Med. Teach. 36 (2), 97–110.

Norcini, J.J., 2003. Setting standards on educational tests. Med. Educ. 37 (5), 464–469.

Norcini, J., Anderson, B., Bollela, V., et al., 2011. Criteria for good assessment: consensus statement and recommendations from the Ottawa 2010 Conference. Med. Teach. 33 (3), 206–214.

Norcini, J., Boulet, J., 2003. Methodological Issues in the Use of Standardized Patients for Assessment. Teach. Learn. Med. 15 (4), 293–297.

Norcini, J., Guille, R., 2002. Combining tests and setting standards. In: Norman, G.R., van der Vleuten, C.P.M., Newble, D.I. (Eds.), International handbook of research in medical education (Part two), vol. 1. Kluwer Academic Publishers, Dordrecht, The Netherlands, pp. 811–834.

Norcini, J., McKinley, D., 2009. Standard Setting. In: Dent, J., Harden, R. (Eds.), A Practical Guide for Medical Teachers (Third). Elsevier Churchill Livingstone, Edinburgh; New York, pp. 311–317.

Popham, W.J., Husek, T.R., 1969. Implications of criterion-referenced measurement. J. Educ. Meas. 6 (1), 1–9.

van der Linden, W.J., Hambleton, R.K. (Eds.), 1997. Handbook of modern item response theory. Springer-Verlag, New York.

van der Vleuten, C., 1996. The assessment of professional competence: developments, research and practical implications. Adv. Health Sci. Educ. 1 (1), 41–67.

Varjavand, N., Greco, M., Novack, D.H., Schindler, B.A., 2012. Assessment of an innovative instructional program to return non-practicing physicians to the workforce. Med. Teach. 34 (4), 285–291.

Written assessments

L. W. T. Schuwirth, C. P. M. van der Vleuten

Trends

- With respect to what an item tests, the content of the question is essential and the question format is not, open-ended questions do not necessarily test higher-order cognitive skills and multiple-choice do not test necessarily only factual recall.

- The most important aspect of item writing is quality control; Staff development and peer review are indispensable in ensuring high-quality assessment.

- There are no question types that are inherently better than others; every method has its own advantages and disadvantages, or put differently; its indications, contraindications and side effects.

Introduction

Despite the increasing popularity of workplace-based assessment, written assessments are still probably the most widely used assessment methods in education. Their popularity is likely to be partly because of their logistical advantages and their cost-effectiveness. In comparison with many other methods they are easy and cost-efficient to construct, and they produce reliable scores. They are not a panacea, though, as no single assessment method is; for comprehensive testing of competence a variety of written and non-written methods would be needed. Currently, the notion of programmatic assessment is gaining popularity rapidly. In this approach different assessment methods are purposively combined to let strengths of one method compensate for the strengths of another. To enable this it is helpful to know strengths and weakness of the various assessment methods. The purpose of this chapter is, therefore, to provide some information about the strengths and weaknesses of written assessment methods.

A variety of written and non-written methods of assessment are required to test medical competence comprehensively.

Question format

Often, a distinction is made between open-ended and closed question formats, and multiple-choice questions are seen as closed formats.

Because of this, multiple-choice items are often deemed unfit for testing higher-order cognitive skills (e.g. medical problem solving) because the correct answer can be found by mere recognition within the options (the so-called cueing effect). From the literature comparing response formats, however, it has become clear that the response format (open-ended or closed) is not so important, but that the stimulus (what you ask) is essential.

 "The positive cueing effect is considered as a disadvantage of the MCQ, and has been documented consistently. However, MCQs apparently also cue in the opposite direction: they can lead the examinee to choose the wrong answer."

Schuwirth et al., 1996

Consider, for example, the following two questions regarding the response format:

You are a general practitioner and you have made a house call on a 46-year-old patient. She appears to have a perforated appendix, and she shows signs of a local peritonitis. Which is the best next step in the management?
and
You are a general practitioner and you have made a house call on a 46-year-old patient. She appears to have a perforated appendix and she shows signs of a local peritonitis. Which of the following is the most appropriate next step in the management?

1. *Give pain medication and re-assess her situation in 24 hours.*

2. *Give pain medication and let her drive to the hospital in her own car.*

3. *Give no pain medication and let her drive to the hospital in her own car.*

4. *Give pain medication and call an ambulance.*

5. *Give no pain medication and call an ambulance.*

In these two questions there is very little difference in what is asked, whereas the way the response is recorded differs.

Now consider these two questions regarding stimulus format:

What is the most prevalent symptom of meningitis?
and

Make a SWOT analysis of the government's regulations to reduce the waiting lists in the healthcare system.

In these questions the response format is similar, but the content of the question is completely different. In the second question the expected thought processes are considerably different to those evoked by the first.

 Stimulus formats: The content of a question will determine the thought processes required to answer it.

For the rest of this chapter we will therefore use the distinction between response formats and stimulus formats.

Quality control of items

No matter which assessment format is used, the quality of the examination is always related to the quality of the individual items. Therefore, it is of no use discussing strengths, weaknesses and uses of various item types if we cannot assume that optimal care has been taken to ensure their quality. One aspect of the quality of an item is its ability to discriminate clearly between those candidates who have sufficient knowledge and those who do not. So, they are a 'diagnostic for medical competence'. This implies that when a student with insufficient knowledge answers a question correctly, this can be regarded as a false-positive result, and the opposite would signify a false-negative result. In quality control procedures, prior to test administration, the diagnosis and elimination of sources of false-positive and false-negative results are essential. In addition, the relevance of the items, the congruence between curricular goals and test content, and the use of item analysis and student criticisms are other important factors in quality control of assessment, but in this chapter we will focus on quality aspects of the individual items.

Response formats

SHORT-ANSWER OPEN-ENDED QUESTIONS

Description

This is an open-ended question type, which requires the candidate to generate a short answer of often no more than one or a few words. For example:

Which muscle origin is affected in the condition 'tennis elbow'?

When to use and when not to use

Open-ended questions generally take some time to answer. Therefore, fewer items can be asked per hour of testing time. There is a relationship between the reliability of test scores and the number of items, so open-ended questions can lead to less reliable scores per hour of testing time. Also, they need to be marked by a content expert, which makes them logistically less efficient and more costly. There might be cases in which spontaneous generation of the correct answer is an essential feature of the knowledge that the test purports to measure.

So, a question such as:

Which kidney is positioned superior to the other one?
is not very sensible as a multiple choice, because there are only two possible answers.

On the other hand, a question like:

In elderly people with vague complaints of fatigue, thirst and poor healing of wounds, which diagnosis should be thought of spontaneously?
would be odd in a multiple-choice format.

Therefore as a rule of thumb it is best to restrict using short-answer open-ended questions to when the content of the question really requires it.

Tips for item construction

Use clearly phrased questions to avoid reading errors by students. Of course, you may not want your students to be bad readers but when this is not what you want to test, it will be a source of error. Use short sentences and avoid double negatives. If in doubt as to whether to use more words for clarity, or fewer words for brevity it is best to opt for more clarity.

Construct a well-defined answer key in which correct and incorrect answers are clarified and possible alternative answers identified (perhaps by a panel of examiners) beforehand. This is especially necessary if more than one person will be correcting the test papers.

Make sure that candidates can be clear about what kind of answer is expected. An open-ended question may be unclear for the candidates as to what kind of answer is expected, or what level of detail. For example, on a question on chest infection, the expected answer could be pneumonia, bacterial pneumonia or even pneumococcal pneumonia. There may also be a lack of clarity about what type of answer is expected, as, for example, in:

What is the main difference between the left and right lung?
is the expected answer here that one is a mirror image of the other, the number of lobes, the angle of the main bronchus, the surface or the contribution to gas exchange?

It is also useful to indicate a maximum length for the answer. Students often apply a 'blunderbuss' approach, which means that they will write down as much as they can in the hope that part of their response will be the correct answer. By limiting the length of the answer this can be prevented.

Use multiple correctors effectively. If more than one teacher is involved in correcting the test papers, it is better to have one corrector score the same item(s) for all students and another corrector score another set of items for all students than to have one corrector score the whole test for one group of students and another the whole test for another group of students. In the latter case a student can be advantaged by a mild corrector or be disadvantaged by a harsh one; in the former the same group of examiners will be used to produce the scores for all students, which leads to a better reliability with the same effort.

 For short-answer open-ended questions, it should be clear beforehand what would be correct answers and what would be incorrect answers.

ESSAY QUESTIONS

Description

Essay questions are open-ended question types that require a longer answer. Ideally, they ask the candidate to describe their reasoning processes, to evaluate a given situation or specifically to apply concepts learnt in one case to a new case. An example is:

John and Jim, both 15 years old, are going for a swim in the early spring. The water is still very cold. John suggests seeing who can stay under water longest. They both decide to give it a go. Before entering the water John takes one deep breath of air, whereas Jim breaths deeply about 10 times and dives into the cold water. When John cannot hold his breath any more he surfaces. Much to his shock he sees Jim on the bottom of the swimming pool. He manages to get Jim on the side, and a bystander starts resuscitation.

Explain at the pathophysiological level what has happened to Jim, why he became unconscious, and why this has not happened to John.

Of course, it is important that the situation of John and Jim is new to the students, and that it has not already been explained during the lectures or practicals. A question such as:

Explain the Bohr effect and how it influences the O$_2$ saturation of the blood.

is therefore less suitable as an essay type of question. Although the knowledge asked for may be relevant, the question asks for reproduction of factual knowledge, which is more efficiently done with other formats.

When to use and when not to use

It is essential to use essay questions only for specific purposes. The main reason for this is the lower reliability and the need for expert hand-scoring. Essay questions are therefore best used when the answer requires spontaneous generation of information and when more than a short text is required. Examples are:

• Evaluating a certain action or situation, for example:
Make a SWOT analysis of the government's new regulations to reduce waiting lists in the healthcare system.

• Application of learnt concepts on a new situation or problem, for example:
During your course you have learnt the essentials of the biofeedback mechanism of ACTH. Apply this mechanism to the control of diuresis.

• Generating solutions, hypotheses, research questions

• Predicting or estimating

• Comparing, looking for similarities or discussing differences.

It can be difficult to score answers submitted as an essay without being influenced by the student's literary style, yet there is no rule whether or not to take this into account. If the purpose of the test is merely to try to gauge the knowledge and understanding the student has literary style is not important, but when the purpose is whether the student can explain it, the style is important. So although there is no general rule, it is important to be clear about the purpose of the assessment both to oneself and to the students.

 It can be difficult to score answers submitted as an essay without being influenced by the student's literary style.

Tips for item construction

For essay questions, essentially the same item construction suggestions apply as for short-answer open-ended questions:

• The question must be phrased as clearly as possible; the candidate should understand what is expected.

• The answer key must be well written and produced before the test, including alternative correct answers and plausible but incorrect answers.

• The maximum length of the answer must be stipulated, to ensure a concise response and avoid the 'blunderbuss' approach.

A special type of essay question is the modified essay question. This consists of a case followed by a number of questions. Often, these questions follow the case chronologically. This can lead to the problem of interdependency of the questions: if candidates answer the first question incorrectly, they are likely to answer all subsequent parts of the question incorrectly also. This is a psychometric problem that can be avoided by test administrations in which the candidates confirm or hand in answers before they are allowed to proceed to the next question.

TRUE–FALSE QUESTIONS

Description

True–false questions are statements for which the candidate has to indicate whether the it is true or false. For example:

Stem: *For the treatment of a Legionella pneumophila pneumonia, a certain antimicrobial agent is most indicated. This is:*

Item: *erythromycin True/False*

The first part, the stem, is always correct information that is given to the candidate. The item is the part for which the candidate has to indicate whether it is true or false.

When to use and when not to use

True–false questions can cover a broad domain in a short period of time, leading to broad sampling. They are often used for testing of factual knowledge, and this is probably what they are most suited for. Nevertheless, they have some inherent disadvantages. First, they are difficult to construct flawlessly. Careful item construction is needed to ensure that the answer is defensibly true or false. This often leads to artificial phrasing. For example:

Stem: *Certain disorders occur together more often than is to be expected on the basis of pure coincidence. This is the case for:*

Item: *diabetes and atherosclerosis True/False*

A second disadvantage is that when candidates answer a false-keyed item correctly, one can only conclude that they knew that the statement was untrue, and not necessarily that they would have known what would have been true. For example, the following question:

Stem: *For the treatment of an acute gout attack in elderly patients, certain drugs are indicated. Such a drug is:*

Item: *allopurinol True/False*

If a candidate answers 'false', one cannot conclude that they would have known which drugs are indicated.

Tips for item construction

Use stems when necessary. It is useful to put all information that is not part of the question in the stem. This way it is clear to the candidate what they have to consider for the answer and what not. Also, with this approach many of the most frequent item-construction flaws can be avoided.

Avoid semi-quantitative terminology. Words such as 'often' and 'seldom' are difficult to define. Different people assign different meanings to those words, so whether the answer is 'true' or 'false' is then a matter of opinion and not of fact. In such cases one has to revert to statements indicating exact percentages, such as:

Stem: *In a certain percentage of patients with acute pancreatitis the disease is self-limiting.*

Item: *This percentage lies closer to 80% than to 50%.*

Avoid terms that are too open or too absolute. Words such as 'can', 'is possible', 'never' and 'always' lead test-wise students to the correct answer. The most probable answer to statements that are too open is 'true', and the most probable answer to statements that are too absolute is 'false'. The same applies to equality, synonymy etc.

Make sure the question is phrased so that the answer is defensibly correct.

Stem: *The cause of atherosclerosis is:*

Item: *hypercholesterolaemia*

In this case, one could argue that there are many causes or that there is a chain of aetiological factors that cause atherosclerosis. In such a case, for example, it would be better to ask for risk factors than causes.

Avoid double negatives. This is especially important in true–false questions, as the answer key 'false' can be seen as a negative also. Unfortunately, this cannot be avoided in all cases.

Stem: *For patients with hypertension, certain drugs are contraindicated. Such drugs are:*

Item: *corticosteroids False*

The double negative 'contraindicated' and 'false' (answer key) cannot simply be removed by using the combination 'indicated' and 'true' because then the question would not be correct.

MULTIPLE-CHOICE QUESTIONS

Description

This is certainly the most well-known item format. It is often also referred to as single-best-option multiple-choice. These questions consist of a stem, a question (called the lead-in) and a number of options. The candidate has to indicate which of the options is most correct.

Stem: *During resuscitation of an adult, compressions of the thorax have to be performed to produce circulation. For this, one hand has to be placed on the sternum and the other has to be placed on this hand in order to give correct compressions.*

Lead-in: *Which of the following options indicates the most correct position of both hands?*

Options:

1. *the junction between manubrium and sternum*
2. *the superior half of the sternum*
3. *the middle of the sternum*
4. *the inferior half of the sternum*
5. *the xiphoid process of the sternum.*

When to use and when not to use

Multiple-choice items can be considered the most flexible question type. Although they may not always be simple to produce flawlessly, they are easy to administer. Answering and scoring are not time-consuming, and they are logistically efficient. They are best used if broad sampling of the domain is required and if large numbers of candidates are to be tested. They yield fairly reliable testing scores per hour of testing time. The two main situations in which multiple-choice questions should not be used are:

- when spontaneous generation of the answer is essential (this is explained in the paragraph on short-answer open-ended questions)
- when the number of realistic options is too large.

In all other cases, multiple-choice questions are a good alternative to open-ended questions.

Tips for item construction

The general tips mentioned in the preceding section all pertain to multiple-choice questions as well (clear sentences, defensibly correct answer key etc.), but there are some tips that apply uniquely to multiple-choice questions. The first is to use equal alternatives.

Sydney is:

a. *the capital of Australia*

b. *a dirty city*

c. *situated at the Pacific Ocean*

d. *the first city of Australia.*

In this case the options all relate to different aspects. In order to produce the correct answer the candidate has to compare apples to oranges. A better and more focused alternative would be:

Which of the following is the capital of Australia?

a. *Sydney*

b. *Melbourne*

c. *Adelaide*

d. *Perth*

e. *Canberra.*

Use options of equal length. Often the longest option is the correct one because often more words are needed to make an option correct than to make it incorrect. Students know this and will be guided by this hint.

Avoid fillers. Unfortunately, it is often prescribed to have four or five options where only three realistic ones can be found, leading to nonsense options (fillers). There is much to be said against this:

- Candidates will recognize the fillers and discard them immediately.
- It is more difficult to estimate the chance of answering the item correctly by random guessing.
- It will take a lot of item-writing time to find an extra option before the author decides to use a

filler (this time would better be used for another question).

- Authors may use combination options ('all of the above' or 'none of the above') instead, which is ill-advised.

Use simple multiple-choice formats only.

The major symptoms associated with cardiovascular disease:

1. *are chest pain, dyspnoea, palpitations*

2. *appear to worsen during exertion*

3. *are fatigue, dizziness and syncope*

4. *appear during rest*

   a. *(1), (2) and (3) are correct*

   b. *(1) and (3) are correct*

   c. *(2) and (4) are correct*

   d. *only (4) is correct*

   e. *all are correct.*

In this case, the question is unnecessarily complicated. Not only can it lead to mistakes in choosing from all the combinations – which has nothing to do with medical competence – but the combinations could also give important clues as to which answer is correct simply by logic. The rule for these formats is simple: do not use them.

Try to construct the question in a way so that, theoretically, the answer could also be given without seeing the answer options. This ensures that there is a clear and well-defined lead-in and that all the alternatives are aimed at the same aspect. So, after a stem or case description the lead- in: *Which of the following is true?* is too open, but the lead-in: *Which of the following is the most probable diagnosis?* is better defined and could theoretically be answered as if it were an open-ended question.

MULTIPLE TRUE–FALSE QUESTIONS

Description

In this question format more than one option can be ticked by the candidate. There are two versions. In the first, candidates are told how many options they should select; in the second, this is left open. The former is used when there is no clear distinction between correct and incorrect, for example:

Select the two most probable diagnoses.

The latter version is used if there is a clear distinction, for example:

Select the drugs that are indicated in this case.

Scoring of such items can be done in various ways. The standard approach is to treat all options as true–false items and then regard a ticked option as 'true' and the others as 'false'. The score on the item is the total of correctly ticked and non-ticked options divided by the total number of options. An alternative scoring system is to indicate a minimum of correct answers for a score of 1 and to score all other responses as 0.

When to use and when not to use

This format is best used when a selection of correct options from a limited number of options is indeed required, and when short-answer open-ended questions cannot be used.

Tips for item construction

There are no specific tips concerning this question type other than those applying to multiple-choice and short-answer open-ended questions.

Stimulus formats

EXTENDED-MATCHING QUESTIONS

Description

Extended-matching items consist of a theme description, a series of options (up to 26), a lead-in and a series of short cases or vignettes.

Theme: *diagnosis*
Options:

a. *hyperthyroidism*

b. *hypothyroidism*

c. *prolactinoma*

d. *hyperparathyroidism*

e. *phaeochromocytoma*

f. *Addison's disease*

g. *...etc.*

Lead-in: *For each of the following cases, select the most likely diagnosis.*

Vignettes: *A 45-year-old man consults you because of periods of extensive sweating. One or two times per day he has short periods during which he starts sweating heavily. His wife tells him that his face is all red. He feels very warm during this period. He has had this now for over 3 weeks. At first he thought the complaints would subside spontaneously, but now he is not sure any more. Pulmonary and cardiac examinations reveal no abnormalities. His blood pressure is 130/80, pulse 76 regular.*

When to use and when not to use

Because the questions ask for decisions and the stimuli are cases, extended-matching items focus more on decision making or problem solving. The large number of alternatives reduces the effect of cueing. Because the items are relatively short and can be answered quickly, extended-matching questions cover a large knowledge base per hour of testing time. They are best used in all situations where large groups of candidates have to be tested in a feasible way.

Tips for item construction

First, determine the theme. This is important because it helps to focus all the alternatives on the same element. To minimize the influence of cueing, it is important that all the options could theoretically apply to all vignettes.

The options should be short. The shorter and clearer the options, the less likely it is that any hints as to the correct answer may be given. It is best to avoid using verbs in the options.

The lead-in should be clear and well defined. A lead-in such as *For each of the following vignettes select the most appropriate option.* is too open and often indicates that the options are not homogeneous or the vignettes are not appropriately related to the options.

In constructing extended-matching questions:

- Determine the theme first.
- Keep the individual options short.
- Ensure that the lead in is clear and well-defined.

KEY-FEATURE APPROACH QUESTIONS

Description

Another format is the key-feature approach. It consists of a short, clearly described case or problem and a limited number of questions asking essential decisions or key-features. Such tests typically consist of many different short cases, enabling a broad sampling of the domain and thus fairly reliable test results per hour of testing time. They have also been demonstrated to be valid for the assessment of medical decision making or problem solving. Some institutes prescribe certain response formats, but key-feature cases can be used with various response formats depending on the content of the question.

For key-feature approach questions:

- All the important information must be presented in the case.
- The question must be directly linked to the case.
- The question must ask for essential decisions.

Tips for item construction

Apart from all the tips concerning the other question types, some tips are specifically pertinent to key-feature tests.

Make sure all the important information is presented in the case. This pertains not only to relevant medical information but also to contextual information (where do you see the patient, what is your function etc.). After you have written the questions, it is a good idea to re-address the case to check whether all the necessary information is provided.

Make sure the question is directly linked to the case. It should be impossible to answer the question correctly if the case has not been read. Ideally, all the information in the case must be used to produce the answer, and the correct answer is based on a careful balancing of all the information.

The question must ask for essential decisions. An incorrect decision must typically lead to an incorrect management of the case. In certain instances the diagnosis may not be the key feature, for example, if a different diagnosis would still lead to the same management of the case. Another way to check this is to see whether the answer key would change if certain elements of the case (such as location of the symptoms or age of the patient) were to be changed.

 "It has proven to be ill-advised to make up cases without consulting others."

Schuwirth et al., 1999

SCRIPT CONCORDANCE TEST QUESTIONS

Description

Based on cognitive theory on development of clinical expertise, Charlin and colleagues (2000) developed the script concordance test (SCT). Such tests use ill-defined problems and a method called aggregate scoring that takes expert variability into account. A clinical scenario is presented in which not all data are provided for the solution of the problem, and a menu of options is presented from which the candidate may score the likelihood of each option in relation to the solution of the problem on a $+2$ to -2 scale. An example is:

A 25-year-old male patient is admitted to the emergency room after a fall from a motorcycle, with a direct impact to the pubis. Vital signs are normal. The X-ray reveals a fracture of the pelvis with a disjunction of the pubic symphysis.

If you were thinking of:
Urethral rupture
And then you find:
Urethral bleeding
This hypothesis becomes:
-2 -1 0 $+1$ $+2$

SCT tests have good reliability per hour of testing time and there are numerous publications supporting validity for their purpose (Lubarsky et al., 2011). SCT has been specifically designed to test clinical reasoning.

Tips for item construction

Many of the tips mentioned above are relevant to constructing SCT items. Clear phrasing of the vignettes is essential as well as careful selection of the considered diagnoses and associated symptoms. The developers of this format recommend the use of expert teams to construct such items and the scoring key.

 "A final piece of advice would be the suggestion ... to look for the possibility of cooperation with other departments or faculties since the production of high-quality test material can be tedious and expensive."

Schuwirth et al., 1999

Summary

It must be stressed again that there is no one single best question format; for a good and comprehensive assessment of medical competence, a variety of instruments is needed. This chapter has provided a brief overview of various written question formats with some of their strengths and weaknesses and some hints for their use. The reference and further reading lists suggest more detailed literature.

References

Charlin, B., Rogh, L., Brailovsky, C., et al., 2000. The script concordance test: a tool to assess the reflective clinician. Teach. Learn. Med. 12 (4), 185–191.

Lubarsky, S., Charlin, B., Cook, D.A., et al., 2011. Script concordance testing: a review of published validity evidence. Med. Educ. 45 (4), 329–338.

Schuwirth, L.W.T., van der Vleuten, C.P.M., Donkers, H.H.L.M., 1996. A closer look at cueing effects in multiple-choice questions. Med. Educ. 30 (1), 44–49.

Schuwirth, L.W.T., Blackmore, D.B., Mom, E.M.A., et al., 1999. How to write short cases for assessing problem-solving skills. Med. Teach. 21 (2), 144–150.

Further reading

Cantillon, P., Hutchinson, L., Wood, D. (Eds.), 2003. ABC of Learning and Teaching in Medicine. BMJ Publishing Group, London.

Case, S.M., Swanson, D.B., 1993. Extended-matching items: a practical alternative to free-response questions. Teach. Learn. Med. 5 (2), 107–115.

Case, S.M., Swanson, D.B., 1998. Constructing Written Test Questions for the Basic and Clinical Sciences. National Board of Medical Examiners, Philadelphia.

Farmer, E.A., Page, G., 2005. A practical guide to assessing clinical decision-making skills using the key features approach. Med. Educ. 39 (12), 1188–1194.

Page, G., Bordage, G., Allen, T., 1995. Developing Key-feature Problems and Examinations to Assess Clinical Decision-making Skills. Acad. Med. 70 (3), 194–201.

Schuwirth, L.W.T., 1998. An Approach to the Assessment of Medical Problem Solving: Computerised Case-Based Testing. University of Maastricht, Maastricht.

Swanson, D.B., Norcini, J.J., Grosso, L.J., 1987. Assessment of clinical competence: written and computer-based simulations. Assess. Eval. High. Educ. 12 (3), 220–246.

Performance and workplace assessment

35

L. Etheridge, K. Boursicot

Trends

- A focus on learning through 'supervised learning events' rather than 'workplace based assessments'
- Increased emphasis on qualitative written feedback rather than quantitative scoring
- Development of tools to explore performance in different settings, e.g. clinical handover, leadership

Introduction

The apprenticeship model of medical training has existed for thousands of years: the apprentice learns from watching the master, and the master, in turn, observes the apprentice's performance and helps them improve. Performance assessment is not, therefore, a new concept. However, in the modern healthcare environment, with its discourse of accountability, performance assessment has an increasing role in ensuring that professionals develop and maintain the knowledge and skills required for practice. A number of international academic and professional bodies have incorporated performance assessment into their overall assessment frameworks for licensing, training and continued professional development. In the United States, the Medical Licensing Examination (USMLE) makes use of a structured test of clinical skills in the second stage of the licensing assessment. In the United Kingdom and Australasia, the main Royal Colleges have assessment frameworks for trainees that include a portfolio of workplace-based assessment (WPBA) tools.

 "Competence describes what an individual is able to do … while performance should describe what an individual actually does in clinical practice."

Boursicot et al., 2011

The terms 'performance' and 'competence' are often used interchangeably. 'Clinical competence' is the term being used most frequently by many of the professional regulatory bodies and in the educational literature. There are several dimensions to competence, and a wide range of well-validated assessments have been developed examining these. Traditional methods focus on the assessment of competence in artificial settings built to resemble the clinical environment. However, more novel methods of performance assessment concentrate on building up a structured picture of how the individual practitioner acts in his or her everyday working life, in interactions with patients and other practitioners, using technical, professional and interpersonal skills. Miller's model (Fig. 35.1) provides a framework for understanding the different facets of clinical competence and the assessment methods that test these.

In this chapter we will look at the different methods used to assess clinical performance, which we will define as the assessment of clinical skills and behaviours in both academic and workplace settings. These methods fall in the top two layers of Miller's pyramid. We will discuss how and why they are used and some of the practical aspects to be considered for educators wishing to make use of them. We will also explore the strengths and weaknesses of the various tools and consider some of the outstanding issues concerning their use.

Choosing the right assessment

When planning assessments, it is important to consider the purpose of the assessment and where it fits into the wider educational programme: a tool is only as useful as the system within which it resides. Considerations would include how to, or indeed whether to, make pass/fail decisions; whether the assessment is 'high-stakes'; how to give feedback to candidates; and effects on the learning of candidates. For example, assessments for the purpose of certification may require different criteria than some medical school assessments, where the primary purpose is to encourage and direct the learning of students (Downing, 2003). In considering the best tools for a particular assessment system, educators should gather information from multiple sources to enable a robust evaluation, as outlined in Box 35.1 (Schuwirth & van der Vleuten, 2009).

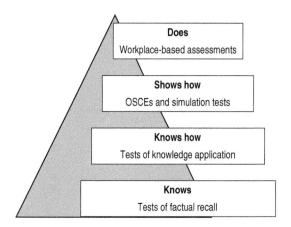

Fig. 35.1 Miller's model of competence. (Adapted from Miller GE: The assessment of clinical skills/competence/performance, Academic Medicine 65(9 Suppl):S63–S67, 1990.)

Educational impact is vital to consider, as inevitably assessments will influence students' learning strategies. Factors such as timing, outcomes (e.g. pass/fail) and format of the assessment will influence student behaviours. Many of the tools previously used for summative assessment are now used instead to structure supervised learning events (SLEs) – interactions between learners and supervisors that lead to immediate feedback and reflective learning. The aim of SLEs is to promote engagement, feedback and development of skills while removing the emphasis on 'passing' or 'failing'.

 Aligning the content of any assessment to the desired learning objectives is a useful way to encourage students to attend to the most important outcomes.

Assessments of clinical competence

Assessments of what a student or doctor is *able to do* can take place in artificial settings and have the advantage of being able to examine a number of individuals at the same time. The best known of these types of assessment is the OSCE.

OBJECTIVE STRUCTURED CLINICAL EXAMINATION (OSCE)

What is it? An OSCE consists of a series of structured stations around which a candidate moves in sequence. At each station specific tasks have to be performed, usually involving clinical skills such as history taking, clinical examination or practical skills. Different degrees of simulation may be used to test a wide range of psychomotor and communication skills, using simulated patients, part-task trainers, charts and results,

Box 35.1   Evaluating assessment tools

Validity – does this assessment tool measure what it is intended to measure?
- Assessment content relates meaningfully to learning outcomes: blueprinting
- Quality of the items has been rigorously appraised
- Results (scores) accurately reflect the candidates' performance
- Statistical (psychometric) properties of the assessment are acceptable; reproducibility and item analyses
- Pass/fail decisions are made fairly and defensibly
- Consequences of the test are considered equitably

Reliability – a measure of reproducibility of the scores, so the outcome would be the same if repeated over time
- Mathematical models calculate a reliability coefficient, the commonest being Cronbach's alpha

Generalizability – a form of reliability measure taking into account different circumstances within the same test form, e.g. in different OSCE circuits
- Allows better scrutiny of sources of variation

Acceptability – do all stakeholders believe in the assessment and find it easy to implement?
- Internal, e.g. teachers and learners
- External, e.g. regulatory bodies, employers, public

Cost effectiveness – does it offer 'value for money'?
- High quality balanced against cost

resuscitation manikins or computer-based simulations. There is a time limit for each station, and the marking scheme is structured and determined in advance.

 When designing an OSCE, the fundamental principle is that every candidate completes the same task in the same amount of time and is marked using the same schedule.

How is it used? The OSCE is typically used in high-stakes summative assessments at both the undergraduate and postgraduate level. The main advantages are that large numbers of candidates can be assessed in the same way across a range of clinical skills. High levels of reliability and validity can be achieved in the OSCE because of four main features:
- Structured marking schedules, which allow for more consistent scoring by assessors

	History	Examination	Health promotion	Practical skills
Cardiovascular	History of palpitations			ECG interpretation
Respiratory	History of breathlessness		Smoking cessation advice	
Gastro		Abdominal examination	Explain high-fibre diet	
Neuro		Gait examination		Lumbar puncture on manikin

Fig. 35.2 Example of an OSCE blueprint.

- Multiple independent observations collected by different assessors at different stations, so individual assessor bias is lessened
- Wider sampling across different cases and skills, resulting in a more reliable picture of overall competence
- Completion of a large number of stations, allowing the assessment to become more generalizable.

Overall, candidate scores are less dependent on who is examining and which patient is selected than in traditional long-case or *viva voce* examinations.

 The key to reliability of the OSCE is the number of stations; the more stations marked by different examiners there are, the more reliable the OSCE will be. However, this has to be balanced with practicality, as clearly the longer an OSCE, the more onerous it will be for all involved.

Organization: OSCEs can be complex to organize. Planning should begin well in advance of the examination date, and it is essential to ensure that there are enough patients, simulated patients, examiners, staff, refreshments and equipment to run the complete circuit for all candidates on the day of the exam. Careful calculations of the numbers of candidates, the length of each complete circuit and how many circuits have to be run need to be made. The mix of stations is chosen in advance and depends on the curriculum and the purpose of the assessment.

 Two of the simplest ways to plan a successful OSCE are to draw up a blueprint well in advance, outlining how the assessment is going to meet its goals, and to follow a standard operating procedure (SOP), describing the activities necessary to achieve these goals.

Development of a blueprint ensures adequate content validity, the level to which the sampling of skills in the OSCE matches the learning objectives of the whole curriculum. An example of a simple blueprint, detailing the different areas of a curriculum and how the stations chosen will cover these, can be seen in Fig. 35.2. It is also necessary to think about the timing of the stations. The length of the station should fit the task requested as closely as possible. Ideally, stations should be practised in advance to clarify this and anticipate potential problems with the setup or the mark sheet. Thought also has to be given to the training of assessors and standardized or simulated patients.

 "To allow insufficient time for the preparation of an OSCE is to court disaster and if the examination is to be successful advanced planning is essential."

Harden & Gleeson, 1979

Outstanding issues: The OSCE has been developed and adapted since it was originally described. The last 10 years has seen an increase in the development of high-fidelity simulation technology for use in medical education. This permits reproduction of complex conditions at any time and allows individuals and teams to practise their skills and management and gain formative feedback. The original description of OSCE marking schemes advocated checklist-style mark sheets, where assessors ticked off the various elements of the task as they were performed. The advantage of this method is the reduction of assessor bias and improvement of inter-rater reliability. However, recent debate has questioned the suitability of this for expert practitioners, who are more likely to have moved away from strictly prescribed and regimented practice (Hodges et al., 1999). Global rating scales are increasingly being developed, which take a more holistic approach to scoring and allow for variation in practice and style.

 The consensus currently is that checklists are more suited to the early, novice stage of practice and that global ratings are better at capturing increasing levels of clinical expertise.

Thought is also being given to who is best placed to do the scoring. In most parts of the world clinician assessors will complete the mark sheets. However, in some countries, such as the United States, scoring by standardized patients is common practice. As with all elements of assessment, consideration needs to be given to the purpose of the test and what is being assessed. If the main goal of the station is to test communication skills with patients, then a patient assessor may be the most appropriate person to judge this. However, if a complex practical task is being assessed, then a clinician with knowledge of the procedure will be better placed. Some institutions will combine clinician and patient assessments in their scoring method.

OTHER ASSESSMENTS OF CLINICAL COMPETENCE

A disadvantage of the OSCE is that candidates only spend short amounts of time at each station and undertake part tasks rather than complete clinical encounters. The Objective Structured Long Case Examination Record (OSLER) attempts to address this by holistic appraisal of the candidate's ability to interact, assess and manage a real patient without the bias and variability associated with the traditional long case. In the OSLER, candidates are assessed throughout history, examination and communication with a standardized patient. Two examiners review the case in advance and use a structured marking schedule. The OSLER is more reliable than the traditional long case, but a large number of different cases are needed to achieve the sort of reliability required for a high-stakes summative assessment.

Assessing performance in the workplace

Assessment of what a doctor *does in practice* requires assessment within the workplace. This raises a number of issues as traditional tests of competence cannot be transplanted easily into busy clinical environments. It is vital that these assessments are feasibly carried out without too much disruption to clinical work or patient care.

 Using a wide range of WPBA tools helps identify strengths and weaknesses in different areas of practice such as technical skills, professional behaviour and teamworking.

The main tools described in the literature and in use in medical education are outlined here, although individual institutions have developed a variety of other tools to fit their own specific needs.

 "There has been concern that trainees are seldom observed, assessed, and given feedback during their workplace-based education. This has led to an increasing interest in a variety of formative assessment methods that require observation and offer the opportunity for feedback."

Norcini & Burch, 2007

MINI CLINICAL EVALUATION EXERCISE (MINI-CEX)

What is it? The Mini-CEX was developed by the American Board of Internal Medicine to assess the clinical skills of residents, particularly focused history taking and physical examination. An assessor directly observes the practitioner's performance in 'real' clinical encounters with patients in the workplace. He or she then discusses diagnosis and management with the practitioner and gives them feedback on the encounter. The practitioner is judged in a number of clinical domains and on his or her overall clinical care. The average Mini-CEX encounter takes around 15–25 minutes. Immediate feedback is then given, which helps identify strengths and weaknesses and improve skills (Norcini, 2003).

How is it used? As part of a programme of WPBA, the Mini-CEX should be performed on multiple occasions with different patients and different assessors. There have been several studies in different clinical specialties looking at the optimum number of Mini-CEX encounters to reliably assess performance. While there is good evidence of its reliability, most studies have looked at use of the Mini-CEX in experimental rather than real-life settings. This makes it possible for one performance to be assessed by multiple assessors, something that is not practical in real clinical settings. Generally, between 10 and 14 encounters over time are needed to show good reliability, if assessed by different assessors and on multiple patients (Boursicot et al., 2011). However, the number of encounters possible in real clinical practice settings needs to be balanced against the need for reliability.

Strengths and weaknesses: High satisfaction rates have been reported by both assessors and assessees. The perceived educational impact of the Mini-CEX is high because of its ability to provide opportunities for structured feedback, giving practitioners the potential to correct their weaknesses and develop as professionals. Increasing the interaction between junior and senior doctors may also enable monitoring of progress and identification of educational needs.

 "Feedback can change physicians' clinical performance when provided systematically over multiple years by an authoritative, credible source."

Veloski et al., 2006

The Mini-CEX appears able to discriminate effectively between junior and senior trainees, with more senior doctors attaining higher clinical and global competence scores. In addition, it is relatively feasible within the workplace, being centred on real patients and clinical encounters. However, scheduling a Mini-CEX does require commitment by both the trainee and the senior doctor. Time constraints and lack of motivation in busy clinical settings may make completing assessments difficult and stressful. The reported inter-rater reliability of the Mini-CEX is variable, even among same assessor groups. There is also variation in scoring across different grades of assessor, with studies showing that trainees tend to score Mini-CEX encounters more leniently than consultants (Kogan et al., 2003). Inter-rater variations can be reduced, with more assessors rating fewer encounters, rather than few assessors rating multiple encounters. Formal assessor training may also help but the evidence for this is variable, with some studies showing that training makes very little difference to scoring consistency and others reporting more stringent marking and greater confidence following assessor training (Boursicot et al., 2011). Finally, the purpose of the Mini-CEX within a programme of WPBA needs to be clarified. If the goal of the programme is to demonstrate satisfactory progress only then fewer encounters will be needed. However, if the goal is to discriminate sufficiently between trainees to allow ranking then a greater number of encounters is required, limiting feasibility.

CASE-BASED DISCUSSION (CBD) OR CHART-STIMULATED RECALL (CSR)

What is it? The CBD in the United Kingdom and Australasia, or CSR in North America, is a structured interview in which practitioners discuss aspects of a case in which they have been involved in order to explore their underlying reasoning, decision making and ethical understanding. It can be used in a variety of settings such as clinics, wards or assessment units, and different clinical problems can be discussed. The practitioner selects suitable cases and gives his or her written records of these to the assessor in advance. It is expected that the practitioner will select cases of varying complexity. He or she then presents the case to the assessor, who asks questions to probe his or her clinical reasoning and professional judgement. The practitioner is scored in a number of domains, mapped to the competencies expected within the programme of training. A CBD will usually take around 15–20 minutes for presentation and discussion with 5–10 minutes afterwards for feedback.

How is it used? As with other WPBA tools, repeated encounters are required to obtain a valid picture of a practitioner's level of development. Again, though, this has to be balanced with the practicalities of a busy clinical setting. The Royal College of General Practitioners in the United Kingdom asks trainees to complete a minimum of six CBDs in each of the first 2 years of training and 12 in the final year, but other Royal Colleges require different numbers. There are data available for the CSR that show good reliability. A comparison with different assessment methods has shown that assessment carried out using the CSR is able to differentiate between doctors in good standing and those identified as poorly performing (Boursicot et al., 2011).

Strengths and weaknesses: As with all WPBAs, the evidence regarding the true costs of the CBD is scarce. Direct costs include training of all assessors and central administration of WPBA records, but there are also costs associated with assessor and practitioner time in theatres, clinics and wards. There is also little published research on the educational impact of the CBD. However, as with other WPBAs, the opportunity for specific and timely feedback is thought to be valuable in helping learners progress.

DIRECT OBSERVATION OF PROCEDURAL SKILLS (DOPS)

What is it? DOPS is a method of assessment developed by the Royal College of Physicians in the United Kingdom specifically for assessing practical skills. The practitioner is directly observed by an assessor while undertaking a procedure on a real patient. Specific components of the procedure are judged and then feedback is given after the event. The mean observation time for DOPS varies according to the procedure assessed and, on average, feedback time takes an additional third of the procedure observation time.

How is it used? Many of the UK Royal Colleges now incorporate DOPS into their programmes of WPBA. Some use a generic score sheet, looking at overall aspects of procedural skill, while others have developed specific score sheets related to the procedure under assessment. There is a wide variety of skills that can be assessed with DOPS, from simple procedures, such as venepuncture, to more complex procedures, such as endoscopy. Again, organizations vary in their expectations of trainees and which type of procedures should be assessed and how often.

Strengths and weaknesses: Scores have been shown to increase between the first and second half of a training year, indicating validity (Davies et al., 2009). In surveys, the majority of practitioners feel that DOPS is a fair method of assessing procedural skills and that it is practical and feasible. There is little current research on the educational impact of DOPS, but again the opportunity for feedback gives it important potential as an educational tool.

 As with the Mini-CEX and CBD/CSR, DOPS needs to be repeated on several occasions for it to be a reliable measure of performance.

MULTISOURCE FEEDBACK (MSF)

What is it? The goal of MSF, or 360-degree assessment, is to collect the structured judgements of those who work with, or have experience of, the practitioner and feed these back in a systematic way, building up a picture of individual practice. Judges can include both senior and junior colleagues, nurses, administrative staff, medical students and patients, depending on the tool used. All judges remain anonymous, and their scores and comments are fed back to the trainee. Comparable assessment tools have been used in industry for nearly 50 years.

How is it used? Two similar instruments have been used in the United Kingdom to evaluate doctors in training. The Sheffield Peer Review Assessment Tool (SPRAT) was validated in paediatric trainees. The mini Peer Assessment Tool (mini-PAT) was developed for more junior doctors based on the SPRAT and has been used by the UK Foundation School. The aim of the mini-PAT is to assess behaviours and attitudes such as communication, leadership, teamworking and reliability (Archer et al., 2008). It is these sorts of attributes that are often best judged by multisource feedback tools. The mini-PAT is primarily meant as a formative form of assessment, allowing the doctor to reflect on the feedback received in order to improve his or her clinical performance.

Strengths and weaknesses: One of the main advantages of MSF is its anonymity, encouraging honest opinions. The main criticisms are that feedback is delayed and lacking specificity because of the anonymous nature. Inter-rater variance has been reported, with consultants tending to give lower scores. However, the longer the consultants have known the doctor, the more likely they are to score them higher. Senior doctors achieve a small but statistically significant higher overall mean score compared to more junior doctors, demonstrating construct validity. There are potential disadvantages to MSF tools as well, including risk of discrimination and potentially damaging feedback, which may need to be managed. However, MSF can be used as part of a programme of WPBA to inform personal development, especially regarding professional and interpersonal skills.

 To be of the most value, assessments within the workplace should capitalize on the rich diversity of clinical practice and build up an authentic picture of the practitioner over time.

Outstanding issues in performance assessment

 "Workplace-based assessment brings a unique set of challenges to medical education and requires fresh thinking about how we consider and construct assessment programmes."

Swanwick & Chana, 2009

WPBA tools are now well-described in many different areas of medicine, and a number of institutions make use of these in their programmes of assessment. However, a number of issues remain poorly resolved, and there continues to be some resistance amongst practising clinicians to their use. Although the goal of WPBA is to assess what a clinician does in practice, formalizing practitioner observation in a structured way does have the effect of reducing practice to the 'shows how' level of Miller's pyramid and may not reflect real life. This, to some extent, seems unavoidable, but as WPBA becomes more integrated into clinical life this effect may be diminished. However, there is still work to be done on how to incorporate the practice of WPBA into busy clinical environments with minimal disruption and maximum benefit and ensure its acceptability to all stakeholders. While most of the research on reliability and validity of WPBA has been done in experimental settings, it remains difficult to determine how it is best used in real-life settings, in different grades and different clinical specialties.

 Institutions need to be clear about the purpose of their programmes of WPBA: are they purely for formative purposes or will the results be used to guide progression? Is their goal to ensure the 'bare minimum' level of performance or are they being used to rank trainees? Without clarity from institutions, both trainees and trainers will feel confusion.

Research so far has been focused on the use of WPBA as formative rather than summative tools, although it is not always clear that this is how they are being used in practice. There is some evidence that trainees are finding the culture shift in assessment hard to adapt to. There is an expectation that all WPBAs should be clearly 'passed' from the start, rather than using them to demonstrate competency progression over time. This can lead to trainees fitting all their assessments into the end of a placement rather than using the assessment and its accompanying feedback as a tool to facilitate improvement over the course of a placement. What is clear is that different institutions have taken the basic frameworks described in the literature and adapted them significantly, using WPBAs summatively rather than formatively, as they were originally intended. There is a growing movement in the medical education world to use WPBAs without numerical or grading scales so the main focus is on performance and feedback rather than any summative or other purpose.

While all the tools described above are widely used in postgraduate assessment around the world, their use is becoming more widespread in the undergraduate arena. The issues here remain largely the same, with a need for clarity of purpose and use of a battery of tools over time to build up a holistic picture of the student's strengths, weaknesses and progression.

Summary

The valid and reliable assessment of performance requires the use of a number of different assessment methods, each with its own strengths and weaknesses, which enable a complete picture of the practitioner to be developed. This is becoming increasingly important in a world where professionals are required to demonstrate competence. In undergraduate and postgraduate academic settings, the OSCE is a well-validated method that is widely used in high-stakes, summative assessments for licensing and progression. In the workplace, a number of instruments have been developed that offer insight into different aspects of clinical performance. In order to maximize the educational potential of these tools for learners and guide professional development, the focus should remain on supervised learning and timely, specific and constructive formative feedback, rather than summative scoring. Institutions need to consider their assessment strategies and goals and make the best use of the different methods available, in order that educators can be trained and guided in their use.

References

Archer, J., Norcini, J., Southgate, L., et al., 2008. Mini PAT: a valid component of a national assessment programme in the UK? Adv. Health Sci. Educ. Theory Pract. 13 (2), 181–192.

Boursicot, K., Etheridge, L., Setna, Z., et al., 2011. Performance in assessment: consensus statement and recommendations from the Ottawa conference. Med. Teach. 33 (5), 370–383.

Davies, H., Archer, J., Southgate, L., Norcini, J., 2009. Initial evaluation of the first year of the Foundation Assessment Programme. Med. Educ. 43 (1), 74–81.

Downing, S., 2003. Validity: on the meaningful interpretation of assessment data. Med. Educ. 37 (9), 830–837.

Harden, R., Gleeson, F., 1979. Assessment of clinical competence using an objective structured clinical examination (OSCE). Med. Educ. 13 (1), 39–54.

Hodges, B., Regehr, G., McNaughton, N., et al., 1999. OSCE checklists do not capture increasing levels of expertise. Acad. Med. 74 (10), 1129–1134.

Kogan, J., Bellini, L., Shea, J., 2003. Feasibility, reliability, and validity of the mini-clinical evaluation exercise (mCEX) in a medicine core clerkship. Acad. Med. 78 (10), 33–35.

Miller, G.E., 1990. The assessment of clinical skills/competence/performance. Acad. Med. 65 (9 Suppl.), S63–S67.

Norcini, J., 2003. Work based assessment. Br. Med. J. 326 (5), 753–755.

Norcini, J., Burch, V., 2007. Workplace-based assessment as an educational tool: AMEE Guide No. 31. Med. Teach. 29 (9), 855–871.

Schuwirth, L., van der Vleuten, C., 2009. How to design a useful test. In: Understanding Medical Education: Evidence, Theory and Practice. Association for the Study of Medical Education, Dundee.

Swanwick, T., Chana, N., 2009. Workplace based assessment. Br. J. Hosp. Med. 70 (5), 290–293.

Veloski, J., Boex, J., Grasberger, M., et al., 2006. Systematic review of the literature on assessment, feedback and physicians clinical performance: BEME Guide No. 7. Med. Teach. 28 (2), 117–128.

Portfolios, projects and theses

E. W. Driessen, S. Heeneman, C. P. M. van der Vleuten

Trends

- Electronic portfolios are used to aggregate assessment information.
- Portfolios are essential in programmatic assessment.
- A qualitative approach works well for the assessment of complex constructs (portfolios, theses, projects).

Introduction

The assessment principles and strategies we will describe in this chapter not only apply to portfolios but have broader applications. They can also be used for other complex assessments, such as assessment of projects or papers, or a master's thesis.

The objectives and contents of portfolios

In less than two decades, portfolios have gained a prominent position in medical education. The portfolio owes its popularity to its suitability for attaining goals that are difficult to achieve with other educational methods: monitoring and assessing competency development and nontechnical skills, such as reflection. In this way the portfolio is in keeping with recent developments in education, such as outcome-based education and competency-based learning. Learners, residents, doctors and teachers are regularly asked to compose a portfolio. The objective of the portfolio, and consequently its format and content, can vary markedly. We distinguish the following main objectives for portfolios:

- *Guiding* the development of competencies. The learner is asked to include in the portfolio a critical reflection on his or her learning and performance. The minimal requirement for this type of portfolio is the inclusion of reflective texts and self-analyses.

- *Monitoring* progress. The minimum requirement for this type of portfolio is that it must contain overviews of what the learner has done or learned. This may be the numbers of different types of patients seen during a clerkship or the competencies achieved during a defined period.
- *Assessment* of competency development. The portfolio provides evidence of how certain competencies are developing and which level of competency has been achieved. Learners often also include an analysis of essential aspects of their competency development and indicate in which areas more work is required. This type of portfolio contains evidential materials to substantiate the level that is achieved.

Most portfolios are aimed at a combination of goals, and therefore comprise a variety of evidence, overviews and reflections (Fig. 36.1). Portfolios thus differ in objectives, and the objectives determine which component of the portfolio content is emphasized. Portfolios can also differ in scope and structure. Portfolios can be wide or narrow in scope. A limited scope is appropriate for portfolios aimed at illustrating the learner's development in a single skill or competency domain or in one curricular component. An example is a portfolio for communication skills of undergraduate students. A portfolio with a broad scope is aimed at demonstrating the learner's development across all skills and competency domains over a prolonged period of education. Portfolios also differ in the degree of structuring or guidance that is provided to the learner in composing the portfolio. This dimension is characterized by the contrast between an open and a closed portfolio. A closed portfolio has to comply with detailed guidelines and regulations and offers relatively little freedom to learners with respect to the format and content of the portfolio. As a consequence, portfolios of different learners are highly comparable and the portfolios are easy to navigate.

A more open portfolio gives general directions, but allows the learners freedom with respect to the actual

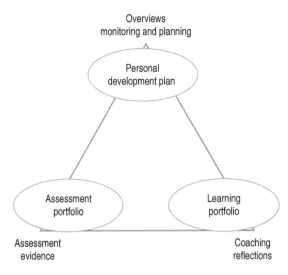

Fig. 36.1 Purpose and content of portfolios.

contents and format of the portfolio. The framework is described in such a way that learners are given a choice about how they present their individual learning process and learning results. A uniform basic structure is nevertheless important because teachers and peers who have to view several portfolios should be able to easily follow the general structure of the materials.

 Portfolios with a closed structure are highly comparable, while portfolios with an open structure allow learners the opportunity to display their individual learning trajectories and competencies.

We have explained that portfolios can contain overviews, evidential materials and reflection. We have located these elements on the corners of a triangle (Fig. 36.1).

Portfolios can contain a variety of materials:

- Products, such as reports, papers, patient management plans, letter of discharge, critical appraisals of a topic
- Impressions, such as photographs, videos, observation reports
- Evaluations, such as test scores, feedback forms (e.g. Mini-CEX), feedback from peers and tutors, certificates, letters from patients expressing appreciation.

The nature and diversity of the materials determine the richness of the picture learners present of their learning and progress. It can be tempting for learners to include a vast amount of materials, leaving it up to the assessor to determine their value. This not only increases the mentors' and assessors' workload, but also can mean that mentors and assessors are unable to see the wood for the trees. It is therefore important

for learners to be selective. A good selection criterion is that materials should provide insight into the student's learning and progress. We will discuss the size and feasibility of portfolios later in this chapter.

 Learners can use captions to indicate the context in which the material was collected or produced, its relevance and why it was included.

REFLECTIONS

Many portfolios contain reflections. These are often organized around the competency framework. Learners can use these reflections as a long-term agenda. Learners support their reflections by referring to materials and overviews in the portfolio. This not only focuses the reflections it also convinces others of the validity of the reflections because learners are likely to aim for consistency of reflections and evidential materials. This makes the reflections less noncommittal. It is, for instance, not acceptable for learners to simply state that they have learned how to give a clinical presentation. They will have to substantiate this statement by evidential materials and overviews demonstrating why and how they have done this.

Electronic portfolios

Most schools use an electronic portfolio (e-portfolio). The e-portfolio can serve three functions: (1) provide a repository for all the materials (dossier); (2) facilitate the administrative and logistical aspects of the assessment process (i.e. direct online loading of assessment and feedback forms via multiple platforms, regulation of who has access to which information, and by connecting information pieces to the overarching framework); and (3) enable a quick overview of aggregated information (such as overall feedback reports). User friendliness is vital. The (e-)portfolio should be easily accessible to whichever stakeholder who has access to it. An example is an electronic portfolio for work-based assessment (http://www.epass.eu/en/about-epass/instructionclips/).

Success factors for portfolios

 Mentoring is of the essence for portfolio use.

Despite the simplicity of the portfolio concept – a learner documents the process and results of his or her learning activities – the portfolio has proved to be not invariably and automatically effective. The literature on portfolios shows mixed results. The key question here is what makes a portfolio successful in one situation and less successful in another situation? A number of reviews have shed light on some key factors (Buckley et al., 2009; Driessen et al., 2007; Tochel et al., 2009).

MENTORING

Mentoring is of the essence for portfolio use. The mentor gives feedback on the portfolio, ensures depth of learning and helps the learner to identify learning needs and formulate learning objectives (Driessen et al., 2010). Learners tend to stop working on their portfolio when they receive no feedback or when they are not questioned about their analyses. In most cases the mentor will be a teacher, but can also be a peer. Mentoring can take place in one-on-one meetings or in mentor groups. It is important that mentors are prepared for their task. Mentoring requires a coaching approach, which is different from the approach customarily taken by teachers when they are teaching and/or supervising patient contacts.

FEASIBILITY

Feasibility should also be considered. Learners and teachers can easily come to see work on the portfolio as burdensome paperwork. Portfolios can be sizeable, and the work for portfolios often comes on top of other tasks. Excessive workload can be prevented by a number of simple precautions. First, learners should be stimulated to be selective in including materials in their portfolio. Portfolio content is only informative if it is relevant to learning and competency development. This requires that it is clearly explained to learners what is expected from them. The competencies to be achieved, the criteria, the content and purpose of the portfolio must be clearly communicated to both learners and teachers. Modern electronic portfolios sometimes aggregate information from the portfolio to the different competencies, giving users a quick overview of competency development. One mouse click suffices to view the original materials.

PERCEIVED USEFULNESS

The learner must experience direct benefit from working on the portfolio. When self-direction is required in a programme, the usefulness of the portfolio will be self-evident to learners. Residents, for instance, are largely responsible for their own learning in the clinical workplace. Using the portfolio as a starting point for discussing their work and progress can support that learning. Residents can ask for feedback and arrange for more time to be scheduled for matters that are relevant to their learning. This will motivate them to work on their portfolio. If little self-direction is required, for instance when the programme consists of lectures and working groups, learners can only too easily come to the conclusion that the portfolio is of little real use to them.

Perceived usefulness also depends on how well the portfolio is embedded in the overall programme. If the portfolio is an integral part of the curriculum and is purposefully used for learning, it will have more value in the eyes of the learners than when it is just another educational activity. A final factor that can contribute to the educational value of the portfolio is the degree to which it accommodates differences between learners. When learners can present their individual profiles in the portfolio, they are more likely to value its usefulness.

 Learners must experience direct benefit from working on their portfolio.

Portfolio assessment

If there is one area in which the portfolio has shown remarkable development in recent years, it is in the way it is assessed. The traditional, psychometric approach to assessment, characterized by standardization and analytical assessment criteria to achieve objective judgements, has proved incompatible with the non-standardized nature of portfolios. Content and format of portfolios vary with the learners, and this runs counter to standardization.

In addition to numerical information (scores), portfolios also contain a variety of qualitative information. Besides technical skills, portfolios are used to assess the softer skills. Weighing the information in a portfolio to assess a competency, such as professionalism, demands of assessors that they use their own judgement to interpret the information. This kind of judgement task is difficult to translate to an analytical assessment procedure using a standardized checklist with numerous strictly defined criteria.

To match assessment with the characteristics of the portfolio, we advocate an approach based on the methodology of qualitative research (Driessen et al., 2005). Qualitative research also requires interpretation of different kinds of qualitative information in order to arrive at meaningful statements about ill-defined problems.

The concept of trustworthiness is at the centre of qualitative research: various procedural measures can ensure that the research is sufficiently rigorous to justify confidence that the conclusions are supported by the data. The principles and methods for evaluating the quality of qualitative research can be translated to principles and procedures for assessing portfolios (Driessen et al., 2005). The following assessment strategies can be used with portfolios.

INCORPORATE FEEDBACK CYCLES

Incorporate in the procedure intermittent feedback cycles to ensure that the final judgement does not come as a surprise to the learners. Since the contents of a portfolio are usually collected over a longer period of time, it is inadvisable to wait until the end of the period to make pronouncements about the quality of the portfolio. Intermediate formative assessments, such as feedback from a mentor, allow learners to adapt and improve their portfolio. Not only from an assessment perspective but also from a mentoring perspective, is it advisable to give feedback at various stages of the portfolio. As we remarked earlier, users will be tempted to stop working on their portfolio if they do not receive feedback.

 Incorporate intermittent feedback cycles to ensure that the final judgement does not come as a surprise to the learners.

OBTAIN MULTIPLE SOURCES OF FEEDBACK

Information for the assessment should be obtained from different people who are involved in the portfolio process one way or another. In addition to the assessors who judge the portfolio at the end of the period, others can be involved in the assessment as well. This enables triangulation of different judgements for the final assessment. We already mentioned that a portfolio is usually the result of work done over a longer period of time. In fact, the portfolio is not just a finished product – a file or web page containing materials – but it is first and foremost a process during which learners document their development over a (prolonged) period of time.

Different people who are involved in the portfolio process can also contribute to the assessment. It is the mentor who first advises about the quality of the portfolio. He or she often knows the learner best, is able to determine the authenticity of the materials and is familiar with the learner's work habits. Peers are another group that can be involved in the assessment. The advantage of peer assessment is that peers know from experience what it means to produce a portfolio, and by engaging in peer assessment they can familiarize themselves with the assessment standards for the portfolio.

Learners can also be asked to judge the quality of their own portfolios. They could, for instance, be asked for their reaction to the mentor's recommendation and/or to self-assess their different competencies. Self-assessment by learners supported by recommendations from the mentor can lead to better validated self-assessments. From the self-assessment literature we know that self-assessments tend to be biased. Eva and Regehr (2008) therefore recommended that learners should be encouraged to actively seek information about their performance to arrive at well-validated self-assessments.

SEPARATE THE ROLE OF THE MENTOR AND ASSESSOR

Separate the multiple roles of assessors by removing the summative assessment decisions from the coaching task. In relation to the previous item, we argued the wisdom of involving the mentors in portfolio assessment because they possess relevant information. However, learners should also have a safe learning climate in which they feel free to discuss the weaknesses of their portfolio with their mentor. It is therefore advisable that mentors should not be required to make the final summative decisions. Such decisions should be the responsibility of a separate assessment committee. In an earlier publication, four scenarios for the role of the mentor in assessment were described (van Tartwijk & Driessen, 2009). This role can range from full responsibility for assessment to a role that is strictly limited to coaching.

- **The teacher** This is the most common assessment scenario in education. Just like most teachers in primary, secondary and higher education, mentors discuss their learners' performance and progress and assess their level of competence at the end of a course.

- **PhD supervisor** In some scenarios the role of the mentors in the assessment procedure of portfolios is comparable to the role of the supervisors of PhD students. In many countries, formal assessment of theses/portfolios is the responsibility of a committee. Supervisors invite their peers to sit on the committee, of which they themselves are not a member. A negative assessment of the thesis/portfolio would harm their reputation among their peers. For this reason they are highly unlikely to invite their peers to sit on the committee unless they are convinced the portfolio meets the criteria. As a consequence, mentors and learners have a shared interest: to produce a thesis or portfolio that merits a positive judgement.

- **Driving instructor** In this model the roles of the mentor and the assessor are strictly separated. The mentor/driving instructor coaches the learner in achieving the required competencies, which are shown in the portfolio. If the mentor thinks the learner is sufficiently competent, he or she invites an assessor from a professional body (e.g. the examiner from the Driver and Vehicle Licensing Agency) to assess the competencies of the learner. It is also possible for learners to take the initiative to approach the licensing agency themselves.

- **Coach** In this model, the learners take the initiative. They can, for instance, ask a senior colleague to coach them until they have achieved the required level of competence. This scenario is appropriate, for instance, when a professional wants to obtain an additional qualification. The assessor would be someone from an external body.

 Separate the multiple roles of assessors by removing the summative assessment decisions from the coaching task.

TRAIN THE ASSESSORS

Organize a meeting of the assessors (before the assessment round and at an intermediate stage of the portfolio period) in which they can calibrate their assessments and discuss the assessment procedure and its results. Assessing the vast amounts of very diverse information in portfolios hinges on professional judgement. Assessors use assessment criteria idiosyncratically. Judgement depends, for instance, on prior experience with assessment and individual notions and beliefs about education and the competencies to be judged. Organizing discussions between assessors can reduce differences between assessors. As a result of discussing a benchmark portfolio, assessors' interpretations of assessment criteria will tend to converge, and a joint understanding of the procedure to be followed can emerge. It is advisable to organize such discussions not only immediately before an assessment round but also at an intermediate stage of the portfolio period when assessors can compare their own portfolio judgements with those of their colleagues and discuss differences of interpretation. After the final assessment the assessors can be given information about all the assessments to gain a better understanding of the entire process.

USE A SEQUENTIAL PROCEDURE

Organize a sequential assessment procedure in which conflicting information necessitates the gathering of more information. At Maastricht Medical School a procedure has been developed to optimize efficient use of the time available for assessment (Driessen et al., 2005). The mentor makes a recommendation for the assessment of the portfolios of his or her students. The learner and an assessor decide whether they agree with this recommendation. If they agree, the assessment procedure is completed. If they do not agree, the portfolio is submitted to a larger group of assessors. In this way, when there is doubt about the assessment of a portfolio, the portfolio is judged more carefully than portfolios whose assessment is straightforward. This gives stronger guarantees of trustworthy assessment because, in cases of doubt, more judges are consulted. The discussions between the assessors will also promote clarity with respect to the application of the criteria (see the section on training of assessors).

REQUEST NARRATIVE INFORMATION

Incorporate in the portfolio requests to provide qualitative, narrative feedback and give this information substantial weight in the assessment procedure. Narrative comments offer learners and judges much richer information than quantitative, numerical feedback. A score of 7 on a 10-point scale, for instance, gives little insight into what a learner has done well and what he or she has not done well. Only when strengths and weaknesses of performance are supported by narrative feedback does assessment become truly informative. An additional problem with workplace assessment is rater leniency. There are various reasons why low scores are rarely given in practice. As a result, scores do not discriminate well, and narrative feedback will often provide better information about the learner's competency development. Narrative feedback can be facilitated by providing a blank space at the top of the assessment form to insert descriptions of strengths and weaknesses.

PROVIDE QUALITY ASSURANCE

Quality assurance must be built into the procedure:
- Offer learners the possibility to appeal against assessment decisions.
- Carefully document the different steps of the assessment procedure (a formal assessment plan approved by an examination board, overviews of results).
- Organize quality assessment procedures with an external auditor.

USE MILESTONES

Education institutions often put a great deal of energy into formulating competency profiles. The important thing is to strike a balance between long lists of concrete criteria detailing all the things a learner must be able to do (can-do statements) on the one hand, and global descriptions offering a general outline but little practical guidance on the other hand. In other words, the trick is to find the right balance between analytical and global criteria. This can be done by giving learners and assessors an idea of the expected level for each global competency. Milestones or rubrics are very useful in this respect (an example is given in Table 36.1). They typically contain descriptions of each competency at different levels, such as the level to be expected from a novice, from a competent professional and from an expert.

Thesis and project circle

Writing a final thesis or dissertation, or a project report is in most cases an individual effort, supervised and assessed by one or two teachers. In most cases the student's learning is limited to his own work and the teacher's feedback. For curricula with a large number of students, teachers are faced each year with a large number of thesis writers, requiring considerable supervision time. In addition, the assessment of a thesis or dissertation is often related to a graduation decision and is used by the student to present oneself with future employees or subsequent education. The criteria for assessment need to be very explicit and the decision itself valid. More and more, an independent second assessor is used in the assessment procedure. To

Table 36.1   Milestones used for the assessment of final-year medical students

	Below expectation	As expected	Above expectation
Clinical performance (for instance, as judged by Mini-CEX)	Slow in taking a history and performing a physical examination. Considers irrelevant aspects. Slow in making a diagnosis. Misses important conclusions. Frequently unable to formulate management plan and needs considerable guidance.	Adequate speed in taking a history and performing a physical examination. Relevant aspects are considered. Adequate speed in making a diagnosis. Diagnosis contains important conclusions. Formulates an adequate management plan for simple clinical presentations. Needs some guidance. Achieves these goals in the second half of the internship.	Conducts an adequate and efficient history and physical examination. Arrives at an accurate diagnosis within adequate time. Formulates an adequate management plan for simple clinical presentations. Needs little guidance. Has achieved these goals at the start of the internship.
Professionalism (for instance, as judged by 360-degree feedback)	Does not keep appointments. Occasionally fails to ask for supervision when this is necessary. Reacts defensively to feedback. Is unable to cope with stress. Does not pay attention to his or her personal appearance. Frequently shows inappropriate behaviour or behaves disrespectfully.	Keeps appointments. Asks for supervision when this is necessary. Needs help in reflecting and considering alternatives and responds adequately to feedback. Occasionally needs help in coping with stress. Appropriate personal appearance; behaves respectfully.	Keeps appointments. Asks for supervision when this is necessary. Is able to reflect critically; responds adequately to feedback and is prepared to acknowledge errors. Is able to cope with stress adequately. Looks well cared for and behaves respectfully.

Source: Maastricht University

overcome the need for extensive input and time from the teacher, and to enable students to learn from each other, 'thesis circles' have been set up. A thesis circle is composed of a number of students and one or two supervising teachers. Teachers and students are jointly responsible for the supervision and assessment of the theses of the students participating in the circle (Romme, 2003; van der Vleuten & Driessen, 2000). Thesis circles get together on a regular basis. Their meetings are conducted according to a fixed pattern: an opening round, setting the agenda, discussion of the content of the theses and a final round. The circle is presided over by an elected chair and a secretary is responsible for minute taking.

The advantage for teachers is greater efficiency through an economy of scale, with less reading time needed because in the conceptual phase reading is divided among several participants, and with less supervision time because the teacher meets with several students at the same time. Furthermore, the thesis circle aims to stimulate cooperative learning and reinforce the feedback function of assessment by stimulating reflection, cooperation and shared responsibility between students on the one hand, and between students and teachers on the other. As to content, discussion of the start and progress of the theses is paramount. The feedback by the members of the circle serves to support the thesis writer. Decisions are taken by consent: upon a grade proposal by the chairman, a decision is taken if none of the members

(either students or teachers) has a reasoned objection. In this way, for instance the chair is elected and the final assessment is given the graduation circle uses a method of assessment that combines teacher assessment and peer-assessment with self-assessment. A condition for ensuring a candid climate is a strict procedure on the basis of formal rules. Each graduation circle is therefore governed by a set of rules and regulations.

The role of supervisor and assessor requires the student to be independent. Experience with other forms of co-operative learning show that students who are used to strong direction by the teacher have trouble studying on their own. They may quickly get the feeling that they are thrown in at the deep end. It is advisable to prepare students by training them in skills needed for the thesis circle. Students who already have experience with self-direction, for example in problem-based learning or other student-centred forms of education, will feel more at home in a thesis circle.

Another condition for the proper functioning of a circle is that the teacher effectively shares responsibility for monitoring and assessment with the students.

Summary

Portfolios serve different purposes in medical education. These purposes can be summarized as guiding, monitoring and assessing the development of students' competencies. Portfolios often combine several objectives.

Apart from differences in objectives, portfolios also differ in scope: a brief versus a long education period, a limited competency domain versus a comprehensive competency profile and an open versus a closed structure. A portfolio is not automatically effective. A number of conditions must be met to ensure that a portfolio makes a meaningful contribution to the learning of students. Mentoring, feasibility and immediate benefits to learners are key factors for portfolio success. Assessing portfolios requires a different approach than is customarily used by most teachers. An approach based on principles from qualitative research is more appropriate than a psychometric one. A number of strategies to ensure rigour of assessment are described: incorporate feedback cycles in the procedure; involve mentor and learners in the assessment; separate the role of the mentor and the assessor; train assessors; use a sequential procedure; use narrative information; provide quality assurance and make use of milestones/rubrics. These strategies are also suited to other complex assessment situations, such as the assessment of projects and theses.

References

Buckley, S., Coleman, J., Davison, I., et al., 2009. The educational effects of portfolios on undergraduate student learning: a Best Evidence Medical Education (BEME) systematic review. BEME Guide No. 11. Med. Teach. 31, 282–298.

Driessen, E., van der Vleuten, C., Schuwirth, L., et al., 2005. The use of qualitative research criteria for portfolio assessment as an alternative to reliability evaluation: a case study. Med. Educ. 39, 214–220.

Driessen, E., van Tartwijk, J., van der Vleuten, C., Wass, V., 2007. Portfolios in medical education: why do they meet with mixed success? A systematic review. Med. Educ. 41, 1224–1233.

Driessen, E., Overeem, K., van Tartwijk, J., 2010. Learning from practice: mentoring, feedback, and portfolios. In: Dornan, T., Mann, K., Scherpbier, A., Spencer, J. (Eds.), Medical Education: Theory and Practice. Churchill Livingstone Elsevier, Edinburgh.

Eva, K.W., Regehr, G., 2008. "I'll never play professional football" and other fallacies of self-assessment. J. Contin. Educ. Health Prof. 28, 14–19.

Romme, S., 2003. Organizing education by drawing on organization studies. Organ. Stud. 24, 697–720.

Tochel, C., Haig, A., Hesketh, A., et al., 2009. The effectiveness of portfolios for post-graduate assessment and education: BEME Guide No 12. Med. Teach. 31, 299–318.

van der Vleuten, C.P.M., Driessen, E.W., 2000. Assessment in Problem-Based Learning (Toetsing in Probleemgestuurd Onderwijs). Wolters-Noordhoff, Groningen.

van Tartwijk, J., Driessen, E.W., 2009. Portfolios for assessment and learning: AMEE Guide no. 45. Med. Teach. 31, 790–801.

Feedback, reflection and coaching: a new model

S. K. Krackov, H. S. Pohl, A. S. Peters, J. M. Sargeant

Trends

- Feedback, reflection and coaching are interconnected components of the learning process and necessary to develop and maintain competence.
- There are four different categories of feedback: feedback about the task, the process, self-regulation and self. Each needs to be used appropriately.
- Reflection enables deeper understanding of the feedback, and coaching enables the learner to use the feedback more effectively.

Introduction

In this chapter, we describe the pivotal and interconnected roles of feedback, reflection and coaching in an experiential competency-based learning model. The model demonstrates the power of the systematic use of these three activities to develop learners' ability to build knowledge, skills and behaviours to become competent healthcare providers. The model is based conceptually on the integration of both competency-based (mastery) learning and deliberate practise. In 'competency-based education' the focus is on learners' achievement of educational outcome objectives, i.e. upon their achievement of competence, irrespective of how long it takes, versus the time spent in the curriculum as in traditional curricula (Cohen et al., 2015). Ericsson (2015) describes 'deliberate practise' as "individualized training activities specially designed by a coach or teacher to improve specific aspects of an individual's performance through repetition and successive refinement". Ericsson's premise is that both mastery learning and deliberate practise allow an individual's knowledge and performance to develop gradually. Commitment to the continuous deliberate practise process with feedback and reflection is necessary to eventually develop expertise.

❝❞ *"Deliberate practice involves repetitively working on well-defined tasks under the watchful eyes*

of a coach who provides informative feedback to help the learners continuously improve and refine their competence."

Holmboe, 2015

Competency-based education

The evolving twenty-first-century healthcare system is characterized by team-based care, and an emphasis on quality and maintenance of competence. To foster this approach to care, educating healthcare workers for the twenty-first century calls for a competency-based (mastery learning) curriculum, where different healthcare professionals learn together to evaluate patients and interact together for the benefit of patient care.

Measuring only competencies, for the most part, limits the measures of knowledge and interpersonal interactions (Aschenbrener et al., 2015). For example, the act of drawing blood seems like a mechanical skill in isolation, but in a clinical situation the healthcare provider would have to have determined the rationale for the blood draw, how the results would affect the possible differential diagnosis of the clinical situation, and the cost-effectiveness of this clinical test versus another one. Actual clinical activities like these that are needed for practice can be measured as EPAs, entrustable professional activities, which are units of professional practice that integrate multiple competencies in a clinical context (Ten Cate, 2013). Recently, the ACGME (2013) introduced the term 'milestones' to measure progressive development in postgraduate education. Milestones are expectations of learners to attain specific competencies or groups of competencies at different levels of professional development. Competencies alone, or in combination within EPAs and milestones, serve as the basis for feedback, reflection and coaching over the continuum of education for practising healthcare providers.

Giving learners feedback to guide their progress has always been viewed as essential to the concept of learning. However, the need to combine reflection and

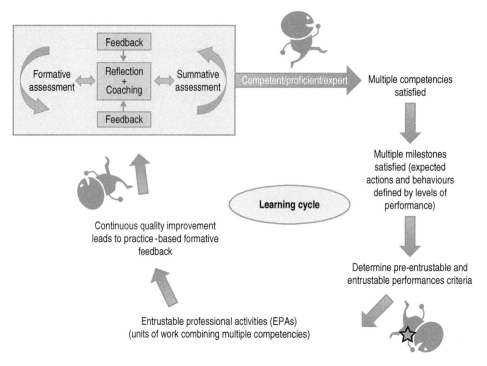

Fig. 37.1 Learning cycle.

coaching with feedback to help learners achieve their learning goals has been under-stressed. As Fig. 37.1 demonstrates, this method enables learners to achieve the required learning objectives through an iterative, stepwise, experiential process, while empowering them to take responsibility for that process with increasing effectiveness.

Description of the curriculum model

Our curriculum model is attuned to the needs of individual learners preparing for the current healthcare system.

The stepwise educational model builds on one described previously (Krackov & Pohl, 2011), and provides an integrated, iterative educational strategy for competency-based education, in which experiential learning is linked with cyclic feedback, reflection and coaching. The model requires clear outcome-based learning objectives and a deliberate practice protocol in which content and instructional methods are matched to the objectives. All educational activities are coupled with formative assessment, feedback, reflection and coaching until competency criteria have been met. Once learners accomplish an objective, they move to the next level, where the cycle is repeated. This curriculum model helps learners achieve competence,

while developing the skills to manage and monitor their own learning agenda.

COMPONENTS OF THE CURRICULUM MODEL

1. **Outcome-based objectives.** Learner-centred, measurable, outcome-based objectives are based on the philosophy outlined by Anderson and Krathwohl (2001) (a revision of Bloom's taxonomy). The objectives should be designed to enable the learner to develop knowledge and skills incrementally. Learners should engage with the objectives and take responsibility for their own learning.

2. **Identification of key content areas.** According to Harden (1986) the criteria for inclusion of content should be that it relates directly to course objectives; constitutes a 'building block' for later, and fosters critical thinking. Opportunities for deliberate practise combined with feedback, reflection and coaching build learners' core knowledge, skills, attitudes and behaviours over time via iterative learning.

3. **Instructional methods.** Instructional methods are learner-centred, foster deliberate practise and iterative learning, and align with the specifically defined outcomes and content. A mixture of learning methods meets all the learners' needs.

4. ***Assessment.*** Through a comprehensive system of formative assessment, feedback, reflection and coaching, learners build ability and competence to achieve the outcome objectives, and identify future learning needs as they progress through the learning cycle (Fig. 37.1). This ongoing process helps them develop the skills to learn continuously – and how to learn through feedback, reflection and coaching – over the course of their careers (Heen & Stone, 2014). Formative assessment helps learners improve performance in order to achieve positive outcomes. Summative assessment occurs at the end of a unit of study and determines whether learners achieved predetermined outcome objectives and are ready to move on. Summative assessment should also be accompanied by feedback, reflection and coaching.

Next, we examine the critical roles of feedback, reflection and coaching, which generally occur during the assessment protocol for both formative and summative feedback.

Feedback

Feedback is specific information about learners' observed performance compared with a previously established standard, given with the intent to increase learners' motivation and to improve their performance (Kluger & DeNisi, 1996). Formative assessment during or after discussions, presentations or observations provides feedback that gives learners the opportunity to improve prior to high-stakes summative assessments (Fig. 37.1). Feedback subsequent to summative assessments facilitates life-long learning and guides learners toward next-step planning, which can help them fill gaps in their learning, hone skills or strive towards expertise.

As we'll discuss here, feedback is complex. To achieve the intended outcomes, instructors will benefit from attending to factors that interact with feedback, and from developing a system of feedback that incorporates the principles of deliberate practise (Ericsson, 2015). Instructors will need to address the outcome-based learning objectives described above in accordance with institutional standards, and in collaboration with their learners, teach with conscious attention to the intended level of cognitive or motor skill learning (i.e. acquisition of knowledge, understanding, evaluation, etc.) (Anderson & Krathwohl, 2001), encourage learners to reflect and self-assess using performance standards; hold interactive feedback dialogues, and gradually transfer responsibility for obtaining feedback to their learners (i.e. coach). We'll explicate this process below. We'll also explore specific factors related to the content and timing of feedback that affect its usefulness.

HOW DOES THE TYPE OF FEEDBACK AFFECT LEARNING?

Hattie and Timperley (2007) define four types of feedback content; the first three affect learning in a positive manner, and the fourth does not.

1. ***Task.*** Feedback that one's answer or performance was right or wrong (i.e. feedback centred on the task) reinforces desired behaviour and reduces mistakes. Such reinforcing or correcting information usually leads to improvement. However, this information tends not to foster transfer of learning – that is, applying previously learned knowledge or skill in new situations to facilitate learning or to solve problems.

2. ***Process.*** Feedback about how one prepared for a task, arrived at the right answer or mastered a skill is embedded in a richer, more memorable context than simple task-based, right versus wrong feedback. When feedback about the process of learning accompanies task-based feedback, transfer of learning is more likely to occur.

3. ***Self-regulation.*** Feedback can foster self-regulation. This can happen when it addresses learners' asking for or acting upon feedback, showing a commitment to learning, or reflecting upon and self-assessing their actions. Through these activities they become better learners in that they gain self-efficacy, develop skills in self-monitoring, and gain a sense of control over their own learning (e.g. confidence that hard work is more likely to lead to success than innate skill).

4. ***Self.*** Feedback at the self level refers to criticism, praise and comments on personal characteristics. As personal characteristics are not readily changed, feedback at this level does not promote learning, and often undermines it. For example, suggesting that learners succeeded or failed because of innate characteristics, such as intelligence, sets them up for a sense of frustration and a lack of control over their own learning; that is, when they fail to master a difficult task quickly, they are likely to feel that they weren't born with the requisite skills for that task and are doomed to failure (Dweck, 2006).

In addition to the feedback types listed above, feedback that is general (good job! or read more) lacks specificity and gives learners no information about what to repeat next time or specifically what they should do. General positive feedback amounts to praise, which feels good momentarily, but does not promote learning (Dweck, 2006).

No discussion of feedback is complete without consideration of the defensive learner. Such learners tend to attribute negative feedback to external factors, such as instructors' bias. In such cases, the content of the feedback must be factual and clear, stated – and sometimes restated – in an unemotional tone (Weeks, 2015). While providing factual feedback on tasks is usually straightforward, discussing failures in process and self-regulation can be challenging since it is more difficult to observe such behaviour. In this case, instructors might focus on outcomes vis-à-vis a learning objective. For example, one might say, "When I gave you feedback on your reliance upon secondary sources last week, you agreed to critically review primary research on tuberculosis for today's class. Your presentation today was not a critical review." Aligning the content of one's feedback with agreed-upon, clear objectives should reduce defensive behaviour and may foster defensive learners' ability to accept and learn from feedback.

WHAT DOES TIMELY FEEDBACK MEAN?

Timely feedback is not necessarily immediate. Instead, the timing of feedback (which, in reality, frequently depends upon context and convenience) should depend upon the nature of the task. A motor skill should be reinforced or corrected quickly so that one can practise procedures again correctly. A lower order cognitive task (e.g. remembering the names of the bones of the hand or indicating that one understands why pain in one part of the body may originate in a different part) also benefits from quick feedback because information at the knowledge or understanding level of learning (Anderson & Krathwohl, 2001) is quickly reinforced (Foerde & Shohamey, 2011), and then becomes the foundation for higher-order tasks (e.g. applying that understanding to the diagnosis of a patient). However, when engaged in higher-order tasks, learners need more time to process their thoughts. This may require retrieving information from long-term memory (Foerde & Shohamey, 2011), for example recalling disparate facts and then thinking about them in novel ways. Quick feedback would disrupt that thought process, which would deprive learners of forming new synaptic connections and establishing deeper learning.

WHY ISN'T GIVING TIMELY AND SPECIFIC FEEDBACK SUFFICIENT TO CHANGE BEHAVIOUR?

It might be. But even well-given feedback may fail because feedback interacts with other factors such as learners' motivation and openness to reflection and feedback. For example, learners' perception of the utility of the feedback depends on their interest in the subject and motivation to succeed as well as their sense of self-efficacy in attaining the goals (Pekrun, 2006). Thus, before engaging in a feedback dialogue, with the intention of planning next steps for improvement, an instructor needs to know what learners' learning goals

are, and whether they see the long-term utility of the skills to be gained (Harackiewicz & Hulleman, 2010) or simply want to learn enough to pass the course. If learners believe the learning objectives for the unit address their own learning goals (and, ideally, seem useful to their career goals), they are likely to be motivated to work hard, to believe themselves capable of the work, and to find feedback helpful.

When the content of feedback appears to lack credibility for the learners or appear irrelevant, it often fails. Learners may reject feedback they perceive to be untrustworthy – perhaps because it was not based on observation, or did not accord with others' feedback. Also, while the instructor's observation of the feedback may be accurate, when it is not concluded with a plan for improvement and a commitment of support from faculty, learners may reject the goal as being undesirable or unattainable (Kluger & DeNisi, 1996).

RECOMMENDATIONS TO FEEDBACK-GIVERS

Feedback is an on-going, repetitive process that engages instructors in cycles of planning, teaching, observing, discussing, giving feedback and coaching, and engages learners in performing, reflecting, responding and planning next steps with faculty coaches (Fig. 37.2). Guidelines to achieving each step are provided in Box 37.1.

Reflection

"Reflection in the context of learning is a generic term for those intellectual and affective activities in which individuals engage to explore their experiences in order to lead to new understandings and appreciations" (Boud et al., 1985). Reflection is critical to experiential learning as it is through the process of reflecting upon and considering one's experiences that one learns from them.

Reflection is integral to feedback for several reasons. First, encouraging reflection inspires learners to think about how the feedback pertains to them and how they might use it for improvement. Second, reflection on feedback can stimulate informed self-assessment, for instance stimulate critical thinking about how they have performed and the new information that the feedback provides about their performance (Sargeant et al., 2010). Finally, fostering reflection on feedback can promote the development of ongoing self-appraisal or self-monitoring skills. In other words, it can teach the self-analytical process required for lifelong learning.

As noted earlier, multiple factors and approaches influence learners' acceptance and use of feedback. One of these is encouraging learners to first reflect upon and assess their own performance in light of their understanding of the performance standard or competency level required, and then to reflect upon the feedback they've received and how it is similar or not to their self-assessment. Such reflection stimulates

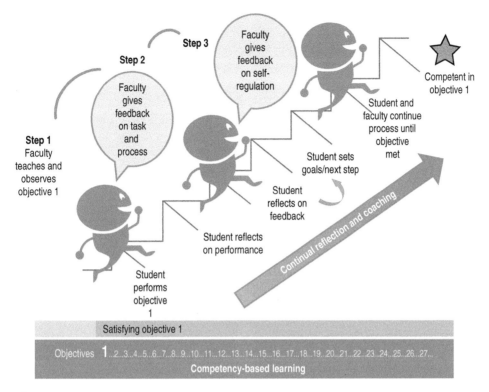

Fig. 37.2 Steps to competence.

Box 37.1 **Key feedback recommendations (see Fig. 37.2)**

Prior to feedback

1. Know the learning objectives and how your teaching will address them.
2. Discuss the objectives with your learners.
3. Determine how the objectives accord with learners' goals and interests.

   "You will be evaluated on your ability to tie suture knots efficiently. I know you plan to be an internist rather than a surgeon so let's think together about the utility of your learning this skill."

Step 1. Teaching and observing an objective

4. Observe students with the learning objective and your shared plan in mind.

Step 2. Giving feedback on task and process

5. Make giving feedback on task (Hattie & Timperley, 2007) common and expected, woven into your teaching. But, two caveats: First, avoid making learners dependent upon constant feedback (e.g. "right, good question"). Second,

time the feedback according to the task at hand: Give students time to think and to reflect when appropriate.

6. Ask learners how they prepared, arrived at an answer etc. Comment upon their process of thinking when it is apparent. Link their process of learning to their performance.

   "The patient's pattern of symptoms could have been misleading had you not drawn upon basic pathophysiology of the lungs, which got you to the right diagnosis."

Step 3. Giving feedback on self-regulation

7. Provide feedback on whether learners acted upon prior feedback and show a commitment to learning.

   "The last time we talked we agreed that you'd research dosages of X for children by age. If you had done that you could have treated that infant much sooner."

learners' critical engagement in their assessment and feedback, and provides instructors with the opportunity to discuss the feedback and share their rationale for it. The latter is especially important if their feedback disconfirms learners' self-assessments of how they are doing and leads to defensive reactions, as noted above (Sargeant et al., 2010).

Over a period of time, multiple sources of feedback and information, and discussion of these with instructors, can heighten learners' awareness of their strengths and weaknesses vis-à-vis a standard. Both the accumulation of evidence and the discussion add to the learners' perceptions of the trustworthiness of the data and make them more difficult to dismiss on the grounds of instructor's bias. Such accumulated evidence also helps learners calibrate their own performance and become more accurate self-assessors. In turn, being willing to reflect upon and assess one's own performance leads not only to greater openness to feedback but a sense of control over one's learning that makes feedback seem desirable and useful.

 "…the process of reflection appeared to be useful as the means through which participants assessed and assimilated not only their feedback but their emotional responses and concerns related to that feedback."

Sargeant et al., 2008

Reflection is generally more effective as a facilitated or guided activity, rather than as a solo activity (Sargeant et al., 2008). An instructor facilitating a learner's reflective process using guiding, open questions can steer the learner towards an objective and specific critique of his or her performance and the feedback received (Box 37.2). Encouraging reflection engages both the cognitive and affective capacities of learners. Reflecting upon one's emotional reactions to a situation or to information is as important for learning as reflecting upon the data or facts. For learners, encouraging reflection upon their performance and upon the feedback they're receiving on their performance can enable understanding, assimilation, and ownership of their progress. In earlier work, "reflection seemed to be the process through which feedback was or was not assimilated and appeared integral to decisions to accept and use the feedback" (Sargeant et al., 2008).

Coaching

Coaching is a term consistent with the central role of feedback in competency-based education. The goal of providing feedback is to enable the learner to use it to develop and improve, and to attain their next milestone or level of achievement. While the term 'feedback' generally connotes appraisal and criticism – i.e. negative activities and feelings – the term

---

Box 37.2   Key questions for reflection

The task/knowledge/performance (done right or wrong?) *Step 2, Fig. 37.2*
1. What was your goal today in performing X?
2. What do you think you did well? What would you like to improve?

The process (how learned) *Step 2, Fig. 37.2*
3. How did you prepare for today's session?
4. Can you tell me what you were thinking when you were doing X?
5. What was your strategy in doing it?

Upon feedback: self-regulation (goal setting/self-assessment) *Step 3, Fig. 37.2*
6. When you compare my observations to your self-assessment, where do we agree and where do we disagree?
7. What might be some reasons for our differing opinions?
8. The purpose of feedback is to point out ways to improve. What would you now like to improve?

Box 37.3   Key questions for coaching

Coaching for improvement
1. Now that we've discussed X, what is your goal for improvement?
2. What do you need to do to reach your goal?
3. How might I (your supervisor) be of assistance?
4. What other resources or learning do you need?
5. When should you hope to achieve this goal?

'coaching' is about helping learners to develop and improve, to become the best that they can be – i.e. positive activities and feelings (Heen & Stone, 2014). Coaching in medical education means providing feedback in a facilitated, reflective manner that encourages leaners to self-assess and reflect upon their feedback and to use it for development (Box 37.3). For instructors, becoming a learning coach means transitioning from providing didactic, directive feedback, to providing performance data in a manner that encourages learners' reflection and planning for improvement.

 "Evaluations tell you where you stand, what to expect, and what is expected of you. Coaching allows you to learn and improve and helps you play at a higher level."

Heen & Stone, 2014

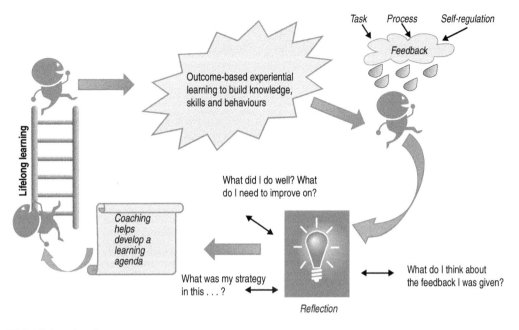

Task   Process   Self-regulation

Feedback

Outcome-based experiential learning to build knowledge, skills and behaviours

Lifelong learning

What did I do well? What do I need to improve on?

Coaching helps develop a learning agenda

What was my strategy in this . . . ?

What do I think about the feedback I was given?

Reflection

Fig. 37.3 Lifelong learning.

The goal of reflection and coaching is also to foster an internal locus of control for one's performance and use of feedback, a self-monitoring and improvement capacity.

Summary

An experiential curriculum that is based on pre-set outcome objectives and linked to strategic feedback, reflection and coaching will support learners' ability to satisfy the competencies that lead to the attainment of expertise and quality healthcare outcomes. Feedback, reflection and coaching form an interdependent, supportive strategy that permits learners to eliminate gaps in their learning and move on to the next phase of their education. As a result, learners gain skills in informed self-assessment and in critiquing their own performance, are better able to take responsibility for their learning process and iteratively strengthen their foundation of knowledge. Feedback, given appropriately, enables learners to determine where they stand with regard to previously established outcome objectives, and to use that information to attain the next level of achievement. With reflection, learners frame, categorize and assess their approach to learning. Coaching encourages reflection on feedback, and fosters planning for improvement. It helps learners develop deliberate strategies to use and to request feedback when they perceive its utility. Effective feedback, reflection and coaching enable learners to develop the insight and skills necessary to ensure lifelong incremental learning, which underpins the maintenance of quality healthcare (Fig. 37.3).

To provide this supportive system and to help learners attain competence, instructors need to develop new skills to effectively communicate timely feedback on task, process and self-regulation. Initiating this comprehensive experiential learning model will entail providing training for faculty in the art of reflection and the nuances of both feedback and coaching.

References

Accreditation Council for Graduate Medical Education (ACGME); American Board of Pediatrics. The Pediatrics Milestone Project, January 2013. Available at: http://peds.stanford.edu/program-information/milestones/documents/Pediatrics_21_Subcompetencies_with_Milestones.pdf. (Accessed 2015).

Anderson, L.W., Krathwohl, D.R. (Eds.), 2001. A Taxonomy for Learning, Teaching and Assessing: A Revision of Bloom's Taxonomy of Educational Outcomes, Complete Edition. Longman, New York.

Aschenbrener, C.A., Ast, C., Kirch, D.G., 2015. Graduate medical education: its role in achieving a true medical education continuum. Acad. Med. 90, 1203–1209.

Boud, D., Keogh, R., Walker, D. (Eds.), 1985. Reflection: Turning Experience Into Learning. Routledge-Falmer, London, p. 19.

Cohen, E.R., McGaghie, W.C., Wayne, D.B., et al., 2015. Recommendations for reporting mastery education research in medicine (ReMERM). Acad. Med. 90, 1509–1514.

Dweck, C.S., 2006. Mindset: The New Psychology of Success. Ballantine Books, New York.

Ericsson, K.A., 2015. Acquisition and maintenance of medical expertise: a perspective from the expert-performance approach with deliberate practice. Acad. Med. 90, 1471–1486.

Foerde, K., Shohamey, D., 2011. Feedback timing modulates brain systems for learning in humans. J. Neurosci. 31, 13157–13167.

Harackiewicz, J.M., Hulleman, C.S., 2010. The importance of interest: the role of achievement goals and task values in promoting the development of motivation. Soc. Personal. Psychol. Compass 4, 42–52.

Harden, R.M., 1986. Ten questions to ask when planning a course or curriculum. Med. Educ. 20, 356–365.

Hattie, J., Timperley, H., 2007. The power of feedback. Rev. Educ. Res. 77, 81–112.

Heen, S., Stone, D. Find the coaching in criticism: The right ways to receive feedback, Boston: Harvard Business Review, 92:108–111, January-February 2014.

Holmboe, E.S., 2015. Realizing the promise of competency-based medical education. Acad. Med. 90, 411–413.

Kluger, A.N., DeNisi, A., 1996. The effects of feedback interventions on performance: a historical review, a meta-analysis, and a preliminary feedback intervention theory. Psychol. Bull. 119, 254–284.

Krackov, S.K., Pohl, H.S., 2011. Building expertise using the deliberate practice curriculum-planning model. Med. Teach. 33, 570–575.

Pekrun, R., 2006. The Control-Value Theory of achievement emotions: assumptions, corollaries, and implications for educational research and practice. Educational Psychology Review 18, 315–341.

Sargeant, J., Armson, H., Chesluk, B., et al., 2010. Processes and dimensions of informed self-assessment: a conceptual model. Acad. Med. 85, 1212–1220.

Sargeant, J., Mann, K., van der Vleuten, C., Metsemakers, J., 2008. Reflection: a link between receiving and using assessment feedback. Adv. Health Sci. Educ. Theory Pract. 3, 399–410.

Ten Cate, O., 2013. Nuts and bolts of entrustable professional activities. J. Grad. Med. Educ. 5, 157–158.

Weeks, H. How to give feedback to someone who gets crazy defensive, Harvard Business Review, Harvard Business Publishing, 15 August, 2015. Available at: https://hbr.org/2015/08/how-to-give-feedback-to-someone-who-gets-crazy-defensive. (Accessed 2015).

The assessment of attitudes and professionalism

38

V. J. Wass, A. Barnard

Trends

- Becoming more human: assessing values-based practice
- Developing reflective professionalism
- Positive continuous formative assessment for learning
- Enactment at individual, team and institutional levels in the workplace
- Increasing national regulatory codes of professional practice

Why assess attitudes and professionalism? Setting the boundaries

The importance placed on the assessment of attitudes and professionalism is growing. This has been partly instigated by demands, following failures in healthcare delivery, for stronger demonstration by clinicians of personal values (e.g. compassion, empathy, integrity), enacted through professional behaviours and reflected in the culture of the workplace. Simultaneously, evidence has emerged suggesting that poor professional behaviour at medical school can relate subsequently to unacceptable performance at work. Internationally, countries are setting up regulatory measures for practising clinicians and developing codes of practice to be applied across the continuum of training and revalidation. There is increasing acceptance that professionalism must be taught explicitly in curricula, and that it is crucial, when assessing professional behaviour, to maximize educational impact. The principle of learning from assessment must be applied and, to ensure the ongoing development of professionalism, formative feedback on performance is fundamental. It is of utmost importance that students are involved in the processes and value the assessments.

 Assessment is not a measurement problem but an instructional design problem: students must learn from it.

The original tendency to focus on 'fitness to practise' procedures and punish negative behaviours has come under review. There has been increasing concern that the focus on poor behaviour detracts from the positive aspects of exploring and developing professionalism. Fitness to practise processes remain absolutely essential, but general acceptance has emerged that the identification and documentation of negative lapses in professional behaviours is better placed in a separate system.

There is now an important trend to strengthen the positive, formative development of professionalism across the continuum of clinical practice. This is key to the instructional design of the assessment programme. Assessments are being used increasingly as formative and reflective exercises to foster high levels of professional practice and concomitantly identify and support struggling students early in training. Clearly, if poor professional behaviour is identified as a definite cause for concern the trainee can be referred into fitness to practise procedures, but the two processes should remain distinct.

There are recognised boundaries to assessing an individual's attitudes. Internal values are personal and lie deep within the individual. They are not easy to access. Health professionals should, without doubt, be aware of their internal attitudes and prejudices, and how these might impact positively or negatively on their interactions with patients and colleagues. Self-awareness and reflection are areas that remain relatively overlooked in medical education. A range of psychological instruments for assessing internal attitudes is available, e.g. the Implicit Association Test (IAT) (https://implicit.harvard.edu/implicit/takeatest.html) and the Consultation and Relational Empathy (CARE) Measure (http://www.caremeasure.org/). Overtly assessing these attitudes is difficult as students are aware that judgements are being made and will modify their responses accordingly.

External attitudinal behaviour is the parameter more open to assessment. This may be only the tip of an 'iceberg' of personal values but is a pragmatic reality. This chapter will focus on attitudes as expressed externally through observable behaviour. Maximizing the formative educational impact of the assessments is the aim. The focus is on assessment FOR learning and not assessment OF learning.

What do we mean by professionalism? Agreeing the definition

The first fundamental principle of any assessment is to achieve clarity on what is being assessed. Herein lies the major challenge. A generic universal definition of 'professionalism' eludes us (Birden et al., 2014). This is perhaps not surprising. Professionalism is a complex multifactorial construct open and sensitive to societal and cultural values within increasingly changing and rapidly globalising healthcare settings. There may be general agreement about the values that underlie professionalism, yet cultural differences (e.g. confidentiality within family structure, consent by minors) must be respected. To date, much of the published literature on professionalism has centred on Western medical education paradigms, although fortunately other cultural perspectives are now emerging. Every institution must therefore produce their own definition and intended learning outcomes (ILOs) to reflect their own local professional values. The training environment should reflect these values to ensure they are transparent and positively role modelled to learners. Faculty training is important to achieve this. Congruence of professional behaviours by all staff is essential if assessments are to achieve the necessary positive educational impact.

 Every institution must agree and enact its own definition of professionalism. It must be transparent to learners what is being assessed and why.

For the purpose of this chapter the definition in Box 38.1 is used.

It highlights the complexity of the subject and the need to select a range of assessment tools designed to promote appropriate learning. There is a knowledge base for professionalism relating to regulatory process

> ### Box 38.1 Definition of professionalism
>
> A concept associated with the education, training, attitudes and ethical practices of a group of workers or practitioners. It includes a regulated educational and training system that has specific standards that are monitored and maintained. It has an ethical framework, concerned with good working practices between practitioners and their clients. Professionalism is characterized by a variety of reflective practices that practitioners engage into maintain their skills (Birden et al., 2014)

and legal and ethical guidelines. Educators must focus not only on the learners' attitudes and behaviours but also ensure trainees know and can apply these ethical frameworks and integrate professional values into practical clinical skills. At the same time, the learner must develop strong reflective practices to develop understanding of their own attitudes and behaviour, and meet the needs of not only patients and their families but also of colleagues across the healthcare team. This is challenging! An international working party on the assessment of professionalism highlighted the multidimensional and multi-paradigmatic approach required when planning how to assess professionalism. It impacts on the health professional at three levels: (1) individual and personal, (2) interpersonal with the healthcare team, (3) at a wider institutional and societal level (Hodges et al., 2011).

 Professionalism is multidimensional and multi-paradigmatic: It impacts on trainees at individual, inter-personal and institutional-societal levels.

When should professionalism be assessed?

Increasingly, it is recognized that professionalism is intrinsic to ongoing training and must be taught and assessed commencing at entry to undergraduate training. A call for medical school selection processes to be based more strongly on personal values is being made, and regular performance appraisal is becoming a norm within career development. It is now mandatory in some countries for doctors to maintain reflective portfolios based on the collation of professional experience for regular revalidation processes through to retirement. Formative continuous assessment along the novice to expert pathway is becoming essential. This represents a very significant move from the past tendency to only identify and address the fortunately rare lapses in professional performance.

 Assessment of professionalism lies across a continuum from entry to exit.

How should professionalism be assessed?

KEY STEPS

Step 1: A fundamental principle

Professionalism is a context- or case-specific attribute; it cannot be assessed as a generic attribute. Professional behaviour is embedded in the context in which it is enacted. This is not surprising. When interacting with patients, the clinician's response is inevitably intertwined with their knowledge, skills, personal feelings, interpersonal interactions and healthcare systems. It can be very different handling a challenging regular patient in the morning outpatient clinic with familiar staff to dealing with an equally challenging emergency in the middle of the night with locum staff. Professional behaviour therefore must be assessed across a range of contexts over time.

 Professional behaviour is not generic or time specific. Assessment requires a range of contexts over time.

Step 2: Curriculum design

Professionalism must have clear, explicitly visible, assessable ILOs. These must be championed from the start of the course using sequential development of increasing complexity along the novice to expert learning pathway. Developing a vertical professionalism strand across all years of the curriculum led by a strong educational advocate can enable horizontal integration across the different clinical contexts and progressive spiralling complexity of learning. The assessment programme should then mirror and support this (O'Sullivan et al., 2012).

Step 3: Consider framing assessments against a published code of conduct

Well-designed codes of conduct are available. These are designed for practising doctors, but there is an international move, in line with the early development of professionalism and professional identity, to publish codes for medical students (e.g. http://micn.otago.ac.nz/wp-content/uploads/micn/2008/03/20151217-medical-student-code-of-conduct-2015.pdf). Although to date these codes mainly originate in Western healthcare systems, they can be adapted to provide a structure for collating and monitoring the positive formative development of professional behaviour. It is not necessary to reinvent the wheel. Adopting or modifying an established code of conduct is acceptable to provide a framework for trainees to plan and gather evidence to build a portfolio of developing professional behaviour. For examples see Box 38.2.

Box 38.2   Examples of published codes of conduct

CanMEDS http://www.royalcollege.ca/rcsite/canmeds-e. (Accessed 28 Jan 2017).
Good Medical Practice http://www.gmc-uk.org/
Medical Board of Australia http://www.medicalboard.gov.au/Codes-Guidelines-Policies/Code-of-conduct.aspx. (Accessed 28 Jan 2017).

Step 4: Blueprinting

As with any assessment, blueprinting is essential to ensure all the ILOs for the vertical professionalism theme are covered at appropriate points in the course. This must mirror the educational intent and be transparent to students. Given the content /case specificity of professionalism (Step 1), blueprinting can ensure it is assessed longitudinally over a wide range of contexts, at increasing levels of complexity, by sufficient different assessors. It should achieve a comprehensive balance across all the defined components (see Section: 'Why assess attitudes and professionalism?'). The horizontal /vertical integration of professionalism within the curriculum (Step 2) offers the opportunity to incorporate professional behaviour either into stand-alone assessments or integrated in clinical scenarios (see Section: 'Tools across the continuum'). To ensure reliability, multiple assessment tools and a range of assessors contextualised across the curriculum must be achieved (Wilkinson et al., 2009).

 For reliability, multiple assessment tools and assessors across the curriculum are needed.

Step 5: Be clear of the purpose of each test

Clarity of purpose is essential when designing the components of any assessment programme. Professionalism is no exception. The selected method must offer validity, i.e. measure what it sets out to measure, and appropriately assess the intended learning and behaviours. It must be clear whether the primary purpose of the assessment is to be formative to provide feedback and set actions for improvement or summative to measure achievement of ILOs. If the assessment is summative and used to determine progression building reliability is also essential.

 Be clear on the purpose of the test and select a valid tool.

Step 6: Choosing a valid assessment tool

Multiple tools are available and a range must be used. Miller's Triangle (Fig. 38.1) offers a helpful framework as outlined below in the Section: 'Tools across the continuum'. A suite of tools is available to progressively test across increasing expertise. Professionalism, as the three-dimensional Miller's model demonstrates, can be intrinsic to them all.

Step 7: Train the assessors

Faculty must aim to ensure assessors own and enact the professional values of the institution (see Section: 'What do we mean by professionalism?'). Positive role modelling is important and not always easy to achieve. Training assessors is essential to ensure consistency of

Increasing
expertise

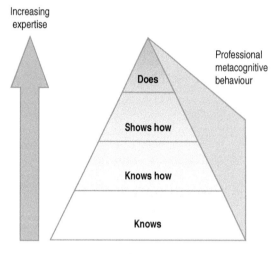

Professional
metacognitive
behaviour

Fig. 38.1 Miller's Triangle (adapted) as a model for competency testing.

Table 38.1 Assessment tools

Miller's assessment level	Assessment tool
Knows: knowledge of legal definitions/regulatory frameworks	written multiple choice question (MCQ)/short answer question (SAQ)/essays/group assignments
Knows how: applies this knowledge in increasingly complex situations	MCQs with scenarios/case studies/modified short essay questions (MEQs)/situational judgement tests/ reflective activities, e.g. critical incident
Shows how: demonstrates skills and behaviours with relevant knowledge	OSPE/OSCE/clinical simulations/standardized professional encounters
Does: observation in practice	multisource feedback (MSF)/peer review (e.g. mini-PAT)/mini clinical evaluation exercise/(mini CEX) professional mini evaluation exercise(P-MEX)/entrustable professional activities (EPAs)/case bases discussion

delivery and judgement in delivering the assessments, and, most importantly, in providing feedback. Agreeing and internalising what is being assessed (see Section: 'What do we mean by professionalism?') is fundamental to making reliable judgements. There has been a tendency to make checklists and dissect out the elements of professional behaviour. Evidence now suggests that assessors can be trusted to judge more globally. This makes sense given the complexity of professional behaviour and its often seamless integration within a clinical context. It is difficult for an assessor to dissect out the components of these constructs, which, with increasing expertise, have become more implicit (unconscious competence) than explicit (conscious competence) in their own professional practice. Assessors need help to unpick this and understand the domains being assessed.

 Beware of atomisation. Value the assessors' expertise to make global judgements.

Step 8: Engage the students

Student engagement at all levels of the process is crucial. Using assessment innovatively to ensure students engage with learning about professionalism and develop the necessary reflective learning skills is essential. All stages of the assessment process need to be transparent and explicit, encouraging formative feedback and ongoing personal development. With increasing awareness of the need to foster the humane side of clinical practice, alongside the scientific learning, assessing professionalism carries an important role as a learning tool for trainees. Students need to understand that faculty seek and value evidence of values-based behaviours (e.g. compassion and empathy) within the working environment, integrity and honesty with patients and peers, and caring interactions with patients. The assessment

programme for professionalism offers the opportunity to build on social behavioural science learning and engage with students to achieve this (Carney et al., 2016)

 "Our great task is to succeed in becoming more human."

Jose Saramago, Nobel Prize Laureate, 1998

THE TOOLS

Miller's pyramid provides a useful framework for categorizing the main tools currently used to assess professionalism. Overviews and reviews can be found in Stern (2006) and Wilkinson et al. (2009). A range of tools exists to assess behavioural competencies; only a small proportion offers strong evidence of validity and reliability. Before selecting the appropriate tool it is important to blueprint (Step 4) and consider the purpose (Step 5). For practical reasons the selection offered here is deliberately limited to account for (1) evidence of reliability, validity and acceptability; (2) emerging new methodology; (3) the balance between formative intent to offer feedback and summative measurement of ILO achievement; and (4) the drive to assess values-based practice at the level of 'does'. Table 38.1 summarizes the tools under discussion. Ongoing development of new assessment methodology should be encouraged as we strive to develop stronger values-based professional identity (Cruess et al., 2016).

Cognition: knows

The factual knowledge base of professionalism can be assessed through conventional written assessments, such as multiple-choice questions (MCQs), short answer questions (SAQs) and essays. Although these formats are arguably easier to deliver, factual answers sit uncomfortably within the complexity of professional practice, except perhaps in the early stages of medical school. At this level there may be a place for questions such as: *What is the age at which a minor can legally give informed consent for an appendicetomy?*

Cognition: knows how

Assessing application of knowledge is strongly recommended. Even at novice level, clinical scenarios can be embedded in MCQs and SAQs or used to focus group assignments. The latter may involve a reflective element and can be useful in interprofessional learning situations. Across the continuum of training, increasingly complex written and reflective tasks can be introduced. These may be based on hypothetical scenarios (modified essay questions [MEQs]), situational scenarios, or real patient case studies that are role relevant at the appropriate training level. An example might be:

A 16 year-old-boy with a learning disability is brought to A&E. He needs an urgent appendicetomy. His parents cannot be contacted. Applying the legal and ethical frameworks you have learnt, how should you proceed?

Situational judgement tests (SJTs) (Patterson et al., 2016) are increasingly used as tests for entry into training. SJT scenarios are designed to assess judgement in increasingly complex clinical work situations, can be written or video based and focus on inter- and intrapersonal dilemmas. Their potential to teach and assess professionalism is promising. Personal reflective activities play an important role and can be designed to apply knowledge to clinical experiences at all three levels of professionalism– individual, interpersonal and institutional. Such activities can be focused and structured for individual reflection or as part of a wider forum, for example through moderated discussion boards. Responsive, supportive feedback is essential for reflective activities.

 Aim to assess cognitive knowledge at a contextually applied level.

Behaviour: shows how

Active observation of a trainee's interaction with a 'staged', clinically relevant simulated scenario enables trainees to demonstrate how they would handle the situation professionally. At this level, scenarios may have an explicit stand-alone professionalism theme or, with increasing complexity, one that integrates attitudinal/professional behaviour into a patient–doctor interaction. Objective structured practical/clinical examinations (OSPEs/OSCEs) with standardized simulated patients in various formats can simulate increasing complexity and are popular. For example:

As the resident on-call doctor, you are asked to see the mother of a 16-year-old boy with a learning disability following an emergency appendicetomy. She is angry about his care and wants to discharge him against medical advice.

When assessing at health-care team and institutional levels, standardized professional encounters (SPEs) using health professionals enacting scenarios centred on interprofessional behaviours are useful. With the increasing focus on professional behaviours at these levels, more complex simulations are gaining favour to reflect actual practice. The consequences of unsatisfactory performance in the 'professional' criteria of an integrated OSCE or clinical simulation need to be carefully delineated.

Behaviour: does

There is now a significant move towards more authentic assessment in the workplace at a 'does' level by direct observation of interactions in the workplace specific or over time. A variety of assessment tools are available (Norcini & Burch, 2007), into which professionalism can be specifically assessed or integrated. Again it is important that assessors understand, personally enact and are trained to implement the institutional parameters set for professionalism when making judgements and giving feedback (Steps 3 and 7).

Multisource feedback (MSF) (or 360-degree review) from a range of work-related colleagues (professional peers or supervisors, associated healthcare workers, patients,) is replacing the more traditional single supervisor assessment of observed behaviours in the clinical setting and workplace. If properly applied, this is proving a valid means of gathering information at the individual and team level within a workplace environment. These reviews are questionnaire-based ratings on selected behaviours extensively used in industry and now, more frequently, health settings (Donnon et al., 2014). There are a number of validated tools, and an increasing number of commercial offerings. Peer review can also be used with pre-clinical student groups, focusing on the professional behaviours relevant to the stage of training, for example teamwork, reliability, and respect for diversity. It is important that these assessments are initially formative, before any summative application, and that feedback, particularly when negative, is supportive.

Tools such as the mini clinical evaluation exercise (MiniCEX) offer specific contextualized observations of professional behaviours and can evaluate clinical performance in real-life settings, and offer feedback building, importantly, actions for improvement. The professional mini evaluation exercise (P-MEX) is designed specifically to evaluate 24 attributes of professionalism, which are grouped into four categories: doctor–patient relationship skills; interprofessional relationship skills; reflection skills and time-management skills (Cruess et al., 2006).

Entrustable professional activities (EPAs) is an emerging tool yet to be fully validated but increasingly used in postgraduate education. EPAs translate competencies, which can map to professionalism frameworks (Step 3), into discrete units of professional work entrusted, or delegated, to a trainee. Like all assessments, EPAs need deliberative selection to cover elements of professionalism (Ten Cate et al., 2015).

Tools across the continuum – a portfolio of professionalism

A professional portfolio, starting at medical school entry, is proving a very useful tool to collate, monitor and strengthen the positive, formative development of professionalism across the continuum of clinical practice. A framework (Step 3) to guide the structure of the portfolio is helpful. The longitudinal and purposive collection of material can effectively demonstrate reflective practice on progress and achievements, and address the disjunction that often appears between undergraduate study and postgraduate training (Buckley et al., 2009).

A professional portfolio may contain:

- Personal and professional development plan
- Results of specific assessments: MSF, peer review, miniCEX, P-MEX
- Reflective assessment tasks
- Critical incident reflections
- Evidence of appropriate self-care activities
- Records of meetings with supervisors
- Sign-off documents for particular skills or competencies.

Summary

Twenty-first-century health-care is demanding more humane values-based professional behaviour. This must be integrated into curricula and assessed formatively, positively and continuously across the spectrum of training from novice to expert, fostering self awareness, reflective practice and the ongoing development of professional identity. One challenge lies in the complexity of professionalism at societal and cultural levels. It must defined at local institutional level, owned and enacted by all staff, and be explicit and transparently shared with students. Professionalism is a contextualized, not generic, attribute and must be assessed using a variety of tools, cases and assessors across time aiming to monitor enactment in the workplace at individual, team and institutional levels. Assessment for learning should underpin the process maximizing educational impact and student engagement. With globalization and changing demands on healthcare,

ongoing development is essential; new tools should be encouraged and robustly validated as we strive to 'become more human'.

References

Birden, H., Glass, N., Wilson, I., et al., 2014. Defining professionalism in medical education: a systematic review. Med. Teach. 36 (1), 47–61.

Buckley, S., Coleman, J., Davison, I., et al., 2009. BEME Guide: No. 11 The educational effects of portfolios on undergraduate student learning: a Best Evidence Medical Education (BEME) systematic review. Med. Teach. 31 (4), 282–298.

Carney, P.A., Palmer, R.T., Fuqua Miller, M., et al., 2016. Tools to Assess Behavioural and Social Science Competencies in Medical Education: A Systematic Review. Academic Medicine 91 (5), 730–742.

Cruess, R.L., Cruess, S.R., Steinert, Y., 2016. Amending Miller's Pyramid to Include Professional Identity Formation. Acad. Med. 91 (2), 180–185.

Cruess, R., McIlroy, J.H., Cruess, S., et al., 2006. The Professionalism Mini-evaluation Exercise: a preliminary investigation. Academic Medicine 81 (Suppl. 10), S74–S78.

Donnon, T., Al Ansari, A., Al Alawi, S., Violato, C., 2014. The reliability, validity, and feasibility of multisource feedback physician assessment: a systematic review. Academic Medicine 89 (3), 511–516.

Hodges, B.D., Ginsburg, S., Cruess, R., et al., 2011. Assessment of professionalism: recommendations from the Ottawa 2010 Conference. Med. Teach. 33 (5), 354–363.

Norcini, J., Burch, V., 2007. AMEE guide: No 31 Workplace-based assessment as an educational tool. Med. Teach. 29 (9), 855–871.

O'Sullivan, H., van Mook, W., Fewtrell, W., Wass, V., 2012. AMEE Guide No 61 Integrating professionalism into the curriculum. Med. Teach. 34 (2), e64–e77.

Patterson, F., Zibarras, L., Ashworth, V., 2016. AMEE Guide: No. 100 Situational judgement tests in medical education and training: Research, theory and practice. Med. Teach. 38 (1), 3–17.

Stern, D.T., 2006. Measuring Professionalism. Oxford University Press.

Ten Cate, O., Chen, H.C., Hoff, R.G., et al., 2015. AMEE Guide: No 99 Curriculum development for the workplace using Entrustable Professional Activities (EPAs). Med. Teach. 37 (11), 983–1002.

Wilkinson, T.J., Wade, W.B., Knock, L.D., 2009. A blueprint to assess professionalism: results of a systematic review. Academic Medicine 84 (5), 551–558.

Programmatic assessment

C. P. M. van der Vleuten, S. Heeneman, L. W. T. Schuwirth

Trends

- A holistic view on assessment is emerging in which formative and summative assessment strategies are combined.
- Competency-based education is spreading both at the undergraduate and postgraduate level of training, but is hampered by an inappropriate assessment approach.
- Programmatic assessment has been proposed as a means to make assessment aligned with a constructivist view on teaching and learning.

Introduction

Programmatic assessment is an alternative way of arranging assessment in a training programme and a different take on how assessment may function to promote learning. Some have called programmatic assessment a paradigm shift in our thinking around assessment. Its origins lie in research and observations in practice. Any individual assessment involves a compromise on quality criteria (van der Vleuten, 1996); it cannot have perfect reliability, validity, educational impact, acceptability and low cost. The choice of compromise depends on the context and purpose of the assessment.

 Any individual assessment is but one data point with limited utility. Consider a data point to be similar to a pixel of an image.

The question is really when to optimize what. The basic tenet of programmatic assessment is to capitalize on the complementarity of different assessment methods by seeking to achieve their most fruitful constellation, rather than pursuing perfection – in terms of fulfilment of all possible quality criteria – in each of these methods individually. When such constellation is reached, its constituent judgements of assessment together will bolster the strength of the assessment as a whole. Such approach requires us to make different choices. In making these choices educational arguments

for maximizing learning by learners weigh heavily. In this chapter we will explain in which respects the traditional approach to assessment can gain from a shift to programmatic assessment. We will then proceed to explaining programmatic assessment itself, illustrated with an example of an existing programme. We will end with some reflections and issues that are found in recent implementations of programmatic assessment.

The traditional approach

The most dominant approach to assessment is to have an end-of-course assessment one has to pass. The performance of the learner is compared with a minimum standard. If a learner fails, then usually he or she has to resit the entire exam. In the event of multiple failures, the learner usually has to redo the course and repeat the assessment. This is how learners navigate through a full training programme. Many training programmes also include a comprehensive assessment at the end: a final exam. When all exams have been passed, the learner is considered qualified to pursue a more advanced programme in the field or to enter professional practice. This classical approach to learning is old and has served us well, but we argue here that there is scope for improvement.

The traditional approach is modular. It assumes that when learners pass, they have mastered the whole domain they were learning, often referred to as 'mastery learning'. Although the learning is triggered by the assessment occasion, the assumption is that learners will have 'mastered' the domain for the remainder of their lives. In most cases, this will likely not hold. Forgetting is quite normal, and the forgetting curves from psychology show that 50% of the learned subject matter is already forgotten after a few weeks. One of the most fundamental problems in education is the issue of transfer. Having the knowledge in no way guarantees that the learner will be able to apply this knowledge when appropriate, i.e. when needed to manage a professional task. Hence, mastery at one moment in time bears little relationship to its use at a later moment. Therefore, in many domains pure mastery learning is an outdated model of learning.

Modern learning programmes are based on 'constructivist' notions: learning occurs more effectively and efficiently if the learner 'constructs' the information or knowledge. Learning in this sense means 'processing information' rather than 'consuming' it. Internalizing information and being able to understand and use it is what makes learning productive. Hence, teaching is not only about transmitting information, but also about enabling learners to make maximum sense of it by allowing them to continuously practise transfer on the basis of professionally authentic tasks. Knowledge, skills and attitudes are integrated by using "whole tasks" (Vandewaetere et al., 2015). Problem-based learning, team-based learning, competency-based learning and outcome-based learning are illustrations of modern education approaches that are founded on this constructivist notion of learning. These approaches enjoy wide currency in undergraduate and postgraduate education in medicine.

A traditional approach to assessment may induce poor learning behaviour as passing the assessment becomes learners' main incentive to learn (Cilliers et al., 2012).

"Better utilization of assessment to influence learning has long been a goal in higher education (HE), though not one that has been met with great success."

Cilliers et al., 2012, p. 40

Learners will wish to maximize their success of passing the assessments and will do anything to pass. In their view, the assessment is what constitutes the curriculum. As a result, learning will be as good as the assessment requires. Many education practices, however, promote poor learning styles. Examples include the rewarding of rote memorization strategies, minimal preparation strategies due to minimal standards or competing exams, or procrastination due to the abundancy of resit opportunities.

Typical of modern programmes is a move beyond the knowledge domain. Many countries in the world have developed competency frameworks. These frameworks have been developed with substantial stakeholder input. What is striking is the commonality across these frameworks: although their descriptions differ, they all emphasize skills such as communication, collaboration and leadership skills, professionalism, reflective abilities, et cetera. Given the overlap across frameworks, there seems to be consensus on what we wish our professionals to be capable of and what skills are needed to improve healthcare. These skills are indeed important because they define success and failure in the labour market. Some therefore call them twenty-first-century skills or 'soft' skills. We choose the term 'domain-independent skills' because they are relevant to any domain of learning, also outside medicine.

Embracing these skills in education has major consequences. First, they cannot be taught and tested in a single course. That is, one cannot have a 4-week course on 'communication', administer a test (e.g. an OSCE) and conclude the learner is a good communicator. These skills are learned longitudinally over longer periods of time. They have to be demonstrated in (daily or habitual) performance and are shaped through on-going feedback. Domain-independent skills therefore have to rely heavily on non-standardized assessment using methods from the top of Miller's pyramid (Miller, 1990). Modern training programmes embracing these competency frameworks typically interweave these competencies as continuous 'learning lines' throughout the curriculum. The longitudinal nature of this approach is not easily reconciled with a traditional mastery-oriented assessment approach.

Traditional assessment systems often lack feedback. For economic reasons many assessment practices do not disclose the content of the assessment (the items, for example) to learners. If anything more than pass or fail is communicated this is usually done in the form of grades. Grades represent a very poor form of feedback (Shute, 2008). When assessing domain-independent skills they are more or less useless because they do not provide information on how to improve. By capturing complex skills in a metric or in so-called objective lists of performance, we often trivialize what is being measured, and induce poor learning strategies as a result. Nothing stimulates learning more than high-quality feedback. Our education practices are frequently feedback deprived.

"The main goal of formative feedback—whether delivered by a teacher or computer, in the classroom or elsewhere—is to enhance learning, performance, or both, engendering the formation of accurate, targeted conceptualizations and skills."

Shute 2008, p. 175

Finally, traditional approaches to assessment do not reward self-directed learning, which is important for lifelong learning. In a traditional mastery-learning assessment approach there is not much to self-direct: everything is fixed and standardized through the stationary set of assessments.

To recap, traditional approaches to assessment can be characterized as rather reductionist. There is little information in the system, whereas promotion is completely based on discrete and stacked performance decisions (on *minimal* performance) often leading to unwanted educational side effects. This is worrisome because whenever there is a friction between the education goals and assessment goals, the latter tend to prevail. Hence, modern education programmes need a different approach to assessment.

Programmatic assessment

Programmatic assessment is based on a set of assessment principles that are derived from the research on assessment (van der Vleuten et al., 2010). Table 39.1 provides a summary.

A curriculum metaphor may help explain the concept of programmatic assessment. Where in the past a curriculum was the amalgamation of teachers' individual contributions, in modern programmes this is no longer the case. Nowadays, the curriculum is governed by a plan, which is implemented and evaluated to be finally rearranged. One makes a deliberate choice to address a topic over here to return to the topic over there. The sum is more than the whole of its parts. Likewise, programmatic assessment is based on an integral plan of assessment. Deliberate choices are made in terms of methods used and when to use them. The result is a variegated mix of methods that have been selected in accordance with their educational purpose at a particular moment in time and in relation to the assessment programme as a whole. Some will require verbalization, others synthesizing information, writing, reporting, performing, etc. The choices are deliberate because of the purposes they serve in the total programme. Like a curriculum, the assessment programme is evaluated and changes are made when needed. Fundamental to programmatic assessment is the elimination of pass/fail decisions from each individual assessment moment to be reintroduced only when sufficient information is gathered.

 Remove pass-fail decision making from individual data points.

Based on the principles of assessment (Table 39.1) and on earlier research on what makes a good assessment programme (Dijkstra et al., 2012), we have formulated the following pillars in programmatic assessment (van der Vleuten et al., 2012):

Each assessment represents but one data point. Recognizing the notion that any single assessment involves a compromise and that no perfect assessment exists that is able to optimize all quality elements of assessment, we regard each assessment as a single data point only.

Each data point is optimized for learning. For a single assessment, no compromise is made on the educational consequences. A single data point is optimized for learning. It is feedback-oriented, rich in nature – either in (profile) scores or words – meaningfully informing the learner, and authentic for the learning task. Sometimes the learning task itself is also assessed. The intent is to support and promote good learning and good learning strategies.

 Maximize meaningful feedback to the learner in individual data points.

The choice for a particular method depends entirely on the educational justification of this method in terms of the purpose it serves at a certain moment in time. There are no 'bad' methods. In the past, some methods were removed from the toolkit because they were considered to be too subjective (e.g. the oral exam or the long case). Subjectivity is not a problem if our prime purpose is to give feedback rather than make decisions (and multiple subjective judgements can be robust also; see principle 2, Table 39.1). When more complex skills need to be assessed, professional judgement is indispensable. Such judgements may also come from peers or patients. Agency and authenticity are essential elements in assessment programmes (Harrison et al., 2016). Any method – old or new – that accommodates these elements and that works educationally and meaningfully in the particular education context can be appropriate.

We advocate both course-related assessment *and* longitudinal or continuous assessment. Traditionally, course-related assessments dominate, but when a training programme relies on competency frameworks, attaching weight to the cultivation of domain-independent skills and personal development, more longitudinal assessment is required. Even knowledge can be assessed longitudinally, such as with progress testing (Wrigley et al., 2012).

Assessment consequences represent a continuum of stakes. In programmatic assessment the terms 'formative' and 'summative' are replaced by a continuum of stakes. This continuum ranges from low-stakes to high-stakes. A pass/fail decision is removed from a single data point, making the assessment low-stakes, which is not to be confused with 'no stakes'. The information from a low-stakes data point may be used later in higher-stakes decisions.

Stakes and number of data points are related. The higher the stakes of the decision, the more robust the information that is giving rise to the decision must be. A distinction is made between intermediate and final decisions. Intermediate decisions are made during the training programme, for example once or twice during the year. They are based on a number of data points. A decision can be expressed as a pass or fail or in any other qualification terminology. What is more important than the qualification is that intermediate decisions are also diagnostic (How is the learner progressing?), therapeutic (What remedies are needed?) and prognostic (What might happen with the learner?). Intermediate decisions may be followed by remediation, which is fundamentally different from re-take or re-sit assessments. Remediation is personal, and the learner will have to demonstrate the remediation has been carried out and has been effective. Final decisions are in order when a progression decision is needed (or selection or graduation decision). Final decisions are high-stakes and therefore based on many data points.

Table 39.1 Principles of assessment derived from past research, categorized into standardized and non-standardized assessment (van der Vleuten et al., 2010).

Standardised Assessment. Assessing 'knows', 'knows how', 'shows how' from Miller's pyramid	Description	Practical implications
1. Competence is context-specific, not generic	Any performance on a test element (item, case, oral, station, patient) is not very predictive of performance on another element, regardless of the method. This has been coined the 'content-specificity problem'. It relates back to the issue of transfer.	• Broadly sample performance across content within each assessment • Combine information across assessment or across time • Avoid high-stakes decision on a single assessment
2. Objectivity is not the same as reliability	Given the content-specificity, problem sampling is the dominant strategy for achieving reproducible test information. Subjective measures can be reliable, objective measures can be unreliable, all depending on the sampling.	• Use holistic professional judgement when it is needed • Use many subjective judgements in combination
3. What is being measured is more determined by the stimulus format than by the response format	The task given to the learner (stimulus format) in a test, much more than the way the response is captured, determines what the test is measuring. Different formats may measure similar or different things all depending on the stimulus format.	• Any method may assess higher-order skills • Produce stimulus formats that are as authentic as possible for the learning task (e.g. scenarios, cases etc.) • Use learning tasks as assessment tasks
4. Validity can be 'built-in'	Quality assurance measures in developing test material have a profound impact on the quality of the test material. Quality assurance can be done prior (e.g. item-writing), during (e.g. good instructions) and post-test (e.g. item and test analysis).	• Organize quality assurance cycles in item and test development • Use peer review • Use psychometric information • Use student input
Non-standardised Assessment. Assessing 'Does'	**Description**	**Practical implications**
5. Bias is an inherent characteristic of professional judgement	Whenever a judgement is made some bias will be introduced. Bias is *not* a reason to not use holistic professional judgement. Professional judgement is indispensable to assessing complex skills. Strategies to reduce bias should be used.	• Use sampling to reduce systematic errors • Use procedural measures of due diligence to reduce unsystematic errors and add to the credibility of the judgement (e.g. committee decisions, multiple cycles of feedback, learner agency in the decision process, etc.)
6. Validity lies in the users of the instruments, more than in the instruments	The seriousness with which the assessment is conducted defines the value of the assessment. Giving and receiving feedback is a skill. The people are therefore important.	• Prepare and train assessors and learners for their role in the assessment • Create working conditions that embed assessment possibilities
7. Qualitative, narrative information carries a lot of weight	For many assessment situations 'words' tell more than '"scores'. This is particularly true for complex skills such as the domain-independent skills.	• Use words for assessing complex skills • Be aware of unwanted side-effects of quantified information
8. Feedback use requires scaffolding	Feedback is often ignored, particularly in summative settings. Feedback use is promoted by the quality of the feedback, the credibility of the source, by reflection and by follow-up.	• Create feedback dialogues • Create feedback follow-up • Create meaningful relations between teacher and learners

Table 39.1 continued

Overall Assessment	Description	Practical implications
9. No single method is perfect	No single assessment method is able to cover all elements of Miller's pyramid. Any individual method will always involve a compromise.	• Vary in use of assessment methods • Combine information from multiple assessment sources
10. Assessment drives learning	The assessment dictates what and how the learner will learn. Any learner will optimize strategies for maximum success in the assessment.	• Verify the effect of assessment on learning • Use the effect strategically to promote desired learning effects

Data points can be compared to pixels in a photograph. Where an individual pixel will not tell you much, a combination of pixels will start to give an image. Sometimes a few pixels suffice to see the image clearly, while in other cases many more pixels are needed to arrive at the image. Information gathering and decision making are purposeful. Information is triangulated. Potential patterns emerge from the information. The stronger the pattern, the clearer the image becomes. Depending on the information, saturation will occur.

 High-stakes decisions should be based on many data points; consider that multiple pixels will provide a clearer image.

Learners are guided in feedback use. Feedback use and self-directed learning are promoted by creating a dialogue through social interaction. One powerful way to achieve this is through mentoring. Creating a trusting relationship with a respected person/teacher with whom all assessment and feedback information is shared and discussed is a very effective strategy for using feedback. Learners prepare meetings. They self-direct their learning through analysis of assessment and feedback data and in some cases set learning objectives to follow-up in subsequent assessment of feedback moments. When done well, learners will actually describe the image emerging from the pixels. Mentors ask questions, probe, stimulate deep reflection, discuss remediation activities, and support the learner in any other way possible. Yet, they are not psychotherapists. The focus is on learning and wellbeing, but there are limits to the personal support given, as mentoring is a resource-intensive activity. Alternative social interaction might be possible as well, such as peer groups and buddy systems (e.g. pairing senior with junior learners). The longer the personal relationship lasts the more effective the mentoring will be.

 Feedback use and self-directed learning require educational scaffolding through the creation of a dialogue between learner and entrusted teacher (mentor).

Aggregation of assessment through meaningful entities. Taking intermediate and final decisions implies that information must be aggregated. The traditional approach is to aggregate by method. For example, we aggregate information across stations of an OSCE. Yet, a meaningful relationship may not exist between these stations (e.g. history-taking and resuscitation), having us combine apples and oranges. Programmatic assessment, by contrast, aims for aggregation *across* methods to meaningful entities. For example, communication-related information is aggregated not only from the OSCE, but also from a multisource feedback (MSF) assessment and set of mini-CEXs. Having meaningful entities requires some overarching framework. This is often found in outcome systems and competency frameworks. They not only help us structure the curriculum, but also lend meaning to the assessment framework. It is important that instruments are structured according to the overarching framework. If not, meaningful aggregation will be complicated.

Due diligence procedural measures add to the trustworthiness of decision making. High-stakes decisions must be made with full confidence. The decision making on all pooled information cannot be a simple automated process. Often, both quantitative and qualitative information are available and simply averaging is not possible. Drawing inferences based on the 'picture' requires another professional judgement. To make this judgement robust or 'trustworthy' several measures can be taken. The first is to invest an appointed committee with decision-making responsibility, its members being sufficiently independent of learner and mentor. The committee weighs the information and deliberates to arrive at a well-founded decision. To be resource-efficient this appraisal process should be efficiently organized. The lion's share of the learners will not require much time or deliberation, but some cases will. Members of the committee may each prepare some of these cases. Basically, the level of expertise and number of assessors is tailored to the available information. When things are clear, little time investment is required, but when things are not, more investment is needed. The level of independence of the mentor will bolster the trustworthiness of decision making but also create a firewall dilemma as the mentor is the one who knows the learner best. Yet, if the mentor also decides on progress, his or her relationship with the learner may be jeopardized. A compromise could be to have mentors submit to the decision-making committee a recommendation that has been annotated by the learner. This will increase the agency of the learner and enrich the decision-making process with more information. Yet another alternative is that the mentor does not give a judgement at all, but merely confirms that the evidence presented is authentic for the learner.

Many other procedural measures can be taken to improve the trustworthiness of the decisions. The size of the committee and audit trail of the processes and assessment information will matter, as will the degree to which decisions can be justified. Also, the preceding intermediate decisions will play a role because they reduce the unpredictability of the final decision. External factors are appeal procedures and the use of standards or milestones available. Finally, calibration of the assessors in the committee by training sessions or by discussing exceptional cases afterwards is pertinent. This is only a dip into the wealth of possible measures for due diligence around the decision making. Together they will bolster confidence in essentially what constitutes a human judgement.

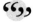

"In making high-stake decisions based on aggregated information, protection could be provided by installing procedures that surpass the 'power' of the individual assessor."

van der Vleuten et al., 2010

The forenamed seven pillars support programmatic assessment with its purpose of optimizing both the learning and the decision-making aspects of assessment. Learning is promoted by focusing on feedback, learner guidance, growth and development, and self-directed learning. The decision making is robust in that it is based on a multitude of data points, significant expertise of the decision makers and richness in the data. Such information is stronger than a single examination, however big. Finally, programmatic assessment optimizes curriculum evaluation including the assessment system. Mentors will have a thorough impression of what is happening where in the curriculum. As such, they are an excellent source of information for curriculum improvement. In this chapter we have deliberately used the term 'optimization' to refer specifically to the optimization of the whole assessment process, as it can hardly be achieved in a single assessment alone.

An example

To demonstrate how programmatic assessment finds expression, in the following we will offer an example

from practice. We will not discuss one of the first programmes, the Cleveland Clinic Lerner College of Medicine programme (Dannefer & Henson, 2007), or the many other practices that have emerged since, both at the undergraduate and postgraduate level and in and outside medicine. Instead, we will describe a programme we have experienced at first hand: the graduate entry programme in medicine at Maastricht University.

This graduate entry programme is a 4-year training programme that leads not only to an MD but also, through a pronounced emphasis on research skills, to a second degree of Master of Science in clinical research. So it is, in fact, a 4-year double-degree programme. The curriculum is structured according to the CanMEDS competencies. Didactically, the first year offers classical PBL, the second year offers a form of PBL based on real patients, the third year contains clinical rotations, and the final year consists of a long-term research participation in the context of a healthcare participation of choice. Students are selected by an MMI-type selection procedure and have at least a bachelor's degree in one of the biomedical sciences. Expectations are high, and students know they have to work hard to be successful.

The assessment programme consists of module-related assessments in the first 2 years and a cross-modular longitudinal assessment. Module-related assessments employ a multitude of different methods: MCQs, open-ended questions, assignments, projects, (mini) OSCEs et cetera. Some modules have a series of mini-tests. In the second year, learners write reports on patient cases and mostly take oral exams that are tailored to their individual experiences. Assessment in the last 2 years is comprised of an elaborate system of work-based assessment using Mini-CEX, OSATS, field notes, and MSF instruments. The longitudinal assessment includes a system of progress testing, which is a kind of final examination in the cognitive domain. It is a written test (200 MCQs) and includes questions from all disciplines and all organ system categories. The test is administered four times per year to all the students in the curriculum. Of course, junior-year students will not be able to answer as many questions as their more seasoned counterparts will, but we do not expect them to. Every 3 months a new test is constructed with new items. For students it is almost impossible to strategically revise for the test, nor do we want them to because anything could be asked. Instead, regular study activity is rewarded because it typically leads to better scores and less stress. For the assessment of the domain-independent CanMEDS competencies, reliance is placed on periodic peer and tutor assessment. The work-based assessment in years 3 and 4 is both module-related and longitudinal. Information is transmitted from one rotation to the other, as in a continuity-of-care approach. Professional behaviour is assessed against end-of-graduation performance.

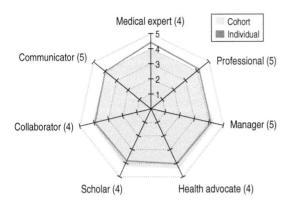

Fig. 39.1 A spider diagram presenting aggregate information from multiple data points on the discrete CanMEDS competencies. Individual performance is related to cohort performance. The number in brackets represents the number of observations.

All assessments are low-stakes; no credit points (European Credit Transfer Accumulation System [ECTS] points in Europe) are awarded to individual assessments. Yet, they are informative, with considerable attention being paid to feedback that may take the form of scores and/or words. For example, learners may review their own performance on an individual progress test or their progress made over the years, as can be gleaned from a series of consecutive tests, online. In doing so, they can select any type of result (e.g. regarding a particular discipline or organ system category). Individual performance is also set against year class performance to enable learners to make thorough analyses of their knowledge base as they progress through the curriculum. The spider diagram in Fig. 39.1 illustrates how feedback is given in years 3 and 4 as part of work-based assessment. In this case, the feedback is presented as a summary of overall performance, while in fact various kinds of graphical overviews can be generated. A student can easily access the underlying individual data points in these graphs and review the original assessment form that reports all quantitative and qualitative information. Finally, summary overviews of narrative information can be generated. All assessment information and all other relevant material are stored in an e-portfolio by the learner or are generated automatically through the e-portfolio assessment services (e.g. in managing an MSF round).

Every learner is assigned a mentor for the entire 4-year study period. This mentor is a regular faculty member overseeing a group of 5 to 10 learners. The mentor has full access to the e-portfolio and has regular meetings with the learners. To prepare these meetings, students write reports reflecting on their progress, and formulate and follow up on study plans or learning objectives based on the evidence included in the portfolio. At the end of the year, the mentor writes a recommendation for promotion to the next year, which is supplemented with a second recommendation put forward by all mentors collectively. In this latter recommendation, however, the learner's personal mentor has no say. The final decision on promotion is taken by an independent portfolio assessment committee. In the event a positive judgement is passed, the student is awarded all credit points (in our case, 60 ECTS per year).

This programmatic approach to assessment has served the programme well. Students have become real feedback seekers and are self-regulating their learning. Results on the progress tests are impressive compared to those of other medical training programmes (Heeneman et al., 2016). Teachers enjoy working with these students. Mentorship is considered a most rewarding role. Many learners publish their research work and some 50% of graduates pursue a PhD. The graduate entry programme has a yearly student intake of 50. We have currently implemented a similar programmatic approach in the much larger undergraduate medical training programme that accepts 340 students per year.

Implementing programmatic assessment

Though programmatic assessment is grounded in research, research has yet to demonstrate if and why it is successful. This research is ongoing. A number of findings have emerged from this research and our experiences so far.

The transition from a traditional system to one that is based on programmatic assessment is a major change comparable to moving from a traditional curriculum to a PBL curriculum. It requires a different mindset of teachers and learners. The prerogative of the individual teacher to fail a learner in the course where the responsibility rests with the teacher is a deeply rooted tradition. Many universities have university-wide assessment regulations and grading systems in place that can often undermine change. Like in any other major education change, good change management is foundational. More specifically, effective change requires appropriate top-down and bottom-up strategies, which, in turn, calls for effective leadership. Faculty training is equally important. Training faculty on the job and just in time can help them make this change effectively. Exposure to programmes that have successfully made such change or following a course on programmatic assessment may accelerate the process. Teachers learn in the same way as our learners do, so all our knowledge on how to facilitate learning equally applies to them. It will not work to just give them the information, as was the case with our learners. Just like PBL can have many manifestations, so might programmatic assessment. Some elements that are easier to implement, or that address a certain need in a particular organization, might create effective hybrids.

 Programmatic assessment is a major innovation that requires a change management policy.

Getting the quality of the feedback right is what poses a challenge in programmatic assessment. The provision of feedback requires time, which is always lacking. Moreover, it is a skill that can be learned and therefore it may help to train learners and teachers alike. Similarly, feedback on feedback may help, as may the application of modern tools (apps) and software that facilitate feedback.

A recurrent finding is that learners do not perceive low-stakes assessment as low-stakes as intended. Programmatic assessment also involves a culture change. Any measure that reduces the 'stick' effect of the assessment is appropriate. This starts with good communication with all stakeholders about the purpose of low-stakes assessment with respect to learners. Some schools that have introduced programmatic assessment include re-take assessment (we have some in our programme), which inherently raises the stakes of the assessment.

Programmatic assessment can be applied to any part of the medical training continuum, although it seems to fit in most naturally with education that stresses experiential learning. This fit can probably be explained by the emphasis that is placed in experiential learning on non-cognitive and complex skills.

As may be clear, we have not used the standard language that often dominates the assessment discourse. Programmatic assessment introduces a take on assessment that differs from the more conventional psychometric view. This does not mean we are antagonistic to psychometric analysis of the assessments being used. As principle 4 in Table 39.1 has demonstrated, quality assurance is integral to good assessment. Psychometricians sometimes play an important role in serving that purpose, but they consider one perspective only. There are at least two other perspectives to programmatic assessment. One concerns education. The purpose is to train qualified professionals in an educationally optimal way. What becomes essential, then, is to foster engagement in learners, which can be achieved by giving them challenging tasks, autonomy, gratifying social relations and personal guidance. Consequently, learning will drive assessment, not the other way around, precisely how it should be. A second perspective is about qualitative inquiry (Govaerts & van der Vleuten, 2013). Qualitative inquiry has its own methodological conventions to deal with complexity. We have used many words that stem from this methodology. One could actually say that programmatic assessment is a mixed-method inquiry into a learner's achievements in a training programme using a multitude of

quantitative and qualitative sources. It involves giving meaning to an individual person's development in an academic trajectory.

 "We should aim for careful balancing of quantitative and qualitative approaches in our assessment programmes, justifying our choices on the basis of assessment purposes as well as conceptualisations of learning and performance/ competence."

Govaerts & van der Vleuten, 2013

Summary

Programmatic assessment considers assessment as an optimization problem. For individual assessments, learning is optimized by selecting a method of assessment that is maximally aligned with the learning task and that provides meaningful feedback to the learner. Decision making is optimized by gathering rich information across many assessment moments in such a way that solid conclusions can be made about the progress of a learner. When implemented well, programmatic assessment may bring substantial benefits. The mushrooming of competency-based education makes it imperative that assessment be closely aligned with education, and we would argue that programmatic assessment can help achieve just that.

References

Cilliers, F.J., Schuwirth, L.W., Herman, N., et al., 2012. A model of the pre-assessment learning effects of summative assessment in medical education. Adv. Health Sci. Educ. Theory Pract. 17, 39–53.

Dannefer, E.F., Henson, L.C., 2007. The portfolio approach to competency-based assessment at the Cleveland Clinic Lerner College of Medicine. Acad. Med. 82, 493–502.

Dijkstra, J., Galbraith, R., Hodges, B.D., et al., 2012. Expert validation of fit-for-purpose guidelines for designing programmes of assessment. BMC Med. Educ. 12, 20.

Govaerts, M.J.B., van der Vleuten, C.P.M., 2013. Validity in work-based assessment: expanding our horizons. Med. Educ. 47, 1164–1174.

Harrison, C.J., Könings, K.D., Dannefer, E.F., et al., 2016. Factors influencing students' receptivity to formative feedback emerging from different assessment cultures. Persp. on Med. Educ. 5, 276–284.

Heeneman, S., Schut, S., Donkers, J., et al., 2016. Embedding of the progress test in an assessment program designed according to the principles of programmatic assessment. Med. Teach. 1–9.

Miller, G.E., 1990. The Assessment of clinical skills/competence/performance. Acad. Med. 65, S63–S67.

Shute, V.J., 2008. Focus on formative feedback. Rev. Educ. Res. 78, 153–189.

van der Vleuten, C.P., Schuwirth, L.W., Driessen, E.W., et al., 2012. A model for programmatic assessment fit for purpose. Med. Teach. 34, 205–214.

van der Vleuten, C.P., Schuwirth, L.W., Scheele, F., et al., 2010. The assessment of professional competence: building blocks for theory development. Best Pract. Res. Clin. Obstet. Gynaecol. 24, 703–719.

van der Vleuten, C.P.M., 1996. The assessment of professional competence: developments, research and practical implications. Adv. Health Sci. Educ. Theory Pract. 1, 41–67.

Vandewaetere, M., Manhaeve, D., Aertgeerts, B., et al., 2015. 4C/ID in medical education: How to design an educational program based on whole-task learning: AMEE Guide No. 93. Med. Teach. 37, 4–20.

Wrigley, W., van der Vleuten, C.P., Freeman, A., Muijtjens, A., 2012. A systemic framework for the progress test: strengths, constraints and issues: AMEE Guide No. 71. Med. Teach. 34, 683–697.

Section 6

Staff

40

Staff development

Y. Steinert

Trends

- Staff development is a critical component in promoting innovation and excellence in medical education.
- Longitudinal programmes, which have increased in prominence in the last decade, yield broader and more sustainable outcomes.
- Learning in the workplace – and belonging to a community of practice – should be recognized as an important aspect of staff development.
- Mentorship plays a key role in the successful development of medical teachers.
- To maximize its benefits, staff development should focus on organizational change and development.

Introduction

Staff development, or faculty development as it is often called, has become an increasingly important component of medical education. Staff development activities have been designed to improve teacher effectiveness at all levels of the educational continuum (e.g. undergraduate, postgraduate and continuing medical education) and diverse programmes have been offered to healthcare professionals in many settings.

For the purpose of this discussion, staff development will refer to that broad range of activities that institutions use to renew or assist faculty in their roles (Centra, 1978). That is, staff development is viewed as a planned activity designed to *prepare* institutions and faculty members for their various roles (Bland et al., 1990) and to *improve* an individual's knowledge and skills in the areas of teaching, research and administration (Sheets & Schwenk, 1990). The goal of staff development in this context is to teach faculty members the skills relevant to their institutional and faculty position, to complement informal learning that occurs in the workplace, and to sustain medical teachers' vitality, both now and in the future.

 "It goes without saying that no man can teach successfully who is not at the same time a student."

Sir William Osler

Although a comprehensive staff development programme includes attention to all faculty roles, including research, writing and leadership, the focus of this chapter will be on staff development for teaching improvement. The first section will review common practices and challenges as well as learning in the workplace; the second section will provide some practical guidelines for individuals interested in the design, delivery and evaluation of formal (structured) staff development programmes.

Common practices and challenges

Knowledge of key content areas, common educational formats, frequently encountered challenges, and programme effectiveness will help to guide the design and delivery of innovative staff development programmes. These topics are discussed below.

KEY CONTENT AREAS

The majority of staff development programmes focus on teaching improvement. That is, they aim to improve teachers' skills in clinical teaching, small-group facilitation, large-group presentations, feedback and evaluation (Steinert et al., 2006). They also target teaching conceptions and learning approaches (Steinert et al., 2016) as well as specific core competencies (e.g. the teaching and evaluation of professionalism), emerging educational priorities (e.g. social accountability, cultural awareness and humility, patient safety), curriculum design and development and the use of technology in teaching and learning. In fact, many of the chapters in this book could become the focus of a staff development programme.

At the same time, less attention has been paid to the personal development of healthcare professionals, educational leadership and scholarship, and organizational development and change. Although instructional effectiveness at the individual level is critically important, a more comprehensive approach to staff development should be considered. That is, we need to develop individuals who will be able to provide leadership to educational programmes, act as educational mentors and design and deliver innovative educational programmes. Staff development also has a significant role to play in promoting teaching as a scholarly activity, and in creating an educational climate that encourages and rewards educational leadership, innovation and excellence. Irrespective of the specific focus, we should remember that staff development can serve as a useful instrument in the promotion of organizational change and that medical schools play a fundamental role in the design and delivery of this essential activity. As McLean and colleagues (2008) have said, "Faculty development is not a luxury. It is an imperative for every medical school."

To date, the majority of staff development programmes have focused on the medical teacher. Staff development initiatives should also target curriculum planners responsible for the design and delivery of educational programmes, administrators responsible for education and practice, and all healthcare professionals involved in teaching and learning (Steinert, 2014). Moreover, although staff development is primarily a voluntary activity, some medical schools now require participation in this type of professional development as they increasingly recognize the 'professionalization' of teaching.

 "The one task that is distinctively related to being a faculty member is teaching; all other tasks can be pursued in other settings; and yet, paradoxically, the central responsibility of faculty members is typically the one for which they are least prepared."

Jason & Westberg, 1982

Staff development also needs to target the organization that supports teaching and learning. For example, staff development can work to promote a culture change by helping to develop institutional policies that support and reward excellence in teaching, encourage a re-examination of criteria for academic promotion, and create networking opportunities for junior faculty members. Clearly, we need to target the organizational climate and culture in which teachers work in order to be successful.

EDUCATIONAL FORMATS

The most common staff development formats include workshops and longitudinal programmes (Steinert et al., 2016). Workshops are one of the most popular formats because of their inherent flexibility and promotion of

active learning. In fact, faculty members value a variety of teaching methods within this format, including interactive lectures, small-group discussions, and experiential learning. Longitudinal programmes typically consist of multiple components, including university courses, monthly seminars, independent projects and participation in a variety of staff development activities, and they have particular appeal because teachers can continue to practice and teach while improving their educational knowledge and skills. Longitudinal programmes also have the ability to enhance educational leadership and scholarship, while promoting a sense of community among programme participants. At the same time, given the ever-changing needs and priorities of medical schools and healthcare professionals, we should consider additional formats for staff development, including decentralized activities, self-directed learning, peer coaching, online learning and mentoring, all of which are outlined below. We should also remember that staff development can occur along two dimensions (Fig. 40.1) from individual (independent) experiences to group (collective) learning, and from informal approaches to more formal ones (Steinert, 2010). Many healthcare professionals learn through experience, by 'doing' and reflecting on that experience; others learn from peer or student feedback, while work-based learning and belonging to a community of practice is key for others. Although the medical school (as an institution) is primarily responsible for the organization of more formal (structured) activities, we must be aware of the powerful learning that can occur in informal settings, most notably the workplace.

 "The greatest difficulty in life is to make knowledge effective, to convert it into practical wisdom."

Sir William Osler

Decentralized activities

Staff development programmes are often departmentally based or centrally organized (i.e. faculty-wide). Given the increasing reliance on community preceptors and ambulatory sites for teaching, staff development programmes should be 'exported' outside of the academic setting. Decentralized, site-specific activities have the added advantage of reaching individuals who may not otherwise attend staff development activities and can help to develop a departmental culture of self-improvement.

Self-directed learning

Self-directed learning initiatives are not frequently described in the staff development literature. However, there is a clear place for self-directed learning that promotes 'reflection in action' and 'reflection on action', skills that are critical to effective teaching and learning

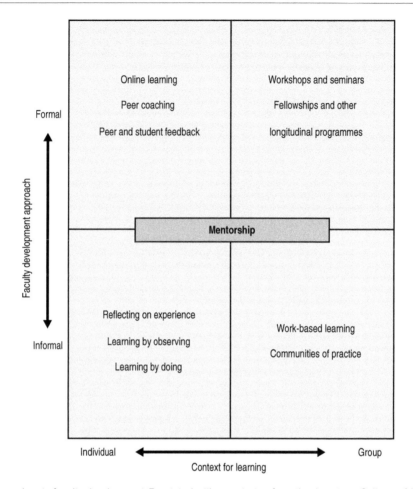

Fig. 40.1 Approaches to faculty development. Reprinted with permission from the American College of Physicians.

(Schön, 1983). As Ullian and Stritter (1997) have said, teachers should be encouraged to determine their own needs through self-reflection, student evaluation and peer feedback, and they should learn to design their own development activities. Self-directed learning activities have been used extensively in continuing medical education (CME); staff development programmes should build on these experiences.

Peer coaching

Peer coaching as a method of faculty development has been described extensively in the educational literature. Key elements of peer coaching include the identification of individual learning goals (e.g. improving specific teaching skills), focused observation of teaching by colleagues, and the provision of feedback, analysis and support (Flynn et al., 1994). This underutilized approach, sometimes called co-teaching or peer observation, has particular appeal because it occurs in the teacher's own practice setting, enables individualized learning and fosters collaboration. It also allows healthcare professionals to learn about each other as they teach together, helping to promote interprofessional education and practice.

Online learning

Online learning and computer-aided instruction is closely tied to self-directed learning. As time for professional development is limited, and the technology to create interactive instructional programmes is now in place, the use of online staff development should be explored. In many ways, online resources could be considered as supplements to centrally organized activities as they enable individualized learning targeting specific needs (Cook and Steinert, 2013); they can also be used in a 'staged approach', later in the development of medical teachers, as long as we do not lose sight of the value and importance of working in context, with our colleagues.

Mentorship

Mentoring is a common strategy to promote the socialization, development and maturation of academic medical faculty (Bland et al., 1990). It is also a valuable, but underutilized, staff development strategy.

Mentors can provide guidance, direction, support or expertise to faculty members on a range of topics, in a variety of settings. They can also help teachers to understand the organizational culture in which they are working and introduce them to invaluable professional networks (Schor et al., 2011). In fact, medical teachers often report that finding a mentor – and being mentored – is critical to personal and academic success; effective mentorship has also been shown to increase career satisfaction and reduce faculty burnout (Boillat and Elizov, 2014). Daloz (1986) has described a mentorship model that balances three key elements: support, challenge and a vision of the individual's future career. This model can serve as a helpful framework in staff development. The value of role models and mentors has been highlighted since Osler's time, and we should not forget the benefits of this method of professional development despite new technologies and methodologies.

 "Mentoring is vital to create new leaders and new kinds of leadership."

Anderson, 1999

 "We must find new ways to help faculty adapt to their new roles and responsibilities while coping with the day-to-day demands that these changes bring."

Ullian & Stritter, 1997

LEARNING IN THE WORKPLACE

The role of informal learning in the workplace is integral to staff development. In fact, it is in the everyday workplace, where teachers conduct their clinical, teaching and research activities, that learning most often takes place (Swanwick, 2008). It is surprising, therefore, that work-based learning is not seen as a common venue for staff development, for it is through teaching in hospital or community settings that teachers acquire new knowledge and refine their approaches to teaching and learning. Staff development activities have traditionally been conducted away from teachers' workplaces, requiring participants to take their 'lessons learned' back to their own contexts. It is time to reverse this trend and think about how we can enhance the learning that takes place in authentic settings; there is also value in rendering this learning as visible as possible so that it can be recognized as an important component of staff development. A pedagogy of the workplace includes individual engagement, sequencing of activities to create pathways for learning, the provision of guidance to promote learning, environmental affordances that enable access to learning, and reflection and role modelling (Billett, 2002). These characteristics also describe key features of staff development.

Closely related to work-based learning is the notion of a community of practice. Barab and colleagues (2002) have defined a community of practice as a "persistent, sustaining, social network of individuals who share and develop an overlapping knowledge base, set of beliefs, values, history and experiences focused on a common practice and/or mutual enterprise." In many ways, becoming a member of a teaching community can be viewed as an approach to faculty development, and we should collectively explore ways to make this community – and the learning that it offers – more accessible to medical teachers. We should also find ways of creating new opportunities for networking and collegial support and valuing the community of which we are a part.

FREQUENTLY ENCOUNTERED CHALLENGES

Staff development programmes cannot be designed or delivered in isolation from other factors that include institutional support, organizational goals and priorities, resources for programme planning and individual needs and expectations. Common challenges faced by faculty developers include defining goals and priorities; balancing individual and organizational needs; motivating faculty to participate in staff development initiatives; obtaining institutional support and 'buy in'; promoting a 'culture change' that reflects renewed interest in teaching and learning; and overcoming limited human and financial resources. As motivating faculty to participate in staff development is one of the key challenges, it will be discussed in greater detail.

Teachers differ from students and residents in a number of ways. They have more life experiences, they have more self-entrenched behaviours, and change may be seen as a greater threat. In addition, motivation for learning cannot be assumed and time for learning is not routinely allocated. Staff development programmes must address these challenges. Teachers do *not* participate in staff development activities for a variety of reasons. Some do not view teaching – or teaching improvement – as important, others do not perceive a need for improvement or feel that their institution does not support or value these activities. Many are not aware of the benefits (or availability) of staff development programmes and activities. We must be cognizant of all these factors in programme planning.

To motivate faculty, we need to develop a culture that promotes and encourages professional development, consider multiple approaches to achieving the same goal, tailor programmes to meet individual and organizational needs and ensure relevant and 'high-quality' activities. We must also build a network of interested individuals, encourage the dissemination of information, utilize student feedback to illustrate need, recognize participation in staff development and, if possible, provide 'release time'. Whenever possible, it is also helpful to link staff development activities with ongoing programmes (e.g. hospital rounds, CME events), to provide a range of methods for learning, and to offer free and flexible programming. Organizational support for staff development is also critical, as are strategies that target organizational norms and values (e.g. recognizing the importance of teaching and learning).

 "The goal of faculty development is to empower faculty members to excel in their role as educators and, in so doing, to create organizations that encourage and reward continual learning."

Wilkerson & Irby, 1998

PROGRAMME EFFECTIVENESS

Despite numerous descriptions of staff development programmes, there has been a paucity of research demonstrating the effectiveness of most faculty development activities (Steinert et al., 2006; Steinert et al., 2016). Few programmes have conducted comprehensive evaluations, and data to support the efficacy of many initiatives have been lacking. Of the studies that have been conducted in this area, the majority has assessed participant satisfaction; some have explored changes in cognitive learning or performance, and several have examined the long-term impact of these interventions. Although most of the research has relied on self-report rather than objective outcome measures or observations of change, methods to evaluate staff development programmes have included end-of-session evaluations; follow-up survey questionnaires; pre- and post-assessments of cognitive or attitudinal change; direct observations of teaching behaviour; student evaluations; and faculty self-ratings of post-training performance. Common problems have included a lack of control or comparison groups, heavy reliance on self-report measures of change, small sample sizes and infrequent use of qualitative methodologies.

Despite these limitations, we do know that staff development activities have been rated highly by participants and that teachers regard the experience as useful, recommending participation to their colleagues. A number of studies have also demonstrated an impact on teachers' knowledge, skills and attitudes, and several have shown changes in student behaviour as a result of staff participation in faculty development programmes (Steinert et al., 2006; Steinert et al., 2016). Other benefits have included increased personal interest and enthusiasm; improved self-confidence; a greater sense of belonging to a community; and educational leadership and innovation (Steinert et al., 2003).

 "My view of myself as a teacher has changed from an information provider to a 'director' of learning."

McGill, Teaching Scholar

The challenge in this area is to conduct more rigorous evaluations of staff development initiatives from the outset, to consider diverse models of programme evaluation, to make use of qualitative research methods and to broaden the focus of the evaluation itself. In no other area is the need to collaborate or transcend disciplinary boundaries greater.

 "I leave rejuvenated and ready to go out and teach a thousand students again!"

McGill, Teaching Scholar

Designing a staff development programme

The following guidelines are intended to help individuals design and deliver effective staff development programmes. They are also based on the premise that the medical school has a critical role to play in providing institutional leadership, appropriate resource allocation and recognition of teaching excellence (McLean et al., 2008).

UNDERSTAND THE INSTITUTIONAL/ ORGANIZATIONAL CULTURE

Staff development programmes take place within the context of a specific institution or organization. It is imperative to understand the culture of that institution and be responsive to its needs. Staff developers should capitalize on the organization's strengths and work with the leadership to ensure success. In many ways, the cultural context can be used to promote or enhance staff development efforts. For example, staff development during times of educational or curricular reform can take on added importance (Rubeck & Witzke, 1998). It is also important to assess institutional support for staff development activities and lobby effectively. Staff development cannot occur in a vacuum.

 Capitalize on the institution's strengths, and promote organizational change and development.

DETERMINE APPROPRIATE GOALS AND PRIORITIES

As with the design of any other programme, it is imperative to clearly define goals and priorities. What is the programme trying to achieve? And why is it important to do so? Carefully determining goals and objectives will influence the choice of activity, programme content and methodology. Moreover, although determining priorities is not always easy, it is essential to balance individual and organizational needs.

CONDUCT NEEDS ASSESSMENTS TO ENSURE RELEVANT PROGRAMMING

As stated earlier, staff development programmes should base themselves on the needs of the individual as well as the institution. Student needs, patient needs and societal needs may all help to direct relevant activities. Assessing needs is necessary to refine goals, determine content, identify preferred learning formats and assure relevance. It is also a way of promoting early 'buy in'. Common methods include written questionnaires or surveys; interviews or focus groups with key informants (e.g. participants, students, educational leaders); observations of teachers 'in action'; literature reviews; and environmental scans of available programmes and resources. Whenever possible, it is worth acquiring information from multiple sources and distinguishing between 'needs' and 'wants'. Clearly, an individual teacher's perceived needs may differ from those expressed by their students or peers. Needs assessments can also help to further translate goals into objectives, which will serve as the basis for programme planning and evaluation of outcome.

 Assess needs to refine goals, determine content, identify preferred learning formats and promote 'buy in'.

DEVELOP DIFFERENT PROGRAMMES TO ACCOMMODATE DIVERSE NEEDS

Different educational formats have been described in an earlier section. Clearly, medical schools must design programmes that accommodate diverse goals and objectives, content areas, and the needs of the individual and the organization. For example, if the goal is to improve faculty members' lecturing skills, a half-day workshop on interactive lecturing might be the programme of choice. On the other hand, if the goal is to promote educational leadership and scholarly activity among peers, a teaching scholars programme (e.g. Steinert et al., 2003) or educational fellowship might be the preferred format. In this context, it is also helpful to remember that staff development can include development, orientation, recognition and support, and different programmes are required to accommodate diverse objectives. Programme content and methods must also change over time to adapt to evolving needs.

INCORPORATE PRINCIPLES OF ADULT LEARNING AND INSTRUCTIONAL DESIGN

Adults come to learning situations with a variety of motivations and expectations about teaching methods and goals. Key principles of adult learning (e.g. Knowles, 1980) include the following:
- Adults are independent.
- Adults come to learning situations with a variety of motivations and definite expectations about particular learning goals and teaching methods.
- Adults demonstrate different learning styles.
- Much of adult learning is 're-learning' rather than new learning.

- Adult learning often involves changes in attitudes as well as skills.
- Most adults prefer to learn through experience.
- Incentives for adult learning usually come from within the individual.
- Feedback is usually more important than tests and evaluations.

Incorporation of these principles into the design of a staff development programme can enhance receptivity, relevance and engagement. In fact, these principles should guide the development of all programmes, irrespective of their focus or format, as physicians and other healthcare professionals demonstrate a high degree of self-direction. They also possess numerous experiences that should serve as the basis for learning.

 Incorporate principles of adult learning to enhance receptivity, relevance and engagement.

Principles of instructional design should also be followed. For example, it is important to develop clear learning goals and objectives, identify key content areas, design appropriate teaching and learning strategies and create appropriate methods of evaluation (of both the students and the curriculum) (Fig. 40.2). It is equally important to integrate theory with practice and to ensure that the learning is perceived as relevant to the work setting and to the profession. Learning should be interactive, participatory and experientially based, using the participants' previous learning and experience as a starting point, and a positive environment for learning should be maintained. Detailed planning and organization involving all stakeholders are also critical.

OFFER A DIVERSITY OF EDUCATIONAL METHODS

In line with principles of adult learning, staff development programmes should try to offer a variety of educational methods that promote experiential learning,

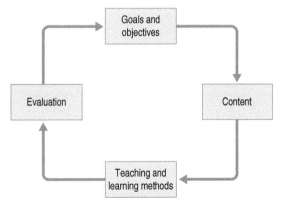

Fig. 40.2 The education cycle.

reflection, feedback and immediacy of application. Common learning methods include interactive lectures, case presentations, small-group exercises and discussions, role plays and simulations, videotape reviews and live demonstrations. (Many of these methods are described in earlier sections of this book.) Practise with feedback is also essential, as is the opportunity to reflect on personal values and attitudes. Online modules, debates and reaction panels, journal clubs, independent study and research projects are additional methods to consider. In line with our previous example, a workshop on interactive lecturing might include interactive plenaries, small-group discussions and exercises and opportunities for practise and feedback. A fellowship programme might include group seminars, independent projects and structured readings. Whatever the method, the needs and learning preferences of the participants must be respected, and the method should match the objective.

 Promote experiential learning, reflection, feedback and immediacy of application.

PROMOTE 'BUY IN' AND MARKET EFFECTIVELY

The decision to participate in a staff development programme or activity is not as simple as it might at first appear. It involves the individual's reaction to a particular offering, motivation to develop or enhance a specific skill, being available at the time of the session and overcoming the psychological barrier of admitting need (Rubeck & Witzke, 1998). As faculty developers, it is our challenge to overcome reluctance and to market our 'product' in such a way that resistance becomes a resource to learning. In our context, we have seen the value of targeted publicity, professionally designed brochures and 'branding' of our product to promote interest. Continuing education credits, as well as free and flexible programming, can also help to facilitate motivation and attendance. 'Buy in' involves agreement on importance, widespread support, and dedication of time and resources at both the individual and the systems level and must be considered in all programming initiatives.

WORK TO OVERCOME COMMONLY ENCOUNTERED CHALLENGES

Common implementation problems such as a lack of institutional support, limited resources, and limited faculty time have been discussed in an earlier section. Faculty developers must work to overcome these problems through creative programming, skilled marketing, targeted fundraising, and the delivery of high-quality programmes. Flexible scheduling and collaborative programming, which address clearly identified needs, will help to ensure success at a systems level.

PREPARE STAFF DEVELOPERS

The recruitment and preparation of staff developers are rarely reported. However, it is important to recruit carefully, train effectively, partner creatively and build on previous experiences. Faculty members can be involved in a number of ways: as co-facilitators, programme planners or consultants. In our own setting, we try to involve new faculty members in each staff development activity and conduct a preparatory meeting (or 'dry run') to review content and process, solicit feedback and promote 'ownership'. We also conclude each activity with a 'debriefing' session to discuss lessons learned and plan for the future. Whenever possible, staff developers should be individuals who are well-respected by their peers and have some educational expertise and experience in facilitating groups. It has been said that 'to teach is to learn twice'; this principle is clearly one of the motivating factors that influence staff developers.

 "I was given new tools to teach. Not only were they described to me in words, but they were also used in front of me and I was part and parcel of the demonstration."

McGill, Teaching Scholar

EVALUATE – AND DEMONSTRATE – EFFECTIVENESS

The need to evaluate staff development programmes and activities is clear. In fact, we must remember that the evaluation of staff development is more than an academic exercise, and our findings must be used in the design, delivery and marketing of our programmes. It has been stated earlier that staff development must help to promote education as a scholarly activity; we must role model this approach in all that we do.

In preparing to evaluate a staff development programme or activity, we should consider the goal of the evaluation (e.g. programme planning versus decision making; policy formation versus academic inquiry), available data sources (e.g. participants, peers, students or residents), common methods of evaluation (e.g. questionnaires, focus groups, objective tests, observations), resources to support assessment (e.g. institutional support, research grants) and models of programme evaluation (e.g. goal attainment, decision facilitation). Kirkpatrick and Kirkpatrick's (2006) levels of evaluation are also helpful in conceptualizing and framing the assessment of outcome. They include the following:

- **Reaction:** participants' views on the learning experience
- **Learning:** changes in participants' attitudes, knowledge or skills
- **Behaviour:** changes in participants' behaviour
- **Results:** changes in the organizational system, the patient or the learner.

At a minimum, a practical and feasible evaluation should include an assessment of utility and relevance, content, teaching and learning methods and intent to change. Moreover, as evaluation is an integral part of programme planning, it should be conceptualized at the beginning of any programme. It should also include qualitative and quantitative assessments of learning and behaviour change, using a variety of methods and data sources.

 Evaluate effectively and ensure that research will inform practice.

Summary

Academic vitality is dependent upon faculty members' interests and expertise. Staff development has a critical role to play in promoting academic excellence and innovation. In looking to the future, we should focus on content areas that go beyond the improvement of specific teaching skills and include educational leadership and scholarship, and academic and career development; adopt diverse educational formats such as workshops and integrated longitudinal programmes, decentralized activities, self-directed learning and peer coaching; consider the benefits of work-based learning and communities of practice in promoting staff development as well as the value of staff development in fostering a sense of community; use staff development programmes and activities to promote organizational change and development; and evaluate the effectiveness of all that we do so that practice informs research and research can inform practice. We should also remain innovative and flexible so that we can accommodate the ever-changing needs of our teachers, our institutions and the healthcare systems in which we work.

 "A medical school's most important asset is its faculty."

Whitcomb, 2003

References

Anderson, P.C., 1999. Mentoring. Acad. Med. 74 (1), 4–5.

Barab, S.A., Barnett, M., Squire, K., 2002. Developing an empirical account of a community of practice: characterizing the essential tensions. J. Learn. Sci. 11 (4), 489–542.

Billett, S., 2002. Toward a workplace pedagogy: guidance, participation, and engagement. Adult Educ. Q. 53 (1), 27–43.

Bland, C.J., Schmitz, C.C., Stritter, F.T., et al. (Eds.), 1990. Successful Faculty in Academic Medicine: Essential Skills and How to Acquire them. Springer Publishing Company, New York.

Boillat, M., Elizov, M., 2014. Peer coaching and mentorship. In: Steinert, Y. (Ed.), Faculty Development in the Health Professions: A Focus on Research and Practice. Springer, Dordrecht, the Netherlands.

Centra, J.A., 1978. Types of faculty development programs. J. Higher Educ. 49 (2), 151–162.

Cook, D.A., Steinert, Y., 2013. Online learning for faculty development: a review of the literature. Med. Teach. 35 (11), 930–937.

Daloz, L.A., 1986. Effective Teaching and Mentoring. Jossey-Bass, San Francisco.

Flynn, S.P., Bedinghaus, J., Snyder, C., Hekelman, F., 1994. Peer coaching in clinical teaching: a case report. Fam. Med. 26 (9), 569–570.

Jason, H., Westberg, J., 1982. Teachers and Teaching in US Medical Schools. Appleton-Century-Crofts, Norwalk, CT.

Kirkpatrick, D.L., Kirkpatrick, J.D., 2006. Evaluating Training Programs: The Four Levels. Berrett-Koehler Publishers, San Francisco.

Knowles, M.S., 1980. The Modern Practice of Adult Education: From Pedagogy to Andragogy. Cambridge Books, New York.

McLean, M., Cilliers, F., Van Wyk, J.M., 2008. Faculty development: yesterday, today and tomorrow. Med. Teach. 30 (6), 555–584.

Rubeck, R.F., Witzke, D.B., 1998. Faculty development: a field of dreams. Acad. Med. 73 (9 Suppl.), S32–S37.

Schön, D.A., 1983. The Reflective Practitioner: How Professionals Think in Action. Basic Books, New York.

Schor, N.F., Guillet, R., McAnarney, E.R., 2011. Anticipatory guidance as a principle of faculty development: managing transition and change. Acad. Med. 86 (10), 1235–1240.

Sheets, K.J., Schwenk, T.L., 1990. Faculty development for family medicine educators: an agenda for future activities. Teach. Learn. Med. 2 (3), 141–148.

Steinert, Y., 2010. Becoming a better teacher: from intuition to intent. In: Ende, J. (Ed.), Theory and Practice of Teaching Medicine. American College of Physicians, Philadelphia.

Steinert, Y. (Ed.), 2014. Faculty Development in the Health Professions: A Focus on Research and Practice. Springer, Dordrecht, the Netherlands.

Steinert, Y., Nasmith, L., McLeod, P.J., Conochie, L., 2003. A teaching scholars program to develop leaders in medical education. Acad. Med. 78 (2), 142–149.

Steinert, Y., Mann, K., Centeno, A., et al., 2006. A systematic review of faculty development initiatives designed to improve teaching effectiveness in medical education: BEME Guide No. 8. Med. Teach. 28 (6), 497–526.

Steinert, Y., Mann, K., Anderson, B., et al., 2016. A systematic review of faculty development initiatives designed to enhance teaching effectiveness: a ten-year update: BEME Guide No. 40. Med. Teach. 38 (8), 769–786.

Swanwick, T., 2008. See one, do one, then what? Faculty development in postgraduate medical education. Postgrad. Med. J. 84 (993), 339–343.

Ullian, J.A., Stritter, F.T., 1997. Types of faculty development programs. Fam. Med. 29 (4), 237–241.

Whitcomb, M.E., 2003. The medical school's faculty is its most important asset. Acad. Med. 78 (2), 117–118.

Wilkerson, L., Irby, D.M., 1998. Strategies for improving teaching practices: a comprehensive approach to faculty development. Acad. Med. 73 (4), 387–396.

Academic standards and scholarship

S. P. Mennin

Trends

- Teachers that guide the preparation of the current and future healthcare workforce are accountable to society to set and maintain standards of practice and professional scholarship in medical education.
- Standards and scholarship must be sufficiently stable to identify, sustain and hold medical educators and practitioners together.
- Standards and scholarship must be flexible enough to respond to the evolving local and regional needs in a rapidly changing dynamic world.

"… scholarship … also means stepping back from one's investigation, looking for connections, building bridges between theory and practice, and communicating one's knowledge effectively to students."

Boyer, 1990

Introduction

Academic standards are what universities, schools, institutes and society mutually agree upon as benchmarks of quality that shape and frame the roles, responsibilities and actions of the professoriate. Standards and scholarship are about measurement, assessment and evaluation and therefore are not neutral. They are political, social and historical (Freire, 1993), and they involve choices about setting the agenda for what and how future health professionals will learn and whom they will serve. Scholarship sets the standards for how teachers live and work in the culture of academia and the greater whole of society.

Standards, like culture, are slow to adapt to changing circumstances. In today's fast-moving world, there continues to be a need for adaptive change in medical education to modernize curricula to be more socially responsible, incorporate different pedagogies, introduce early and sustained clinical experiences, promote viable community-based education and use new technologies in the learning/assessment process. At the same time, many of the cultures in which medical education operates today exist in strained economies and have to deal with the migration of health professionals further disrupting already overburdened health systems. The pressures on medical and health professional faculty and staff to do more with less are greater than ever. Limited resources, especially financial pressures, are pushing leadership at academic medical centres, teaching hospitals and clinics to adopt values and fiscal policies more attuned to the entrepreneurial world of business than to the primary goals of caring, health, learning and scholarship. The number of private medical schools has increased rapidly in recent years and, in the present climate, there is a palpable risk that the core values of learning and scholarship may be subjugated to profit-oriented pressures.

The Internet, diseases without borders, conflicts and other international events emphasize the essential role of collaboration in the face of seemingly intractable regional and transnational issues. The call for international or global standards in medical education that respect the integrity of regional cultures grows stronger. Outcome-based medical education is becoming the norm (Frank et al., 2010), although not without problems. Nevertheless, it seems paradoxical that with the push for defined and measured outcomes, one observes in medical curricula less attention and time devoted to discussion, reflection and problem solving related to more global outcomes such as the failure of healthcare systems and the millions of people who are without access to basic attention and healthcare.

Double standard: research, patient care and teaching

"It would be nice if all of the data which sociologists require could be enumerated because then we could run them through IBM machines and draw charts as the economists

do. However, not everything that can be counted counts, and not everything that counts can be counted."

William Bruce Cameron, 1963

The reality of practice in academic life reveals a double standard for success: one for research and patient care and another one for education. Research and patient care have clear, well-established rules, expectations, standards, and a clear formal pathway to prepare for professional roles and responsibilities. The ability to generate outside funding from research and/or clinical care confers influence and status in academic, institutional and political processes. The culture of research and patient care is highly developed and almost universally accepted. Not so for scholarly work in medical education.

Unlike research and patient care activities, teachers in the health professions rarely receive formal preparation for their educational roles: teaching, assessment of learners and educational planning, and collaboration. Poor teaching performance is tolerated much more than is poor quality in research and substandard patient care. Peer review is well established for research and patient care activities, and comparatively under-developed in teaching and related educational activities. Teachers at medical schools and healthcare institutions are well aware that the rewards and recognition for research and patient care are substantive and those for teaching and education much less so, if at all.

The absence of a common language in education and related shared values is a major barrier to achieving integration of the scholarship of teaching, research and patient care. Few medical teachers can describe how people learn, what is known about the development of expertise, or the application of basic concepts and approaches to the assessment of learning. Even fewer can formulate and pursue research questions related to health professions education. It is a disturbing observation that those who are entrusted with the care and preparation of their successors are ill-informed about contemporary approaches to learning, teaching, education and research in education for the health professions. We are concerned with professional behaviour among practitioners and students. We profess, but are we professional?

Professionalizing teaching

Experience informs the professional identity of teachers. We recognize that experience must include holding each other to shared standards of scholarship in education as part of, rather than separate from, day-to-day clinical care and inquiry. How can this be accomplished in a sustainable way? One approach is to expand the institutional values of academic merit to include

educational work measured by peers according to established standards of scholarship (Boyer, 1990; Glassick, et al., 1997). For example, new methods of teaching are developed (discovery), and tested (applied) and integrated with existing pedagogies. It is feasible and necessary to articulate and reward excellence in all forms, and to support an enriched culture of inquiry in medical education and teaching in health professions schools.

Broadening the definition of scholarship

 "What we urgently need today is a more inclusive view of what it means to be a scholar – a recognition that knowledge is acquired through research, through synthesis, through practice and through teaching."

Boyer, 1990

The practice, theory and standards of medical education continue to evolve and expand over time. How we perceive and understand the work of medical teachers influences what we define as success in educational change and innovation. A broader and more inclusive definition of scholarship promotes inquiry-based medical education (Table 41.1) (Boyer, 1990; Glassick et al., 1997). A broader approach to scholarship is *inclusive. It strengthens and extends* established criteria that recognize the value of teaching as foundational to the merit and promotion process; especially at a time when much needed change in medical education is emerging (McGaghie, 2009; Mennin, 2015).

Criteria for scholarship in teaching and education

 "Almost all successful academics give credit to creative teachers – those mentors who defined their work so compellingly that it became, for them, a lifetime challenge. Without the teaching function, the continuity of knowledge will be broken and the store of human knowledge dangerously diminished."

Boyer, 1990

Meeting criteria for scholarship (Boyer, 1990; Glassick et al., 1997; Hutchings & Schulman, 1999) suggest some simple rules. Simple rules guide individual local actions at all levels in in a complex adaptive system. Examples for scholarship in education could include: teach and learn in every exchange; practise with understanding (theory) and put theory into practise; stand in inquiry that is open and accessible to the public; participate in

Table 41.1   Four arenas of scholarship

Category of scholarship	Description	Questions posed
Discovery	Knowledge for its own sake	What is known? What is yet to be found?
Integration	Making connections across disciplines, illuminating data in a real way, interpreting, drawing together and bringing new insight to bear on original work	How do these findings fit together … with what is already known? So what does this mean for us? For others?
Application	Engagement with society to apply what is known	How can what is known be responsibly applied to consequential problems? How can it be helpful to individuals, society and institutions?
Teaching	To make accessible, and to participate in the transformation of what can be known with others	Now what can we do? How can what is known be shared? How can what is known be transformed?

From Boyer EL: *Scholarship reconsidered: priorities of the professoriate. The Carnegie Foundation for the Advancement of Teaching, San Francisco, 1990, Jossey-Bass.*

peer review and evaluation of educational work; and share work in a form accessible to others (Holladay and Tytel, 2011)

The demands of day-to-day activities in health institutions leave little time to consider the scholarship of teaching. Some strategies have been suggested that link everyday educational activities and scholarship (Morahan and Fleetwood, 2008). Two levels of scholarship have been named and described: a scholarly approach and educational scholarship (Simpson et al., 2007).

1. *A scholarly approach* occurs when an anatomist or a paediatrician reads recent literature on a topic, adds relevant contemporary findings to their teaching and places his or her work in an authentic context relevant to the learners' capacities. By extending shared knowledge and building on the work of others, these educators are engaged in *a scholarly approach* to teaching. This is an important step for many teachers.

2. *Educational scholarship* occurs when a teacher documents and produces a product that is shared publicly with the education community in a form upon which others can build. *Educational scholarship* is work that is in the public domain and therefore subject to peer review using accepted criteria. When a teacher makes his or her work available to other teachers, presents it at a peer reviewed professional meeting, has it accepted by an approved peer reviewed clearing house such as MedEdPortal (https://www.mededportal.org/), or disseminates it on a website, he or she has demonstrated *educational scholarship*. The teacher has engaged with and contributed to the broader educational community. Other examples of educational scholarship include the production and sharing of syllabi, web-based instructional materials, fellowship programmes, continuing medical education programmes, performance data about learners, accomplishments of advisees and educational leadership programmes (Simpson et al., 2007; Morahan & Fleetwood, 2008).

Recognizing and evaluating a scholarly approach to teaching and educational scholarship

 "Academics feel relatively confident about their ability to assess specialized research, but they are less certain about what qualities to look for in other kinds of scholarship, and how to document and reward that work."

Glassick, et al., 1997

Academic standards for recognition and promotion require credible documentation that includes: (1) the quantity and (2) the quality of the educational activities, and (3) a description of the nature of the person's engagement with the wider educational community (Simpson et al., 2007). Quantity refers to the types and frequencies of educational roles and activities (Simpson et al., 1994). Quality refers to measures of the effectiveness and excellence of the educational activity (Bleakley et al., 2014). Engagement with the education community occurs when the educational activity is informed by what is accepted as known in the field (scholarly approach) and when the teacher contributes to the knowledge in the field (educational scholarship.) Table 41.2 illustrates the application of these criteria from Glassick et al. (1997), to scholarship in lecturing, precepting, small-group facilitation and educational administration (Fincher et al., 2000).

Increasing support for a scholarly approach to teaching and educational scholarship

Compared to the end of the twentieth century, there is today much more access to, and support for, peer reviewed

Table 41.2 Comparison of criteria for assessing scholarship and quality teaching. Teaching is taken to mean any activity that fosters learning, including lecturing, tutoring, precepting or creation of associated instructional materials.

Six criteria for scholarship (Glassick et al., 1997)	Criteria for quality teaching (Fincher et al., 2000)	Documentation of evidence (Simpson et al., 2007)			
		Quantity	Quality	Draws from field to inform own work *(scholarly approach)*	Contributes to field to inform others' work *(educational scholarship)*
Clear, achievable goals that are important to the field	Establish clear, achievable, measurable, relevant objectives	Teaching role, how long (duration and frequency)	Awards with criteria, evaluation by students, peers, consultants	How teaching approach is informed by the literature	List of interactive learning exercise is accepted in peer-reviewed repository
Adequate preparation, including an understanding of the existing work in the field	Identify and organize key materials appropriate to audience level and objectives	Where (required courses, venue)	Evidence of learning (self-reports, performance on standardized tests)	Impact of colleague discussions on subsequent practice	List of invitations to present teaching approach at regional, national and/or international conferences
Appropriate methods relative to goals	Select teaching methods and assessment measures to achieve and measure objectives	Formats, number and level of learners			
Significant results that contributes to the field	Assess learner performance				
Effective communication of work to intended audiences	Assess quality of presentation – instruction				
Reflective critique to improve quality of future work	Critical analysis of teaching that results in change to improve it				

publication of scholarship in medical education. There are excellent online, easy to search opportunities such as MedEDPORTAL (https://www.mededportal.org/) and MedEd Publish (http://www.mededworld.org/MedEdWorld-Papers.aspx). Many print and electronic journals provide public venues for scholarly work in medical education (http://guides.library.stonybrook.edu/medical-education/journals). Medical, dental and discipline-based specialty journals devote space to education. Professional associations and organizations such as the International Association of Medical Educators (https://iamse.site-ym.com/), invite basic science teachers to publish and share their work. The educator's portfolio is an institutional strategy for clinical teachers to meet the criteria for promotion by providing acceptable evidence of scholarship in teaching (Simpson et al., 1994). Additional institutional infrastructure supportive of the scholarship of teaching includes defined positions,

offices, committees and resources for medical education, and access to relevant journals, websites and books. Faculty and staff development, new faculty orientation to education programmes, handbooks, and educational fellowships are important. Transparency in policies for promotion, leadership positions, for example chairs of committees are essential. Finally, educational ceremonies recognizing excellence, and education as a regular part of the routine agenda for faculty meetings help to set conditions to optimize the scholarship of teaching (Fincher et al., 2000).

Leadership: promoting the scholarship of teaching

 "In so far as one role of education is to perpetuate and stabilize our way of life, it is necessarily

biased. The problem is that if we see education, or changes in education, only as a process of replication, then we will continue to be plagued with the cultural disparities that we abhor or deny today. On the other hand, adaptive education is, by nature, sensitive to individual or local or cultural differences."

Eoyang, 2012

Experience teaches us that the role of leadership is critical for change and innovation in medical education. A practical and theoretically informed approach to leadership inclusive of both the educational institution as a whole and the individual teacher promotes and sustains scholarship in teaching. Leadership is a process of adaptive action in which people make meaning in iterative cycles of inquiry that leads to understanding and informed action (Eoyang & Holladay, 2013). Fundamentally, leadership is about recognizing patterns in the environment and engaging in multiple cycles of adaptive action (pattern logic, www.hsdinstitute.org).

Leadership, then, is about setting conditions so that new teaching patterns and productivity can emerge; patterns that optimize the fitness for purpose, sustainability and resilience of learners, teachers, administrators, institutions as a whole and the health systems in which they are co-embedded.

Tradition privileges a hierarchical *top-down leadership* structure in medical education that expresses itself as command and control in contemporary sociology of a medical school or health practice (Bloom, 1988; Mennin & Krakov, 1998). *Bottom-up leadership* emerges when individuals share information, make meaning between and among themselves, and take actions that promote self-organization into communities of practice (Wenger et al., 2002; Mennin, 2010). Both forms of leadership (top-down and bottom-up) are necessary for scholarship and both depend on the local conditions. Wise top-down leadership relaxes constraints to create space and provide resources for bottom-up innovation, pilot projects, new methods, etc. Individuals and small groups have more flexibility in their style and approach to patient care and teaching than do leaders at the top of the organization.

Conditions at a larger scale in the region influence leadership at the local level and vice versa as society grants substantial autonomy to physicians to practise the art and science of healing based on recognized expertise, individual licensing and institutional certification (standards, peer review, response to criticism, institutional transparency). Autonomy includes responsibility for the education of future physicians. Interestingly, the best physicians, the best athletes and performers don't necessarily make the best teachers or coaches. Expertise as a physician is necessary but not sufficient for effective medical education. A major challenge for leadership in medical education in general, and specifically in the adoption and adaptation of the scholarship of teaching, is to promote and embrace the development of adaptive capacity among teachers that is grounded in scholarship.

For many biomedical experts and specialists, learning new and collaborative educational methodologies and practices is very challenging. Going from expert to novice can raise issues of fear of loss of control. For some medical educators, effective collaborative teaching and teamwork can be uncomfortable as they are uncertain when it's appropriate to step forward and when it's more appropriate to step back into a supportive role. Fortunately, the culture of autonomy in practice, independent research, specialization-based status and self-directed learning is amenable to leadership and change through cycles of adaptive action.

Adaptive action: leadership for scholarship

Society demands a safe, sensitive and responsive health system in which changes in medical practice and education emerge from disturbances in the status quo that could be as simple as new information or as complex as a periodic institutional self-study and review. In either case, and especially in more complex circumstances, effective leadership with adaptive action is an iterative inquiry process informed by three deceptively simple and yet powerful questions: What? So What? Now What? (Eoyang & Holladay, 2013).

1. **What?** What is the data? What do we know and how do we know it?

   For example, to what extent is the scholarship of teaching consistent with existing individual and institutional values, past experiences, the needs of potential adopters as well as societal values? To what extent does expanding the definition of scholarship to include application, integration and teaching in addition to discovery create a more inclusive environment without lowering the standards of the 'traditional' scholarship of discovery? What we perceive is that promotion criteria based on a narrow interpretation of scholarship (restricted to publications in prestigious journals, grants and awards) are inconsistent with the rising demands of day-to-day clinical work and can result in the loss of outstanding clinicians and educators.

   Observability. To what extent will the results of implementing a scholarship of teaching be observable and measurable? If faculty can see and feel it working in their department or with someone they respect (an opinion leader), they will be more likely to accept an invitation to consider trying something different. Visibility (peer review, accessible to the public) stimulates peer discussion and helps leadership to promote scholarship to others.

2. **So What** does this mean for me? For us? For the Department? For our clinical practice? For others?

What does it mean for a group, a department, a practice to embed changes related to the scholarship of teaching at multiple levels in the health system? So what does it mean when a medical school introduces community-based medical education in service of regional health needs and at the same time improves health professions education? (Petroni Mennin, 2015).

Degree of difficulty. What does it mean for us and how difficult is it for us to grasp and implement the idea of the scholarship of teaching? (McGaghie, 2009) For some faculty and staff, education is not the most important part of their day-to-day activities. Few people give their best effort to activities for which they are insufficiently prepared, do not fully understand and for which they receive insufficient recognition. Teaching, when perceived as not being appropriately rewarded, can result in teachers choosing not to pursue their interests in the educational process. For example, the University of Louisville found itself in economic difficulty: the administration was using a research-focused promotion and reward system to evaluate clinician educators (Schweitzer, 2000), a mismatch of expectations and evaluation; they adopted the Boyer approach and had difficulty understanding how that approach to scholarship applied to a variety of faculty activities; the model was too difficult and burdensome and was not adopted by the faculty (Schweitzer, 2000).

3. **Now What?**

Trialability. Now what will we do? Educational approaches that can be pilot tested have a much better chance of succeeding compared to those for which a small-scale trial is not possible. Adopting criteria for scholarship in teaching promotes a shared understanding among teachers and leadership. Teachers can produce educational materials and innovations that are recognized and meet the criteria of scholarship.

The University of Kentucky School of Medicine found that its faculty recruitment, development, retention and promotion processes were not working optimally (Nora et al., 2000). Most faculty perceived that only the scholarship of discovery (publication of 'scientific' research) mattered for promotion. A broad representative task force collected data, developed procedures, examined policies and perceptions, kept in close contact with the larger faculty community, the

university administration and governing bodies and reported findings publicly to the general faculty. Subsequently, promotion guidelines were clarified and new mechanisms to support faculty were implemented, reaffirming support for all forms of scholarship, including teaching (Nora et al., 2000).

The results of taking informed action as in "now what will we do?" create a new situation that becomes a new "what?" Curiosity, inquiry (sampling), making meaning and taking action are fundamental features of nature and living systems. Adaptive action helps medical educators and leadership to be resilient as fit for purpose. It gives resilience and sustainability to both the practice and theory of standards and the scholarship of teaching in medical education.

Summary

The definition of scholarship is expanded to include the scholarship of discovery, integration and application to embrace teaching for medical education. The criteria for educational scholarship, like other forms of scholarship, require that activities be informed by both the latest ideas in the subject field; be open and accessible to the public; be subject to peer review critique and evaluation; and be in an accessible form upon which others can build. Teachers engaged in routine teaching activities can take a scholarly approach when they draw from the established literature and known practices in their subject area. Going further, teaching becomes educational scholarship when teachers make original contributions to the existing peer-reviewed resources related to medical education.

Academic standards for recognition and promotion based on educational scholarship and scholarly activities require credible documentation that includes the quantity and the quality of the educational activities, and a description of the nature of the person's engagement with the wider educational community. The challenge is to support the development and acceptance of documentation of scholarship as an important part of an educator's portfolio in support of merit and promotion.

Successful movements in medical education, such as the current expansion of the definition of scholarship and the refinement of documentation of evidence for recognition and promotion, depend upon an understanding of the practical and theoretical aspects of adaptive action and leadership. Inquiry founded on three simple, yet deep questions, What? So What? Now What? informs the actions of both top-down and bottom-up leadership.

The sustainability and resilience of standards for medical education and the scholarship of teaching require dedicated staff and teachers capable of expanding the boundaries of education, together with a system capable of recognizing and supporting those who do so. Academic health science centres, teachers and teaching practices in all forms are co-embedded in complex healthcare systems. It is up to each one of us to engage with those around us and create a shared understanding and practice of educational scholarship. In this way, a 'new traditional' institutional fabric supportive of academic careers in health professions education serve to stay relevant and responsive to the priority health needs of society.

References

Bleakley, A., Browne, J., Ellis, K., 2014. Quality in medical education. In: Swanwick, T. (Ed.), Understanding Medical Education: Evidence, Theory and Practice, second ed. Wiley Blackwell, Oxford, p. 48.

Bloom, S.W., 1988. Structure and ideology in medical education: an analysis of resistance to change. J. Health Soc. Behav. 29, 294–306.

Boyer, E.L. Scholarship reconsidered: priorities of the professoriate. The Carnegie Foundation for the Advancement of Teaching, San Francisco, 1990, Jossey-Bass.

Eoyang, G.H., Holladay, R., 2013. Adaptive Action: Leveraging Uncertainty in Your Organization. Stanford University Press, Stanford, California.

Fincher, R.M.E., Simpson, D.E., Mennin, S.P., et al., 2000. Scholarship as teaching: an imperative for the 21st century. Acad. Med. 75, 887–894.

Frank, J.R., Mungroo, R., Ahmad, Y., et al., 2010. Toward a definition of competency-based education in medicine: a systematic review of published definitions. Med. Teach. 32, 631–637.

Freire, P., 1993. Pedagogy of the Oppressed. The Continuum International Publishing Company, New York.

Glassick, C.E., Huber, M.T., Maeroff, G.I., 1997. Scholarship Assessed: Evaluation of the Professoriate. Jossey-Bass, San Francisco.

Holladay, R., Tytel, M., 2011. Simple Rules: A Radical Inquiry Into Self. Gold Canyon Press, Apache Junction.

Hutchings, P., Shulman, L.S. The scholarship of teaching: new elaborations, new developments, 1999. Change September/October:11-15.

McGaghie, W.C., 2009. Scholarship, publication, and career advancement in health professions education: AMEE Guide No. 43. Med. Teach. 31, 574–590.

Mennin, S., 2010. Self-Organization, integration and curriculum in the complex world of medical education. Med. Educ. 44, 20–30.

Mennin, S., 2015. How can learning be made more effective in medical education? In: Bin Abdulrahman, K.A., Mennin, S., Harden, R.M., Kennedy, C. (Eds.), Routledge International Handbook of Medical Education. Routledge, London, pp. 207–220.

Mennin, S.P., Krackov, S.K., 1998. Reflections on relatives, resistance, and reform in medical education. Acad. Med. 73 (Suppl.), S60–S64.

Morahan, P.S., Fleetwood, J., 2008. The double helix of activity and scholarship: building a medical education career with limited resources. Med. Educ. 42, 34–44.

Nora, L.M., Pomeroy, C., Curry, T.E. Jr., et al., 2000. Revising appointment, promotion, and tenure procedures to incorporate an expanded definition of scholarship: The University of Kentucky College of Medicine experience. Acad. Med. 75, 913–924.

Petroni Mennin, R.H., 2015. Benefits and challenges associated with introducing, managing, integrating and sustaining community-based medical education. In: Bin Abdulrahman, K.A., Mennin, S., Harden, R.M., Kennedy, C. (Eds.), Routledge International Handbook of Medical Education. Routledge, London, pp. 157–170.

Schweitzer, L., 2000. Adoption and failure of the 'Boyer model' in the University of Louisville. Acad. Med. 75, 925–929.

Simpson, D., Morzinski, J., Beecher, A., Lindemann, J., 1994. Meeting the challenge to document teaching accomplishments: the educator's portfolio. Teach. Learn. Med. 6, 203–206.

Simpson, D., Fincher, R.M.E., Hafler, J.P., et al., 2007. Advancing educators and education by defining the components and evidence associated with educational scholarship. Med. Educ. 41, 1002–1009.

Wenger, E., McDermott, R., Snyder, W.M., 2002. A Guide to Managing Knowledge: Cultivating Communities of Practice. Harvard Business School, Boston.

Section 7

Students

Student selection

I. C. McManus, H. M. Sondheimer

Trends

- Selection should aim at a relatively small number of what can be called 'canonical traits' – the three or four stable characteristics that are likely to predict future professional behaviour and can be assessed reliably at medical school application.

- If schools currently select almost entirely on academic ability, then they will inevitably lower their academic standards in order to select effectively on non-academic criteria.

- Selection should be recognized as being limited in its power. The really powerful tools for affecting change are education and training (McManus & Vincent, 1993).

Introduction

Selection seems deceptively easy: if there are more applicants than places, simply choose the best applicants. In practice, things are far more complicated. Selection may be:

- of dubious validity
- statistically unreliable
- a vulnerable process legally and ethically
- open to challenge on grounds such as discrimination
- criticized by society at large
- under-resourced, given the implicit expectations of society, the profession and medical schools.

Although student selection is traditionally concerned with entry to medical school, recent years have seen a growing interest in postgraduate selection, where similar problems apply and similar principles and methods can be used.

 "For a man to be truly suited to the practice of medicine, he must be possessed of a natural disposition for it, the necessary instruction, favourable circumstances, education, industry and time. The first requisite is a natural disposition, for a reluctant student renders every effort vain."

Hippocrates

Why select?

Selection programmes must clearly state their reasons for selecting. If the *only* reason were reduction of numbers then a lottery would suffice. In reality, selection has multiple components occurring at different stages.

SELECTION OF STUDENTS BY THE MEDICAL SCHOOL

The straightforward reason is to choose the best students. Although seemingly simple, that little word 'best' hides many subtleties and complexities. Increasingly in the United States, medical schools are utilizing mission-based admissions (Kirch & Prescott, 2013). For those whose mission is to create future researchers and academic physicians, they aspire to choose applicants who have the traits that will lead to academic careers. Conversely, those medical schools who wish to train physicians to practice within their own state in primarily clinical settings are looking for applicants with a different set of attributes.

SELECTION BY APPLICANTS OF MEDICINE AS A CAREER

The pool of medical school applicants only contains those who have selected medicine as a career. The many individuals who did not apply cannot be selected, even if they might have made excellent doctors.

IMPLICIT SELECTION OF THE MEDICAL SCHOOLS BY APPLICANTS

While schools are selecting students, students are also selecting medical schools. A school's excellent selection system is of little use if the best applicants apply elsewhere. Effective selection begins by encouraging the right students to apply.

EXPLICIT SELECTION OF MEDICAL SCHOOLS BY APPLICANTS

When applicants receive offers from two or more medical schools, it is they who select medical schools, not vice versa.

SELECTION FOR A PARTICULAR ACADEMIC CURRICULUM

Increasingly, medical schools are developing curricula with different emphases. Schools with a curriculum with large components of problem-based learning in small groups might prefer students who work together cooperatively rather than competitively.

SELECTION BY STAFF FOR STAFF

Staff who are actively involved in selection feel ownership of the process, developing a relationship with future students who themselves feel that by staff selection they have become accepted into membership of the institution.

The limits of selection

 "Unfortunately the qualities which count for most in medicine are not precisely measurable. The measurable – examination performance at school – neither necessarily relates to these quantities nor guarantees intellectual potential. ... In this sea of uncertainty it is not surprising that selection processes are imperfect and open to criticism or that the remedy is not immediately apparent."

Richards, 1983

A common misconception is that medical schools receive numerous applications. In practice, particularly in the United Kingdom and the United States, the ratio is typically about two and a half total applicants for every place, although admissions officers often feel the ratio is much higher as each candidate makes multiple applications. The power of selection ultimately depends on the 'selection ratio', the number of applicants for each place. As the ratio grows, selection will be more effective. A decline in the ratio below 1.5:1 would represent a severe weakening in the overall pool and the possibility that medical schools would have to consider applicants who they feel are academically under-qualified. The current 2.5:1 ratio allows all medical schools to feel that they are seriously considering only academically qualified students.

The limits of selection are easily shown mathematically. If selecting on a single criterion (such as intellectual ability) that has a normal distribution of ability, and with a selection ratio of two applicants per place, the optimal selection places the candidates in order, and those above the median are selected (see Fig. 42.1).

The limits of selection become particularly apparent when two or more criteria are introduced, for example intellectual ability and communication skills, which are essentially uncorrelated. The distribution is bivariate normal (Fig. 42.2), and the aim is to select the best 50% of candidates on the joint criteria. The dashed

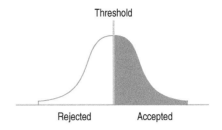

Fig. 42.1 A simple model of selection when there is a single characteristic on which selection is taking place; those above the threshold are accepted, and those below are rejected.

lines indicate the median for each of the separate distributions.

Selecting candidates to be above a particular threshold on *both* criteria means they are in the top right-hand corner of the figure. The key point to realize is that the threshold on either criterion will be substantially below the median. In fact, with two independent criteria, selected candidates are only in the top 71% of the ability range, rather than the top 50%, and hence are less able on average than if either criterion alone had been used. The same conclusion applies if one allows compensation between the separate abilities (McManus & Vincent, 1993). If medical student selection is based predominantly on academic achievement, then for non-academic factors to be taken substantially into account, academic standards will be reduced.

Medical schools considering non-academic attributes for selection rapidly develop long lists of desiderata, often containing 5, 10, 20 or even 50 components. The model of Fig. 42.2 can easily be extended to three, four, five or many criteria, when the limits of selection appear with a vengeance. Assuming the criteria are statistically independent, then as the number of criteria rise, so the proportion of candidates eliminated *on any single criterion* becomes ever smaller. To put it bluntly, 'if one selects on everything, one selects on nothing' (Table 42.1).

Which are the canonical traits in selection?

Attempts have been made to identify canonical traits for selection (McManus & Vincent, 1993).

INTELLECTUAL ABILITY

Doctors probably cannot be too intelligent. Meta-analyses of selection in many different occupations show that general mental ability is the best predictor both of job performance and of the ability to be trained (Schmidt & Hunter, 1998). Although claims are often made for some minimum threshold ability level that is 'good enough', systematic research suggests that 'more is better' (Arneson et al., 2011).

LEARNING STYLE AND MOTIVATION

Students study for many different reasons, and those motivations mean they adopt particular study habits and learning styles. In Biggs's typology (Table 42.2), both deep and strategic learning (but not surface

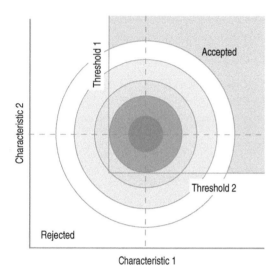

Fig. 42.2 Example showing two criteria.

learning) are compatible with the self-directed, self-motivated approach to learning that is required in the lifelong learning needed in medical practitioners.

COMMUNICATIVE ABILITY

Many complaints about doctors involve communication problems, and so it makes sense to include communication in selection. Assessment is not straightforward, but interviews, multiple mini interviews, questionnaires and situational judgement tests can all assess communication.

PERSONALITY

Many studies have examined the 'big five' personality traits of extroversion, neuroticism, openness to experience, agreeableness and conscientiousness. Schmidt and Hunter's (1998) meta-analysis showed that the best predictor of job performance and trainability, after intellectual ability, was integrity or conscientiousness, not least because highly conscientious people tend to work harder and be more efficient and so gain more and better experience. Conscientiousness may, though, not be a good predictor when creativity or innovation is important. At medical school, conscientiousness better predicts achievement in basic medical sciences, rather than clinical studies or postgraduate activities such as research output.

SURROGATES FOR SELECTION

Although intelligence, learning style, communication and personality should probably form the basis of

Table 42.1 The effects of selection on the basis of multiple criteria (assuming two applicants for every place)

Number of independent selection criteria	Proportion of applicants rejected on any single criterion
1	Bottom 50%
2	Bottom 29.3%
3	Bottom 20.6%
4	Bottom 15.9%
5	Bottom 12.9%
6	Bottom 10.9%
10	Bottom 6.7%
20	Bottom 3.4%
50	Bottom 1.4%
N^*	Bottom $100 \cdot (1 - r^{(-1/N)})\%$

$^*N$: number of criteria; r: selection ratio (e.g. if $r = 3$, there are 3 applicants for each place and 1/3 applicants are accepted).
Reproduced from McManus IC, Vincent CA: Selecting and educating safer doctors. In Vincent CA, Ennis M, Audley RJ, editors: Medical Accidents, Oxford, 1993, Oxford University Press, pp 80–105.

Table 42.2 Summary of the differences in motivation and study process of the surface, deep and strategic approaches to study

Style	Motivation	Process
Surface	Completion of the course	Rote learning of facts and ideas
		Focusing on task components in isolation
	Fear of failure	Little real interest in content
Deep	Interest in the subject	Relation of ideas to evidence
	Vocational relevance	Integration of material across courses
	Personal understanding	Identification of general principles
Strategic/ Achieving	Achieving high grades	Use of techniques that achieve
	Being successful	Highest grades

Based on the work of Biggs, 1987, 2003.

selection, it is often sufficient to select on measures that correlate highly with them. School-leaving examinations are such a surrogate, as high grades represent the resultant of adequate intelligence, appropriate learning styles and a systematic approach to study (and hence school-leaving exams are better predictors of career outcomes than pure tests of intelligence [McManus et al., 2013]). A person of lower intellect may pass exams by prodigious rote learning, conscientiously carried out, but that becomes increasing difficult at higher levels of achievement. Playing in an orchestra or for a sports team also implies conscientiousness at practising, good communicative ability when collaborating and an interest in the deeper aspects of a skill (intrinsic motivation). Good selection processes do not use such surrogates uncritically, but must ask what underlying psychological traits are being assessed by such biographical data (biodata).

Methods and process of selection

 "If selectors are trying to do too much too well, they will end by failing to do anything properly."

Downie & Charlton, 1992

The process of selection and the methods used to carry it out are entirely separate (Powis, 1998). Medical schools should have a selection policy that clearly states how selection takes place, what traits and attributes are of most significance to that school, how information is collected and how decisions are based on the information, including the weighting of the various components. Decision making should, in the end, be an entirely administrative process, as that ensures good practice and avoids suggestions of discrimination, unfairness, or apparent inconsistencies in selection. Academic and educational inputs to the system should be in deciding the protocol and, where necessary, making subtle judgements about the information (such as evaluating aspects of the application form or interviewing). An important corollary of this principle is that the separate items of information should be assessed separately. If interviewers are asked to judge a candidate's knowledge of medicine as a career then that is what they should do; information about interviewees' examination results, hobbies etc. may result in a 'halo effect'.

ASSESSING METHODS OF SELECTION

The many methods of selection each have their strengths and weaknesses. Each should be assessed in terms of:

- **Validity.** All selection assessments should be implicit predictions of a candidate's future behaviour. If there is no correlation with future behaviours, then methods are not useful, however much assessors may like them.

- **Reliability.** If different selectors disagree about a characteristic, or reassessment gives different answers then the information is probably unhelpful.

- **Feasibility.** If an assessment involves too great a cost, either financially or in staff effort, the gain may not be worth the expenditure.

- **Acceptability.** Candidates and their teachers, friends and relations, and the public in general, must feel selection methods are appropriate.

Assessing selection needs data, and, fortunately, eventual outcomes can now be tracked, for example what percentage of a school's graduates enter research or academic careers, what percentage of the graduates practice in a primary care or rural setting. In addition, big data will soon tell us who is a better physician in relation to ordering of tests, prescribing drugs etc. Clear delineation of personality and other variables assessed during selection may identify correlations with future practice variables. In a major project, the UK Medical Education Database (UKMED, http://www.ukmed.ac.uk/) is integrating data across multiple UK databases to allow research at the level of individual students and doctors and medical schools.

DIFFERENT METHODS OF SELECTION

Open admissions and lotteries

Systems for avoiding the hard decisions of selection are the former Austrian 'open admissions' system and the weighted lottery in Holland. Each of these has been abandoned. Recent comparisons showed that selected students performed better academically and were better motivated than those admitted by an open system or lottery (Reibnegger et al., 2010; Urlings-Strop et al., 2011). Such findings are probably the death knell for solving problems of selection by not selecting.

Administrative methods

These are typically carried out by office staff who assess relatively objective information from application forms, primarily for rejecting unsuitable candidates. While usually reliable, cheap and acceptable, its validity depends on the information being used.

Assessment of application forms

Unstructured personal statements and referees' reports on application forms (so-called 'white-space boxes') are often assessed by shortlisters who try to determine a candidate's motivation and experience of medicine as a career.

Like interviewing, this is subjective and often of moderate or even poor reliability and of dubious validity. It is, however, cost-effective and acceptable to applicants. Reliability is improved by training, and the use of structured assessment protocols, clear criterion referencing and carefully constructed descriptors of the various characteristics to be identified. The rise of the Internet, however, does mean that statements can be heavily plagiarized, to wit:

 "Ever since I accidentally burnt holes in my pyjamas after experimenting with a chemistry set on my eighth birthday, I have always had a passion for science."

Plagiarized quotation used by 234 UK medical school applicants in 2007, detected using specialist software (http://news.bbc.co.uk/1/hi/education/6426945.stm).

Biographical data (biodata)

Biodata can be assessed from an open-ended application form (e.g. the 'personal statement') or from a semi-structured questionnaire. Its utility derives from the psychological principle that the best predictor of future behaviour is past behaviour. Generally, it is reliable, valid (Cook, 1990), cost-effective and acceptable, although verification may be needed to present dis-simulation. Background can also predict practice area, as in the United States and Australia, where candidates from rural areas are more likely eventually to practice in such areas.

Referees' reports

If honest, these can be useful, but referees often feel greater loyalty to the candidate (whom they know) than to the medical school (whom they don't know). Experienced head teachers say that medical schools should 'read between the lines', so that what matters is not what is said, but what is left unsaid or under-stated. Reliability is inevitably low, validity dubious and acceptability ambiguous. Attempts at standardiza-tion using grading scales in referees' reports have led to almost uniformly high scores, negating the value of these efforts.

Interviewing

 "The personal character, the very nature, the will, of each student had far greater force in determining his career than any helps or hindrances whatever. … The time and the place, the work to be done, and its responsibilities, will change; but the man will be the same, except in so far as he may change himself."

Sir James Paget, 1869

Although most UK and US medical schools conduct interviews, that has not always been the case. The reliability and validity of one-on-one interviews depend heavily on interviewer training and a clear structure. Behavioural interviewing, which emphasizes the can-didate's actual previous behaviour in concrete situations, is typically more effective than questions about hypothetical unknown situations in the future. Although expensive in terms of staff time, interviews are highly acceptable to the general public, who are not happy with doctors being selected purely on academic grounds, but are often criticized after the event by candidates and teachers, and may not actually be effective (Goho & Blackman, 2006). One argument for interviews is that they are at least in part a recruiting tool for the medical schools as well as an opportunity for the applicant to show her or his value.

Multiple mini-interviews (MMIs)

MMIs are effectively OSCEs (objective structured clinical examinations) used for selection, typically with 12 or so short stations. Reliability is certainly better than for conventional interviews, and claims are made for predictive validity (Eva et al., 2009). MMIs are virtually universal in the Canadian medical schools and increasingly utilized by US and UK schools. Candidates experiencing an MMI for the first time need to be thoroughly briefed on the format. A recent review of 30 studies (Pau et al., 2013) showed MMIs to be acceptable to candidates, while not favouring those with previous MMI coaching. MMI scores correlated well with subsequent performance on OSCEs during medical school and were predictive of performance on qualifying examinations in spite of not correlating with pre-entry academic performance.

Psychometric testing

Psychometric tests are of several types. Measures of motivation and personality, and of psychomotor char-acteristics such as manual dexterity, are often used in industry where they can have good predictive validity, but are little used at present in medicine. In medicine, psychometric tests can be time-consuming and expen-sive to administer and can be unpopular with candidates who worry that there are 'trick' questions and that the content does not seem relevant to a career in medicine. Tests of attainment, such as the biological sciences scale of the American MCAT, have good predictive validity (Donnon et al., 2007), but inevitably correlate with school-based measures of educational attainment. Tests such as BMAT, UMAT, GAMSAT and UKCAT have become popular in the United Kingdom, Australia and elsewhere, despite being introduced without evidence of predictive validity. Studies of UMAT (Mercer & Puddey, 2011) and GAMSAT (Wilkinson et al., 2008) suggest that predictive validity is low, particularly when educational attainment is taken into account. When psychometric tests are predictive, it mainly seems to be due to assessing attainment rather than ability or aptitude (McManus, Ferguson, et al., 2011).

Situational judgement tests

Situational judgement tests are multiple-choice assess-ments in which a range of options are ranked in order, often involving not merely factual knowledge but also an holistic awareness of the social processes and organizational needs of modern health care (Weekley & Ployhart, 2006). Their use is rapidly increasing in selection for postgraduate training, and they are being considered for selection into medical school (Lievens & Sackett, 2012). An interesting theoretical question concerns why they may work. One possibility is that they demonstrate candidates' ability imaginatively to place themselves in novel situations and anticipate the consequences so that perhaps they are assessing situational empathy.

Assessment centres

Assessment centres are the core selection method of the army, civil service and major companies. Candidates are brought together in groups of 4–12, for 1 to 3 days, and carry out a series of novel exercises, often involving group work. They are particularly appropriate if the emphasis is upon assessing ability under competitive time stress or when collaborating in group activities. At this time, we are not aware of any medical schools that have committed the time and resources to a full testing centre.

The costs of selection

The direct costs of selection for a medical school are difficult to assess, but are probably about £2000/$3000 per entrant, mostly accounted for by staff time. The unstated and unmeasured criterion of success is that graduates practise high-quality medicine until retirement, perhaps 40 years later. The issue is that student selection is currently an 'open-loop' system, without feedback/accountability to the medical schools. Bad doctors cost society dearly, but none of that cost comes back to the medical school. If the loop were closed, so that graduates incurred costs and/or provided rewards to their medical school throughout their careers, then selection and subsequent training would be at the core of a medical school's activities, instead of at its margins.

Routine monitoring of selection

Selection is vulnerable to criticism and even to legal challenge, making it essential that clear policies are in place, and that routine data are collected for monitoring the process, particularly of what the UK Equality Act of 2010 refers to as 'protected characteristics' (age/ disability/gender reassignment/marriage and civil partnership/pregnancy and maternity/race/religion or belief/sex/sexual orientation). Simple head counts are not sufficient since groups may differ in relevant background factors, making multivariate techniques necessary for identifying possible disadvantage and understanding its locus.

Widening access

Monitoring of the demographics and social background of medical students and doctors has resulted in concern about widening access to the medical profession, with attempts to increase participation of students from low socioeconomic backgrounds or particular ethnic or geographical groups. There can be tension if it is perceived that candidate selection is based on quotas rather than quality or ability as such. Prideaux et al. (2011) have suggested the importance of 'political validity' in selection. Witzburg and Sondheimer (2013) have noted how holistic review of each applicant can widen access while in no sense reducing academic standards. For those doing holistic review of applicants, there is a recent publication outlining an ongoing method of evaluation (Roadmap to Excellence, 2013).

"Widening access is a values question, not a technical question of choosing one selection method over another. Widening access is driven by socio-political concerns. These are real concerns. … Social accountability requires responsiveness to the communities the medical school serves and ensuring that the communities are represented in the student population. From this derives the concept of political validity."

Prideaux et al., 2011

Studying selection and learning from research

Medicine can be notoriously insular. Research and experience outside of medicine are often ignored. There are medical schools that will not even consider experience gained at other medical schools, never mind in industry, commerce and the public sectors in general. Personnel selection has been much studied and there is a vast literature. A good place to start is the regular series of articles in the *Annual Review of Psychology*, which are frequently updated (see Sackett & Lievens 2008).

EVIDENCE-BASED MEDICINE AND THE SCIENTIFIC STUDY OF SELECTION

Evidence-based medicine is the current dogma in medicine, and student selection should be no different. However, the limitations of the purely evidence-based approach should be recognized. If only 'gold-standard' randomized controlled trials were accepted as evidence then most of medical education would have no evidence base, and the inevitable result is that opinion, prejudice and anecdote become the bases for action. Observational studies and epidemiology's powerful methods are also useful, as elsewhere in the social sciences, particularly when embedded in robust theories developed in psychology, education and other basic sciences. A particularly infuriating error occurs in evaluating methods of selection, when arguments of the following form are used simultaneously:

- "These students have only been followed up for 5 years, but our selection process was assessing who would become good practising doctors in the future. These results do not look far enough into the future."
- "This study was carried out over 5 years ago, and since then we have changed our selection process and our undergraduate curriculum, and the doctors will be working in a medical system that has also changed. These results are only of historical interest."

Put thus, the sophistry is obvious: prospective, longitudinal studies for N years must, of necessity, have been started more than N years ago. Of course, the same arguments are not used in medical practice: chemotherapeutic regimens looking at 5-year survival must be subject to the same problems, but the trials are still done.

A further problem with studying selection is the vulnerability of the egos of those doing the selection. No one wants to feel that their actions have been wasted or their best-considered schemes are worthless. Nor do institutions want to publish results suggesting they are not doing a perfect job. A typical reflex response is to demand an unreasonably high criterion of evidence that is a paragon of perfection. The best is, however, the enemy of the good. The scientific study of selection is no different from any other science. One is not searching for proof of absolute truth, but identifying working explanatory hypotheses, compatible with evidence, which have acceptable methodology, take known problems into account and are therefore robust against straightforward refutation and make useful predictions. That is then a basis for practical action and further research. Just like medicine, in other words.

Summary

"Medical schools are picking individuals who will ultimately enter the health service as doctors. This means that factors other than academic attainment have to be considered; medical schools have to judge whether applicants have the necessary core skills, values and attributes which can be developed during their time at medical school in order to become a good doctor."

Selecting for Excellence (Medical Schools Council, 2014)

Selection is an important but under-resourced aspect of medical school activity. Medical schools select applicants but also applicants select medical schools.

Many selection methods can be used by schools, from a purely administrative review, reading of application forms, assessment of biodata, psychometric testing, interviews, multiple mini-interviews, situational judgements tests and assessment centres.

Whatever process is used, it will have its costs and its benefits and needs to be routinely monitored, evaluated and compared with examples of best evidence-based practice.

References

Arneson, J.J., Sackett, P.R., Beatty, A.S., 2011. Ability-performance relationships in education and employment settings: critical tests of the more-is-better and good-enough hypotheses. Psychol. Sci. 22, 1336–1342.

Biggs, J.B., 1987. Study Process Questionnaire: Manual. Australian Council for Educational Research, Melbourne.

Biggs, J.B., 2003. Teaching for Quality Learning at University. SRHE Open University Press, Milton Keynes.

Cook, M., 1990. Personnel Selection and Productivity. John Wiley, Chichester.

Donnon, T., Paolucci, E.O., Violato, C., 2007. The predictive validity of the MCAT for medical school performance medical board licensing examinations: a meta-analysis of the published research. Acad. Med. 82, 100–106.

Downie, R.S., Charlton, B., 1992. The Making of a Doctor: Medical Education in Theory and Practice. Oxford University Press, Oxford.

Eva, K.W., Reiter, H.I., Trinh, K., et al., 2009. Predictive validity of the multiple mini-interview for selecting medical trainees. Med. Educ. 43, 767–775.

Goho, J., Blackman, A., 2006. The effectiveness of academic admission interviews: an exploratory meta-analysis. Med. Teach. 28, 335–340.

Kirch, D., Prescott, J., 2013. From Rankings to Mission. Acad. Med. 88, 1064–1066.

Lievens, F., Sackett, P.R., 2012. The validity of interpersonal skills assessment via situational judgment tests for predicting academic success and job performance. J. Appl. Psychol. 97, 460–468.

McManus, I.C., Dewberry, C., Nicholson, S., et al., 2013. Construct-level predictive validity of educational attainment and intellectual aptitude tests in medical student selection: meta-regression of six UK longitudinal studies. BMC Med. 11, 243.

McManus, I.C., Ferguson, E., Wakeford, R., et al., 2011. Predictive validity of the BioMedical Admissions Test (BMAT): An evaluation and case study. Med. Teach. 33, 53–57.

McManus, I.C., Vincent, C.A., 1993. Selecting and educating safer doctors. In: Vincent, C.A., Ennis,

M., Audley, R.J. (Eds.), Medical Accidents. Oxford University Press, Oxford, pp. 80–105.

Mercer, A., Puddey, I.B., 2011. Admission selection criteria as predictors of outcomes in an undergraduate medical course: a prospective study. Med. Teach. 33, 997–1004.

Pau, A., Jeevartnam, K., Chen, Y.S., et al., 2013. The Multiple mini-interview (MMI) for student selection in health professions training – a systematic review. Med. Teach. 35, 1027–1041.

Powis, D., 1998. How to do it: select medical students. Br. Med. J. 317, 1149–1150.

Prideaux, D., Roberts, C., Eva, K., et al., 2011. Assessment for selection for the health care professions and specialty training: consensus statement and recommendations from the Ottawa 2010 conference. Med. Teach. 33, 215–223.

Reibnegger, G., Caluba, H.-C., Ithaler, D., et al., 2010. Progress of medical students after open admission or admission based on knowledge tests. Med. Educ. 44, 205–214.

Richards, P., 1983. Learning Medicine: An Informal Guide to a Career in Medicine. British Medical Association, London.

Roadmap to Excellence: Key Concepts for Evaluating the Impact of Medical School Holistic Admissions. AAMC online publication, 2013.

Sackett, P.R., Lievens, F., 2008. Personnel selection. Annu. Rev. Psychol. 59, 419–450.

Schmidt, F.L., Hunter, J.E., 1998. The validity and utility of selection methods in personnel psychology: practical and theoretical implications of 85 years of research findings. Psychol. Bull. 124, 262–274.

Urlings-Strop, L.C., Themmen, A.P.N., Stijnen, T., Splinter, T.A.W., 2011. Selected medical students achieve better than lottery-admitted students during clerkships. Med. Educ. 45, 1032–1040.

Weekley, J.A., Ployhart, R.E., 2006. Situational Judgment Tests: Theory, Measurement, and Application. Psychology Press, Hove.

Wilkinson, D., Zhang, J., Byrne, G.J., et al., 2008. Medical school selection criteria and the prediction of academic performance: evidence leading to change in policy and practice at the University of Queensland. Med. J. Aust. 188, 349–354.

Witzburg, R., Sondheimer, H., 2013. Holistic review – shaping the medical profession one applicant at a time. N. Engl. J. Med. 368, 1565–1567.

43 Student support

B. Barzansky, G. H. Young

Trends

- Distress and burnout can negatively impact students' learning and their development as caring professionals.
- To prevent and mitigate distress, medical students need access to an array of services offered in the context of a supportive and non-stigmatizing learning environment.
- Services to promote learning and psychological and physical well-being should be made available, and students should be encouraged to utilize them.
- Overcoming student resistance to admitting a need for help is a major challenge, and requires that students be educated about the sources of assistance and, if relevant, their confidentiality.

Medical school is a time of intense mental and physical effort. Regardless of the differences in the structure and characteristics of medical education around the world, studies in a number of countries have shown that a percentage of medical students experience psychological distress, including burnout and depression (Dyrbye et al., 2006; Hope & Henderson, 2014; Sreeramareddy et al., 2007). Such distress can, in turn, hamper students' ability to learn and to develop as future professionals (Dyrbye et al., 2006; Dyrbye et al., 2010).

The purpose of medical education is to assist students in acquiring the knowledge, skills and attitudes that prepare them for the eventual practice of patient care. Therefore, medical schools should take steps to create a learning environment that supports student learning and professional development. This means identifying and mitigating the conditions that can potentially lead to distress.

The actions that the administration and faculty of medical schools can take fall into several key categories: supporting student learning; supporting student mental and physical wellbeing; and creating a comprehensive student services system. Some of these actions are preventive of future problems and others are designed to assist students experiencing distress from academic and personal issues, ranging on a continuum from concern and worry to psychiatric symptomology.

The published evidence for the prevalence of medical student distress is strong and there are many descriptions of its causes. However, there is less evidence for the success of various types of interventions in addressing the underlying problems. We will describe examples of strategies found in the literature. While there are published studies from around the world, they often involve a single institution with a limited number of participants and so may have limited generalizability. In describing potentially successful strategies to support students and mitigate distress, we will summarize the results of similar individual reports and include anecdotal observations by the authors. Those individuals at medical schools who are responsible for developing student support programmes should adapt the suggested approaches to fit the characteristics of their medical education system, of their specific medical school, and of their student body, taking into account such things as student age and university and national culture.

While the varieties of actions to support students that schools can take are described in distinct categories, there can be significant overlap in implementation. Each benefits from the presence of an underlying 'system', defined as the coordinated actions of people and the interactions of people and programmes/activities that is grounded in organizational policies and supported by organizational resources.

 A positive learning environment is a key contributor to an effective student support system and requires the support of institutional leadership and the participation of all members of the medical education community.

Ideally, a culture of teaching and learning is rooted in respect for all and fosters resilience, excellence, compassion, and integrity. A positive learning environment allows health professionals to carry out patient care, research, and learning environments built upon constructive collaboration and mutual respect. Addressing the learning environment is the foundational element to student support.

The 'learning environment' encompasses the sites where students learn; the professionals, faculty, administrators, staff, and beginning and advanced learners who interact within those sites; and the policies and processes that guide the interactions. A given student will experience many such learning environments, including classrooms, clinics, and hospital wards, as well as the office(s) that manage and execute policies and/or provide support and resources. The characteristics of the learning environment may act to mitigate medical student stress or to enhance it.

There are aspects of the learning environment within the control of the medical school, so it is useful to identify areas that could be modified to support student wellbeing. For example, how students are evaluated, including the grading system used, can be a stress point for students. The results of a multi-institutional cross-sectional study in the United States among first and second-year (pre-clerkship) medical students showed that a pass-fail grading system resulted statistically in less burnout and stress than a grading system with three or more categories. There was no statistical relationship between hours spent in class or the balance between clinical and didactic time on indicators of student wellbeing (Reed et al., 2011).

Medical students also may be subject to harassment, abuse and discrimination from faculty, residents/postgraduate trainees, other students, and others in the learning environment. This has been identified as a broad problem that occurs in medical schools around the world and can result in depression, anxiety and emotional health problems (Fnais et al., 2014).

Mistreatment can include behaviours such as verbal or physical abuse, harassment based on gender or race/ethnicity, or denial of opportunities for learning. There should be mechanisms to prevent the occurrence of such behaviours and to respond to incidents when students believe that they have been subject to mistreatment. As noted previously, institutional policies and codes of conduct set expectations for learner and faculty behaviour. There also should be clear processes that allow students to report incidents of mistreatment. Students, faculty, and others need to be informed about these policies and processes. The institution also should have ways to gather information about the learning environments to identify sites where negative events, including mistreatment, may be occurring. Such information may be collected through students' evaluations of their courses and clinical experiences, reports from individual students about mistreatment, or observations of faculty or others. Once incidents have been investigated and confirmed, steps should be taken to address the issue and to prevent recurrence. This will need the support of institutional leadership, who may need to exert authority to remediate or discipline the responsible individual(s).

The responsibility for cultivating a positive learning environment is institution-wide. However, the management of the student services component may, for example, be centred in a medical school office with responsibility for student affairs (Drolet & Rodgers,

2010), or one that combines the resources based in both student affairs and educational/curricular affairs (Slavin et al., 2014). Reliance upon isolated programmes in individual units (departments, offices) can result in duplication of effort and has the potential to result in gaps in services due to the lack of coordinated planning.

 An effective student support system requires the coordinated efforts of many members of the medical education community.

A centralized and coordinated system that combines the efforts of medical school administrators, faculty, and relevant counsellors and support staff can make efficient use of available institutional resources. A breadth of resources assembled as a comprehensive system is especially important since an individual medical student may have needs or experience distress arising from interacting sources and so need multiple sources of support.

Members of the medical education community, including administrators, faculty, counsellors/learning specialists, physicians/psychologists, and students have roles within a medical school to support medical student wellbeing. We are using the definition of wellbeing articulated by Vanderbilt Medical School in the United States, which includes intellectual, psychological, physical, and environmental components (Drolet & Rodgers, 2010). The members of the medical education community can have multiple and interrelated roles within student support systems. These roles will be described in the following sections.

 Medical students should be informed of the availability of support services and encouraged to make use of them, as needed.

Students should be made aware of the availability of support services. Ideally, this should take place early in the curriculum, for example during an orientation prior to the start of formal classes. Such an orientation can be used to describe support services and to introduce students to individuals who deliver these services. It is equally important to provide informational sessions to students during their clinical years, where the stressors are different. Some studies have found that anxiety, attentional, and depressive symptoms were highest in medical students during their clerkship (clinical) years (Chandavarkar et al., 2007).

Orientations alone may not be sufficient since students likely will not retain the information. It is helpful to provide the information about student support resources in a written and/or online format, such as in a hard copy student handbook or on the school's website, and to regularly remind students of where and how to access needed information.

Supporting student learning

 Medical schools should have resources to identify and remediate the multiple causes of academic risk and failure.

Strategies to support student learning may have as a goal the prevention of future academic failure or the remediation of current academic difficulty. Numerous studies have identified that academic difficulties may be the result of a variety of factors including poorly developed study or time-management skills, learning disability, insufficient knowledge and pre-medical preparation, personal or health-related problems, and a learning environment that does not support students' accomplishment of educational goals. Medical schools should have resources to 'diagnose' the root cause(s) of a given student's academic risk or failure and to develop a tailored plan for his or her academic support.

ENHANCING STUDY AND LEARNING SKILLS

Medical students may enter with deficits in the skills needed for mastery of the breadth and depth of information in the medical curriculum. A study of entering students in the United States indicated that adequate study skills (i.e. time management and self-testing) were strong predictors of academic performance early in medical school (West & Sadoski, 2011). Test anxiety was also identified as a problem leading to poor academic performance in a study from India (Mysorekar, 2012). Medical students also may enter with a previously undiagnosed learning disability, since they were able to compensate during their previous educational experiences.

Medical schools should have processes for early identification of problems in these areas, since students may not be aware of deficiencies or know how to overcome them. Specialized expertise at the level of the medical school/medical education programme and/or university is essential. For example, learning specialists are needed to deliver sessions on study and time-management skills and to diagnose and create an accommodation plan for students with a learning disability. Regardless of their organizational locus, specialists should have sufficient time allocated to medical students.

Sessions to identify deficits in learning skills can be offered prospectively, for example during the orientation to medical school to identify students with potential academic challenges, and also to set the expectation that students should access needed resources. Students then can be referred to appropriate specialists. There also should be tailored programmes for students who have already experienced an academic failure and for those who have been identified as having deficits in their learning skills.

PROVIDING SUPPORT FOR KNOWLEDGE DEFICITS

Risk for sub-optimal academic performance or academic failure may be a result of inadequate academic preparation. Based on the characteristics of their pre-medical education, students may have knowledge deficits in specific subject areas that could affect their performance during the medical curriculum. These deficits could be identified prospectively from reviews of pre-medical coursework, pre-medical grades, or performance on tests used for admission. Including such reviews ensures that the admissions process and staff are integrated into the student support system. Deficits in pre-medical preparation may be remediated through short pre-entry programmes for newly-admitted students, which include introductory preparation in medical school subject areas (Office of Educational Programs, 2015) or through longer courses based at medical schools or universities for students who have not yet applied to medical school and need prerequisite coursework (Andriole & Jeffe, 2011).

There are various support services that can benefit enrolled medical students who have concerns about their academic performance or have identified knowledge deficits in specific subject areas. For example, review sessions in specific subjects can be provided for groups of students, or one-on-one tutoring sessions can be made available for students with specific needs. Remedial tutoring may be provided by the faculty responsible for an individual course or by more senior students familiar with the course material. Peer teaching, in general, has been shown to be useful, with benefits for both learners and teachers. Even students very early in the curriculum, for example first-year medical students in the United Kingdom, found teaching by near-peer tutors to be an effective means to support their learning (Jackson & Evans, 2012).

MONITORING STUDENT PERFORMANCE

Student academic performance during medical school should be monitored by the student himself or herself and by school personnel. Ideally, students should be able to judge their academic performance before academic failure occurs, so as to obtain tutoring and/or counselling for their study or learning skills if the need is identified. Monitoring student performance before failures occur is facilitated by the availability of formative assessments, defined here as tests or study questions that are provided for the purpose of student learning, not for grading purposes. Courses should include such formative assessments early enough to allow students to identify and strengthen their knowledge base. Even with the results of formative assessments, students may be unable to recognize or unwilling to admit that they have academic deficits, as many will have been successful previously and are failing academically for the first time. Therefore, results of the formative assessments also should be used by students' faculty advisors and/or medical school administrators, who may invite (or require) participation in remedial activities.

A more structured system to identify students at academic risk could be created by performing a retrospective analysis of variables that are correlated with academic difficulty. For example, the University of Nottingham Medical School identified a series of markers during years 1 and 2 of the curriculum that were associated with later severe academic problems (Yates, 2011). Such a set of variables could be used to monitor student performance and to develop tailored remediation plans.

Supporting student mental and physical wellbeing

As with academic performance, student wellbeing should be facilitated through both preventive and interventional measures carried out by a variety of trained experts.

MENTORING

 Mentors are important participants in a system of student services. They must be trained for this role and provided with sufficient time and information for their duties.

Medical school faculty members can have various roles within a student support system. We already have described their roles as content experts in monitoring student performance and in providing tutorial assistance. In this section we will use the term 'mentor' to cover the role of the faculty member as a 'guide' who helps support the "personal and professional development" of the student (Frei et al., 2010). A systematic review of the literature completed in 2008 identified that reports of mentoring programmes for medical students originated mainly from the United States and were relatively rare from other countries (Frei et al., 2010).

Mentoring may be organized as episodic or longitudinal relationships between a single student or a group of students and a faculty member. In group mentoring, students may be from a single year of the curriculum or there may be students from each curriculum year. The latter organization allows both faculty and peer mentoring to occur, as students from later years in the curriculum serve as support for more junior students (Drolet & Rodgers, 2010).

Mentorship programmes may have specific goals and objectives or may be less structured, with topics to be covered arising from student and faculty interests. For example, mentorship programmes that include student professional development as a goal often include career advising, where the mentor helps students consider specialty options and directs them to faculty advisors and informational resources for their chosen specialty (Frei et al., 2010). There often are school-set expectations that students have a minimum number of meetings with their mentors so that the expected 'curriculum' of the mentorship programme is covered.

Regardless of the specific purpose(s) of the mentorship programme, it is important that mentors be carefully selected; trained on such things as academic, career and wellness advising; and supplied with appropriate informational and other resources to support their work with students (Drolet & Rodgers, 2010). Mentors also should be familiar with relevant institutional policies and resources, so that they can appropriately direct students to people and information to meet their needs. Conflicts of interest must be avoided so that students feel free to consult with their mentors about issues of current concern to them. For example, students may be less willing to talk freely with a mentor who has a role in their assessment or promotion. Mentors should have sufficient release time from their teaching, research and/or clinical roles to spend with the students so as to accomplish the goals of the mentorship programme.

SUPPORTING HEALTH AND WELLNESS

Stress and its sequelae, such as burnout, occur among medical students throughout the world and can have serious consequences for student health and wellbeing. A study from Brazil indicated that burnout, including emotional exhaustion and sleep difficulties, had negative effects on students' physical and psychological health (Pagnin & de Queiroz, 2015). Medical schools should have programmes to prospectively address the sources of student stress and to support student wellbeing.

Mentoring programmes, as described above, can be one important tool to support student wellness. The medical school administration, especially the leadership and staff in the student affairs office, can serve important roles, including providing financial and staff support for wellness activities as well as a triage function to direct students to resources. To support the triage function, the student affairs staff should be readily available by e-mail or phone in the case of emergencies. Medical students can organize wellness activities for their peers and, with appropriate training, serve as peer counsellors. Finally, schools can include wellness topics within the formal curriculum to help students develop realistic expectations and learn how to deal with stressors (Benbassat et al., 2011).

The medical school and/or the university can supply additional resources to support wellness. A gym or exercise facility can help students to maintain physical fitness and to relax from academic pressures. Classes in relaxation, mindfulness-based stress reduction, and meditation techniques can be made available. Also, activities that bring students together for sports or social events can be organized, often by the student body leadership and supported by the medical school administration.

PROVIDING HEALTH AND PSYCHOLOGICAL SERVICES

Medical students need access to healthcare for preventive and curative purposes. Depending on how healthcare is organized and financed in a given country, the mechanisms to ensure that students have accessible and appropriate care will vary. Providing healthcare may be the responsibility of the institution. For example, a university may have an onsite student health service, where physicians and other healthcare personnel are available at a set schedule. Where such onsite care is not available, medical schools should help students find a location for care, especially if students are not from the region of the medical school. In any case, the medical school should have policy that students can be excused from classes or clinics to access needed health services.

Students also should have information about and access to psychological and psychiatric services.

 Medical schools should ensure that students are not stigmatized for seeking needed psychological and psychiatric services.

As noted earlier, a proportion of medical students experience psychological distress, including burnout and depression (Dyrbye et al., 2006; Hope & Henderson, 2014), and depression has been associated with suicidal ideation (Givens &Tija, 2002). However, medical students may be reluctant to recognize and seek treatment for depression because of a number of factors, including concerns about confidentiality and the perceived stigma associated with mental illness that may come from other students or faculty (Givens &Tija, 2002; Schwenk et al., 2010). A supportive learning environment and culture enables students to freely discuss their mental health concerns without fear, thus reducing resistance to seeking support (Schwenk et al., 2010). Access to psychiatrists and psychologists and other qualified mental health counsellors who have no role in student assessment or promotion is important in creating such a safe environment. Students also should be counselled about the importance of seeking care and about the options that are available for confidential access.

During their time in the clinical setting, students may be exposed to infectious and environmental hazards, such as blood-borne pathogens or communicable diseases. The medical school should ensure that students are taught about how to prevent such exposures before they first work with patients. In addition, students should be informed of the steps to take in case of an environmental exposure, such as a needlestick injury, including the process for reporting such an injury and the site(s) they should go for care. It is helpful to provide students with a laminated card or other easily carried document, so that the information is readily available should an accidental exposure occur.

Providing other support services

 There should be knowledgeable individuals available to provide career and financial aid counselling. These counsellors should understand the specific needs of medical students related to these areas.

Medical students need assistance to manage their decision making in areas such as career choice and finances. Such support should include counselling from knowledgeable individuals and access to informational materials.

SUPPORTING STUDENT CAREER CHOICE

The type of career counselling a medical student needs will depend on how the transition from medical school to postgraduate/graduate medical education or practice occurs in a given country. Many countries with a 6-year medical curriculum where the medical student enters after high school require a 1-year internship after medical school graduation during which a specialty is selected for further training. For example, in Saudi Arabia, medical students do a year of internship after medical school graduation and then apply to enter specialties based on performance in an examination and medical school grades. In the United States and Canada, in contrast, students typically enter medical school after graduation from university and medical students enter residency directly after medical school.

In either model, students need help selecting a specialty and understanding the requirements and expectations for entry. As described previously, faculty mentors can be a valuable source of general information about specialty and career choice. In addition, students could benefit from presentations by faculty about training and practice in various specialties and by school personnel about the process of and requirements for residency selection. Students can learn about practice by observing ('shadowing') physicians in various specialties. School personnel should decide which of these opportunities should be optional and which mandatory, and when specific types of sessions should take place. For example, in the United States, shadowing is valuable for students in the pre-clerkship phase of the curriculum, while specific sessions on application to residency may better occur when students are in their clinical training. In countries where there is an internship year, students should be counselled about the general requirements for entry into residency early in the clinical phase of the curriculum, but specifics might be more suitable for the internship period when applications are or soon will be in process.

PROVIDING FINANCIAL AID SERVICES AND COUNSELLING

The mechanisms to finance a medical education vary by country. In some countries, there is no charge for education to the first medical degree in public medical schools, while in other countries medical education can be costly. In addition to the education costs, if any, students may attend medical school far from home and have living expenses as well as costs for books and student fees. Financial support to cover tuition and living expenses may come from scholarships or bursaries, which may or may not have a service requirement attached, and/or from loans originating in the private or public sectors. Medical students need to understand the implications of how their own medical education is being financed. For example, they should be aware before making a commitment that loans will need to be repaid after graduation and scholarships may obligate the student to specific specialty or practice location. Counselling related to financial aid should be available through formal sessions and opportunities for one-on-one interaction with experts, such as a director of financial aid or the dean for student affairs. The formal informational sessions should begin early, perhaps even before the student enters the programme. This will allow students to make informed choices about borrowing and budgeting. If loans are a major source of financial aid, there should be ongoing information provided to students about the debt that they are accruing. Whether or not students borrow to finance their education, they should be provided with information about managing their finances.

Creating a comprehensive student services system

We have detailed the elements of a comprehensive student services system and an approach to providing the requisite services.

Developing a comprehensive system of student support requires the efforts of individuals from many groups within a medical school/university, including faculty, members of the medical school administration, healthcare providers, and counsellors. These individuals will be responsible for specific components of the student support system, but should not function in isolation. Instead, there is a need for coordinated planning and implementation to ensure that all student needs can be met in an efficient delivery of services.

There are planning considerations and barriers that must be anticipated and overcome in order to implement a coordinated student support system. These fall into general categories.

IDENTIFYING AND MAINTAINING ADEQUATE RESOURCES

Planning for a student services system should take into account the total number of students from the medical school or other schools who may need services, the number and types of personnel available to supply each of the needed services, and the additional resources to support the system, such as information technology. Individuals may need to be hired if not already available and to be provided with adequate time to contribute to the student support system. This can be problematic if, for example, the faculty already have time commitments to be involved in teaching, research and/or clinical care. Release time from other duties is critical, since students will not utilize resources that they cannot easily access. Individuals who have specialized expertise, such as learning specialists, may be shared among a number of colleges and programmes.

The faculty, administrative staff, and counsellors who provide various services should be conveniently located and should have 'office hours' that take into account students' schedules, especially when they are in the clinical years or away from campus. Willingness to respond to e-mail and telephone calls 'after hours' is much appreciated by students.

OVERCOMING STUDENT RESISTANCE

Students may be reluctant to access services for a number of reasons. Services may not be readily available or conveniently located. Students may believe that, as future physicians, they should not give in to what they see as weakness, or they may fear being stigmatized by faculty members or peers, which may negatively impact their career. There may be a lack of trust that counselling and psychological and psychiatric services truly are confidential.

These barriers can be overcome through a variety of strategies. Students should be informed at the time of admission and throughout their curriculum about the potential for and frequency of burnout and depression and the importance of self-care (Benbassat et al., 2011). The confidentiality of counselling and health services should be closely monitored and student satisfaction with these services collected. Problems should be identified and acted upon, so that students know that the services are trustworthy. Students should also be provided space and time during their education to talk with mentors and other students regarding their experiences.

Policies and procedures should readily be available to all in the learning environment with clear expectations of how issues and reports of unprofessionalism and/or mistreatment will be managed. Perhaps the best advocates for student support services are the students themselves, as more senior students inform their junior peers about the need for and utility of the services.

Helping students develop the skills to monitor and maintain their wellbeing will likely benefit their resilience and their professional and personal development, as well as their ability to ultimately deliver patient care.

Summary

The institutions that sponsor medical education programmes should recognize their responsibility to provide student services and should organize these services to maximize their efficiency and effectiveness. This requires the allocation of personnel and other resources that support both student learning and overall student wellbeing. Students also have an important role to play. They should be encouraged and willing to become partners in creating and utilizing a system that serves their needs.

References

Andriole, D.A., Jeffe, D.B., 2011. Characteristics of medical-school matriculants who participated in postbaccalaureate-premedical programs. Acad. Med. 86, 201–210.

Benbassat, J., Baumal, R., Chan, S., et al., 2011. Sources of distress during medical training and practice: suggestions for reducing their impact. Med. Teach. 33, 486–490.

Chandavarkar, U., Azzam, A., Mathews, C.A., 2007. Anxiety symptoms and perceived performance in medical students. Depress. Anxiety 24, 103–111.

Drolet, B.C., Rodgers, S., 2010. A comprehensive medical student wellness program - design and implementation at Vanderbilt School of Medicine. Acad. Med. 85, 103–110.

Dyrbye, L.N., Massie, F.S. Jr., Eacker, A., 2010. Relationship between burnout and professional conduct and attitudes among US medical students. JAMA 304, 1173–1180.

Dyrbye, L.N., Thomas, M.R., Shanafelt, T.D., 2006. Systematic review of depression, anxiety, and other indicators of psychological distress among U.S. and Canadian medical students. Acad. Med. 81, 354–373.

Fnais, N., Soobiah, C., Chen, H., et al., 2014. Harassment and discrimination in medical training: a systematic review and meta-analysis. Acad. Med. 89, 817–825.

Frei, E., Stamm, M., Buddenberg-Fischer, B., 2010. Mentoring programs for medical students-a review of the PubMed literature 2000–2008. BMC Med. Educ. 10, 32.

Givens, J.L., Tija, J., 2002. Depressed medical students' use of mental health services and barriers to use. Acad. Med. 77, 918–921.

Hope, V., Henderson, M., 2014. Medical student depression, anxiety and distress outside North America; a systematic review. Med. Educ. 48, 963–979.

Jackson, T.A., Evans, D.J.R., 2012. Can medical students teach? A near-peer-led teaching program for year 1 students. Adv. Physiol. Educ. 36, 192–196.

Mysorekar, V.V., 2012. Need for mentorship to improve learning in low-performers. Natl Med. J. India 25, 291–293.

Office of Educational Programs, UT-Houston Medical School: Pre-entry program, 2015. Available at http://med.uth.edu/oep/medical-education/student-programs/pre-entry-program. (Accessed 29 December 2015).

Pagnin, D., de Queiroz, V., 2015. Influence of burnout and sleep difficulties on the quality of life among medical students. Springerplus 4, 676.

Reed, D.A., Shanafelt, T.D., Satele, D.W., et al., 2011. Relationship of pass/fail grading and curriculum structure with well-being among preclinical medical students: a multi-institutional study. Acad. Med. 86, 1367–1373.

Schwenk, T.L., Davis, L., Wimsatt, L.A., 2010. Depression, stigma, and suicidal ideation in medical students. JAMA 304, 1181–1190.

Slavin, S.J., Schindler, D.L., Chibnall, J.T., 2014. Medical student mental health 3.0: improving student wellness through curricular changes. Acad. Med. 98, 573–577.

Sreeramareddy, C.T., Dhankar, P.R., Binu, V.S., et al., 2007. Psychological morbidity, sources of stress and coping strategies among undergraduate medical students of Nepal. BMC Med. Educ. 7, 26.

West, C., Sadoski, M., 2011. Do study strategies predict academic performance in medical school? Med. Educ. 45, 696–703.

Yates, J., 2011. Development of a 'toolkit' to identify medical students at risk of failure to thrive on the course: an exploratory retrospective case study. BMC Med. Educ. 11, 95.

Student engagement in learning

44

S. Ambrose, D. M. Waechter, D. Hunt

Trends

- Learning is enhanced when the stages of mastery are taken into account for a lecture, discussion or for the curriculum design.
- Knowing how to identify what we do not know is an important step in becoming a lifelong learner.
- Designing educational programmes that engage the student in the management and improvement enhances the overall learning process.

Why is it that sometimes our very high achieving medical students struggle with aspects of our medical school curriculum? What can we as medical educators do to address their struggles and promote deeper learning? How much of the learning process do we control? How can we better motivate medical students to be active participants in the learning environment? How do we engage our students in curriculum management and faculty evaluation systems so that they feel ownership of their education?

These are common questions with a variety of different answers, and this chapter describes aspects of learning and student engagement that can help us as teachers address these issues. We possess the power, as teachers and educators, to create conditions that can help students learn a great deal – or keep them from learning much at all (Palmer, 1998). But we can only create these conditions if we both engage them in the learning process and understand our own and our medical students' level of competence and consciousness about what we and they know, and how that impacts the teaching and learning process. Let's begin with an examination of us, as experts in our discipline.

 "Teachers possess the power to create conditions that can help students learn a great deal – or keep them from learning much at all. Teaching is the intentional act of creating such conditions."

Palmer, 1998

Expertise

Teaching to help a student master content should be easy for those who are content experts, right? Not exactly. It is precisely *because* we are experts that helping our students develop mastery is so difficult. The more expert we are, the less conscious we are about our competence because many of the strategies, processes, protocols, procedures, etc. that we engage in on a daily basis have become automated or semi-automated, and/or we often skip or combine steps, both a blessing (for our own work) and a problem (for us as teachers/educators). It only makes sense, then, that when experts are 'teaching' to non-experts, they do the same thing they do when engaging with a task, for example skip or combine steps. This is part of the reason we often hear from medical students how much they value learning skills such as review of systems or differential diagnosis from residents to complement the information provided by the attending physician. There is more common ground between students and residents in terms of how they organize, represent, and interpret information about the patient than there is between students and attending physicians. Attending physicians are at a state of "unconscious competence", which is sometimes referred to as "expert blind spot" (Nathan & Koedinger, 2000), and this can work against us as we strive to help our students learn.

Sprague and Stuart (2000) shed light on this phenomenon in their illustration of the stages of mastery, ending in the state of unconscious competence, i.e. expertise (Fig. 44.1). As mastery develops and students gradually gain competence within a domain, they first gain and then lose conscious awareness of the skills they are developing and using. As a result, experts eventually find themselves in a state of unconscious competence, executing procedures and processes etc. without thinking much about how they actually engage in the procedure and process etc., and totally unaware of the 'shortcuts' they take as they combine and/or skip steps. Think of how often, during your routine drive to work, you don't even notice how you got there because it is so routine (both the actual driving

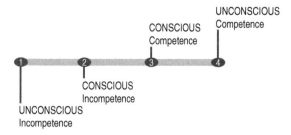

Fig. 44.1 Stages in the development of mastery.

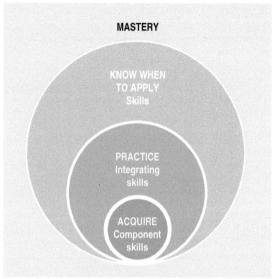

Fig. 44.2 Elements of mastery.

From Ambrose et al.: How learning works: 7 research-based principles for smart teaching, San Francisco, CA: Jossey-Bass, 2010.

and the route), and yet many complex cognitive and motor skills were on autopilot to you, the 'expert' driver. You were in the state of unconscious competence, and yet think about how more challenging it would be to explain how to drive to a beginner.

Because of this expert blind spot, when we as teachers are at the state of unconscious competence level, we also over-estimate what novices know and can do, and under-estimate how long novices will take to complete a task. We can fail to anticipate where novices will have difficulty, and presume that novices do things the way the expert does (Hinds, 1999; Nathan & Koedinger, 2000).

As we design our small group sessions, lectures, and ultimately the curriculum as a whole, these blind spots in both the teacher and the learner can negatively impact the learning environment. When the student is in the unconscious incompetence stage, they are not yet aware of what and how much they do not know, which often makes it difficult for them to even ask questions. Soon, however, they develop the basic sets of information or skills and can use them consciously with concentration, energy, and effort (so they are consciously competent), although they still might not be able to identify gaps or integrate and synthesize the information (per the development of mastery, discussed below).

It is at precisely this stage that residents, being just a few years ahead of students in their own training, can exert catalytic impact for the medical student because the residents are still in touch with the logic or steps in procedures that lead to competence. The residents who are still, in their own mind, going through the steps of logic to carry out the skill or to arrive at a diagnosis are able to explain the connections of otherwise isolated data in the student's mind. With the more experienced physician, who has passed through these stages long ago, it takes a conscious effort to recapture those connections in order to explain them in a way that fits the student's needs. Being aware of these factors can greatly contribute to the learning environment of our students.

So, what does this mean for helping our students to learn/develop mastery?

Mastery

No matter what we are teaching, our goal is for students to master the content, whether the content is a concept (e.g. patient safety), a discrete skill (e.g. auscultate the lungs), a process (e.g. formulate a patient problem list), a system (e.g. accessing pharmaceutical formularies), a procedure (e.g. perform a venipuncture), etc. In order to develop mastery, learners must acquire component knowledge and skills, practise integrating them, and know when to apply them (Fig. 44.2) (Ambrose et al., 2010).

The initial stage in mastery is the acquisition of component skills, which at first pass one would assume would be easy for experts to teach. But as noted above, experts may have difficulty even recognizing the component parts of a process or procedure because what appears simple and easy to them often includes a complex combination of components or sub-skills that they are no longer conscious of. For example, knowing when to see past 'demoralization' and explore the underlying depression to determine the lethality of the self-destructive tendencies, or understanding how carbohydrates are metabolized in order to anticipate the best medication for a diabetic patient. These are complex skill sets that link several different sets of information in order to arrive at the best solution.

The importance of clearly articulating and modelling each of the steps in a process or procedure is twofold:

it allows both the learner and the teacher to identify areas of struggle with or lack of understanding of a particular step in the process, which then enables the learner to focus his or her practise where necessary. While practise of component skills is important to assure that certain components become automatic (such as how people learn multiplication tables), it is equally important for students to learn to use those skills in combination with other skills that are necessary to perform complex tasks.

This leads to the next stage of mastery, which is the opportunity to practise using the component skills in combination, which requires executing and coordinating multiple skills at the same time. Experts are experts in part because they have a level of fluency and automaticity of the component parts that allows them to perform complex tasks by combining a number of component skills, something that took years to master. Experts can tend to forget how they themselves struggled to achieve this mastery level.

The final stage of mastery occurs when learners are able to use the skills they've learned in the appropriate context – they recognize the combination of skills that are necessary to complete a task. This, of course, is one of the main goals of education – to enable students to apply the skills and knowledge they have to new situations in the real world.

We can also connect these three elements of mastery to three types of knowledge that are equally important: declarative, procedural, and contextual (Anderson & Krathwohl, 2001). Declarative, or factual knowledge, is often thought of as 'knowing what' – it is knowledge of facts, concepts, terminology, symbols, etc. For example, being able to describe the circulatory system, define hypernatremia, recite a patient history, or list the warning signs of cardiac arrest represent declarative knowledge.

Procedural knowledge, or 'knowing how', is the ability to enact what one knows – the procedures, techniques, and methods of the discipline. For example, it is easier to describe the laparoscopic procedure for removing all or part of the colon, but another level to actually perform a laparoscopic colectomy.

Contextual knowledge, 'knowing when', is closely connected to procedural knowledge, and represents the ability to know when to use what you know, including the criteria/conditions of applicability. For example, the choice of treatment to eradicate squamous cell carcinoma is based on the tumour's type, size, location, and depth of penetration, as well as the patient's age and general health. At a minimum, if you cannot apply your knowledge effectively in the 'right' situation, it is useless; in medicine, it can be dangerous. Contextual knowledge is covered in more detail next, but below are some strategies to address expert blind spot and student mastery because, if we can be intentional about designing our learning experiences with the elements of mastery in mind, we should see

learners who are able to use their knowledge and skills fluently and flexibly in new situations.

Addressing our expert blind spot and developing student mastery

Now that our consciousness is raised about how expertise can interfere with teaching and learning, and how mastery is developed, we turn to how experts can mitigate expert blind spot and help students to master content more efficiently and effectively.

- Utilize 'intermediaries' in your courses – those individuals who are somewhere in between expert and novice, such as residents and basic science postdoctoral students – both during the design phase of the course as well as the teaching phase, for example to review your lecture notes and identify 'gaps', indicate areas where students often struggle, suggest where more or varied examples might be useful. (Addresses expert blind spot.)
- Decompose complex tasks into their component parts (intermediaries may be particularly helpful with this by assuring that you are identifying every step or sub-component of a process). (Addresses expert blind spot.)
- Create different explanations of the same principle, system, theory, protocol, etc. for those students who need to hear multiple explanations to process the information effectively. (Addresses the 'your students aren't you' phenomena that comes with expert blind spot.)
- Identify appropriate analogies to help make new material more understandable and to aid students in connecting new knowledge to prior knowledge. (Address same issue as above.)
- Provide as much opportunity for learning in context as possible – so that students understand the conditions of applicability of what they're learning. (Addresses 'transfer' issue in mastery, using knowledge and skills in new contexts.)
- Balance isolated practise with whole task practise so that students can integrate knowledge and skills toward solving a problem, making a diagnosis, completing a task, etc. (Addresses mastery.)
- Gather data to use as you plan assignments, exams, projects, etc., for example on how long it takes your students to do tasks, and the different ways they engage with tasks. (Address expert blind spot per us over-estimating and under-estimating.)
- Model expert performance by 'thinking out loud' as you engage in a task. This allows students to 'see' the steps you go through, the issues you consider, the questions you ask yourself, etc. as

you work towards solving a problem. (Addresses mastery.)

Contextual learning and thinking

 "When I ask my students at the beginning of the clinical year to explain symptoms, they seem to go blank … I feel like I have to teach it all over again for them."

Commonly heard among attendings in the hospitals and clinics

As a clinician on the wards, have you had the experience of asking a student to explain the underlying cause of an illness, such as diabetes, and then watched the blank (and sometimes panicked) look come over the student's face as he or she struggles to articulate an answer? Do you sometimes ask your colleagues what they are teaching in those pre-clinical years because it seems like we have to teach it all ourselves? This common phenomenon is in part a result of the context in which the student learned the information and developed the skills. As many schools around the world retain the division between the basic science years, referred to here as the pre-clinical years and the clinical training years, the issue of contextual learning is another important learning principle to be aware of and apply in the design of our curricula.

The application of skills or knowledge learned in one context and then applied to a different context is referred to as 'transfer' (Ambrose et al., 2010). Transfer is said to be 'near' if the learning context and transfer context are similar, and 'far' when the contexts are dissimilar. We especially need to prepare our students for far transfer as most often they will be using their knowledge and skills in very different contexts from which they originally learned them. For example, when a series of basic science courses, such as physiology and biochemistry etc., are taught separately as 'building blocks' in the pre-clinical phase, even though clinical examples and cases are provided, the students will learn what is likely to be on the test, which will be more about the Krebs cycle of carbohydrate metabolism rather than the context of clinical presentation of diabetes. The context here is far apart and leads to the observation of the clinician in the hospital that students have not learned this material. The student may have the information but it is not activated or organized in way that leads to easy access and use when presented with the patient problem.

As described in Chapters 2 and 3 of this book, there has been an evolution of how information is taught to allow transfer to the clinical setting to be easier for students. An organ systems curriculum design integrates the information better than separate basic science courses but still leaves the contexts apart. Patients don't present with a 'cardiovascular' event.

Patients present with arrhythmias and congestive heart failure.

Problem-based learning (Chapter 18) reduces the contextual distance but can have limited generalizability because of the increased demand for resources. The clinical presentation model, introduced by the University of Calgary Cumming School of Medicine, uses 120 clinical presentations to organize the pre-clinical information needed by the student for clinical problem solving (Mandin et Al., 1995). Because the diagnostic schema for each of the clinical presentations drives the organization of the basic science and clinical skill teaching, the information is mentally organized in a way that allows them to apply what they know to situations that don't present in their clinical training and practice of medicine. Here the context is 'near' and, when presented with that clinical situation in the clinic or hospital, the information is more readily accessible.

 Let students hear you 'talk out loud' as you describe the way you would assess the task and assess your own strengths and weaknesses in relation to the task. ("I have a pretty good handle on the basic concepts, but I don't yet know what recent research has been done on the subject.")

Ambrose, 2010

Strategies for developing medical students' contextual thinking

- **Show application of knowledge in different contexts.** Teach more than just knowledge – teach when to apply it. Clearly and explicitly explain the conditions and contexts within which particular knowledge is applicable. For example, don't just teach students sharp debridement procedures for wound healing, teach students to recognize which patients are good candidates for the procedure. Chapter 3 of this book describes curriculum design concepts that emphasize this area.
- **Provide opportunities for application of knowledge and skills to various contexts.** Teaching students to apply knowledge and skills across diverse contexts can prepare them to transfer those to novel situations. To assist in this, present students with a problem, case or scenario and ask them to address or solve it. For example, if you are teaching students how to write a treatment plan, assign multiple cases to provide students the opportunity to apply this skill in the context of different patient diagnoses. Or provide students with a case about a patient with hyperthyroidism and ask them to determine the underlying causes, diagnosis and appropriate treatment.

- **Ask students, through discussion and on assignments, to move from specific contexts to larger principles.** Students should have opportunities to practise generalizing from specific contexts to abstract principles in order to increase the flexibility of knowledge and its transfer to multiple/new situations. For example, you might ask, "Given this patient's reported symptoms, what additional information would you gather to determine a diagnosis?"

- **Provide practice for students to identify key information.** Students may not transfer knowledge or skills appropriately if they do not recognize the significant features of the problem. Providing students with structured comparisons – of problems, cases or scenarios – can assist them in learning to differentiate the pertinent features of the problem from surface characteristics. For example, you could present students with two cases in which the initial complaint is chest pain or headache but the underlying causes are different.

- **Require students to generate situations where specific skills or knowledge could be applied.** Another approach to help students effectively apply their knowledge and skills across a variety of contexts is to specify a skill or piece of knowledge and ask students to generate contexts in which the skill or knowledge would apply or not apply. For example, after the student has learned how to examine the external canal of the ear with an otoscope, they should be provided with the information of the likelihood of finding any abnormalities in the absence of symptoms.

- **Use prompts to assist student learning.** Sometimes students do not realize they have skills or knowledge relevant to a situation or problem. A prompt from the teacher can provide the stimulus that helps students make the connection between the situation and their skills and knowledge. Examples of prompts include "Where have we seen this cluster of symptoms before?" or "Think back to the treatment options we discussed last week."

Student engagement in the management of the learning environment

As we incorporate these concepts into our interactions with students, it is equally important to engage them in the process of their own learning. Providing students the opportunity to contribute to the design, management and evaluation of the curriculum is an important aspect of adult learning principles. Ensuring that students see the result of their course and faculty evaluations closes the loop to help them be engaged learners, and reduces the distance between the teacher and the learner when it is a partnership to maximize the learning potential. The Bologna Process for the European Higher Education Area recommended that schools should:

 "Establish conditions that foster student-learning, innovative teaching methods and a supportive and inspiring working and learning environment while continuing to involve students and staff in governance structures at all levels."

(EHEA, 2012:5)

One key phrase from this consensus paper is the importance of involvement of students in the governance of the educational programme. Engaging students with this process fosters their sense of ownership and provides them with an opportunity to step back from the day-to-day learning and both see and contribute to the improvement of the overall design. The more that students can be involved in the creation of the design of the curriculum and engaged in the quality improvement of the courses and the teaching, the more the student gains the sense of ownership for their own learning. Student engagement at this level encourages a form of metacognition that allows the learner to think about the learning process, and thereby make it more effective.

But how do we know when a school has the best form of student engagement? This question can now be answered with the information that is starting to emerge from the ASPIRE to Excellence project, which is an initiative of the Association for Medical Education in Europe (AMEE). The ASPIRE project brings together experts from around the world to develop accreditation-like standards that describe the evidence that would be required to document an exemplary programme in a specific field of medical education. Unlike typical accreditation standards that define minimum standards, these ASPIRE standards describe levels of excellence. The topics that have been developed as of the printing of this book are criteria for excellence in faculty development, student engagement, student assessment, and simulation. Schools submit their evidence to AMEE and panels made up of international experts in these five areas judge them and give the school feedback (http://www.aspire-to-excellence.org/). For student engagement, the general criteria and the number of supporting elements are as follows:

1. Student engagement with the management of the school, including matters of policy and the mission and vision of the school. (Seven supporting elements.)

2. Student engagement in the provision of the school's education programme. (Eight supporting elements.)

3. Student engagement in the academic community. (Two supporting elements.)

4. Student engagement in the local community and the service delivery. (Four supporting elements.)

Beginning in 2013, schools from around the world submitted evidence that includes surveys of students for their opinions for each of these four domains. International panels of experts independently review the school's data and reach consensus on whether a school has, indeed, met these high standards and deserve ASPIRE recognition. During the first 3 years of this project, 25 schools submitted evidence, and 13 schools have been recognized for their excellence in student engagement. Underlying the international nature of this effort, these 13 schools are located in 12 different countries. This speaks to the universal recognition of the importance of involving students in the governance and evaluation of the educational programme.

Key issues that these panels look for is evidence that students have significant representation and full voting privileges on curriculum and other decision-making committees. The panel has enjoyed impressive descriptions of major curricular change as a result of the student voice.

It is also important that student evaluations of the faculty are not just for awards but are used as a basis for faculty promotion as well. Peer teaching, peer evaluation, self-directed learning, and access to research opportunities are also part of a strong student engaged learning environment.

An aspect of self-directed learning that is particularly important is one that is associated with learning skills to prepare for lifelong learning. It is common to observe in all professions that people tend to focus their learning later in life in the areas that they are already familiar with. Thus, in medical school it is important to expose students to the self-directed learning skills that include the students' self-assessment of learning needs; independent identification, analysis and synthesis of relevant information; and appraisal of the credibility of information sources. This can be most easily done in the context of problem-based learning that is described in Chapter 18.

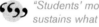 *"Students' motivation generates, directs, and sustains what they do to learn."*

Ambrose, 2010

One school that won the ASPIRE award for student engagement, the University of Leeds Faculty of Medicine and Health in the United Kingdom, was especially noted for the very high response rate for course and faculty evaluations even at the end of the years of training. It became clear to the panel that this high response rate was a result of an annual report that the school sent to each class as it was ready to move on to the next year of the programme. The letter was called their *You said…we did* report. It let the students

know exactly how their comments and feedback had been used. For example, "You said that the biochemistry exam was too close to the physiology exam. We have moved them one week apart." This feedback to the students allows them to see that the information on their course evaluation forms are being heard, thus closing the loop and leading to a strong engagement between students and teachers.

Summary

As experts, because we have achieved the state of unconscious competence, we must work especially hard to recapture the logical steps that lead us to a diagnosis or allow us to carry out a complex procedure. Residents who are able to carry out these procedures or arrive at these conclusions are closer to the student because they still consciously think about these steps as an important contribution to the learning environment. Being aware of the stages of mastery can help us to prepare our lectures as well as help us as we design the entire curriculum. Then, as we design our educational programmes, it will be important to learn from the lessons provided through the ASPIRE programme that has identified standards of excellence and specific schools that are exemplary in student engagement. When students perceive that it is 'their' educational programme and not just something being done for them for their own good, they learn deeper and faster.

References

Ambrose, S.A., Bridges, M.W., DiPietro, M., et al., 2010. How Learning Works: 7 Research-Based Principles for Smart Teaching. Jossey-Bass, San Francisco, CA.

Anderson, L.W., Krathwohl, D.R., 2001. A Taxonomy for Learning, Teaching, and Assessing: A Revision of Bloom's Taxonomy of Educational Objectives. Longman, New York, NY.

Hinds, P.J., 1999. The curse of expertise: the effects of expertise and debiasing methods on predictions of novice performance. J. Exp. Psychol. Appl. 5 (2), 205–221.

Mandin, H., Harasym, P., Eagle, C., Watanabe, M., 1995. Developing a "clinical presentation" curriculum at the University of Calgary. Acad. Med. 70 (3), 186–193.

Nathan, M.J., Koedinger, K.R., 2000. An investigation of teachers' beliefs of students' algebra development. Cogn. Instr. 18 (2), 209–237.

Palmer, P.J., 1998. The Courage to Teach: Exploring the Inner Landscape of a Teacher's Life. Jossey-Bass, San Francisco, CA.

Sprague, J., Stuart, D., 2000. The Speaker's Handbook. Harcourt College Publishers, Fort Worth, TX.

Peer-assisted learning

M. T. Ross, T. Stenfors-Hayes

Trends

- Peer-assisted learning (PAL) is increasingly being formalized as part of the core curriculum in medicine and other disciplines.
- Current research seeks to measure and maximize the potential benefits of PAL for peer tutors, tutees and the institution.
- PAL tutoring experiences are often part of a range of activities aimed at helping students and trainees learn to teach.

Introduction

There has been a considerable increase in the number of medical schools incorporating various kinds of peer teaching, peer assessment and medical teacher-training into their undergraduate curricula in recent years. There has also been a noticeable increase in the number of teacher-training courses, qualifications and formalized teaching opportunities available to junior medical staff. These are reflected in the growing literature and supporting evidence for teaching and learning approaches that we will collectively refer to here as 'peer-assisted learning' (PAL). This chapter outlines the principles of PAL and its relationship to 'collaborative learning', the potential applications of PAL in medical education with examples from the literature, and a practical approach to planning and developing new PAL initiatives that may help readers anticipate and avoid common pitfalls and maximize benefits for participants and the institution.

Medical students and postgraduate trainees have a long history of supporting and assisting the learning of their peers and colleagues. Examples in the literature can be found as far back as Aristotle. The origins of the phrase see one, do one, teach one are obscure, but the legacy lives on – although generally now with much more consideration of patient safety and quality assurance. Consultants and other experienced healthcare professionals have long been expected to take on teaching responsibilities, and this is increasingly reflected in professional standards for practice and contractual

agreements. Only relatively recently, however, have medical undergraduates and junior doctors been required to learn about teaching and gain some practical teaching experience as part of their formal curriculum. Many learning outcome and competency frameworks for undergraduate and postgraduate medical training now include something about teaching, and medical job applications at all levels typically enquire about teaching experience and training. PAL approaches represent practical and effective ways for medical students and postgraduate trainees to gain experience in teaching, to undertake focused teacher-training, and to receive constructive feedback on their teaching skills.

 "One who has just acquired a subject is best fitted to teach it."

Quintillian, c. 80 AD

Defining PAL

PAL can be defined as "people from similar social groupings who are not professional teachers helping each other to learn and learning themselves by teaching" (Topping, 1996). Using this definition, 'peers' share certain characteristics but are not necessarily from the same course or year of study, so may include students and trainees from different healthcare disciplines, although should not be significantly different in status or qualification. The term 'near-peers' is sometimes used if there is a larger difference between otherwise similar groups. For example, junior doctors teaching senior medical students, or occasionally senior medical students teaching much more junior students. The term PAL is a broad umbrella term, covering a wide range of teaching and learning situations, and also many teaching-related activities. Because it has been developed in different ways across a spectrum of educational fields, the terminology is diverse and sometimes conflicting. PAL approaches are sometimes referred to as peer teaching or tutoring; near-peer teaching; peer-supported learning; peer-assisted study; peer assessment; cooperative learning; peer group learning; students helping students; student tutoring or facilitation; student mentoring; study advisory schemes; teaching assistant schemes;

supplemental instruction; *parrainage* and proctoring. Terminology is not standardized, and sometimes these terms are also used to describe learning and teaching situations that are not PAL. A confusing variety of terms have also been used to describe PAL participants, activities and learning and teaching situations depending upon local preference and context. For clarity in this chapter and elsewhere, we attempt to standardize terminology so that in any organized PAL 'project', 'tutors' assist the learning of 'tutees' through a variety of PAL 'interactions' or 'sessions'. It is recognized, however, that in some instances, as in the production of PAL learning resources or curriculum development, there may be no direct interaction between tutors and tutees. Also in 'reciprocal PAL' each participant will at different times be tutor and tutee.

PAL and collaborative learning

Collaborative learning can be defined in many ways, the broadest of which is 'a situation in which two or more people learn or attempt to learn something together' (Dillenbourg, 1999). Undergraduate medical students and postgraduate trainees commonly work, study and learn together in groups, share experiences and stories and offer mutual support and advice. Informal collaborative learning is very commonly seen in friendship or study groups, 'coffee room' discussions and team meetings. More formal collaborative learning includes small-group tutorial activities, problem-based learning and 'buddy' systems. Whilst some types of PAL involve collaborative learning and vice-versa, they are often very different. Also, PAL tutors and tutees typically learn, or attempt to learn, very different things from the experience.

Theoretical basis for PAL

Most PAL participants report the experience to be enjoyable and beneficial in a variety of ways, and some of these benefits have been demonstrated in empirical studies and systematic reviews (e.g. Burgess et al., 2014). The findings suggest that the interactions and relationship between PAL tutor and tutee can be qualitatively different to that between student or trainee and 'expert' teaching staff. Many theories have also been proposed to explain the success and appeal of PAL. Topping and Ehly (2001) offer an accessible introduction to this literature, highlighting cognitive, communication, affective, social and organizational factors.

COGNITIVE FACTORS: CHALLENGE AND SUPPORT

PAL typically involves tutors and tutees being challenged in their understanding, beliefs and assumptions, leading to 'cognitive conflict', which Piaget and others consider

crucial to learning. Topping and Ehly note that tutors derive less academic benefit from PAL if there is low cognitive challenge, although they suggest that the cognitive demands of monitoring learner performance and of detecting, diagnosing and correcting tutee errors in PAL are typically high (Topping & Ehly, 2001). PAL tutors are closer to the academic level of tutees than 'expert' staff and so may be better able to understand their difficulties, sometimes referred to as 'cognitive congruence' (Ten Cate & Durning, 2007). For tutees, supported or 'scaffolded' learning within what Vygotsky described as the 'zone of proximal development' (the distance between what a learner can achieve independently and what he or she can achieve with more experienced assistance), through interaction with more experienced peers, is thought to be very significant (Topping, 1996). In a classic study, Bargh and Schul (1980) demonstrated that learning content in order to teach it results in better understanding and recall than learning the same content for an assessment. Such goal-oriented information processing, content learning and structuring are thought to offer significant cognitive benefits to PAL tutors (Ten Cate & Durning, 2007), although further research is required to explore under what circumstances the learning of content can be maximized through PAL tutoring (Burgess et al., 2014).

COMMUNICATION FACTORS

All participants, whether tutor or tutee, may be called upon to recall, explain and structure their understanding of content, perhaps for the first time. Verbalization is considered to be of key importance to the success of PAL, with both tutors and tutees gaining significant benefit from listening, explaining, questioning, clarifying, simplifying, summarizing and hypothesizing during PAL interactions (Topping, 1996).

 "How do I know what I think until I see what I say?"

E. M. Forster

AFFECTIVE AND SOCIAL FACTORS

Tutor enthusiasm and competence are likely to motivate tutees and enhance role-modelling. Because of their similarity, PAL participants are likely to establish a relaxed relationship with their peers. Ten Cate and Durning (2007) outline current thought on the impact of this 'social congruence' in motivating and reducing anxiety in tutees and of PAL as a vehicle for transmitting the 'hidden curriculum'. They also discuss affective aspects of PAL for tutors, including Maslow's need for esteem, role theory and self-determination theory. This suggests that by 'acting' as a relative expert, tutors are likely to feel, and then become, more like an expert in terms of competency, autonomy, esteem and motivation.

"The authority of those who teach is often an obstacle to those who want to learn."

Cicero

ORGANIZATIONAL FACTORS AND THE PAL PROCESS

PAL is often voluntary and supplemental to core programme learning activities. As such, it may result in increased time and engagement with content for tutors and tutees, and may add variety and interest to their studies. In some cases tutors also receive additional teaching from staff as preparation for PAL interactions. Group sizes are typically small, resulting in more individualized and immediate feedback for tutees than may be possible from staff. Intrinsic rewards from tutoring PAL, such as satisfaction and learning, are thought to have a significant effect on tutor attitudes and motivation, as may extrinsic rewards such as payment, privilege and evidence of participation for job applications.

All the above factors feed into the PAL process in which participants may extend, modify and rebuild their knowledge and skills; develop shared understanding; rehearse and consolidate core skills; generalize specific concepts; and give and receive feedback and reinforcement. This may lead to increased self-awareness, metacognition and self-confidence in both tutors and tutees.

Evidence for PAL

The medical and healthcare education literature now contains a substantial body of project evaluations, discursive papers and research on PAL. Together with research from school and post-compulsory education in other disciplines (Topping, 1996), there is much evidence to support and guide the use of PAL. It must be remembered, however, that PAL is not one single approach. Although there is evidence for the utility, acceptability and effectiveness of PAL with certain types of content in particular situations, it will not be appropriate in all situations.

PAL can also have disadvantages and unintended consequences, particularly if used indiscriminately or inappropriately. For example, it would probably be detrimental to PAL tutees for a tutor to give a didactic lecture on a topic about which they knew little, or try to teach them how to diagnose or manage cases that are too complex for the tutors themselves. It may, however, be very effective to have a PAL tutor facilitate a discussion and question-generating session on such topics or cases, lead a problem-based learning tutorial or teach specific well-defined clinical skills (such as shoulder ultrasound in Knobe et al., 2010). Commonly cited advantages of PAL for tutors, tutees and the host

institution, along with potential disadvantages, are discussed below.

 "PAL strategies are very well researched, with a substantive evidential basis for effectiveness in terms of raising achievement, fostering social and emotional gains, and often also developing transferable interpersonal skills."

Topping & Ehly, 2001

ADVANTAGES FOR TUTORS

Many PAL approaches encourage tutors to reflect upon and revise their own prior learning, to become more self-directed in identifying and addressing any learning needs they may have in relation to the topics being taught and to increase their self-confidence in content knowledge and skills. They may be motivated to learn new content and find new ways of thinking about and structuring content. They gain practical experience and greater understanding of teaching in relation to peers, which helps prepare them for teaching students and trainees in the future, and can result in a greater sense of engagement with the educational programme. PAL tutoring is also likely to enhance their ability to deliver patient education, although further research is required to explore the relationship between these two related activities.

Development of skills in communication, verbalization, observation, assessment and the giving and receiving of feedback have all been reported from PAL, as have teamworking, taking responsibility, organizational skills and empathy. In follow-up surveys many years later, PAL tutors often report that the experience had a significant and lasting impact on their clinical practice, teaching skills and attitudes. There is a lack of more rigorous evaluation of the longer-term impact of PAL, however, not only on the learning of content and its application to clinical practice for tutors and tutees but also on the development of tutor competencies in teaching, assessment and giving feedback (Burgess et al., 2014).

 "I think being able to teach is a crucial part of being a doctor in the future."

PAL tutor in O'Donovan & Maruthappu, 2015

ADVANTAGES FOR TUTEES

If PAL is supplemental to the core curriculum, tutees effectively gain additional teaching; provided the content does not conflict with or take too much time away from core teaching. They may also gain opportunities to ask questions and receive detailed feedback on their knowledge and skills. If PAL is used to deliver core teaching, as an alternative to professional teachers, then the question arises, how do PAL tutors compare to 'expert' teachers? In situations where tutees would be better served by core teaching from experts, it would be hard to justify replacing this with PAL.

The small number of studies directly comparing PAL tutors with experts suggest that they can, in certain situations, achieve similar outcomes in terms of tutee evaluation and assessment scores (e.g. Knobe et al., 2010; Perkins et al., 2002). It has also been suggested that in certain situations PAL tutors may be more effective than expert teachers in helping tutees attain defined outcome measures, for example by providing more individualized feedback, whilst in other situations PAL tutors will be less effective (Burgess et al., 2014; O'Donovan & Maruthappu, 2015). Selection of outcome measures and many other factors will affect such comparisons. Caution must therefore be exercised when interpreting sweeping over-generalizations such as 'peer tutors are as good as or better than staff', which are commonly seen in the literature. Peer and expert teaching do seem to result in qualitatively different learning experiences for tutees, which in itself makes PAL a very fruitful area for further empirical research.

PAL interactions are often relatively relaxed and informal, providing tutees with opportunities to formulate and ask even apparently 'silly' questions. They seem more likely to disclose ignorance or misconception without intimidation or concern that this may affect their assessment. PAL tutors are felt to be more aware of problem areas than expert tutors, as they are, or have recently been, in the same situation themselves. PAL tutors can often help tutees by talking about their own strategies and study skills and can act as role models and motivators for tutee learning.

 PAL may be particularly useful to ease the transition and cultural change when the context of learning changes acutely, for example new students or those moving from a pre-clinical to a clinical environment.

 "It was a good way for us to benchmark our performance in clinical skills."

PAL tutee in O'Donovan & Maruthappu, 2015

ADVANTAGES FOR THE INSTITUTION

PAL approaches can also offer significant advantages to the institution in helping address curricular outcomes and external requirements for students and trainees to gain experience in teaching. PAL may also be used to address other content gaps in core curricular teaching, to encourage a culture of collaborative learning rather than competitiveness between peers and to stimulate student engagement in the educational programme. From a quality assurance perspective, it has been observed that compared to staff it may be easier to

train PAL tutors and standardize their teaching. PAL may sometimes result in cost savings when students deliver teaching that would otherwise be delivered by salaried staff. However, as many PAL projects are supplementary to the curriculum and require additional training, supervision or reward for tutors, PAL can often generate additional costs to the institution.

Potential disadvantages and concerns about PAL

A number of authors have expressed concerns that PAL tutors may have inadequate depth of content knowledge and so may teach 'the wrong thing' or give incorrect information to tutees. They lack the experience of professional teachers and may not be able to adequately teach the knowledge and skills that they possess. They may lack experience in facilitating small groups and have difficulty retaining focus and discipline. They may overload tutees with information, teach in a way that conflicts with the rest of the curriculum and leads to confusion, or there may be personality clashes or personal relationships that interfere with the tutee–tutor interaction.

If a PAL project involves peer physical examination (PPE), there may also be increased potential for peer pressure, embarrassment and inappropriate behaviour. These are real and important issues, which have been reported from various institutions, although it should be noted that similar issues have also been reported for staff teaching. Concerns have been raised about PAL tutors being used as 'cheap labour' to teach on established courses because there are insufficient staff, where there are limited benefits for tutors, or where tutees would be better served by staff teaching. Concerns have also been expressed about the time and effort required to organize supplemental PAL projects, train tutors and monitor outcomes - all of which may take resources and efforts away from 'core' teaching. When developing a new PAL it is worth considering how these potential disadvantages can be minimized and how advantages can be maximized. A structured approach for this is presented in the next section.

Components and choices in PAL

PAL has been developed in many different ways for a wide variety of applications, including face-to-face teaching and tutoring; mentoring and support; assessment and feedback; resource development; and some types of curriculum evaluation, research and development (Furmedge et al., 2014). Irrespective of the type of PAL initiative being proposed, there are a number of common issues to consider at an early stage of the planning process, which can be summarized under the following eight themes (from Ross & Cameron, 2007).

BACKGROUND

PAL projects are developed within the context of wider educational programmes and should be considered in relation to programme learning outcomes, opportunities and progression. The opportunities and constraints, acceptability and potential applications of PAL will depend upon local institutional factors and the structure, processes and principles of the curriculum. PAL may be mandatory or supplemental to core teaching. Multiple PAL projects may be linked to provide teaching experience for all students in a particular year group. It is important to be clear about why PAL is being considered, be aware of the wider context and identify who will lead the project. Sometimes PAL projects are entirely student-led or staff-led, although in many cases they involve a combination of both.

AIMS

There are many reasons why PAL approaches may be considered, including educational, social, organizational and financial. It is helpful to consider these separately in terms of aims for tutors, tutees and the institution. Aims often relate to the reported advantages of PAL detailed above. Ensuring that PAL projects have clear aims and learning objectives and well-defined and structured subject areas can increase tutor familiarity with material and also provide a structure and focus to sessions. It is also important to define aims so that the PAL project can be properly evaluated.

 Think carefully about programme learning outcomes and how to maximize benefits for both PAL tutors and tutees.

TUTORS

Tutors can be recruited compulsorily as part of a course, on a voluntary basis or on the basis of high achievement. There have also been a few reports of PAL in which tutors are recruited on the basis of low achievement, in recognition of the potential cognitive benefits of tutoring, although more examples of this in medicine with objective measures of improvement in tutor learning are required. Tutors are usually drawn from the same year as tutees or from a more advanced year and so generally have a similar or more advanced level of ability compared to tutees in relation to the content. Very occasionally, tutors have even been drawn from a lower year. Some reciprocal PAL programmes involve tutors becoming tutees and vice versa. It is important that the tutors feel confident enough to undertake the task well and understand what is expected of them. Tutors may have to complete supplementary tutor training on content or educational approaches prior to PAL interaction. This might, for example, include learning how to facilitate a small group, teach practical skills or provide feedback. Tutors may also be required

to research a topic, prepare learning materials or generate a lesson plan in advance of PAL sessions.

 Try to ensure that tutors know what is expected of them and are sufficiently prepared, for example by giving them an opportunity to practise and gain confidence in their teaching through simulation before the PAL interaction.

TUTEES

Most PAL projects are offered as supplemental teaching for all students in the target group on a voluntary basis. Less often, PAL is used to deliver or help deliver core compulsory teaching, or is only available to selected students such as those with poor academic achievement. In all cases it is important to consider tutees' prior learning and experience. Most PAL projects involve no specific additional tutee preparation, although they may sometimes be asked to read preparatory material or even to participate in training prior to the PAL interaction.

INTERACTION

PAL sessions can be incorporated into the curriculum, timetabled outside normal working hours or held on an ad hoc basis depending upon the availability or needs of participants. There is wide variation in the frequency of sessions, where they are held, how long they last, how tutors and tutees are matched together and how many tutors are present (from one-to-one dyads to large-group lectures). Involving more than one tutor per session increases the breadth of tutor knowledge, dilutes the impact of an individual tutor's personality and may reduce idiosyncratic teaching. Sessions can be organized by staff or by students themselves at a variety of locations.

The commonest form of PAL in the medical education literature is the peer-led supplementary small-group tutorial, typically for revision (exam practice, past papers or discussion), remediation (help with content or study skills) or the practice of clinical skills (observed practice and reflection or review of videos). Some forms of PAL involve more didactic tutorials or lectures in which new content is presented to tutees (e.g. Knobe et al., 2010), or a less-structured approach, such as peer mentoring and support. Other forms of PAL do not involve face-to-face contact at all, but rather involve interaction using social networking tools such as blogs and asynchronous discussion boards, email and synchronous audio or video calls (e.g. O'Donovan & Marthappu, 2015).

Some PAL may not involve direct 'interaction', but instead tutors may help tutees to learn via the production of resources such as written summaries, revision aids and computer-aided learning programmes, or even occasionally through curriculum evaluation, research and development (e.g. Furmedge et al., 2014).

Curriculum developers may want to explore different types of PAL to provide tutors with a variety of teaching experiences, including large-group, small-group and individual teaching, assessment, giving feedback, creating resources, course organization and student support.

EVALUATION

Numerous approaches to evaluating and researching PAL can be found in the literature, from simple participant questionnaires to randomized controlled trials. PAL tutors and tutees are almost invariably positive about their experiences in feedback questionnaires. Interviews with participants, focus groups or observational studies by staff or simulated patients can be more revealing about how well PAL interactions have functioned. Studies of outcome measures, such as assessment results, comparisons between different types of PAL interaction or tutor training, or the reliability and usefulness of peer assessment and feedback, are less common in the literature but are fertile ground for further research (Burgess et al., 2014).

INSTITUTION

The administration and financial implications of PAL projects vary considerably depending upon the content being taught, the amount of training and support given to tutors, and whether sessions are timetabled and organized by staff or students. Staff involvement and contribution to PAL initiatives will depend upon the content being taught, the PAL approach and the local context.

As with planning any other teaching and learning initiative in higher or continuing education, it is recommended that PAL is undertaken in a considered, logical and reflective manner, aligning content and processes with learning outcomes for the educational programme and seeking approval and stakeholder engagement as appropriate. If tutees are to select from a list of available PAL sessions, the administrative time required will be greatly reduced with the use of an online sign-up tool.

REALIZATION

A number of potential pitfalls and unintended consequences of PAL have already been highlighted in this chapter, most of which can be avoided with careful planning. Simply thinking in advance about these potential problems and early recognition may be all that is required to minimize them. A timeline and action points will also facilitate communication between different stakeholders and ensure that important deadlines are not missed.

Table 45.1 presents three questions for each of these eight themes, the answers to which will form the basis of a draft PAL project plan and can help ensure the important issues have been considered (Ross &

Cameron, 2007). We suggest anyone seeking to develop a new PAL initiative, whether staff or students, work through these 24 questions, and then send the resulting draft plan to other stakeholders for feedback and approval before implementation.

Applications and examples of PAL in healthcare education

Many teaching modalities and strategies have been used in PAL, including revision tutorials, PBL facilitation, student support, various types of summative and formative assessment, lectures and the production of learning resources. Multiple examples and approaches to research in the literature can be found by following the references at the end of this chapter (particularly Ross & Cameron, 2007 and Burgess et al., 2014). Three practical illustrative examples of PAL projects in medical education are also outlined below.

 "The involvement of medical students as educators extending through a range of educational activities offers significant profit for both student and medical school alike."

Furmedge et al., 2014

SKILLS TRAINING IN SHOULDER ULTRASOUND (KNOBE ET AL. 2010, GERMANY)

One of the commonest forms of PAL described in the literature is face-to-face teaching and tutoring. There are innumerable examples in which PAL has been used to help students learn communication skills, history-taking, physical examination, practical procedures, evidence-based medicine, interpretation of X-rays or ECGs and prescribing. Most of these include self-reported benefits for tutors and tutees. In this example, nine willing medical students in years 3 and 4 were selected and trained in shoulder ultrasound, and the remaining students in their year groups were randomly assigned into two groups to be taught either by their trained peers or by experienced staff. There was no difference in scores between peer-taught or staff-taught groups in theoretical MCQs and practical OSCE assessments, but the trained peer tutors scored significantly higher in both assessments. Peer tutors were, however, evaluated lower than staff tutors for perceived competence and for not answering all tutee questions.

ONLINE FORMATIVE ASSESSMENT AND FEEDBACK IN CLINICAL EXAMINATION (O'DONOVAN & MARUTHAPPU, 2015, UNITED KINGDOM AND MALAYSIA)

Many PAL approaches in the literature describe peer assessment and feedback, most commonly in a

Table 45.1 PAL planning framework

Domain	Question
Background	What is the current situation and context in the curriculum? Why is this PAL project being considered now? Who is responsible for the project, and who will lead it?
Aims	What are the aims and objectives of the project for tutors? What are the aims and objectives of the project for tutees? What are the aims and objectives of the project for the institution?
Tutors	Who will be tutors, and how will they be recruited? What training will tutors require, and how will this be provided? How else will tutors prepare themselves and reflect afterwards?
Tutees	Who will be tutees, and how will they be recruited? What related prior knowledge and experience will tutees have already? What information and preparation will tutees require before the interaction?
Interaction	What will be the format of the interaction, and what resources are required? What would be a typical plan of activities during the PAL interaction? When and where will PAL interactions occur, and how will they be arranged?
Evaluation	What feedback will be collected from participants, and how will it be used? How else will the project be piloted and evaluated? What are the academic hypotheses, and how will they be tested?
Institution	Who are potential stakeholders in the project? What are the staff time and funding implications of the project? How could the project be developed, and how might it affect the curriculum?
Realization	What are the potential pitfalls or barriers to the success of this project? What are key points on the timeline for this project? What actions need to be taken to develop the project, and by whom?

From Ross MT, Cameron HS: AMEE Guide 30: Peer assisted learning: a planning and implementation framework. Medical Teacher 29:527–545, 2007.

face-to-face mock-OSCE format. By contrast, in this example, junior medical students in Malaysia were paired with senior medical student PAL tutors in the United Kingdom and expected to learn one aspect of clinical examination per week using open-access online videos. At the end of each week they would video-call their PAL tutor using a tablet computer and demonstrate the skills they had learned. The PAL formatively assessed them using an OSCE mark scheme, provided individualized feedback and encouraged further discussion. Participant numbers were small, but tutees seemed highly satisfied with the approach and all indicated they would recommend it to others. The feedback provided by tutors was rated particularly highly, and both tutees and tutors felt that good rapport was established.

RESEARCHING AND DEVELOPING AN UNDERGRADUATE MENTAL HEALTH CURRICULUM (FURMEDGE ET AL., 2014)

Many short courses and events developed by PAL tutors have been described in the literature, but it is less common for PAL tutors to undertake more formal evaluation, development or research of their core

curriculum. In one of the examples of PAL presented in this article (as 'Case study 4'), PAL tutors reviewed the way mental health was taught across each year of their undergraduate medical curriculum; undertook interviews, focus groups and questionnaires to explore the attitudes of other students; and then made recommendations for curriculum change. Their recommendations informed significant restructuring of the curriculum, which we are told improved student feedback, confidence and perception of mental health issues. Whilst not directly 'tutoring' face-to-face in this example, the PAL tutors were undertaking an educational role in relation to their peers, and so it still fits within our broad definition of PAL.

Conclusions

There is increasing evidence in the literature to support the efficacy and acceptability of PAL for a variety of situations and applications. PAL is particularly useful for well-defined subject areas such as the teaching and assessment of basic sciences or practical clinical and communication skills, but has also been successfully applied to more complex areas of training such as helping support students in difficulty, facilitation of self-directed learning, curriculum evaluation, educational research and development. The literature suggests that PAL may be less suitable for subjects where teachers need a broad general knowledge or considerable experience, such as advanced consultation skills and complex decisions about patient management, but further research in this area is required.

Development of a new PAL initiative should be undertaken with care and attention to detail, adequate resourcing and support, appropriate tutor training and educational scholarship – consistent with the development of any other component of an undergraduate or postgraduate curriculum. It is particularly important to ensure alignment with programme learning outcomes, to carefully plan the approach in consultation with all relevant stakeholders and to engage in ongoing evaluation and development.

Summary

PAL is a collective term for interactions between similar people, who are not professional teachers or 'experts', in which one helps the other to learn through some form of teaching. The concept dates back to ancient times, but has come to the fore recently in medical education; particularly in countries where all graduates are now expected to have teaching skills and experience.

There is a growing literature on PAL in medical and allied healthcare education. This includes using PAL to teach and assess knowledge-based subjects and clinical skills; revision and help with study skills; student support; course organization and development; resource preparation; and the facilitation of self-directed and problem-based learning. Many of these programmes report considerable benefits for student tutors, tutees and the institution, although further research is required to objectively measure them. There are potential pitfalls and drawbacks of PAL, but with careful planning these can be minimized.

References

Bargh, J.A., Schul, Y., 1980. On the cognitive benefits of teaching. J. Educ. Psychol. 72 (5), 593–604.

Burgess, A., McGregor, D., Mellis, C., 2014. Medical students as peer tutors: a systematic review. BMC Med. Educ. 14, 115.

Dillenbourg, P. (Ed.), 1999. Collaborative-Learning: Cognitive and Computational Approaches. Elsevier, Oxford.

Furmedge, D.S., Iwata, K., Gill, D., 2014. Peer-assisted learning – beyond teaching: how can medical students contribute to the undergraduate curriculum? Med. Teach. 36, 812–817.

Knobe, M., Münker, R., Sellei, R.M., et al., 2010. Peer teaching: a randomized controlled trial using student-teachers to teach musculoskeletal ultrasound. Med. Educ. 44, 148–155.

O'Donovan, J., Maruthappu, M., 2015. Distant peer-tutoring of clinical skills, using tablets with instructional videos and Skype: a pilot study in the UK and Malaysia. Med. Teach. 37, 463–469.

Perkins, G.D., Hulme, J., Bion, J.F., 2002. Peer-led resuscitation training for healthcare students: a randomised controlled study. Intensive Care Med. 28 (6), 698–700.

Ross, M.T., Cameron, H.S., 2007. AMEE Guide 30: Peer assisted learning: a planning and implementation framework. Med. Teach. 29, 527–545.

Ten Cate, O., Durning, S., 2007. Dimensions and psychology of peer teaching in medical education. Med. Teach. 29, 546–552.

Topping, K.J., 1996. The effectiveness of peer tutoring in further and higher education: a typology and review of the literature. Higher Education 32 (3), 321–345.

Topping, K.J., Ehly, S.W., 2001. Peer assisted learning: a framework for consultation. J. Educ. Psychol. Consult. 12 (2), 113–132.

Section 8

Medical school

Chapter 46

Section 8: Medical school

Understanding medical school leadership: medical teachers as agents of change

J. Gold, H. Hamdy, D. Hunt

Trends

- Everyone involved in the medical education programme needs to be an agent of change.
- Change is hard enough but becomes impossible if one does not understand organizational structure and how decisions are made.
- Decision making in complex organizations is less a top-down phenomena and more often driven by policies and relationships.
- It is important to remember that the *raison d'être* of a medical college is to educate medical students to become trustable doctors.

Everyone in a medical school has an important role and responsibility to participate in the quest for quality improvement. The title of this book, *A Practical Guide for the Medical Educator*, guides the perspective of this chapter to first provide an introduction in how to anticipate where and how decisions will be made in a complex organization such as a medical school, and then to use that understanding to know if the influence or information should be at the individual, committee, or affiliated group level. This is how one becomes an effective change agent.

While medical schools are organized differently, even within the same country, they almost always have in common three basic organizational structures to keep in mind as one traces how decisions are made and change is implemented. Understanding these basic models and knowing when one is more dominant than the other sets the stage for individuals to participate in and influence the changes that are essential for the rapidly changing dynamics of healthcare education and healthcare delivery.

As people move through the role of student, junior faculty, and ultimately to senior faculty and into administrative roles, experiences with increased authority is accrued and critical leadership skills can be nurtured, but these valuable insights can be lost or diminished if incorrectly applied.

Where and how decisions are influenced in complex organizations

 "If we could convince the dean on this issue then all would be settled."

A commonly heard refrain that often underestimates the complexity of medical school.

TOP-DOWN DECISIONS

Change can certainly happen based on a directive from the dean or the leader of the organization, but, in most cases, there is more to the process. In complex organizations such as medical schools one must consider the policies and committees that contribute to the outcome, and take into account the influences of the affiliated partners. These complexities are not represented in a medical school's typical organizational chart (Fig. 46.1), with its portrayal of a top-down reporting chain of command with the top of the pyramid being the dean. Assistant and associate deans, department chairs (sometimes numbering in the dozens), hospital and ambulatory care leaders, and research centre directors, are portrayed with direct and/or indirect reporting relationships to the dean (Northouse, 2004). While it is easier to portray it this way, it is not always this simple.

Fig. 46.1 does not adequately portray the complexities of these relationships nor does it clearly reflect how information flows and decisions are made. This typical organizational chart contributes to the common misconception that complex organizations such as medical schools have a pure top-down decision-making culture. While the dean does typically hold considerable influence, decisions are rarely as simple as the dean telling those below him or her what to do.

Individuals who underestimate the true complexity of these relationships can be heard lamenting that if they could only get to the dean and explain the situation or present them evidence of a better way to proceed then issues could be resolved. Sadly, these are the same people who get discouraged and may even give up trying to improve the educational programme because the strategy of "convincing the dean" fails to anticipate the other systems that are in play.

MATRIX-MODEL DECISIONS

The pure top-down model of decision making can work reasonably well in smaller organizations with single missions and fewer employees, but in medical schools with multiple missions that range from education, healthcare delivery, wellbeing of the community, research, and population health issues, decisions are rarely this one dimensional. Decisions in medical schools require an appreciation of the underlying systems that are in place, such as the committees that are governed by policies and bylaws. Then, if the decision involves resources such as access to clinical settings or research institutes, the needs of the affiliated partners must be accounted for. Thus, the challenge for an effective change agent is knowing when to mobilize consensus, how to use evidence, and how best to understand the relationships of different groups and anticipate how they will in turn use their influence on any given change event.

Knowing how policies evolve and how they are interpreted by the committees that are convened to use them is of utmost importance when the issue in question primarily involves resources directly under the control of the school. Knowing the composition of the curriculum committee and the scope of that committee's charge is essential when considering a proposal for change, such as introducing longitudinal integrated clerkships (Chapter 12), changing the admissions system to include mini-multiple

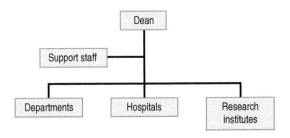

Fig. 46.1 The top-down representation of a medical school's organization is an over-simplification.

interviews (MMIs, Chapter 42), or proposing new systems to monitor professionalism in the clinical settings (Chapter 26).

A visual model of how various sub-groups contribute to the decision-making model is to think of it as a matrix. Here, as shown in Table 46.1 the different service units are shown across the top of the matrix and the different missions are shown on the vertical axis. Where these intersect in the matrix represent where the different policies of one or the committees of the other are the key points where change can take place. This matrix indicates that even though the curriculum committee might have the authority to make a change in the curriculum, such as introducing the MMI, the decision does not end there. In this situation, the decision to introduce a new way to select students for admission to the school will require interactions with the faculty development unit and its committees to secure time to train faculty in this new model (Steinert et al, 2006). It may also require the involvement of the human resource unit to create new categories for employment for the standardized patients, and, of course, the financial unit will always need to be closely consulted to get the pay structures in place for the new venture.

The awareness of these overlapping areas that intersect with the decision is useful for all decisions, and is most important when the decision only involves resources that are under the direct authority of the school. The effective change agent will have done their homework at the beginning as to how flexible the faculty development unit is and what kind of timing it might take to get their programmes imitated. Having the dean's buy-in is always helpful/important but the job to get the change implemented does not end with that first step. The work at this level requires the identification of the appropriate policy or committee that needs to reach consensus, and then an anticipation of the various other groups within the school that will need to support the change.

VENN DIAGRAM DECISIONS

Training a physician requires partnerships with clinics, hospitals and research institutions that, while affiliated, are not directly accountable to the dean. A decision to implement longitudinal integrated clerkships as described in Chapter 12 requires more than just the consensus of the faculty and the approval of the appropriate committees. Here the change will likely

Table 46.1 The intersection of mission and service can be fertile grounds for change agents

	Faculty development	Human services	Financial services
Research	Committee/policy	Committee/policy	Committee/policy
Patient Care	Committee/policy	Committee/policy	Committee/policy
Education	Committee/policy	Committee/policy	Committee/policy

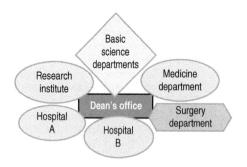

Fig. 46.2 Overlapping areas of authority and control complicate the change process.

involve clinical partners who often as not are not under the direct authority of the medical school dean.

When change involves these affiliated partners, a Venn diagram provides a visual model to help capture the relationships that need to be taken into account. Figure 46.2 illustrates this with the different sizes and shapes of the various contributing units which exert influences that vary depending on the topic that is being considered for a change. The degree of influence over specific decisions will vary based on the nature of the issue. For example, the introduction of longitudinal clerkships will likely have a reaction from some of the clinical partners but little reaction from the research affiliates. The switch to a different selection process for the admission of medical students is likely to have much less reaction from either of the groups.

 "Both forms of leadership (top-down and bottom-up) are necessary for scholarship and both depend on the local conditions. Wise top-down leadership relaxes constraints to create space and provide resources for bottom-up innovation, pilot projects, and new methods."

(Mennin, 2017)

A medical school with its many affiliated partners with different missions and different degrees of influence at times is like a group of loosely allied and relatively independent units that occasionally have a common objective. Fortunately, the work of medical education can be one of those common objectives, and often serves as a unifying mission.

The challenge for the medical educator is that all three of these decision-making models are in play at same time for most issues. A dean may initiate a study group or issue a mandate. Committees will work within their charge to examine and hopefully improve outcomes. Influential partnerships will gauge their role and exert their influence. There will be times when, in order to understand why a decision was made or failed to be implemented, one must not only understand the priorities of the dean but also anticipate the

influence of the committee structure, and the influence of key partners. As medical educators with a responsibility to influence, improve and at the same time survive, understanding these dimensions is critical.

As one matures in academic medicine through experience and study there are increased opportunities for leadership. With that increased authority, the need to read and understand the implications of the 'topography' of the college, university and community landscape becomes ever so important. Awareness and understanding of the relationships with various key aspects of a medical school, parent university and clinical learning environment are critical. Thus, the next portion of this chapter is devoted to describing these important relationships that operate on the decisions of many medical schools.

Relationships with the medical school departments

The relationship with the clinical and basic science departments is particularly important given that the majority of the faculty are organized into these units and answer to their department chair. In these units and through their chairs, the faculty must be integrated into the school's clinical and research missions. Increasingly, in medical schools, significant time commitments of faculty are allocated to the delivery of clinical care and to peer-reviewed, grant-funded research science. In these instances, faculty members need dedicated time to carry out their role in the educational mission. This is typically facilitated through the office of the department chair. In most institutions, the department chairs report directly to the dean, and in many countries they are recruited, evaluated and compensated based upon criteria that are consistent with their ability to effectively use resources. The academic promotion system and the funds flow model for each of the medical school departments may vary, and how much they take into account the medical education activities and scholarly activity in education is important.

The challenges in this area typically relate to the effectiveness of the chairs and division chiefs to work with each other, and the medical school leadership to balance the components of the mission as pressure for more research and increased demand for clinical care. Key to this balance is the personal leadership of the department chairs and their skill in clearly articulating commitment to the educational mission.

 "Many observers still see the topic of money in medicine as taboo—after all, the primary goal for many organizations is to help patients, not make profits. Yet it is important to acknowledge the cost of health care has been rising at unsustainable rates."

Wartman, 2015

Relationships with the clinical learning sites

Relationships with both inpatient and outpatient clinical training sites are particularly important for the experiential and assessment components of the medical school curriculum. The opportunity to assure quality learning settings in acute medical/surgical care, critical care, emergency services, and procedural experience for students as well as meaningful outpatient experience across a wide spectrum of settings depends not only upon faculty and chair willingness but agreement with the clinical institution is also key. Therefore, a mission driven focus on quality educational experiences is key for those clinical learning sites in which students rotate. In most instances, a binding affiliation agreement sets the legal framework for this relationship. However, the day-to-day management and overall effectiveness of the learning environment depends largely on the clinical service chiefs and clinical centre directors that are responsible for the area of clinical care in the specific sites in which the learners gain their experience.

In many instances, there is a wide spectrum of clinical site relationships that vary from single practitioner clinical settings through small group practices up through multi-specialty group practices, government supported clinics and ultimately university outpatient and inpatient centres. Because of this wide variation and the typically large number of such relationships, standardized affiliation agreements that span many years result in long-term stable clinical relationships. These affiliation agreements should contain language that ensures that the clinical affiliate and the medical school have a shared responsibility for creating and maintaining an appropriate learning environment.

The challenges in this area relate to inefficiencies caused by the learners in the clinical setting and the perception and/or the reality of diminished productivity and related revenue. In most instances, these concerns are balanced by the mission driven commitment to educating future colleagues and the potential workforce that can be recruited and retained as a result of these relationships. From the institutional side, having learners in the clinical environment can enhance recruitment and retention.

Relationship with the graduate medical education programmes

Given the need for mentoring of medical students by residents and fellows, the relationship with the graduate medical education programme is critical. Medical students are routinely taught, mentored, counselled, advised, and, in many instances, evaluated by the residents and fellows. Medical students readily identify with residents and fellows and, as noted in Chapter 44. The residents are only one step further along on mastery and they are better than the more experienced attending in "unbundling" the step-by-step logic that underlies complex skills and the synthesis of information. As such, there must be didactic and experiential instruction of residents to help them know both what and how to teach, but also to help them learn how to provide assessment of the student performance.

Challenges in these relationships typically stem from time constraints, and from the role transitions from student to resident and as such from the 'pure' learner to the hybrid learner/teacher/mentor.

Relationship with the research institutes and research centres

Many medical schools and universities have research institutes and research centres that are either part of or are affiliated with the medical school. These institutes and centres provide important sites not only for research experience for future physician scientists, doctoral students and others but they often provide portions of the pre-clinical curriculum.

When these research institutes and centres are tightly affiliated with the parent university or the medical school, the research and, in some instances, the clinical faculty are typically jointly appointed. This makes the assignment of their time through the basic science department chair and/or through the institute director, a relatively straightforward matter.

Greater challenges arise when the research institute or centre is independent or loosely affiliated. As extramural research funding becomes increasingly competitive and the pressures for academic productivity and commercialization increase, securing dedicated quality research experiences for medical students may become more difficult. The agreements/relationships with these institutes and centres may be as individualized as a separate one for each learner or global enough to cover the broadest of relationships. Strong leadership and experienced mentors as well as the opportunity to shape the next generation of physician scientists provide effective conditions to offer quality research experiences.

 "Thought of as a relationship, leadership becomes a process of collaboration that occurs between leaders and follows."

Rost, 1991

Relationships with the parent university administration

In many instances, the medical school is one of many schools within a parent university. This parent university may be dedicated purely to the health sciences or be made up of traditional undergraduate and graduate disciplines of study. These may exist on a single campus or they may be in a distributed campus system, within close proximity or scattered across hundreds of miles. If the medical school is a part of a public university system, there may be an elected or appointed government agency or leader involved as well.

The direct reporting relationship of the medical school dean to the parent university administration is particularly important, not only for advice and counsel but also as it relates to the distribution of resources and relationships with the community. In most instances, the basic science and clinical programmes within the medical school form a major part of the foundational infrastructure of the business aspects of the parent university, given the extensive funds flow that is connected to the research grants and the clinical care delivery aspects of the mission. In addition, the health sciences tend to be responsible for a significant portion of commercialization and intellectual property transfer as well as connections to the philanthropic community.

The challenges in this area relate to maintaining effective communication, particularly when distance and busy schedules create barriers. Active participation with the university and hospital leadership and their governing bodies helps to communicate expectations. Active participation by the dean of the medical school will often optimize the outcomes of these critical university system-wide decisions in maintaining core aspects of the medical school's mission and the critical resources necessary to support it.

Summary

Change within a medical school involves complex matrix systems for internal decisions and consensus building among affiliated partners when the decisions depend on resources outside of the direct control of the school. In order to understand how a decision came about or how to influence a decision, one must see more than a 'top-down' decision-making model. It is critical to understand how policies or bylaws drive committee behaviour, and then to take into account the perspectives of the affiliated partners in order to be an effective change agent. The dean serves as a 'translator of meanings' in the mission and vision for the guidance of strategic direction and actions. It is important to remember that the *raison d'être* of a medical college is to educate medical students to become trustable doctors.

Many of the chapters in this book describe new and exciting medical education innovations and strategies that are waiting to be adopted but to do so requires everyone to take part in the change process. Whether it is integration of behavioural science into a curriculum that lacks that subject matter, a new way to approach interprofessional education, or a pilot programme to try out longitudinal integrated clerkships, change is difficult and soon becomes impossible unless the complexities of a typical medical school are taken into account. A culture of quality improvement requires all participants from student to dean to at least respect, if not understand, these complexities in order to accommodate the inherent and realistic limitations when change is needed.

References

Mennin, S., 2017. Academic standards and scholarship. In: Dent, J.A., Harden, R.M., Hunt, D. (Eds.), A Practical Guide for Medical Teachers, fifth ed. Elsevier, Edinburgh.

Northouse, P., 2004. Leadership: Theory and Practice, third ed. Sage, London.

Rost, J.C., 1991. Leadership for the Twenty-First Century. Praeger Publishers, New York.

Steinert, Y., Mann, K., Carteno, A., et al., 2006. A systemic review of faculty development initiatives designed to improve teaching effectiveness in medical education. BEME Guide No. 8. Med. Teach. 28 (6), 497–526.

Wartman, S.A., 2015. The Transformation of Academic Health Centers: Meeting the Challenges of Healthcare's Changing Landscape. Elsevier, Edinburgh.

Medical education leadership

J. McKimm, S. J. Lieff

Trends

- Medical educators need good leadership, management and followership skills – the 'leadership triad'.
- These skills are essential for organizational, team and individual success.
- There is no 'perfect' leadership style or approach – leaders need to work adaptively and flexibly.
- Understanding systems thinking and complexity is vital to effect sustainable change.

Introduction

Medical educators are involved in a wide range of activities including teaching, facilitating learning, curriculum design and development, assessment, evaluation and managing teams, departments and programmes. All these activities require some form of leadership, whether this is leading a project team, ensuring the right clinical learning environment or leading new programme development. Effective leaders have followers, take responsibility, do the right things and achieve results (Drucker, 1996). We often think of 'leadership' as associated only with formal senior management positions but this is not the case. Medical educators can take both 'big L' (big projects, senior positions) and 'little l' (teams, classrooms) leadership roles, and individuals switch between leadership, management and followership roles depending on context and demands (Bohmer, 2010; Till & McKimm, 2016).

No matter the sector, the evidence shows that good leadership is essential for organizational success. Conversely, poor leadership or management plays a major part in failing organizations (Kotter, 1990). Internationally, doctors are being called upon to be more engaged in the leadership and management of clinical services, which has led to an increased emphasis on learning leadership in education and training programmes. This requires medical educators to be much more aware not only of their practice as leaders but

also providing education that includes leadership concepts.

A massive leadership literature has discussed whether specific qualities, attributes, knowledge or skills are more effective in different organizational situations. And whilst many leadership attributes and skills are generic, identifying the unique issues, challenges and opportunities in medical education helps to strengthen capacity of educational organizations to improve individual leaders' performance, thereby enhancing the experience of faculty, learners and ultimately patients.

Medical education leadership involves:

- Roles played out in a highly visible, regulated and complex environment: a 'crowded stage'
- Working across multiple organizational boundaries (higher [tertiary] education environments, community settings and complex health services), which are constantly changing
- Producing highly skilled, socially accountable professionals.

The 'leadership triad'

 "No-one is terribly enthusiastic about managers who don't lead: they are boring, dispiriting. Well, why should we be any more enthusiastic about leaders who don't manage: they are distant, disconnected. Hence I shall argue for leading embedded in managing, by recognizing its true art and respecting its true craft."

Mintzberg, 2009

Leadership, 'management' and 'followership' are interrelated activities – the 'leadership triad' (McKimm et al., 2016). Whereas many writers in the past clearly differentiated between the three activities, this somewhat artificial distinction promotes the idea that it is preferable to lead rather than manage or follow. Contemporary theory emphasizes the equal value of these roles embodied within the same individual.

In terms of management, this ensures that vision is supported by implementation and that valued operations and accountabilities are maintained and monitored while change and innovations are enabled. For example, if the vision cannot be translated into activities that work on the ground and make a difference to improving the performance of an organization or a learner, then the vision is illusory. Similarly, in the context of change, the management of important structures and processes must be attended to as well as new ones developed.

The followership literature moves away from leader-centric theories, which can have the disadvantage of over-attributing a leader's activities to outcomes and minimizing or ignoring the contribution of followers. Instead, outcomes are seen as the result of a dynamic, fluid, co-creative process between leader and follower in which followers and leaders influence one another.

"Our understanding of leadership is incomplete without an understanding of followership."

Uhl-Bien et al., 2014, p 84

When followers are engaged and active, they can help and support even relatively poor or inexperienced leaders; however, followers can also have a negative effect and undermine a leader's authority and effectiveness, despite positional or other power. This can be partly explained by the implicit leadership theories (Derler & Weibler, 2014), which suggest that people, groups and organisations have beliefs about 'good' or 'bad' leadership. These beliefs are culturally derived and often rest on historical factors, unconscious bias or characteristics of individuals unrelated to actual leadership performance or capabilities. Such characteristics include gender, age, ethnicity and professional background (Mannion et al., 2015). An inclusive leadership approach recognizes these issues, celebrates and welcomes diversity and challenges biases in self and others. Inclusive leadership also helps generate new perspectives and creativity and provides a sense of belonging that followers need (Hollander et al., 2008).

Our current understanding of medical education leadership

In academic medicine, practising and aspiring leaders identify knowledge of academic role-related and health professional practice, interpersonal/social skills, vision and organizational orientation as desired abilities of academic physicians (Taylor et al 2008). Rich and colleagues' (2008) literature review of desirable qualities of medical school deans identifies a variety of management and leadership skills and attitudes as well as specific knowledge regarding academic medical governance, medical education processes, legal issues and challenges and faculty expectations. Leithwood et al. (2009) found that successful school leaders engaged in the core practices of setting directions, developing people, redesigning the organization and managing the teaching programme.

The literature surrounding medical education leadership is, however, still in its infancy. Bland et al. (1999) were among the first to empirically study specific education leadership behaviours for successful university–community collaborations related to curricular change. The successful leaders in this study most frequently used participative governance and cultural value-influencing behaviours: communicating vision, goals and values, creating structures to achieve goals, attending to members' needs and development, and creating and articulating symbols and stories representing dominant values. Lieff and Albert (2011) extended these findings by studying the leadership practices (what they do and how they do it) of a diversity of medical education leaders in a faculty of medicine. They categorized medical education leaders' practices into four domains: intrapersonal (e.g. role modelling, communication), interpersonal (e.g. value relationships, soliciting support), organizational (e.g. sharing vision, facilitating change), and systemic (e.g. political navigation, organizational understanding).

This framework of practices aligns with the primarily relational and complex nature of leadership work in a medical education system that must simultaneously attend to education and healthcare service needs.

Bordage et al (2000) set out to identify the desirable competencies, skills and attributes of prospective educational programme directors in a variety of health professions as judged by potential employers. They identify educational, decision-making, communication, interpersonal, teamwork and fiscal management skills as important, but also being a competent practitioner, that is, having credibility. The top personal attributes were being visionary, flexible, open-minded, trustworthy and value-driven. McKimm's (2004) study of health and social care education leaders in the United Kingdom describes similar skills and attributes, and adds self-awareness, self-management, strategic and analytic thinking skills, tolerance of ambiguity, being willing to take risks, professional judgement and contextual awareness.

"Managing is a tapestry of the threads of reflection, analysis, worldliness, collaboration and proactiveness, all of it infused with personal energy and bonded by social integration."

Mintzberg, 2009

Mintzberg's 'threads' require deliberate attention in order to be effective. Effective leaders know how to think and make decisions in dynamic complex environments, which are constantly evolving in response to internal processes as well as unpredictable external demands. For complex issues, leaders are encouraged to act and learn at the same time by conducting small experiments with tight feedback loops that illuminate the path forward (Snowden & Boone, 2007). Education leaders must keep their eye on the central focus of student learning and look for ideas that will further the thinking and vision of the school as a whole (Fullan, 2002).

Lieff and Albert's study of medical education leaders' mindsets shows that, while these leaders employed the 'four frames' technique (Bolman & Gallos, 2011) for understanding organizational work, they favour the human resource frame followed closely by the political and symbolic frames. The human resource lens encourages education leaders to invest in valuing, supporting and caring for faculty and students and think carefully about engaging people by aligning faculty member interests with organizational needs. From the political perspective, they recognize, understand and engage with stakeholders' interests in order to be informed, advocate and cultivate support. They identify and leverage diverse sources of influence and appreciate that resource and political issues can underpin tensions in educational work. From a symbolic perspective, they work at ensuring a vision or direction that people can commit to. They attend to the importance of credibility and modelling important values and messages in their behaviours and programme, activities and policies. They also appreciate that traditions and belief systems can impede or enable change. Additionally, they deliberately appraise others' interpersonal and work style in order to understand how to socially situate people in the organization so they can work to their strengths (Lieff & Albert, 2010).

Leadership theory and practice

In this section we describe some leadership theories and models that are most relevant to medical education with practical examples. Table 47.1 summarizes a wider range of leadership theories and their key features found in the literature. Leadership theories provide lenses and explanatory frameworks for understanding situations and reflecting on and improving practice. Just as in education, some theories are more prominent than others at various times, but being able to take these different perspectives provides opportunities and ideas for leadership practice and development.

Personal qualities and attributes

Early theories of leadership saw leadership as a concrete phenomenon, focused primarily on personality traits and personal qualities, with the (stereo)typical leader being a charismatic, inspiring individual. In many

societies, reflecting patriarchal structures, historical traditions and storytelling that downplayed women's role, the term 'leader' equated with both being a man and with masculine characteristics (McKimm et al., 2015). These early theories are therefore sometimes called the 'great man' or 'hero-leader' theories and still have resonance today. Effective leaders understand themselves well, continue to learn and develop, seek feedback and can communicate well with others. This reflects the move away from the charismatic hero leader. For example, the 'authentic leader' is someone who is deeply aware of how they think and behave. They demonstrate a passion for their purpose and lead from the basis of their personal convictions and values. They are aware of others' values, perspectives and strengths, establish long-term meaningful relationships connected through a common purpose and are resilient, fallible and humble (George et al., 2007).

Authentic leaders are equally aware of the context in which they operate (Shamira & Eilam, 2005). In the unpredictable and ever-changing world of medical education, a transactional leadership approach that relies on extrinsic motivators such as material reward and recognition will not motivate and engage people (Bass & Avolio, 1994). Authentic leaders attend to people's search for meaning and connection, genuinely relate to others, support optimism and display resilience that contributes to the building of trust, engagement and commitment in others (Avolio & Gardner, 2005; George et al., 2007). Members of this leader's team are motivated by the leader's example, support of authenticity and self-determination in others as well as emotional contagion and positive social exchanges.

The 'relational leader' takes a 'leader as therapist' role, an approach derived from the human relations movement (Western, 2012).

 "A focus on individual personal growth and self-actualisation was readily translated to the workplace, through techniques to motivate individuals and teams, through job re-design and job satisfaction to make work more satisfying and produce group cohesion."

Western, 2012

The leaders' personal qualities include values of moral purpose and spirituality. The relational leader works with people in an authentic way, displays emotional congruence, humility, emotional intelligence and quiet authority. Much of the recent focus of leadership development activities on coaching and personal development reflects this approach.

The theories we have described so far emphasize the qualities that 'good' leaders display, but many leaders have a 'dark side' to their personality and can be toxic or destructive within teams and organizations (Jonason et al., 2012). Whilst some leaders are destructive

Table 47.1 Leadership theories and approaches

Leadership theory	Key features	Indicative theorists
Adaptive leadership	This leader facilitates people to wrestle with the adaptive challenges for which there is no obvious solution.	Heifetz et al., 2009
Affective leadership	Involves expressed emotion, the 'dance of leadership'. Leaders rapidly assess the affective state of the other, analyze their affective state and select the appropriate affect to display in order to achieve the desired (or best achievable) outcome.	Denhardt & Denhardt, 2006; Newman et al., 2009
Authentic leadership	Extends from authenticity of the leader to encompass authentic relations with followers and associates. These relationships are characterized by transparency, trust, worthy objectives and follower development.	Luthans & Avolio, 2003
Charismatic leadership Narcissistic leader	Hero leader, strong role model, personal qualities important, 'leader as messiah'. Organization invests a lot in one senior person, often seen as rescuer, doesn't recognize human fallibility. Leader fails to distribute/share power and can lead organization to destruction.	Maccoby, 2007
Collaborative (shared, collective) leadership	Ensure all those affected are included and consulted. Work together (networks, partnerships) to identify and achieve shared goals. The more power we share, the more power we have.	Archer & Cameron, 2013; West et al., 2015
Contingency theories	Leadership varies according to (contingent on) the situation or context in which the leader finds him- or herself.	Goleman, 2000
Destructive (toxic) leadership The Dark Triad	Leaders' personalities make them less effective or inappropriate as leaders. Extreme personality traits lead to highly toxic behaviours.	Kaiser et al., 2015; Furnham et al., 2013
Dialogic leadership	Promotes inquiry and advocacy practices in order to explore possibilities and stimulate creative thinking.	Isaacs, 1999
Distributed, dispersed leadership	Informal, social process within organizations, open boundaries, leadership at all levels, leadership is everyone's responsibility.	Kouzes & Posner, 2002
Eco leadership	Connectivity, interdependence and sustainability. Socially responsive and accountable.	Western, 2012
Emotional intelligence (EI)	Comprises self-awareness; self-management; social awareness; social skills: can be learned.	Goleman, 2000
Engaging leadership	Nearby leadership, based on relationship between leaders and followers. Effective style for public services.	Alimo-Metcalfe & Alban-Metcalfe, 2008
Followership	Followers are as important as (if not more than) leaders. All have different styles and behaviours that impact on leadership. A mix of followers is helpful; take care not to stereotype.	Kelley, 2008; Collinson, 2006; Uhl-Bien et al., 2014
Inclusive leadership	Welcomes diversity, surfaces unconscious bias	Hollander et al., 2008
Leader-member-exchange (LMX) theory	Every leader has a unique, individual relationship with each follower. These relationships differ in terms of the quality of the interactions based on whether the follower is part of the 'in-group' or 'out-group'.	Graen & Uhl-Bien, 1995; Seibert et al., 2003
Ontological leadership	'Being' a leader is central, in terms of process, actions and impact on others and self.	Erhard et al., 2011
Relational leadership	Emerged from human relations movement. Leaders motivate through facilitating individual growth and achievement.	Binney et al., 2004
Servant leadership	Leader serves to serve first, then aspires to lead; concept of stewardship is important.	Greenleaf, 1977

Table 47.1 continued

Leadership theory	Key features	Indicative theorists
Situational leadership	Leadership behaviour needs to adapt to readiness or developmental stage of individuals or the group, e.g. directing, coaching, supporting, delegating.	Hersey & Blanchard, 1993
Trait theory 'Great man' theory	Based on personality traits and personal qualities, e.g. 'big five' personality factors: extraversion, agreeableness, conscientiousness, neuroticism, openness to new experience.	Judge et al., 2002; Maccoby, 2007
Transactional leadership	Similar to management, relationships seen in terms of what the leaders can offer subordinates and vice versa. Rewards (and sanctions) contingent on performance.	Burns, 1978
Transformational leadership	Leads through transforming others to reach higher order goals or vision. Used widely in public services	Bass & Avolio, 1994
Value-led Moral leadership	Values and morals underpin approaches and behaviours.	Collins, 2001

because they do not have the skills or knowledge to do the job, or are unlikable, research is ongoing into personality factors and toxic leadership. Furnham et al. (2013) reviewed the empirical evidence around the dark triad, the three overlapping personality traits of narcissism, Machiavellianism and psychopathy. When these traits are extreme, this type of manipulative, self-serving, forceful, self-aggrandizing leadership is highly damaging and can lead to bullying and other toxic behaviours. However, Kaiser et al. (2015) suggest that all leaders need 'a right amount' of these characteristics (toughness, social influence, self-confidence, political 'savvy') combined with emotional resilience and stability in order to succeed.

Leadership is context dependent

In the late 1980s, the idea that leadership behaviours could be learned (rather than leadership being bestowed or earned) gained prominence. As their names suggest, the contingency or situational leadership approaches propose that how a leader behaves should depend on the situation or context. Hersey and Blanchard (1993) suggest that leaders should flexibly shift amongst four behaviours: directing, coaching, supporting and delegating in response to the follower's or group development. If followers are less confident, capable or willing, a directing or coaching approach is appropriate. With increased capability and confidence, leaders need to shift to more supporting or delegating styles. Laiken (1998) proposes that these behaviours map onto Tuckman's stages of group development. In the early stages of a team's work, leaders need to be more directive to facilitate forming. As the group moves into storming and norming, leaders shift to a coaching style and so on. This model can be useful for leaders in appreciating the need for flexibility in their leadership of individuals,

committees, task forces or teams. Often, medical education leaders prefer the coaching and supporting roles, where they still have a hand in the work; however, delegating to a willing and capable group or individual is essential and enables succession.

The contingent leader also assesses the context to determine the most appropriate leadership style. Goleman (2000) proposes that the emotionally intelligent leader can adapt to the context by drawing from six leadership styles:

- Coercive
- Authoritative
- Pacesetting
- Affiliative
- Democratic
- Coaching.

Leaders who use the authoritative, affiliative, democratic and coaching styles outperform those who use fewer and other styles. The authoritative style has the most strongly positive impact on organizational climate. The authoritative leader presents a compelling future vision and direction, maximizes engagement and commitment to the organization's goals and generates trust. The affiliative, democratic and coaching styles emphasize emotional harmony, consensus and support and development, respectively. Often medical education leaders have little formal power or authority, so engaging people around aspirations, valuing them and ensuring that voices are heard can be effective.

Importantly for medical education leaders (who are often high-performing clinicians or academics), pacesetting leadership can have a negative impact on organizational performance, leading to the leader becoming alienated and resented by colleagues as they struggle to keep up to (sometimes) unrealistic standards or pace of work.

Leading groups and teams

Leadership is often about effecting change through team- and group working. Drawing from humanistic psychology, 'transformational leadership' (a widely cited theory) focuses on stimulating the followers in the organization to transcend their own self-interest for a perceived greater organizational good (Bass & Avolio, 1994). This approach emphasizes motivating group members by raising their awareness of and motivation for idealized goals and values. This is achieved through role modelling, influencing skills and providing leadership tailored to enabling people to see the alignment of their own personal and professional goals with those of the organization to effect positive change.

In a similar vein, Kouzes and Posner (2002) describe five leadership practices: model the way, inspire a shared vision, challenge the process, enable others to act and encourage the heart. Both these approaches align closely with findings on the mind-sets and practices of medical education leaders, suggesting that this is a popular implicit model (Lieff & Albert 2010, 2011). These leaders role-model their values and moral standards, leading others to trust and respect them, creating a shared vision that arises from the collective, which then inspires participation. They foster a supportive climate by nurturing, coaching and developing people to achieve these goals. It can be exciting for people to have the opportunity to stretch themselves (with appropriate development) to create and contribute to something that is greater than the local and immediate needs. Such enterprises include curriculum development, or other educational innovations or adaptations that feel meaningful.

In the knowledge-based and networked world of medical education, the ability to communicate and think together well is critical to team and organizational effectiveness. Dialogic leadership evolved from the field of dialogue. The dialogic leader uncovers, through conversations, people's untapped wisdom, insights and creative potential (Isaacs, 1999). The leader's role is to ensure that people transparently share their ideas, and do not judge others' ideas. Inclusive leaders facilitate a broadening of peoples' perspectives and promotes creative problem solving by leading themselves (through candid conversations and being open to learning), building strong relationships and building a safe culture (Morrow, 2014). In medical education, this leader would try to ensure that working group members share responsibility for:

* initiating ideas and offering direction
* supporting and helping others clarify their thoughts
* respectfully challenging what is being said
* providing perspective on what is happening.

A systems perspective

Medical schools, their curricula and linked health services are a complex adaptive system (Mennin, 2010) that includes collections of independent–minded individuals who can act unpredictably (Westley et al., 2006). Consequently, medical education leaders need to let go of notions of control, tolerate uncertainty and ambiguity, and collaborate with others to identify the issues and potential solutions to try. A collaborative, shared or collective leadership approach (West et al., 2015) recognizes that programmes need to adapt to the environment, and that solutions will emerge from experiments and pilot projects whose results (failures and successes) will inform further design of initiatives. They collect team members with a diversity of perspectives to ensure the generation of innovative ideas and approaches.

For the adaptive leader, discerning whether challenges can be solved with known expertise (technical problems, which reside in the head) or whether new learning and behaviours are required (adaptive problems, which reside in the stomach and heart) is foundational to their work (Heifetz et al., 2009).

Changing curricula demands that require new designs and assessments of clinical capabilities and identities (such as competency-based education) are adaptive challenges that require new learning. The leader's work is to mobilize and facilitate people wrestling with these issues in order to be able to solve challenges, while keeping the picture of the whole education system in mind. The adaptive leader maintains focus on issues by asking difficult ('wicked') questions that enable conflicts and sensitive issues to be surfaced and addressed. Rather than telling people how to manage the problem, they assist the team in receiving the information they need to know and facilitate discussion of the difficult questions to enable them to make decisions.

In reality, leaders often fulfil many roles and operate within multiple discourses and realities as situations demand. The challenge for the current medical education leader is to achieve balance whilst operating in complex and constantly changing environments, managing as well as leading, and doing all this with compassion, authenticity and efficiency.

Western (2012) offers us the paradigm of eco-leadership, which has elements of other approaches and takes an ecological perspective. The eco-leader works within open systems, within networks and connectedness.

"Eco-leadership is about connectivity, inter-dependence and sustainability, underpinned by an ethical, socially responsible stance ... it is fuelled by the human spirit, for some this is underpinned by spirituality, for others not."

Western, 2012

Summary

 "Educators carry the double burden of managing and leading teams and institutions in a rapidly changing educational environment whilst working in close collaboration with a range of healthcare professionals to deliver safe and high-quality patient care."

McKimm & Swanwick, 2011

Medical educators at all levels provide leadership to their learners, colleagues and others that is characterized by its ultimate goal: to benefit today's and tomorrow's patients. This leadership is played out in a complex system that includes university environments, healthcare organizations and other regulatory and professional bodies. Leaders also manage and follow; they understand how to move within these roles seamlessly as they navigate through complexity. This requires understanding of policy agendas, strategy, systems and organizations as well as knowledge of operational management processes and procedures, without which change and quality improvements will not happen. Effective leaders are change agents who are comfortable with working in uncertain and rapidly changing environments, holding onto and communicating core vision and values, adapting strategy to external and internal change. Being able to negotiate across and within organizational, professional, department and team boundaries and to work within the 'spaces between' (which is where change is effected) is a vital characteristic.

But leadership is also about knowing yourself and 'people work': emotional labour (Held & McKimm, 2011). So authentic and consistent personal leadership and 'modelling the way' is vital. This is where leadership most closely intersects with where medical education and the practice of medicine are moving: into an arena where the social accountability role of medical schools is being questioned and co-created, where the concept of being and becoming a doctor and a professional is debated, researched and challenged, and where the importance and impact of emotional labour is acknowledged. Here is where the most recent discussions of leadership in terms of values, relations, authenticity, inclusivity, complexity and eco-leadership can inform the day-to-day practice of all medical educators, whether or not they are in formal leadership roles.

References

Alimo-Metcalfe, B., Alban-Metcalfe, J., 2008. Engaging Leadership: Creating Organizations that Maximise the Potential of Their People. CIPD, London.

Archer, D., Cameron, A., 2013. Collaborative Leadership: Building Relationships, Handling Conflict and Sharing Control, second ed. Routledge, London.

Avolio, B.J., Gardner, W.L., 2005. Authentic leadership development: getting to the root of positive forms of leadership. Leadersh. Q. 16, 315–338.

Bass, B.M., Avolio, B., 1994. Improving Organisational Effectiveness Through Transformational Leadership. Sage, Thousand Oaks, NJ.

Binney, G., Wilke, G., Williams, C., 2004. Living Leadership: A Practical Guide for Ordinary Heroes. Pearson Books, London.

Bland, C.J., Starnaman, S., Hembroff, L., et al., 1999. Leadership behaviours for successful university-community collaborations to change curricula. Acad. Med. 74, 1227–1237.

Bohmer, R., 2010. Leadership with a small 'l'. BMJ 340, c483.

Bolman, I., Gallos, J., 2011. Reframing Academic Leadership. Jossey Bass, San Francisco.

Bordage, G., Foley, R., Goldyn, S., 2000. Skills and attributes of directors of educational programmes. Med. Educ. 34 (3), 206–210.

Burns, J.M., 1978. Leadership. Harper & Row, New York.

Collins, J., 2001. Good to Great. Random House, London.

Collinson, D., 2006. Rethinking followership: a poststructural analysis of follower identities. Leadersh. Q. 17, 179–189.

Denhardt, B., Denhardt, V., 2006. The Dance of Leadership: The Art of Leading in Business, Government, and Society. M.E. Sharpe, Armonk, NY.

Derler, A., Weibler, J., 2014. The ideal employee: context and leaders' implicit follower theories. Leadersh. Organ. Dev. J. 35, 386–409.

Drucker, P., 1996. Foreword: not enough generals were killed. In: Hesselbein, F., Goldsmith, M., Beckhard, R. (Eds.), The Leader of the Future. Jossey Bass, San Francisco.

Erhard, W.H., Jensen, M.C., Granger, K.L. Creating leaders: an ontological model. Harvard Business School Negotiation, Organisations and Markets Research Papers No. 11-037, 2011. Available at: http://ssrn.com/abstract=1681682. (Accessed 27 January 2017).

Fullan, M., 2002. The change leader. Educ. Leadersh. (May), 16–20.

Furnham, A., Richards, S.C., Paulhus, D.L., 2013. The dark triad of personality: a 10 year review. Soc. Personal. Psychol. Compass. 7, 199–216.

George, B., Sims, P., McLean, A.N., Mayer, D., 2007. Discovering your authentic leadership. Harv. Bus. Rev. (Feb), 129–138.

Goleman, D., 2000. Leadership that gets results. Harv. Bus. Rev. (March), 78–90.

Graen, G.B., Uhl-Bien, M., 1995. The relationship-based approach to leadership:

development of LMX theory of leadership over 25 years: applying a multi-level, multi-domain perspective. Leadersh. Q. 6 (2), 219–247.

Greenleaf, R.K., 1977. Servant Leadership: A Journey Into the Nature of Legitimate Power and Greatness. Paulist Press, Mahwah, NJ.

Heifetz, R.A., Grashow, A., Linsky, M., 2009. Leadership in a (permanent) crisis. Harv. Bus. Rev. (July).

Held, S., McKimm, J., 2011. Emotional intelligence, emotional labour and affective leadership. In: Preedy, M., Bennett, N., Wise, C. (Eds.), Educational Leadership: Context, Strategy and Collaboration. The Open University, Milton Keynes.

Hersey, P., Blanchard, K., 1993. Management of Organizational Behaviour: Utilizing Human Resources, sixth ed. Prentice Hall, Englewood Cliffs, NJ.

Hollander, E.P., Park, B.B., Elman, B. Inclusive leadership and leader-follower relations: concepts, research and applications, The Member Connector, 2008, International Leadership Association.

Isaacs, I., 1999. Dialogic leadership. Syst. Thinker. 10 (1), 1–5.

Jonason, P.K., Slomski, S., Partyka, J., 2012. The dark triad at work: how toxic employees get their way. Pers. Individ. Dif. 52, 449–453.

Judge, T.A., Bono, J.E., Ilies, R., Gerhardt, M.W., 2002. Personality and leadership: a qualitative and quantitative review. J. Appl. Psychol. 87 (4), 765–780.

Kaiser, R.B., Lebreton, J.M., Hogan, J., 2015. The dark side of personality and extreme leader behavior. Appl. Psychol. 64, 55–92.

Kelley, R.E., 2008. Rethinking followership. In: Riggio, R.E., Chaleff, I., Lipman-Blumen, J. (Eds.), The Art of Followership: How Great Followers Create Great Leaders and Organizations. Jossey-Bass, San Francisco, CA, pp. 5–15.

Kouzes, J.M., Posner, B.Z., 2002. The Leadership Challenge, third ed. Jossey-Bass, San Francisco.

Kotter, J.P., 1990. A Force for Change: How Leadership Differs From Management. Free Press, New York.

Laiken, M., 1998. The Anatomy of High Performing Teams: A Leader's Handbook, third ed. University of Toronto Press, Toronto.

Leithwood, K., Day, C., Sammons, P., et al. Successful school leadership: what it is and how it influences pupil learning. Research report 800. National College for School Leadership, 2009, University of Nottingham.

Lieff, S.J., Albert, M., 2010. The mindsets of medical education leaders: how do they conceive of their work? Acad. Med. 85, 57–62.

Lieff, S.J., Albert, M. What do I do? Practices and learning strategies of medical education leaders.

Abstract from the Proceedings of the International Conference on Faculty Development, Toronto, 2011.

Luthans, F., Avolio, B.J., 2003. Authentic leadership: a positive developmental approach. In: Cameron, K.S., Dutton, J.E., Quinn, R.E. (Eds.), Positive Organizational Scholarship. Barrett-Koehler, San Francisco, pp. 241–261.

Maccoby, M., 2007. Narcissistic Leaders: Who Succeeds and Who Fails. Harvard Business School Press, Boston.

Mannion, H., McKimm, J., O'Sullivan, H., 2015. Followership, clinical leadership and social identity. Br. J. Hosp. Med. 76, 230–234.

McKimm, J. Special Report 5. Case studies in leadership in medical and health care education, York, 2004, The Higher Education Academy.

McKimm, J., O'Sullivan, H., Jones, P.K., 2016. A future vision for health leadership. In: Curtis, E.A., Cullen, J. (Eds.), Leadership and Change for the Health Professional. Open University Press & McGraw Hill Education, Maidenhead. (in press).

McKimm, J., da Silva, A., Edwards, S., et al. Women and leadership in medicine and medical education: International perspectives. In Emerald Publishing: Gender, Careers and Inequalities in Medicine and Medical Education: International Perspectives. Published online 25 September 2015, pp 69–98. http://www.emeraldinsight.com/doi/abs/10.1108/S2051-233320150000002005. (Accessed 6 April 2017).

McKimm, J., Swanwick, T., 2011. Educational leadership. In: Swanwick, T., McKimm, J. (Eds.), The ABC of Clinical Leadership. Wiley Blackwell, London.

Mennin, S., 2010. Self-organisation, integration and curriculum in the complex world of medical education. Med. Educ. 44, 20–30.

Mintzberg, H. Managing San Francisco, 2009, Berett-Koehler.

Morrow, C., 2014. The linkage inclusive leadership model, www.diversityjournal.com/13313-moving-dial-measuring-inclusive-leadership. (Accessed 4 February 2016).

Newman, M.A., Guy, M.E., Mastracci, S.H., 2009. Beyond cognition: affective leadership and emotional labour. Public Adm. Rev. 69, 6–20.

Rich, E.C., Magrane, D., Kirch, D.G., 2008. Qualities of the medical school dean: insights from the literature. Acad. Med. 83, 483–487.

Seibert, S.E., Sparrowe, R.T., Liden, R.C., 2003. A group exchange structure approach to leadership in groups. In: Pearce, C.L., Conger, J.A. (Eds.), Shared Leadership: Reframing the Hows and Whys of Leadership. Sage Publications, Thousand Oaks, CA.

Shamira, B., Eilam, T., 2005. What's your story? A life-stories approach to authentic leadership development. Leadersh. Q. 16, 395–417.

Snowden, D.J., Boone, M.E., 2007. A leader's framework for decision-making. Harv. Bus. Rev. (Nov), 68–76.

Taylor, C.A., Taylor, J.C., Stoller, J.K., 2008. Exploring leadership competencies in established and aspiring physician leaders: an interview-based study. J. Gen. Intern. Med. 23 (6), 748–754.

Till, A., McKimm, J. Leading from the frontline, BMJ, March 2016 (in press).

Uhl-Bien, M., Riggio, R.E., Lowe, K.B., et al., 2014. Followership theory: a review and research agenda. Leadersh. Q. 25, 83–104.

Western, S., 2012. An overview of leadership discourses. In: Preedy, M., Bennett, N., Wise, C. (Eds.), Educational Leadership: Context, Strategy and Collaboration. The Open University, Milton Keynes.

West, M., Armit, K., Loewenthal, L., et al., 2015. Leadership and Leadership Development in Healthcare: The Evidence Base. Faculty of Medical Leadership and Management, London.

Westley, F., Zimmerman, B., Patton, M., 2006. Getting to Maybe: How the World Has Changed. Random House, Toronto.

Additional reading

Doyle, M.E., Smith, M.K. Classical leadership. In The encyclopedia of informal education, 2001. http://www.infed.org/leadership/traditional_leadership.htm. (Accessed March 2017).

The medical teacher and social accountability

J. Rourke, C. Boelen, R. Strasser, B. Pálsdóttir, A. J. Neusy

Trends

- Social accountability forms the essential foundation for medical practice and medical education.
- Excellence should be the goal of both.
- The medical teacher's role is key.

Introduction

The medical teacher is at the intersection of providing medical care today and educating the doctors of tomorrow, with the fundamental goal to improve the health of patients and communities now and into the future. Through these vital medical care and education dual roles, medical teachers can demonstrate social accountability by role modelling and actively involving learners in their medical practices and healthcare and community advocacy. Medical teachers can play a key role in developing their medical school's vision, mission and curriculum, and especially in keeping it connected to the communities, regions and nation that it serves.

 Medical teachers connect their communities, medical schools and students.

Using practical examples from around the world, this chapter will provide an overview of the concept of social accountability of medical schools and the contributions that medical teachers can make.

The concept of social accountability of medical schools

Social accountability is a public commitment to respond as best as possible to society's priority health needs and challenges – keeping quality, equity, relevance and effectiveness of healthcare as reference values – and to report back progress to society. For a medical school, it implies the adaptation of its education, research and service programmes accordingly, and the demonstration that it makes or is likely to make a significant difference to the quality of graduates, to the performance of the health system and ultimately to people's health status.

Social accountability has emerged as the core principle for medical school and health workforce education reform (Box 48.1, Rourke, 2013). This is reflected in national initiatives such as the Future of Medical Education in Canada (2010, 2012), international collaborations (THEnet; Pálsdóttir et al., 2008), the World Health Organization's new Global HRH Strategy 2030 (WHO, 2016) and is becoming embedded in evolving accreditation standards (WFME, 2015) and aspirational goals (ASPIRE).

 "The medical school must: ... consider that the mission encompasses the health needs of the community, the needs of the healthcare delivery system and other aspects of social accountability".

World Federation for Medical Education, 2015

From an educational point of view, a socially accountable school has the triple and intricate obligation to identify determinants of health in society, to produce graduates who are well prepared to address those determinants, and to ensure the best use is made of those graduates in a health system. Consequently, the socially accountable medical school contributes to a more efficient and equitable healthcare delivery system, in part through collaboration with other health stakeholders (Boelen & Heck, 1995). For instance, if the reduction of health disparity is a commonly agreed target, the school will partner with potential employers of graduates to design appropriate educational programmes and create attractive job opportunities in areas of greatest need.

 The essence of social accountability of medical schools is how they engage, partner with, and respond to the needs of their communities.

The notion of impact is essential in social accountability, as confirmed by the Global Consensus for Social Accountability of Medical Schools (Global, 2010) (Box 48.2). Guided by the uninterrupted thread from

Box 48.1 Social accountability conceptual foundation

- Medical doctors (MDs, physicians) have served humanity's needs since the earliest of times.
- As members of the medical profession, doctors are inherently given the privilege and responsibility of caring for patients through an implicit trust created by society and an explicit need structured through legislation and regulation.
- Medical schools, by permit of legislation, regulation and accreditation are entrusted with the education and graduation of future doctors and must take responsibility to provide appropriate medical education that will produce competent doctors ready to meet society's needs.
- Socially accountable medical education extends from the mission of the medical school to its organization, function, curriculum and learning experiences, and outcomes.
- Medical teachers connect the community with the school and the learners at every level.

Adapted from Rourke J: 2013.

Box 48.2 Socially accountable medical schools

- Have an education, research and service delivery vision, mission, and strategic plan inspired by the current and prospective needs of its immediate society including current and future health system challenges and requirements.
- Recruit, support, and promote faculty that are aligned with its social accountability mission, who reflect the demographic and geographic diversity of the medical school's region/nation and will model, teach and develop social accountability.
- Actively engage and partner with their community, health system and other key stakeholders in designing, implementing and evaluating their education, research and service programmes.
- Select medical students who reflect the demographic and geographic diversity of the medical school's region/nation on basis of their potential.
- Provide a curriculum that reflects the priority health needs of the medical school's community/region, with emphasis on clinical service learning in partnership with the region's health service organizations.
- Produce graduates with the knowledge, skills and commitment to practice how and where they are needed in the medical school's region/nation.
- Provide professional development/continuing education based on its region's identified health needs for practising physicians and healthcare workers in its region.
- Engage in ethical research activities inspired by and responding to the health needs of their region/nation and world health priorities, and promote this research and evidence-based policy and practice changes to improve health and health service delivery.

identification of health needs in society to health service delivery, a socially accountable school keeps its focus on desired impacts, i.e. improving coverage, promoting people centeredness, enhancing healthy life styles, preventing risks and avoidable deaths, and reducing acute relapses in chronic patients. To this end, the school must seek to establish sustainable partnerships with key health actors: public authorities, health service organizations, health insurance schemes, and professional associations and communities to ensure the greatest relevance for its work. These partnerships will help the school to be more knowledgeable of people's specific characteristics living in a given territory, be it a district or an entire nation, and of their health concerns; this will help with recognition of health priorities that need to be addressed by doctors in collaboration with other professionals in the health and social sectors. The partnerships and identified health priorities help provide the basis for counselling graduates in making rewarding career choices.

Medical teachers and social accountability

The transition from traditional medical education to socially accountable medical education may require a major change in medical school orientation and organization, and the medical teacher is right at the crossroads (Ventres & Dharamsi, 2015). As medical schools are important players in people's health development, markers of social accountability are being integrated into accreditation norms for recognition of excellence, which provides incentives to faculty, particularly medical teachers, to bring social accountability to life. Medical teachers can indeed be instrumental as they plan, implement and assess educational programmes. As planners, regardless of their specialty, medical teachers imbued with the concept of social accountability can argue cogently for the essential competencies to be acquired by graduates. Similarly, on an educational committee, by referring to what is collectively perceived as the role of the doctor in a future health system, they can moderate debates in favour of a more relevant, balanced and integrated curriculum. Greater coherence and synergy among medical teachers can therefore be expected.

 Demonstrating social accountability improves medical teachers' practices, communities and medical schools and provides a positive role model for medical students.

As implementers, medical teachers can be advocates for early and longitudinal immersion of medical students in the social milieu to enable them to grasp the complexity of determinants of health, identify populations at risk, follow up patients within their families, and prepare them to make more relevant decisions in health promotion and preventive care. In so doing, medical teachers will imbue students with a critical approach to causal effects that should guide them throughout their educational experience.

Medical teachers have an invaluable influence on students as role models in demonstrating the concrete implications for a socially accountable practice, eventually by spending more time in primary care settings, by working with multi-professional teams, by applying people-centeredness approaches, by caring for the most vulnerable populations, by engaging and partnering with community leaders. Without compromising their specialized field of expertise, medical teachers can also be health advocates by addressing health issues from a wider economic, cultural and environmental angle and advocating for improving policy and practice towards greater equity, relevance, quality, effectiveness and efficiency.

Finally, medical teachers can stress the added value of social accountability to the evidence-based paradigm as proof of impact is sought on targeted health problems in society (Box 48.3). They can persuade students of the usefulness of practices inspired by health needs and their multiple causation and guide them in making professional choices most consistent with their ideals. Medical teachers have the potential to be true champions of social accountability and promoters of purposeful changes in the academic institution.

Medical teachers comprehensive roles in socially accountable medical schools

The Northern Ontario School of Medicine (NOSM) and Patan Academy of Health Sciences in Nepal are two medical schools that were developed to embody

Box 48.3 Socially accountable medical teachers

- Weave social accountability into the fabric of their medical school's vision, mission, strategic plan, organization and function.
- Participate in their medical school's community engagement and partnership building.
- Bring a community perspective to the medical schools selection/admission process.
- Infuse social accountability into their medical school's curriculum and medical student experiential learning.
- Develop their own medical practice as a social accountability role model based on their community needs.
- Involve learners in socially accountable medical practice and community activities including research projects that focus on community engagement, partnership and responding to priority health needs.
- Inspire their learners to choose career paths relevant to society's priority challenges and needs.
- Assess their impact in terms of meeting community/society's priority needs.

social accountability from the beginning and illustrate medical teachers vital and comprehensive roles.

In 2005, NOSM opened as a stand-alone medical school in a rural under-served region of Canada, with a social accountability mandate focused on improving the health of the people of Northern Ontario (Strasser et al., 2013). Distributed Community Engaged Learning, NOSM's distinctive model of medical education and health research, ensures that students and residents are learning to practice in the Northern Ontario context. This involves over 90 sites in which local physicians are the medical teachers.

During the 8-month Comprehensive Community Clerkship (CCC), each third-year student is placed in one of 15 large rural or small urban communities to learn core clinical medicine from a family practice and community perspective. Students follow patients and their families encountered in the primary care setting over an extended period of time, engaging with a range of community medical specialists and health professionals, so as to experience continuity of care in family practice, while also studying different clinical specialty disciplines. Much of the CCC programme is devised by and in partnership with the host communities.

The medical teachers have a pivotal role in this community engaged, socially accountable education. They provide much of the local clinical and classroom teaching, as well as acting as role models and mentors for the students during their clerkship year. Socially accountable medical teachers challenge students to: consider the social determinants of health in each patient and family interaction; undertake research that addresses the health issues in the CCC community; and focus always on responding to the health needs of the patients and families under their care.

In addition, medical teachers help connect the community with the medical school. They have made an essential contribution to the development and implementation of the NOSM programme. Examples include: bringing the community perspective to strategic planning; participation in the selection and admissions process; curriculum development, including case writing for case-based learning; small-group classroom and clinical skills teaching; and faculty development through peer teaching.

Between 2009 and 2015, 62% of NOSM graduates chose family medicine (predominantly rural) training, almost double the Canadian average. Since 2009, 70% of NOSM residents (both NOSM graduates and those from other medical schools) have chosen to practice in Northern Ontario after completing their training (including 22% choosing small rural communities), and some have become NOSM faculty members. Ninety-four percent of the physicians who completed MD and residency education with NOSM are practising in Northern Ontario.

Patan Academy of Health Sciences' (PAHS) community-based learning and education is implemented in partnership with communities and Nepal's national health system. The primary goal of the medical school is to improve healthcare delivery in the region by producing well-educated graduates with a community health development orientation who are able and committed to work in the rural areas of the Nepal.

The school uses an innovative curriculum focusing on the region's highest priority health needs, teaching pedagogy to foster students' problem-solving and independent thinking skills, and a community health development orientation that stresses health development capacity for enhancing community health status alongside individual medical care skills and knowledge. Local leaders and service providers as medical teachers are engaged as preceptors and in assessing student performance.

Initially, students at rural sites are given the opportunity to analyse simple problems and over time are exposed to complex issues – technical, managerial and societal in nature – as they advance to higher-year postings. Medical teacher role modelling is emphasized through supervisory visits to rural training sites, where faculty members provide clinical services and help build the capacity of local providers. Community members are involved in the student-selection process, especially as assessors of communication skills and of sensitivity, compassion and empathy.

Practical examples of medical teacher social accountability

In their practices, communities and medical schools, medical teachers demonstrate and role model social accountability all over the world. Here are some practical examples.

- At Tours Faculty of Medicine (France), *practising physicians (medical teachers) were invited by the dean to be part of a meeting of all main health stakeholders* from the centre of France and the Loire Valley Region where the school is the only one for a population of two million inhabitants. Political leadership, regional health authorities, health professional associations, patient associations and representatives of the public assembled to identify key health issues in the territory and best ways for the medical school to contribute. A list of priority areas and recommendations for action emerged. A committee representing all the partners is charged to prepare an annual meeting for follow-up. Major priorities for the school will be the retention of graduates in under-served areas and the involvement of regional health stakeholders in the medical school's community work. The school experience is viewed by the French association of medical school deans as a model.

- At Memorial University of Newfoundland (Canada) Faculty of Medicine, over *150 physician part-time and full-time faculty of medical teachers volunteer as interviewers in an admission process* that recognizes that rural, indigenous and economically disadvantaged students may have had different sociocultural and educational experiences but also are more likely to practice in those communities of need. To ensure broad representation, the admissions selection committee includes members from indigenous communities, rural communities, general public, allied health professions, medical students, biomedical scientists, university, administration, provincial medical association and provincial departments of health and community physicians.

- At Hull York Medical School (UK), *all problem-based learning (PBL) facilitators are practising clinicians (medical teachers) and two thirds work in primary care.* PBL problems are constructed from general practice 'list' of common patient presentations. The 'patient's perspective' is emphasized alongside the 'doctor's perspective'.

- At Memorial University of Newfoundland (Canada) Faculty of Medicine, *family physicians as medical teachers work with either a social worker or psychologist to facilitate the year 1 small-group clinical skills sessions.* Case study discussions involve the determinants of health at the levels of the individual and the community incorporating the relationships between socio-economic deprivation and health. Discussions are often student led and peer evaluated.

- At Ghent University Faculty of Medicine and Health Sciences (Belgium), medical teachers emphasize research and training in Community Oriented Primary Care (COPC), and the school has a chair in equity in healthcare. *Family physicians as medical teachers bring medical students into their practices beginning in the students' first year.* In the second year students have a 2-week clerkship in a nursing home, in the third year they have 1 week of clerkship in family medicine and a 1 week block as part of health and society inter-professional Community Oriented Primary Care experience in a deprived area of the city of Ghent. During the second and the third year, students are attached to a family anticipating the birth of a child. They follow-up the development of the child, and interact with the family members. The students interview three primary care providers involved in the care of that family and pay particular attention to social determinants of health. By combining observation from community experiences and epidemiological data on the community, students, with teacher support, formulate a community diagnosis. They then look for ways to improve the social conditions in the community.

- *Medical teachers* at Ghent University *also model social accountability by having their medical practice in community clinics in neighbourhoods with underserved urban populations and by taking care of vulnerable populations such as refugees.* In 2016, the Department of Family Medicine and Primary Health Care took responsibility for coordinating the care of 250 refugees from Syria, Afghanistan and Iraq. It put together a volunteer team of family physicians, nurses, mental health workers, dentists and pharmacists to organize comprehensive care for the asylum seekers. This project will endeavour to combine service with research and educational opportunities, contributing to increasing social accountability at Ghent University.

- At University of New Mexico School of Medicine (USA), *community-based preceptors as medical teachers provide medical students with social accountability experiential learning in continuity clinics* one afternoon per week for their first 2 years of medical school, giving students the opportunity to develop ongoing relationships with both patients and practitioners that help them gain an understanding of the social determinants of health. There are patient care and educational activities in more than 155 communities in New Mexico, many focused on under-served disadvantaged communities. The Pajarito Mesa project created by one medical student and now an ongoing programme for faculty, residents and students is an example.

- Flinders University School of Medicine with facilities in Adelaide, rural South Australia and Victoria, and the Northern Territory (Australia) values its reciprocal links with indigenous communities and with the wider Australian and international communities. *Indigenous medical teacher academics are involved in recruitment, admissions and support of indigenous students* and the school established the Poche Centre of Indigenous Health and Well-Being in Adelaide and the Indigenous Transition Pathways Unit in Darwin to provide support and mentoring.

- At Southern Illinois University School of Medicine (USA), *physician faculty as medical teachers provide multiple elective opportunities for students to work alongside them in community service*, which can include providing cost-free care at both the primary care and specialty levels for uninsured patients.

- At Memorial University of Newfoundland (Canada) Faculty of Medicine, the Gateway project began in 2005 as a medical–student-led community initiative to help newly arriving refugees in the St. John's area. Most year 1 and year 2 students volunteer for this service-learning activity that affords experiences with under-served and disadvantaged patients, communities and populations. They carry out a medical interview and history taking aided by an interpreter for all participating refugees (adults and children) as well as performing an initial screening. *Students work directly with a family doctor as medical teacher who is the faculty advisor* and a public health nurse at each session. Gateway has become a strong partnership between the faculty, regional health services, and local communities including the Association for New Canadians (ANC), the settlement agency, aiming to improve access to healthcare and other services that determine health for refugees in the province.

- At Southern Illinois University School of Medicine (USA), special individually designed electives (IDEs – design your own elective) *allow students with creative service ideas, with the approval of supervising medical teacher faculty members*, to receive elective credit.

A recent example was a group of eight students, accompanied by a clinical faculty member as medical teacher, spent 2 weeks in Haiti providing free medical care there.

- The Faculty of Medicine at the University of Gezira (FMUG) was established in 1975 to serve rural communities in Sudan's Gezira region. FMUG *medical teachers developed a field training research and rural development programme through which students train and work with more than 1500 families in over 300 villages.* Students are involved in such diverse activities as establishing and developing water resources and sanitation facilities as well as health and TB units; introducing electricity in villages; and conducting health education and environmental health outreach programmes. Facilitated by faculty members, these interventions are evaluated to measure the outcomes of each using typical indicators based on project objectives. These might include increased use of insecticides in homes; decreased incidence rate of malaria or other diseases; increased use of antenatal care services; and increased use of latrines.

- At the FMUG *medical teachers model approaches and behaviours that will help students in their future practice.* For example FMUG's Safe Motherhood project was initiated by faculty members to improve the health status of rural communities in collaboration with health authorities. FUMG's faculty trained village midwives and facilitated their absorption into the government-funded health system. This initiative led to a remarkable reduction in the maternal mortality ratio (MMR) and in the neonatal mortality ratio (NMR) in Gezira state. The project helped lower the MMR from 469 per 100,000 live births in 2005 to 106 in 2011, and the NMR from 43 per 1,000 live births in 2005 to 10.2 per 1,000 in 2011. Many strategies were applied, including the training and provision of jobs for village midwives in collaboration with Gezira State.

- The University of New Mexico School of Medicine (USA) uses social determinant prescription pads for health to help students make the connection between education and service to the school's social mission. *Students and residents in primary care work with their preceptors (medical teachers) and community health workers in addressing social determinants of health of patients by 'prescribing' resources* for: hunger and food insecurity, prescription benefits, housing, employment, education, workforce training and health insurance coverage options.

- James Cook University (JCU) in Northern Queensland (Australia), established to help address the rural doctor workforce shortage, delivers the Australian General Practice Training (AGPT) programme for the Australian Government Department of Health. This postgraduate vocational training programme for medical graduates allows vertical integration of training, producing a cohort of doctors with knowledge, skills and aptitude to meet community need. The Rural Generalist Pathway provides a supported training and career pathway for junior physicians to train in rural and remote medicine, combined with financial and professional recognition. Teaching in both the undergraduate and postgraduate programmes is provided by *a distributed network of committed rural and regional preceptors as medical teachers, each modelling social accountability through their skills, service and commitment to community.*

- *The medical and nursing teachers* at the University of the Philippines Manila School of Health Sciences in Leyte (UPM-SHS) and the Ateneo de Zamboanga University School of Medicine (ADZU-SOM) in the Philippines *work closely with communities and other health system stakeholders to design, implement and evaluate their programmes. They also build the capacity of their partners to improve health.* For example, they developed and implemented a Municipal Leadership and Governance Program in their respective regions. It is a 1-year, two module programme for mayors, municipal health officers and Department of Health officials, which offers training and leadership coaching on local health system development for officials who are committed to supporting health reforms. The programme was developed in collaboration with local authorities and trainees have to be endorsed by the Department of Health's Center for Health Development.

Research

Medical schools that are socially accountable conduct research that is inspired by and responds to their community's and region's priority health needs. This may range from biomedical discovery to clinical to population health research. A socially accountable medical school actively engages the community in research, including developing the agenda, partnering and participating in research and knowledge translation/mobilization/application. The research gives priority to activities that create beneficial effects upon its community/region including a positive impact on the healthcare for and the health of the population served.

Medical teachers can play a significant bidirectional role, engaging with the community to conduct community needs inspired research and then integrating research findings into medical practice, and involving students in both directions from practice to research and back again.

For example, Newfoundland and Labrador, a large province (400,000 km) with a small population of 500,000 people, has a very distributed founder population with clusters of genetic disease. *Medical teachers in Newfoundland and Labrador have this additional layer of genetic knowledge about patients from different communities* that they teach medical students. This population need has inspired Memorial University of Newfoundland Faculty of Medicine to do breakthrough genetic research needed for the province's population, but with worldwide significance, as these diseases are not confined to Newfoundland and Labrador. One such example is arrhythmogenic ventricular cardiomyopathy (ARVC), a disease in which the first symptom is usually sudden death in young men and women from ventricular fibrillation. Researchers at Memorial first identified that this often struck down every other person in the families affected. Initial treatment with implantable defibrillator pacemakers in all family members was found to stop the sudden deaths. The genetic riddle was solved and a genetic test developed for at-risk families to determine exactly who had the gene, and put the defibrillator pacemakers into those who really needed them.

With a clearly defined mission to serve rural, indigenous and tropical Australia, JCU is engaged in research related to its social accountability mission. In addition to more traditional biomedical and basic science investigations, JCU centres its research on rural health, medical education and health workforce and primary healthcare. For example, JCU's Anton Breinl Research Centre for Health Systems Strengthening conducts research related to health system development, workforce capacity and development, education and training, populations, equity and engagement, Aboriginal and Torres Strait Islander health and responding to priority health challenges in the region. *Medical teachers conduct graduate tracking and retention research; health workforce modelling; and collaborative health services research with indigenous, rural, and remote populations.* The research not only informs strategy and policy making, but feeds directly back into the education process.

Flinders University School of Medicine (Australia) Centre for Point-of-Care Testing *has responded to the needs identified by medical teachers who care for populations in very dispersed rural Australia* by developing point-of-care devices and training a range of practitioners including indigenous health workers to conduct tests for chronic, acute and infectious diseases, particularly in indigenous communities and rural and remote settings nationally and internationally.

This generates a test result that can be used to make an immediate informed clinical decision.

The Philippines suffers from significant health inequities with rural and poor regions lacking access to health workers, especially physicians. In the country, 68% of Filipino medical graduates end up practising overseas. Two health professional schools – ADZU-SOM and UPM-SHS – were established to address these challenges. *Medical teachers at both schools are involved in various efforts to assess the impact their schools are having.* The medical teachers participate in tracking graduates of their school. Both socially accountable schools have retention rates of more than 90% remaining in the Philippines, with more than 80% of graduates working in under-served or rural regions. Their research questions focus on determining whether their graduates address the needs of the local health system in terms of location and their practice; whether they contribute to a more functional local health system, and whether the presence of faculty, students and graduates in rural communities ensures better population health outcomes.

Summary

Over the past 20 years, the concept of social accountability of medical schools has become firmly established. Medical teachers are the socially accountable medical school's key linkage to the community, playing a vital role in how it engages, partners with and responds to its communities and region. Medical teachers provide medical care needed by the population, live in communities they serve, and can help shape the policies and services affecting the people who live in their communities and regions. They can also shape their medical school's mission, education and research to be more socially accountable. Through curriculum development, teaching and role modelling, medical teachers have their greatest impact: developing future medical doctors to best meet the needs of society.

References

ASPIRE: International Recognition of Excellence in Education. Available at: www.aspire-to-excellence.org.

Boelen, C., Heck, J., 1995. Defining and Measuring the Social Accountability of Medical Schools. WHO, Geneva.

Future of Medical Education in Canada: A collective vision for MD education in Canada, 2010. Available at: https://www.afmc.ca/pdf/fmec/ FMEC-MD-2010.pdf.

Future of Medical Education in Canada: A collective vision for postgraduate medical education in Canada, 2012. Available at: https://www.afmc.ca/future-of

-medical-education-in-canada/postgraduate-project/phase2/pdf/FMEC_PG_Final-Report_EN.pdf.

Global Consensus for Social Accountability of Medical Schools, 2010. Available at: www.healthsocialaccountability.org.

Pálsdóttir, B., Neusy, A.-J., Reed, G., 2008. Building the evidence base: networking innovative socially accountable medical education programs. Educ. Health 21 (2).

Rourke, J., 2013. Social accountability of medical schools. Acad. Med. 88 (3), 430.

Strasser, R., et al., 2013. Transforming health professional education through social accountability: Canada's Northern Ontario School of Medicine. Med. Teach. 35, 490–496.

THEnet: Training for Health Equity Network. Available at: www.thenetcommunity.org.

Ventres, W., Dharamsi, S., 2015. Socially Accountable Medical Education—The REVOLUTIONS Framework. Acad. Med. 90 (12), 1728.

World Federation for Medical Education: Basic Medical Education WFME Global Standards for Quality Improvement: The 2015 Revision, Copenhagen, 2015, World Federation for Medical Education. Available at: http//wfme.org. (Accessed 22 Janaury 2017).

World Health Organization (2016). Global strategy on human resources for health: Workforce 2030. Available at: http://who.int/hrh/resources/globstrathrh-2030/en/. (Accessed 22 June 2016).

Further reading

Larkins, S., Preston, R., Matte, M., et al., 2013. Measuring social accountability in health professional education: development and international pilot testing of an evaluation framework. Med. Teach. 35 (1), 32–45.

Larkins, S., Michielsen, K., Iputo, J., et al., 2015. Impact of selection strategies on representation of underserved populations and intention to practise: international findings. Med. Educ. 49, 60–72.

Ross, S., Preston, R., Lindemann, I., et al., 2014. The training for health equity network framework: a pilot study at five health professional schools. Educ. Health 27 (2), 116–126.

Strasser, R., Neusy, A.-J., 2010. Context counts: training health workers in and for rural areas. Bull. World Health Organ. 88 (10), 777–782.

Chapter

49

Section 8:
Medical school

The educational environment

L. D. Gruppen, M. E. Rytting, K. C. Marti

Trends

- There is a growing concern about the impact of the educational environment on learner performance.
- Efforts to understand the impact of the educational environment require a multi-level perspective.
- Interventions to improve the educational environment need to be evaluated with strong research designs.

Introduction

There is a growing interest in defining the educational environment in medical education, which includes efforts to measure it and to improve it. The impetus for this interest is the research evidence that the educational environment has an impact on learning, wellbeing (e.g. burnout, stress), student involvement, faculty and learner satisfaction, successful performance, and faculty teaching (Schönrock-Adema et al., 2012). Although there has been longstanding concern with the educational environment in individual schools and hospitals, there is an emerging emphasis on assessing and monitoring the quality of the learning environment from accrediting agencies (e.g. the US Accrediting Council on Graduate Medical Education and the Liaison Committee on Medical Education). Attention to the educational environment is growing in other health professions (dentistry or nursing) and in countries around the world.

Interest in the educational environment may also reflect the increased diversity of the student population in many health professions schools (Roff & McAleer, 2001). This diversity reflects age and gender differences as well as increased representation from minority groups. It is reasonable to expect that diverse student groups will experience the educational environment in different ways.

 In many ways, every learner experiences a unique educational environment defined by personal experiences, social connections and individual characteristics.

The educational environment, or educational climate, is complex. It includes both the formal curriculum and the 'hidden' curriculum. It encompasses the social relationships among faculty, learners and administrators, as well as the physical environment and resources. Although it may be convenient to talk about the educational environment at a given school, the reality is that every learner has a unique educational environment, different from his or her peers because he or she interacts with different people, learns in different settings, has different schedules, and directs his or her own learning in different directions – all within the apparent uniformity of the same institution.

What is the educational environment?

Because of the variation in how students and faculty perceive the educational environment, we need to identify the elements or parts of the educational environment in order to evaluate these learner or teacher perceptions (Harden, 2001; Roff & McAleer, 2001). Defining the educational environment is a complex task. First, there are a number of alternative terms that are used as virtual synonyms, for example learning climate, learning environment. Then there are related constructs, such as psychological climate, social environment, work environment, and the climate in specific settings (clinical environment, classroom climate). We use educational environment in this chapter to highlight the fact that the environment affects both teaching and learning, viz. the entire educational enterprise.

 The educational environment is incredibly complex, and any definition or measurement of these environments must recognize what is being left out, as well as what is being included.

Context is another related term that can add to the confusion. In many situations, such as socioeconomic contributors to health or illness, the context of the patient is a key part of what needs to be learned. However, in terms of the educational environment, 'context' refers to the numerous factors that influence

Table 49.1 A few things that can be considered part of the educational environment

Physical facilities	The faculty
Hospital and clinic characteristics	Fellow learners
Clinical team members	Patient population
Class size	Leisure time
Teaching methodologies	Assessment procedures
Timetabling	Student support
Group sizes	'Ambience' or culture
Teacher's competencies	Learning resources
Learning and teaching methodologies	Relations with peers
Relations with faculty	Ethical climate of the institution
Class composition	Well-defined learning outcomes

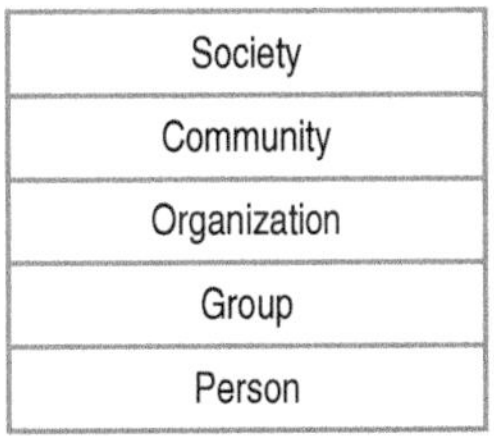

Fig. 49.1 The educational environment as a hierarchy of levels of living systems.

(Schönrock-Adema et al., 2012), they accounted for over 90% of the items on these measures.

Genn (Genn, 2001b) takes a more concrete approach to sorting educational environment components into faculty, students, administration, and physical features as key components of the educational environment. Each of these categories interacts with the others in complex ways and reflect both social and physical dimensions of the educational environment.

Another way to structure the complexity of the educational environment is to think of it in terms of a hierarchy of levels based on Miller's levels of living systems (Miller, 1978) (Fig. 49.1). The most basic level that would be relevant to the educational environment would be the individual learner (Person). The next level, Group, encompasses the social interactions that are so important in the educational environment. The Organization level includes physical features as well as cultural characteristics. The Community level can reflect regional geographic characteristics as well as additional cultural variables. Finally, the Society level may encompass national characteristics, policies and values.

We will use Miller's hierarchy to organize a consideration of how teachers can better understand the dynamics of the educational environment and how they can adapt their teaching activities to both adapt to the environment and to change it.

The person level

In most efforts to quantify the educational environment, the data are derived from learner perceptions and judgements, typically gathered by means of a questionnaire. The result is that the educational environment is operationally defined at the level of Person in Fig. 49.1. This means that anything that might influence the perceptions and judgements of individual learners could impact their assessments of the educational environment.

Indeed, it is common to observe that what constitutes a hostile and stressful environment for some learners may be regarded as routine or even stimulating for others. Not all learners regard an academically rigorous teaching hospital with high anticipation, or

education but are not its focus. In other words, we must distinguish between the context that students learn *about* and the context that students learn *in*. The context students learn about is part of the curriculum; the context students learn in is part of the educational environment.

Genn (Genn, 2001a) provides a very expansive treatment of the educational environment and the curriculum, noting that virtually anything can be included in the description to the extent it has an impact on the educational process. However, elucidating all of the factors and variables that could be considered as part of the educational environment leads to a sprawling mass of possibilities (Table 49.1).

This expansiveness is conceptually helpful only to the extent it can be organized into categories or classes of influences. However, there are few conceptual frameworks in the health education literature to help guide our thinking about the scope of the educational environment or how it influences teaching and learning (Schönrock-Adema et al., 2012).

One framework (Moos, 1974) posits three key categories of educational environment components: (1) *Personal Development/Goal Direction*, which relates to educational goals, relevant learning content, and constructive criticism; (2) *Relationships*, which focus on the extent to which learners and faculty support each other, communicate openly, and demonstrate affiliation and emotional support; and (3) *System Maintenance and System Change*, which characterizes the extent to which the environment has clear expectations, is orderly and organized, reflects innovation, and allows student influence. When these categories were used to sort the individual items from nine different educational environment measurement instruments consider regimented case presentations with extensive differential diagnoses and fierce competition among learners as hostile. Other learners may find the so-called friendly general hospital setting to be boring and devoid of necessary academic rigor.

Person-level variables can influence how learners perceive (and judge) the educational environment. These variables include personality characteristics and individual preferences, such traits as introversion and extraversion, tolerance for ambiguity, personal and professional goals, engagement in reflection and the like. One illustrative trait that could influence how learners view the educational environment is that of resilience. Evidence suggests that more resilient students judge their quality of life and educational environment to be higher than less resilient students.

Person-level variables also provide points at which interventions can be mounted to improve the educational environment. Again, resilience provides an example to the extent that developing resilience in learners may be a strategy to minimize emotional distress, improve quality of life, and enhance medical training. Similarly, efforts to encourage student reflection on their learning and the educational environment can be valuable means for both changing the environment itself and the learners' evaluation of it.

In addition to long-term variables, short-term events can also influence how individuals perceive the environment and how it affects them. Personal life crises, adverse (or positive) academic feedback, and just having a good or bad day can influence judgements about the educational environment. Similarly, for interventions to improve the educational environment, faculty must be sensitive to the possibility of making short-term gains but little longer-term effect.

 Most studies of the educational environment are a snapshot in time, so there are few data about how stable or constant the educational environment might be in a given situation.

The group level

At the Group level of analysis, the focus shifts to the interactions that learners have with others, both directly and indirectly. For educational environments, these interactions tend to focus on other learners or on faculty members, although interactions with patients and healthcare professionals are central to many clinical educational environments.

LEARNER–LEARNER INTERACTIONS

The educational environment depends greatly on interactions among learners. Peers influence how one sees the world through shared observations, complaints and celebrations, but peers also ARE a major part of one's environment. Peers who are cooperative,

supportive, fun to be with, hold high standards but encourage each other, create a very different environment for learning compared with peers who are competitive, disgruntled, antisocial, and lax in academic standards.

Interventions that influence learner–learner interactions can be fruitful vehicles for improving the educational environment. The recent proliferation of learning communities at many medical schools can be seen, in part, as an effort to improve the quality of learner–learner interactions and thus improve the educational environment. Similarly, efforts to move from a multi-level grading system to pass-fail has often included an argument that this change would reduce competition among students, and thus, improve the educational environment.

LEARNER–FACULTY INTERACTIONS

Learner–faculty interactions are similarly critical to the quality of the educational environment. When looking at the faculty side of these interactions, one theme has been to identify desirable characteristics of faculty members. Naturally, faculty are expected to be knowledgeable and to possess significant clinical experience. They should be excellent role models and dedicated to the teaching of young doctors. In the aggregate, they need to be diverse, sufficiently numerous, and varied in specialty and level of specialization. Ideally, the faculty should also be attuned to the community being served. A faculty cohort with these characteristics is more likely to engender a positive educational environment.

Teaching behaviours are also relevant. It is difficult to make universal statements about effective teaching behaviours because some learners react strongly towards or against a particular teaching style. For example, small-group sessions with a particularly demanding instructor may leave some learners in tears, while others wonder what the big deal is. Nonetheless, there are some general relationships that have broad support. Learner centredness is one attribute of teaching that seems to promote more positive educational environments. It is not clear whether the benefits of learner centeredness arise out of a better fit between teaching and learning that is fostered by more learner input into the educational process, or if it stems from more positive interpersonal interactions between faculty and learners.

Effective mentoring also encompasses a broad set of issues in learner–faculty interactions. There is extensive literature on mentoring skills that guide learners in a supportive and encouraging environment that fosters the achievement of important professional and personal goals. Similarly, role modelling is extremely important, particularly in the clinical environment. Good and bad role models are a major part of the hidden curriculum and have a major impact on the quality of the educational environment for their learners.

Beyond direct teaching, learner–faculty interactions around feedback and assessment are also relevant to the educational environment. The lack of timely and useful feedback as well as (perceived) unfair and arbitrary assessments are common complaints about poor educational environment.

Improving teaching skills is one potential means for improving the educational environment. The need to measure, develop and promote faculty teaching ability is a key part of the larger faculty development community in medical education. Explicit rewards and incentives for excellence in education may also contribute to an improved educational environment. However, the repeated calls for better faculty teaching speaks to the fact that, despite its desirability, it is not routinely met and still is not materially recognized in accordance with its importance to the educational environment.

LEARNER–PATIENT/STAFF INTERACTIONS

 Particularly in clinical environments, it is very important to include nursing and other healthcare professionals in defining and modifying the educational environment. An inter-professional perspective provides a more comprehensive view of the current environment and potential improvements.

The educational environment for clinical teaching is very distinct from that for classroom learning. It adds the influence of learner interactions with patients and staff in the context of providing healthcare services, not just learning. The clinical environment is focused first on patient care and only secondarily on education, so there are additional issues in developing a positive educational environment. Because learners are no longer the primary focus, clinical faculty must make sure that learners are clearly welcomed and oriented to this new environment or risk the common learner perception that they are 'the lowest of the low' on the hospital ward (Soemantri et al., 2010).

Differences in patient population, such as those between private physician offices and clinics that care for under-served populations, contribute to different educational environments. Different patient populations may lead to the development of physicians with different priorities for treating diverse populations and different levels of learner autonomy. Learners vary in the value they place on these environmental attributes, but this is an area in which further research is very much needed to compare the impact of the social medicine environment.

The organization level

The influences on the educational environment at the Organizational level can be grouped into physical and cultural factors.

PHYSICAL FACTORS

Although the physical environment where learning takes place is given relatively little attention in educational research, it is the most visible element, and the element that is most consistent from one learner's experience to the next. The physical environment may also be where changes in the educational environment can be implemented rapidly and on a broad base of learners.

Much has been written about the physical environment for education, but most often from a perspective of architecture and facilities planning. Well-lit, comfortable learning spaces with flexible furniture arrangements that foster group collaboration and interaction between the teacher and the audience are now the norm. Support for technology is a key element of these physical spaces, but even with electronically facilitated learning, physical spaces for social connections, teaching and assessment are still necessary. These needs extend from the classroom and laboratory to the clinic and hospital ward.

The clinical setting poses some additional concerns related to the physical environment. An appropriate workspace is an outstanding need if learners are part of the care team. Much of the learning in the clinic takes place in the examination rooms, learners need a space to rest, an on-call room, and access to computers where they will not feel that they are invading or obstructing the workings of the clinical staff. They need a place to interact with faculty and to formulate plans for patients.

In the physical environment of the clinic, space is at a premium. Organizations that lack such physical spaces may be perceived as unfriendly and difficult places to work. Conversely, organizations that have invested in such spaces are quick to highlight that fact to learners.

CULTURAL FACTORS

Cultural factors that influence student learning also play a role in the educational environment, according to sociocultural theory (Schönrock-Adema et al., 2012). Organizational culture is more often the focus of leadership theory, but it is clearly a part of the educational environment, as well. Empirical work on the effects of different organizational cultures is minimal, but anyone who has changed jobs or educational programmes between different organizations likely has a good idea of the impact of changing organizational cultures.

For academic institutions, the intellectual culture may reflect the extent to which the medical school functions within a university campus, participating in campus-wide events that promote a more holistic, creative and 'forward-thinking' environment. Synergies with non-science programmes such as law, ethics, drama, communications, religion, and public policy may also foster a vibrant intellectual environment.

The lack of scholarship about Organization-level factors in the educational environment makes it difficult to identify relevant characteristics empirically, but there are likely candidates. One is the degree to which the organization emphasizes scholarship and research versus clinical productivity or a specific healthcare mission. Another might be the balance between specialty and generalist care, or the size of the organization, or whether non-profit or for-profit. Organizations that are part of a national healthcare system are likely to have very different cultures from those in the private sector.

The community and society levels

Influences on the educational environment that represent the Community or Society levels of Miller's hierarchy (Fig. 49.1), are largely speculative, given the fact that this level is relatively further from that of the individual person, where most of the definition of educational environment originates. Also, there are few, if any, direct comparisons of educational environments that would enable distinctions among communities or societies. However, as a part of our conceptual model, this level would encompass such factors as national differences in culture, societal values, governmental policies and systems, community resource levels, socio-economic impact on disease distribution, and others that operate on large groupings of people.

How is the educational environment measured?

 Maintaining an excellent educational environment requires regular monitoring. This is a responsibility that the faculty should take seriously.

Because the educational environment is a key component in medical education, it is essential to have tools to evaluate the educational environment. Any faculty member or institution concerned about their educational environment would want trustworthy data on both the current state of that environment and the impact of any attempts to improve it. Thus, there is considerable interest in developing assessment instruments to quantify the quality and characteristics of the educational environment.

Unfortunately, as described above, any effort to measure the educational environment is likely to be fraught with difficulty because of the challenges in defining it and the variability in how it is manifested and experienced. Almost all methods for measuring the educational environment depend on learner judgements or ratings, typically to items in a questionnaire. Some qualitative studies have sought to explore the dynamics of the educational environment, but

quantitative assessments are almost exclusively based on learner questionnaires. This method is appropriate to the extent that the educational environment is different for each individual, but it has serious problems for anyone seeking to measure the educational environment at higher levels in Miller's hierarchy (Fig. 49.1).

Even within the set of learner questionnaires, there is substantial variation in content, sub-scales, intended focus, and questionnaire rigor. It is important to point out that, in the same way that there is no agreed upon definition of the educational environment, there is no 'right' instrument for measurement of it. Each instrument operationally defines the educational environment in its own way, and users need to make sure they agree with this definition before selecting and using a given instrument. Selecting the 'wrong' one will still give you data, but its meaning and interpretation may not be suited to what you want to focus on. Fortunately, several recent reviews of the numerous instruments designed to assess the educational environment provide a central source for considering alternative instruments (Schönrock-Adema et al., 2012; Colbert-Getz et al., 2014; Soemantri et al., 2010). Table 49.2 provides a listing of many of the existing instruments included in these reviews; others are included with relevant citations. As the names indicate, many are modifications of the Dundee Ready Education Environment Measure, to be used in specific educational settings.

Suffice it to say that measuring and assessing the educational environment is not easy and is fraught with difficulties. Almost certainly, there will be deficiencies in any assessment measure with which learners or teachers might take issue. It is also just as certain that regular assessments must be done to build and to maintain an excellent learning programme.

Teaching with the educational environment in mind

The practical importance of having a solid conceptual framework for understanding the educational environment and sound measures for assessing it is to help faculty be more thoughtful and effective in their teaching. We believe it is simply good educational practice to consider the impact of the educational environment on one's teaching and the impact of one's teaching activities on the environment. Towards that end, we offer some illustrative examples of the connection between the educational environment and teaching practice. Several connections appear amenable to alteration in order to improve the learning environment.

ADDRESSING STUDENT MISTREATMENT

Student mistreatment has emerged as a major concern in connection with the educational environment. Indeed,

Table 49.2 Some instruments for measuring the educational environment

Instrument	Setting
Dundee Ready Education Environment Measure (DREEM)	Medicine (undergraduate and postgraduate (PG), other health professions
Johns Hopkins Learning Environment Survey (JHLES) (Shochet et al., 2013)	Medical (undergraduate)
Learning Environment Questionnaire (LEQ)	Medicine
Medical School Learning Environment Scale (MSLES)	Medicine
Course Valuing Inventory (CVI)	Medicine
Medical School Environment Questionnaire (MSEQ)	Medicine (undergraduate)
Medical School Environment Inventory (MSEI)	Medicine
Surgical Theatre Educational Environment Measure (STEEM)	Medicine (undergraduate and PG)
Assessment of Medical Education Environment by Teachers (AMEET) (Shehnaz et al., 2014)	Medical faculty members' perceptions
Postgraduate Hospital Educational Environment Measure (PHEEM)	Medicine PG Dentistry PG
Ambulatory Care Learning Education Environment Measure (ACLEEM) (Riquelme et al., 2013)	Resident (PG) ambulatory environment
Undergraduate Clinical Education Environment Measure (UCEEM) (Strand et al., 2013)	Medical undergraduate Clinical education
Anaesthetic Theatre Educational Environment Measure (ATEEM)	Medicine (PG)
Practice-Based Educational Environment Measure (PEEM)	GPs in training
Pololi & Price Instrument	Medicine

in the United States, it has become a focus of national concern and programme accreditation review. Physical or psychological mistreatment of students is clearly a manifestation of an educational environment that has problems that need to be addressed. Not only are such environments potential obstacles to effective learning, they are also detrimental to the reputation of these institutions. Such high-profile problems with the educational environment garner attention and interventions to improve the environment. The extent to which the interventions help remains to be evaluated in many cases.

CURRICULUM CHANGE AND THE EDUCATIONAL ENVIRONMENT

Changes to the curriculum of a training programme frequently lead to changes in the educational environment – sometimes intentionally, but sometimes unintentionally (Genn, 2001a). Changing from a traditional lecture-based curriculum organized by departmental specialties to a small-group, problem-based curriculum organized around organ systems creates numerous changes in the educational environment. Some, such as greater student interaction and collaboration, may be intentional. Others, such as a greater demand on faculty time, the upheaval of change,

and shifting resource allocation, may have adverse and unintended impact on the environment.

Rigorous study of interventions to improve the educational environment are difficult to conduct, in part because of ethical issues in allowing sub-optimal environments to persist but also because it is extremely difficult to change any one part of the complex, interconnected educational environment without changing other parts. The interconnectedness of the educational environment is illustrated in one study (Robins et al., 1996) of the effects on the educational environment of a multi-faceted curriculum revision that included reduced number of lectures, pass-fail grading, more active learning and weekly quizzes for formative feedback. These changes produced a moderate to large effect size improvement in the perceived learning environment, but it is impossible to tease apart the independent contributions of multiple concurrent changes.

FACULTY BEHAVIOURS

Faculty are a major component of the educational environment, both in the aggregate and individually. Inadequate numbers of faculty who are overextended and frustrated will tend to damage the educational environment, whereas accessible, enthusiastic and dedicated faculty will augment it. Individual faculty are also important as influences on large numbers of learners in classroom settings or more intensively on individual learners in clinical settings. The clinic attending is a useful example of how much impact a faculty member can have on creating an educational environment that may motivate or disenchant learners. The attending can select interesting and willing patients to meet individual learner needs or can disenfranchise learners from having an authentic role in the clinic. Clinic attendings can foster tremendous independence and autonomy in learners or maintain their dependency. The attending must be able to relate to the learners as not just an instructor and critic, but as a team member with a stake in maintaining a non-threatening, efficient work environment.

 It is important to recognize that the educational environment affects faculty as much as it does learners; however, faculty perspectives on the educational environment are rarely examined.

Given the influence of faculty behaviours on the educational environment, a significant intervention may consist in supporting and developing these faculty. Too often, formal training in key teaching skills occurs only sporadically, but a growing number of institutions are investing substantively in programmes and interventions to coach and improve the educational and community-building skills of faculty as a way to improve the clinical educational environment.

Similarly, the selection of faculty is a potential pressure point for influencing the environment. Recruiting excellent teachers and removing those who prove to be toxic can benefit the educational environment. However, the criteria for identifying exemplary and problematic faculty still rest too heavily on learner evaluations, with all of the limitations that go with them.

THE EFFECT OF THE EDUCATIONAL ENVIRONMENT ON FACULTY

Most of the literature views the educational environment from the perspective of the learners, using learner perceptions to quantify it, and to judge its impact. However, faculty are also influenced by the educational environment and, as longer-term residents of that environment, may have more to gain or lose in efforts to change the environment. Understanding faculty satisfaction and motivation is a concern not only for the human resources department but also for the educational mission of the institution. One study suggests that faculty motivation is heavily influenced by the environment, as reflected in such things as noticeable appreciation for teaching by one's direct superior, teaching small groups, feedback on teaching performance, and freedom to determine what one

teaches (van den Berg et al., 2013). Addressing these kinds of factors as well as experimenting with incentive structures for teaching may improve the educational environment for faculty and, by extension, for learners as well.

TIME AND SPACE

The educational environment is not just a socio-psychological phenomenon, but depends on physical space and time as well. A lack of space for learning activities or even for the learners themselves will adversely affect the educational environment. Old, undesirable, dark and dingy spaces for learning convey an impression about the value of education as does cramped and overcrowded facilities.

The importance of time for the educational environment is very visible in the multiple efforts to limit work hours for learners in numerous countries. There is growing recognition that learning (and teaching) takes time and that education needs to be viewed in the context of all the other responsibilities of the learners. Educators and administrators need to carefully assess practical experiments in balancing education with clinical care in allocating time to foster education while balancing efficiency.

 "The most rewarding clinic I encountered in my education functioned using nurses and residents only. The clinic attending was available to answer questions, but mainly came to clinic at the end of the week to review charts and to review resident presentations on ambulatory medicine topics. Treatment decisions were made by the residents and the experienced nurses, and the length of the clinic was determined by the efficiency of the resident. This is perhaps the best motivator for working with alacrity."

COMMUNITY BUILDING

The social nature of much of the educational environment suggests that one class of interventions to improve the environment would focus on building supportive, dynamic educational communities. Such communities can take many forms and be embedded in many situations. The clinical community of learners, faculty, staff and patients constitutes a community that is primarily focused on clinical care, but which also has significant educational impact. Communities more specifically focused on education can be nurtured or created around key components of the curriculum, shared interests, or periods in the training process. Such communities can be as small as a team following an attending or as large as a medical school class. Building such communities requires attention to the interpersonal relationships within the community, both among learners and between learners and faculty. Indeed, peer-to-peer learning is an extremely valuable component of such communities, leading to a sense of 'safety' in exposing learning needs. It must also consider the educational purpose for the community and the external support that will be needed to give the community a healthy start.

Summary

The educational environment is a very complex phenomenon that functions at multiple levels of systems and affects both learners and faculty members. Understanding the overall nature of the educational environment is a first step towards being able to thoughtfully develop interventions that may improve the environment. Such interventions require well-designed measurement procedures, for which there exist numerous tools for quantifying the educational environment. It is important to recognize that the dynamic complexity of the environment means that it will change continuously and that any intervention will very likely have unintended consequences. Nonetheless, the pervasive impact of the educational environment on almost all goals and outcomes of medical education makes it a critically important area for study and for experimentation.

References

Colbert-Getz, J.M., Kim, S., Goode, V.H., et al., 2014. Assessing medical students' and residents' perceptions of the learning environment: exploring validity evidence for the interpretation of scores from existing tools. Acad. Med. 89, 1687–1693.

Genn, J.M., 2001a. AMEE Medical Education Guide No. 23 (Part 1): Curriculum, environment, climate, quality and change in medical education–a unifying perspective. Med. Teach. 23 (4), 337–344.

Genn, J.M., 2001b. AMEE medical education guide no. 23 (Part 2): Curriculum, environment, climate, quality and change in medical education—a unifying perspective. Med. Teach. 23 (5), 445–454.

Harden, R., 2001. The learning environment and the curriculum. Med. Teach. 23 (4), 335–336.

Miller, J.G., 1978. Living Systems. McGraw-Hill, New York.

Moos, R.H., 1974. The social climate scales: an overview. Consulting Psychologists Press, Palo Alto, CA.

Riquelme, A., Padilla, O., Herrera, C., et al., 2013. Development of ACLEEM questionnaire, an instrument measuring residents' educational environment in postgraduate ambulatory setting. Med. Teach. 35 (1), e861–e866.

Robins, L.S., Alexander, G.L., Oh, M.S., et al., 1996. Effect of curriculum change on student perceptions of the learning environment. Teach. Learn. Med. 8 (4), 217–222.

Roff, S., McAleer, S., 2001. What is educational climate? Med. Teach. 23 (4), 333–334.

Schönrock-Adema, J., Bouwkamp-Timmer, T., van Hell, E.A., Cohen-Schotanus, J., 2012. Key elements in assessing the educational environment: Where is the theory? Adv Heal Sci Educ 17, 727–742.

Shehnaz, S.I., Premadasa, G., Arifulla, M., et al., 2014. Development and validation of the AMEET inventory: An instrument measuring medical faculty members' perceptions of their educational environment. Med. Teach. 26, 1–10.

Shochet, R., Colbert-Getz, J., Wright, S., 2013. The Johns Hopkins Learning Environment Survey (JHLES): Development of an efficient tool to assess student perceptions of the medical school learning environment. J Gen Int Med 28, S206–S207.

Soemantri, D., Herrera, C., Riquelme, A., 2010. Measuring the educational environment in health professions studies: a systematic review. Med. Teach. 32 (12), 947–952.

Strand, P., Sjöborg, K., Stalmeijer, R., et al., 2013 Dec 1. Development and psychometric evaluation of the undergraduate clinical education environment measure (UCEEM). Med. Teach. 35 (12), 1014–1026.

van den Berg, B.A.M., Bakker, A.B., ten Cate, O.T.J., 2013. Key factors in work engagement and job motivation of teaching faculty at a university medical center. Perspect Med Educ 2 (5-6), 264–275.

50

Medical education research

J. Cleland, S. J. Durning

Trends

- Research in health professions education is emerging, and often '"borrows"' from other related fields.
- Select your research paradigm—qualitative and quantitative research differ on several key aspects.
- Qualitative research is growing in health professions education.
- Use of theory is key to studying our complex environments.
- Grant funding opportunities are growing yet are still not on par with biomedical sciences.

Research in medicine and the health professions is critical to the future of education and patient care. By encouraging thinking, discovery, evaluation, innovation, teaching, learning and improvement via research, the gaps between best practice and what actually happens can be optimally addressed. Ideally, research should inform and advance education and practice, while education and practice should inform and advance future research. In other words, health professions education research is grounded in the real world of education practice. This is analogous to applied clinical research, where research yields actionable knowledge.

It is helpful to illustrate what we mean with relevant examples. The field of assessment is a good illustration of how health professions education research has informed health professions education. Assessment has changed dramatically in just a few decades, from a reliance on essays and long cases, to understanding and widespread adoption of more reliable and valid measures such as the mini clinical evaluation exercise (mini-CEX) and the objective structured clinical exam (OSCE). Both of these assessment methods have the benefit of much research to ensure not just their psychometric properties but also their relevance to particular health professions settings and stages of training (e.g. undergraduate versus postgraduate). Secondly, some excellent examples of how education research has impacted patient care come from the field

of research into expert performance. This approach focuses on measuring performance on clinical tasks to isolate features of expert performance, to identify the mechanisms that underpin these, and then use this information to create educational environments that facilitate its acquisition.

Expert performance, and its components of deliberate practise and mastery learning, have been very well researched, and found to lead to improved and safer care practices, and better patient outcomes (for further explanation of these concepts and an overview of research in the area, see McGaghie and Kristopaitis, 2015). Although we use assessment and expert performance as examples of good research that informs both education practice and patient care, note that these are not 'out-of-date' areas of research – far from it. There is much we still need to know about both processes, and ongoing research to advance knowledge and practice provides exciting opportunities to progress knowledge and collaborate.

If one delves into assessment and expert performance, one sees that research and practice in these approaches draw from other fields of knowledge, from broader educational, sociological, cognitive and psychological literatures. Why? In part because this research (i.e. in the field of health professions education) is still relatively new and in part because the context of this work draws heavily on the theories, study designs, methods and analytic techniques of other more established disciplines. We shall discuss each of these points.

 Research and practice in health professions education often draw from other fields outside of medicine.

Like many relatively 'young' areas of research, the early years of health professions education research were characterized by studies drawing on the scientific tradition and without an obvious philosophical or theory base. This is illustrated well by looking chronologically at research in any one field of health professions education. In relation to assessment, for example, this is evident from initial work that focused typically on correlation of measures from convenience samples from single institutions and addressed limited view of validity evidence (e.g. predictive validity); even this work now entails more comprehensive views (e.g. Kane's validity framework) with specific theoretical underpinnings and reporting of results.

Another example is that of clinical communication skills. In this area, papers published in the 1980s tended to be descriptive, sharing with readers how one institution taught communication skills to medical students, usually in a pre-clinical context, and perhaps describing outcomes in the form of student acceptability and satisfaction with the course. Our brief historical review of this literature indicated that studies in this area have progressed notably over time, first towards examining if particular ways of teaching made an impact on performance on examination, but then towards more nuanced explorations of the social, emotional and contextual variables that might influence not just student performance but also assessor behaviour in communication skills teaching and assessment, with the most recent studies providing possible theoretical reasons to help frame their study findings.

Quantitative and qualitative research

As the field has matured, the importance of being explicit about the philosophy behind a piece of work is reflected in the reporting of studies. How this is done is fundamentally different between quantitative and qualitative research. The differences between these two approaches are not just about how data is collected – for example, the randomized controlled trial (RCT) versus the exploratory interview – but rather about very different assumptions of the world and how science should be conducted. In short, quantitative research assumes knowledge is observable and measurable, and hence the method, approaches and procedures of the natural sciences can be used for the study of individual and objective findings (e.g. knowledge acquisition from this view as an object in memory). On the other hand, the premise of qualitative research is subjectivity.

Reality is relative and multiple, perceived through socially constructed and subjective interpretations, and hence different designs, methods and data analysis approaches are required in research. Interestingly, it is commonplace for those working in the qualitative tradition to report their philosophical stance explicitly in their papers (e.g. along the lines of "this study was underpinned by social constructionist epistemology, and employed interpretivism as its theoretical perspective"). This type of statement is not seen typically in quantitative studies, perhaps because the stance of the researcher is assumed because of the nature of the research questions and approaches.

 Research approaches often fall into two broad camps: quantitative and qualitative. These

approaches differ in terms of their philosophies, designs, methods and analysis techniques but can be amalgamated in the same programme of research, with care.

Many people carrying out health professions education research are from scientific backgrounds, such as medicine or biomedical sciences. Their training is in the scientific method, of proving or disproving hypotheses and controlling for confounding variables. That approach is what they are inherently comfortable with, and it can work very well in some areas of health professions research (for example, the area of expert performance given as an example earlier). However, it is just not appropriate for other areas of study, specifically when the research question is concerned with more social or cultural factors. Examples of this would include how students or trainees experience a particular clinical learning environment, placement, situation or role, and how these experiences may impact on their learning and personal development. Table 50.1 gives a useful overview of the assumptions, purpose and approach of quantitative and qualitative philosophies.

It is critical to select the right research philosophy, design, methods and analysis approach for the right question. This is likely to require drawing on the theories, study designs, methods and analytic techniques of other more established disciplines such as education, psychology and sociology. To do so makes common sense – why reinvent the wheel? A breadth of theories, from computing science, psychology, sociology, education and other fields, may be used to help design a research question, guide the selection of relevant data, interpret the data and propose explanations of the underlying causes or influences of the observed phenomena in health professions education research.

 It is critical to select the right research philosophy, design, methods and analysis approach for the right question.

There are debates in the wider literature as to whether theory is a product (in other words, where the aim of the research is to develop or refine a theory, to test it out in some way) or a tool (something that helps explain what we are researching or our findings). For most of us, it will be the latter – using theory as a tool to draw ideas together, to make links and offer explanations (Bourdieu & Wacquant, 1992). The following example shows how theory was used in practice in one of Cleland's programmes of research.

One of Aberdeen's three medical education research themes is selection and widening access to medicine. Widening access refers to policies and practices designed to ensure that no group of individuals are disadvantaged or face barriers into professions such as a medicine, to ensure equality of opportunity to education. This is

Table 50.1 Key characteristics of quantitative and qualitative research (reproduced with permission, from Cleland (2015))

Approach or philosophy	Quantitative	Qualitative
Assumptions	• Positivism/post-positivism • Social phenomena and events have an objective reality • Variables can be identified and measured The researcher is objective and 'outside' the research	• Constructivism/interpretivism • Reality is socially constructive • Variables are complex and intertwined The researcher is part of the process
Purpose	• Generalisability • Prediction • Explanation	• Contextualisation • Interpretation • Understanding
Approach	• Hypothesis testing • Deductive, confirmatory, inferential – from theory to data • Manipulation and control of variables • Sample represents the whole population so results can be generalised • Data is numerical or transformed into numbers • Counting/reductionist • Statistical analysis	• Hypothesis generation • Inductive and exploratory – from data to theory • Emergence and portrayal of data • The focus of interest is the sample (uniqueness) • Data is words or language, minimal use of numbers • Probing/holistic • Analysis draws out patterns and meaning

linked to diversifying the medical student body on the basis of social class, ethnicity, gender and other demographic characteristics (the particular issues tend to vary by country although low income tends to be a common denominator for those groups that are not well represented in medical education.

Widening access to medical education is the focus of much political rhetoric, national and local activities across the developed world. However, the statistics indicate that, despite much investment, in the United Kingdom at least, nothing has changed for those from lower socioeconomic groups who remain underrepresented in medicine. (Selection is equally topical, both in terms of 'fairness' to those from certain groups but also in terms of measurable factors such as the predictive validity of different approaches to selection.) National statistics indicated that the impact of much policy and investment for widening access to medicine has differed by sub-group: the issue of widening participation (WP) in terms of social economic background, status or 'class' remains an issue in the United Kingdom.

What became clear during a study where we interviewed all the UK medical admissions deans, is that individual medical schools interpret and put WP policy into practice very differently (Cleland et al., 2015). This finding was not in itself new – publically available information from medical schools admissions webpages indicated a variety of approaches to widening access, such as extended medical programmes, specific foundation to medicine programmes, student-led mentoring of non-traditional applicants and so on. However, through our knowledge of the literature and an openness to considering education theory, we identified the concept of policy enactment, which helped

explain how putting macro-level WP policy into micro-level (local) practice was a complex, interpretative process.

Institutions, in this case medical schools, must interpret policy, drawing on their own culture, within the limitations and possibilities of their context, such as available resource. Using this theory, we identified that a number of contextual dimensions interact to influence the enactment of WP policy in UK medical schools. We did not aim to identify which dimension was most important but rather used the theory to illustrate that how WP policy processes are played out varies on the basis of contextual dimensions. This provided a more nuanced account of the processes of WP within medical schools that had been previously available. Thus, the use of the theory clarified a complex phenomenon. It also facilitated a cumulative programme of research where we were able to gain funding to explore WP in much more detail, in order to make recommendations for policy and practice change. Our outputs have already changed practice and policy.

In summary, theory can help to identify the appropriate study question and target group, clarify methods, provide more details and informative descriptions of the intervention or phenomena, uncover unconsidered effects and assist in analysis and interpretation of results.

 Theory strengthens the practice of research.

These examples illustrate how useful it is to learn from other fields where there is cross-fertilization, then consider how best to combine knowledge from these fields to guide and enrich what we do, opening our minds to different ways of thinking and working. As further examples, consider using biologic measures from heart rate variability combined with validated surveys (from cognitive psychology and education) to better understand mental effort (cognitive load) or use of functional magnetic resonance imaging (MRI) scanning with validated multiple-choice questions to assess clinical reasoning. By being open to the use of different theories and approaches in this way, and in time, it is likely that health professions education research will develop its own novel theories and approaches, which other disciplines may, in turn, borrow and adapt.

 Being open to the use of different theories and approaches can be exciting and informative.

One point of caution. Whatever be your question and natural inclination towards particular schools of theory, consider different theories and methods carefully. Do not jump too quickly, consciously or not, onto a single option without exploring others. The time spent in reflecting on which theory and methods are appropriate for your purposes early in the research process is time well spent – and can be fun to discuss and debate with your collaborators and co-authors. For example, we have both benefited from working with colleagues with different backgrounds from our own, who introduced us to theories and perspectives common in their disciplines, but quite new and novel to us. Exploring and discussing these in terms of their potential relevance to the proposed studies was stimulating and thought provoking and opened our eyes to new ways of thinking and working. Indeed, many of the problems and questions that need to be explored are not unique to any one area. Some require the bringing together of resources and knowledge from different fields and disciplines to understand and perhaps even solve complex, real-life problems.

Before leaving this point about the importance of selecting the right approach for your research question, it is also worth being aware that different types of research are judged differently in terms of their quality and rigour. For example, it would be very appropriate to look for a power calculation when evaluating a funding proposal or reviewing a paper for publication that involves a randomized controlled trial in health professions education. This would not be the case in a qualitative interview study, where it is usual to just give an approximation of how many participants will be required (e.g. 12–18 people). In both cases, a description of the sample is equally important so the readers know the population/participants are appropriate to the research question.

 Different types of research are judged differently in terms of their quality and rigour. Being aware of the different criteria can help you plan good quality research.

Mixed-methods research

Many people take the pragmatic stance of a mixed-methods approach – where a programme of work may encompass quantitative and qualitative designs, methods and data collection. This can be very useful in terms of answering research questions, but it is important to be clear about the relationships between different approaches within a programme.

As stated earlier, one of Aberdeen's education research themes is selection and widening access to medicine. The projects within this theme vary from quantitative studies examining patterns in 'big' national data sets, to small qualitative projects, which use education and linguistic theories to give insight into the complex topics of selection and widening access. We (Cleland and colleagues) used Bourdieu's concept of reflexive sociology as the theoretical basis for this mixed-methods programme of research (Bourdieu, 1990). This approach allowed us to reflect on the differences between qualitative and quantitative approaches.

The objective database studies provided the picture of what was going on in terms of objective patterns or class, gender, ethnicity and attainment in relation to medical application and selection. At the same time, the qualitative studies provided insight into how different groups of applicants and medical students act, which in turn produces and reproduces the social phenomena of limited social (class) diversity in medical education and training in the United Kingdom. In this way we articulated how and why we integrated quantitative and qualitative methods in our programme. This approach may seem a tad esoteric but these are the kind of things that help in terms of planning, justifying and reporting mixed-methods approaches.

 If using mixed-methods research, be clear about the relationships between different approaches within the research programme.

If the mixed-methods approach seems appropriate for your research, Creswell and Plano Clark provide an excellent guide.

Reflection

It is important to consider how your preconceptions about the world might influence your research. As mentioned above, you may have been trained in an objective, quantitative approach and thus feel more comfortable working in that way. Equally, you may be a social scientist working in health professions education research, and be less than enthusiastic about quantitative approaches as your own training leads you to consider the world as social and subjective. Both stances are valid, but it is important to actually reflect on assumptions about knowledge and reality, and to consider what worldview would provide the most suitable lens and tools for understanding the particular health professions education issue under investigation.

Consider how your preconceptions about the world might influence your research in terms of your assumptions and preferred methods.

Reflexivity is a way of doing so. This involves thoughtful analysis self-reflection of assumptions, and a continuous checking that these assumptions are aligned with and appropriate for the research situation, the research question, and the methodologies and methods adopted. There are various ways of doing this. An audit trail, tracking decisions made during the research process, is useful, particularly if this also contains notes on the thinking processes, which were integral to the study design and its implementation and subsequent analysis and reporting (see McMillan, 2015, for a full discussion of reflexivity, or "worldview"). By being reflexive, you consider issues such as why one approach rather than another (because it was not appropriate, rather than because you did not know how to conduct a particular approach), and ensure that your enquiry was conducted well, and without unacknowledged assumptions or pre-conceptions. You may well use reflection in your clinical practice, and so have the necessary skills to transfer to your research work.

Building capacity

For many people, education research is part of a portfolio of activities that include clinical service, teaching, administration and research – possibly clinical as well as education research. There are few people who have the luxury of focusing on only one of the above on a week-to-week basis. Given this, it is important to be realistic about what you can achieve by focusing on one topic or theme. If you can develop a programme of research, or a research theme (e.g. workplace-based assessment, selection, deliberate practise, or focused topics within these broad areas), you are more likely to produce a series of studies that flow logically from one to another – the questions raised by one study decide the focus of the next, and so on. This approach to (clinical or education) research increases your chances of success in terms of publication and grants (see later), and in terms of developing a team of collaborators with whom you have common interests.

If setting out on this journey, the first step is to look at the literature for evidence on your topic of interest. It may be that your original research question has already been answered, but equally your review is likely to identify other questions and avenues for future research – indeed, it is commonplace for academic papers to finish with a section outlining directions for future research, policy and practice. Do the unanswered research questions fit with your interests, knowledge and skills? Are there people who would willingly work with you to answer these questions? Is this something that would be useful locally (in which case you may find your colleagues are more supportive of your ideas)?

Do not neglect the basics – always do a literature review in the early stages of planning your research.

These are all questions to ask oneself, and it is also important to recall where we started in this chapter. There is a shift away from researching how do we do x at y institution, or in such-and-such a context, towards bigger picture studies, including regional, national and international studies and collaborations. This might seem too ambitious if you are new to health professions education research. Consider, then, a pilot quantitative study or a context-dependent qualitative study that is positioned beyond the local.

Think "who else will be interested in this", but at the same time do not underestimate the importance of demonstrating the value of your work to local institutional practice.

Our own experiences have also taught us the importance of acknowledging our own limits. We all have our areas of expertise – no one is an expert in everything. Working with others opens the mind to other ways of thinking, different theories, different ways of seeing the same problem, and different methodological and analytic tools. We could not do what we do without colleagues from medical statistics, health economics, sociology, linguistics and psychology. The research is so much the better as group effort. But to build this group, we have had to network in our own institutions as well as externally – to pursue casual chats by email to firm up ideas and potential alliances. Some potential collaborations have not materialized, for whatever reason (people are busy and/or do not have common interests), but where they have worked, all involved have gained.

Being focused in terms of a theme or topic, and collaborating appropriately to ensure a wide skills set in the research team, will increase your chances of success.

Related to this, many of the problems and questions require the bringing together of resources and knowledge from different fields and disciplines to understand and perhaps even solve complex, real-life problems. It is important to stress the need for interdisciplinary in addition to than multidisciplinary research. In the latter, research problems are investigated from different disciplines, while in the former, theories, insights and methods from different disciplines are integrated to investigate a jointly defined problem. Interdisciplinary collaboration has the potential to forge new research fields. Collaboration of this type is, however, not always easy – different disciplines have different assumptions, language, methods and viewpoints, as well as different journals, publication norms and standards. On a practical note, funders often like – and look for – multidisciplinary collaborations. Indeed, the right team is a core feature of a successful grant application.

Funding

Finding grant funding for health professions education can be challenging. Opportunities are growing, however, to include AMEE grants, funding through the medical education meeting sponsored by the AAMC in the United States and equivalent funding in other countries. Critical to the success of any grant project includes having a team, being adaptable (e.g. where one searches/ considers for funding), and speaking with (and following) grant guidelines of the funder – in addition to demonstrating clarity of one's ideas and rigor in the approach to planned research. Given that opportunities are limited, one will need to be both creative about where to send ideas as well as resilient if one receives a rejection. Our experience is that health professions education grant funding typically requires multiple attempts. For additional reading, we would recommend the reader reviews the recent AMEE Guide on Grant Funding (Blanco et al., 2015).

 Grant funding requires patience, resilience with the process, creativity and building a strong team.

Summary

In this short chapter, we cannot give readers more than a flavour of the basic building blocks of research. However, the references give a broad introduction to health professions education research and introduce how to use a theory to underpin research, as well as

providing examples and illustrations of a diversity of methods and their use. We hope that this chapter stimulates fresh thinking and new ideas for educational research in medical and health professions, and encourages you to engage further with the many exciting theories, models, methodologies and analysis approaches available, the use of which will progress your field of study. If so, we refer you to the textbook *Researching Medical Education*, for a good introductory text (Cleland and Durning, 2015).

References

Blanco, M.A., Gruppen, L.D., Artino, A.R. Jr., et al., 2015. How to write an educational research grant: AMEE Guide No. 101. Med. Teach. 2015 Nov 2:1-10.

Bourdieu, P., 1990. Other Words: Essays Towards a Reflexive Sociology. Harvard University Press, Palo Alto, CA.

Bourdieu, P., Wacquant, L., 1992. An Invitation to Reflexive Sociology. University of Chicago Press, Chicago.

Cleland, J.A., 2015. Exploring versus measuring: considering the fundamental differences between qualitative and quantitative research. In: Cleland, J.A., Durning, S.J. (Eds.), Researching Medical Education. Wiley, London, pp. 3–14.

Cleland, J.A., Durning, S.J., 2015. Researching Medical Education. Wiley, London.

Cleland, J.A., Kelly, N., Moffat, M., Nicholson, S., 2015. Taking context seriously: explaining widening access policy enactments in UK medical schools. Med. Educ. 49, 25–35.

McGaghie, W.C., Kristopaitis, T., 2015. Deliberate practice and mastery learning: origins of expert medical performance. In: Cleland, J.A., Durning, S.J. (Eds.), Researching Medical Education. Wiley, London, pp. 219–230.

McMillan, W., 2015. Theory in healthcare education research: the importance of worldview. In: Cleland, J.A., Durning, S.J. (Eds.), Researching Medical Education. Wiley, London, pp. 15–24.

Index

Page numbers followed by "*f*" indicate figures, "*t*" indicate tables, and "*b*" indicate boxes.